BEDSIDE MEDICINE
WITHOUT TEARS

BEDSIDE MEDICINE
WITHOUT TEARS
(Second Edition)

SN Chugh

MD MNAMS FICA FICP FICN FIACM FIMSA FISC
Senior Professor of Medicine and
Pro Vice Chancellor
Pt BD Sharma University of Health Science
Rohtak, Haryana, India

JAYPEE BROTHERS MEDICAL PUBLISHERS (P) LTD

**New Delhi • St Louis (USA) • Panama City (Panama) • London (UK) • Ahmedabad
Bengaluru • Chennai • Hyderabad • Kochi • Kolkata • Lucknow • Mumbai • Nagpur**

Published by

Jitendar P Vij

Jaypee Brothers Medical Publishers (P) Ltd

Corporate Office

4838/24 Ansari Road, Daryaganj, **New Delhi** - 110002, India, Phone: +91-11-43574357, Fax: +91-11-43574314

Registered Office

B-3 EMCA House, 23/23B Ansari Road, Daryaganj, **New Delhi** - 110 002, India
Phones: +91-11-23272143, +91-11-23272703, +91-11-23282021, +91-11-23245672, Rel: +91-11-32558559
Fax: +91-11-23276490, +91-11-23245683
e-mail: jaypee@jaypeebrothers.com, Website: www.jaypeebrothers.com

Offices in India

- **Ahmedabad**, Phone: Rel: +91-79-32988717, e-mail: ahmedabad@jaypeebrothers.com
- **Bengaluru**, Phone: Rel: +91-80-32714073, e-mail: bangalore@jaypeebrothers.com
- **Chennai**, Phone: Rel: +91-44-32972089, e-mail: chennai@jaypeebrothers.com
- **Hyderabad**, Phone: Rel:+91-40-32940929, e-mail: hyderabad@jaypeebrothers.com
- **Kochi**, Phone: +91-484-2395740, e-mail: kochi@jaypeebrothers.com
- **Kolkata**, Phone: +91-33-22276415, e-mail: kolkata@jaypeebrothers.com
- **Lucknow**, Phone: +91-522-3040554, e-mail: lucknow@jaypeebrothers.com
- **Mumbai**, Phone: Rel: +91-22-32926896, e-mail: mumbai@jaypeebrothers.com
- **Nagpur**, Phone: Rel: +91-712-3245220, e-mail: nagpur@jaypeebrothers.com

Overseas Offices

- **North America Office, USA,** Ph: 001-636-6279734, e-mail: jaypee@jaypeebrothers.com, anjulav@jaypeebrothers.com
- **Central America Office, Panama City, Panama,** Ph: 001-507-317-0160, e-mail: cservice@jphmedical.com Website: www.jphmedical.com
- **Europe Office, UK,** Ph: +44 (0) 2031708910, e-mail: info@jpmedpub.com

Bedside Medicine: Without Tears

© 2011, Jaypee Brothers Medical Publishers (P) Ltd.

This book has been published in good faith that the material provided by author is original. Every effort is made to ensure accuracy of material, but the publisher, printer and author will not be held responsible for any inadvertent error (s). In case of any dispute, all legal matters are to be settled under Delhi jurisdiction only.

First Edition: **2007**

Second Edition: **2011**

ISBN 978-93-5025-028-0

Typeset at JPBMP typesetting unit
Printed at Sanat Printers, Kundli.

Preface to the Second Edition

With great success of the first edition of this book, I am pleased to introduce the mega and enlarged second edition with addition of some new cases and illustrations. I admit that it is not easy to write a book in the form of questions and answers, because a question may be asked in many forms though the answer may be the same. I have tried to compile as many questions as I can on a single case discussion, therefore, repetition of question is unavoidable.

Before the publication of the second edition, I have interacted with my undergraduate and postgraduate students to find out the shortcomings of the first edition. This way shortcomings of the first edition have been removed in this edition.

On the request of the students and residents, I have introduced a few more cases in the second edition. I have tried to put the questions and answers in simple form. I have made this book complete so that it can help the students in quick revision of the subject after theory examination and before appearing in practical examination. I have covered some important theoretical questions also so that students should not have to consult any theory book because of shortage of time between the theory and practical examinations.

I have deleted the ECG portion of the book as students usually read the ECG book separately. I have fully explained the X-rays and instruments. Some instruments have also been added to complete the list of instruments. The common drugs, which are kept in the drugs tray in the examination have also been discussed in details.

Lastly, I must say that medicine is an ever changing subject; it is not possible to keep oneself updated. I am aware of my capabilities as well as shortcomings. I have tried my best to present the updated questions and answers, however, any lapse or deficiency from my part may be excused.

I extend my sincere thanks to M/s Jaypee Brothers Medical Publishers (P) Ltd. for valuable suggestions as well as guidance to make the book more informative. The publisher has taken special care to project the clinical material in excellent way. I am delighted to see the format of the book.

Mere words are not sufficient to express my thanks to my family members and friends who have helped me during this endeavor. I can say that it was impossible for me to bring out this book without their moral support.

Lastly, I request the readers to send their suggestions or comments regarding the second edition directly either to the publisher or to me.

SN Chugh

Preface to the First Edition

I have realised over the years that the students are not oriented well to practical examinations and face difficulty in the interpretation of clinical signs. They lack basic sense to analyse the symptoms and signs probably because either they do not attend the clinical classes or they lay more stress on theoretical discussion. In clinical case discussion, the questions are asked according to the interpretation of clinical symptoms and signs, and the students find difficulty in answering them because they are not ready to face practical examination immediately after the theory examination. The students prepare the subject for theory paper from the Textbook of Medicine but they do not have too many books on practical aspects of medicine. After the theory papers, the time given to the students is short to prepare for practical examination. They want to revise the subject as a whole for practical examinations because the examiners in practical examination do not limit themselves only to practical aspects but also can forward questions on theoretical aspects of medicine.

Today, the students want such a book which can orient them not only to clinical examination but also prepare them to face theoretical discussion about the case. Keeping in view the dire necessity of a book which can cater the needs of the students to their satisfaction and allow them to face the examination "without tears in their eyes", I am bringing out the first edition of this book after consultations with students, residents and my teacher colleagues. I hope this book will not disappoint them at the hour of need.

The medicine being an ever-changing science, it is difficult to cope with the recent advances. I have attempted to include all the available informations in the literature, so as to present this book as updated. However, "to err is human", and I am conscious of my deficiencies, therefore, I may be excused for any lapse or deficiency in this book as this is written by a single author.

I extend my sincere thanks to M/s Jaypee Brothers Medical Publishers (P) Ltd., for bringing the excellent first edition of the book. The publisher has taken special care to depict the clinical material provided to him clearly and carefully for which I am highly indebted. My special thanks to Mr Atul Jain of Jain Book Depot, Rohtak who had played vital role in the preparation of this book.

Mere words are not sufficient to express appreciation for my wife and children who have supported me during this period. I can say that it was impossible for me to bring out this book without their moral support.

At last, I request the readers to convey their suggestions or comments regarding this book to the publisher or author.

SN Chugh

Contents

$$\boxed{\text{SHORT CASES AND SPOT CASES}}$$

UNIT 2: BEDSIDE PROCEDURES AND INSTRUMENTS

UNIT 3: COMMONLY USED DRUGS

UNIT 4: RADIOLOGY

1

Clinical Case Discussion

Respiratory Diseases

CASE 1: CHRONIC OBSTRUCTIVE PULMONARY DISEASE (COPD) WITH OR WITHOUT COR PULMONALE

The patient (Fig. 1.1A) presented with cough with mucoid sputum for the last 8 years. These symptoms intermittently increased during windy or dusty weather. No history of hemoptysis, fever, pain chest. The sputum is white, small in amount with no postural relation.

Clinical Presentations

- Initially, the patients complain of repeated attacks of productive cough, usually after colds and especially during winter months which show a steady increase in severity and duration with successive years until cough is present throughout the year for more than 2 years.

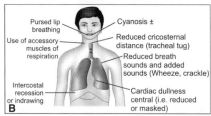

Figs 1.1A and B: Chronic obstructive pulmonary disease (COPD): A. Patient of COPD demonstrating central cyanosis. B. Clinical signs of COPD (Diag)

- Later on with increase in severity of the disease, patient may complain of repeated chest infections, exertional breathlessness, regular morning cough, wheeze and occasionally chest tightness.
- Patient may present with acute exacerbations in which he/she develops fever, productive cough, thick mucopurulent or purulent sputum, often streaked with blood (hemoptysis) and increased or worsening breathlessness.
- Patient may present with complications, the commonest being *cor pulmonale*, characterized by right ventricular hypertrophy with or without failure. The symptoms of right ventricular failure include, pain in right hypochondrium, ascites (swelling of abdomen) and swelling of legs (edema).

Points to be Noted in History

- *Cigarette smoking.* Exposure to smoke from cigarette or biomass and solid fuel fires, atmospheric smoke is important factor in pathogenesis as well as in acute exacerbation of COPD. The smoke has adverse effect on surfactants and lung defence.

Fig. 1.1C: Chest-X-ray PA view showing hyper-inflated (hyper-translucent) lungs and tubular heart

- *Precipitating factors,* e.g. dusty atmosphere, air pollution and repeated upper respiratory tract infections. They cause acute exacerbations of the disease.
- *Family history:* There is increased susceptibility to develop COPD in family of smokers than non-smokers.
- *Hereditary predisposition.* Alpha-1-antitrypsin deficiency can cause emphysema in non-smokers adult patients.

Physical Signs (See Table 1.1)

General Physical

- Flexed posture (leaning forward) with pursed lip breathing and arms supported on their knees or table.
- Central cyanosis, may be noticed in severe COPD.
- Bounding pulses (wide pulse pressure) and flapping tremors on outstretched hands may be present is severe COPD with type 2 respiratory failure. These signs suggest hypercapnia.
- Disturbed consciousness with apnoeic spells (CO_2 narcosis-type 2 respiratory failure).
- Raised JVP and pitting edema feet may be present if patient develops cor pulmonale with congestive heart failure.

Edema feet without raised JVP indicate secondary renal amyloidosis due to pulmonary suppuration, e.g. bronchiectasis, bronchitis, chest infections.

- Respiratory rate is increased (hyperpnea). There may be tachycardia.

Examination

Inspection

Shape of the chest
- AP diameter is increased relative to transverse diameter.

- *Barrel-shaped chest:* The sternum becomes more arched, spines become unduly concave, the AP diameter is > transverse diameter, ribs are less oblique (more or less horizontal), subcostal angle is wide (may be obtuse), intercostal spaces are widened.

Movements of the chest wall
- Bilaterally diminished

Respiratory rate and type of breathing
- Pursed-lip breathing
- Intercostal recession (indrawing of the ribs)
- Excavation of suprasternal, supraclavicular and infraclavicular fossae during inspiration
- Widening of subcostal angle
- Respiratory rate is increased. It is mainly abdominal. The alae nasi and extra-respiratory muscles are in action.

All these signs indicate hyperinflation of lung due to advanced airflow obstruction.

- Cardiac apex beat may or may not be visible.

Palpation
- Movements of the chest are diminished bilaterally and expansion of the chest is reduced.
- Trachea is central but there may be reduction in length of palpable trachea above the sternal notch and there may be tracheal descent during inspiration (tracheal tug).
- Intercostal spaces may be widened bilaterally.
- Occasionally, there may be palpable wheeze (rhonchi) during acute exacerbation.
- Cardiac apex beat may not be palpable due to superimposition by the hyperinflated lungs.

Percussion
- A hyperresonant note on both sides.
- Cardiac dullness is either reduced or totally masked
- Liver dullness is pushed down (below 5th intercostal space).
- There may be resonance over **Kronig's isthmus** and **Traube's area** (splenic dullness is masked).

- Diaphragmatic excursions are reduced on tidal percussion.
- Tactile vocal fremitus may be reduced bilaterally. It can be normal in early cases.

Auscultation
- Breath sounds may be diminished in intensity due to diminished air entry.
- Vesicular breathing with prolonged expiration is a characteristic sign of COPD.
- Vocal resonance may be normal or slightly diminished on both sides equally.
- Rhonchi or wheeze are common especially during forced expiration (expiratory wheeze/rhonchi). Sometimes crackles may be heard during acute exacerbation of chronic bronchitis.
- Check for forced expiratory time (FET). Ask the patient to exhale forcefully after full inspiration while you are listening over the trachea. If patient takes > 6 sec, airway obstruction is indicated.

Common Questions and their Appropriate Answers

Q. What is your provisional diagnosis?

Ans. Chronic obstructive pulmonary disease.

Q. Summarize findings in your case. What are points in favor of your diagnosis?

Ans. A 45 yr male presented with history of chronic cough and expectoration with exacerbation on exposure to dust and smoke with no positive history of such disease in the family. Examination revealed physical signs of *bronchitis*, i.e. cyanosis wheezing, rhonchi, vesicular breathing with prolonged expiration and signs of *emphysema* (e.g. barrel-shaped chest, purse lip breathing, excavation of suprasternal and supraclavicular fossae, diminished movement, and chest expansion, diminished vocal fremitus on both sides, hyperresonant note, obliteration of liver dullness, central apex indicate hyperinflated lungs. Hence my case has features of both chronic bronchitis and emphysema (COPD).

Q. What is your differential diagnosis?

Ans. Based on the symptoms and signs, other two conditions that come into differential diagnosis are:

1. Bronchial asthma
2. Chronic asthmatic bronchitis
For physical signs, read Table 1.1

Q. What is COPD?

Ans. Chronic obstructive pulmonary disease is the internationally recognised term, includes chronic bronchitis and emphysema.

By definition, COPD is a chronic progressive disorder characterised by airflow obstruction (FEV1 <80% predicted and FEV1/FVC ratio <70%) which does not change markedly over several months.

Q. What is tidal percussion?

Ans. Read Clinical Methods in Medicine by Prof SN Chugh.

Q. How do you define chronic bronchitis?

Ans. Chronic bronchitis is a condition characterised by cough with or without expectoration on most of the days in a week for at least 3 months in a year for 2 consecutive years (WHO). Chronic bronchitis simply denotes mucoid sputum production. Chronic bronchitis with acute exacerbation means, fever, persistent or recurrent mucopurulent sputum in the absence of localised suppurative lung disease, e.g. bronchiectasis.

3

Table 1.1: Important differential physical signs in various respiratory disorders

Sign	Lobar consolidation	Lobar collapse	Fibrosis/ bronchiectasis	Cavity or lung abscess	Pleural effusion	Pneumo- thorax	Acute or chronic bronchitis	Bronchial asthma	Emphy- sema
1. Shape of the chest	N	Retraction on the side involved	Retraction on the side involved	N or slight retraction on the side involved	N	N	N	N	Hyper- inflated or barrel-shaped
2. Chest wall movement	Reduced on the side involved	Reduced on the side involved	Reduced on the side involved	Slightly reduced on the side involved	Reduced or absent on the side involved	Reduced or absent on the side involved	N	Bilateral diminished	Bilateral diminished
3. Expansion of chest	Reduced on the side involved	Reduced on the side involved	Reduced on the side involved	Slightly reduced on the side involved	Reduced or absent on the side involved	Reduced or absent on the side involved	N	B/L reduced	B/L reduced
4. Activity of extrarespira- tory muscles	A	A	A	A	A	A	P	P	P
5. Position of trachea and mediastinum	N	Shifted to the side involved	Shifted to the side involved	Shifted to the side involved	Shifted to opposite side	Shifted to opposite side	N	N	N
6. AP and trans- verse diameter	N	N	N	N	N	N	N or abnormal	N	Abnormal AP > T
7. Vocal fremitus	Increased on the side involved	Reduced or absent on the side involved	Increased over the area involved	Increased over the area involved	Reduced or absent on the side involved	Reduced or absent on the side involved	N	N	N or reduced on both sides
8. Percussion note	Dull on the side involved	Dull on the side involved	Impaired over the area involved	Impaired over the area involved	Stony dull on the side involved	N or hyper- resonant on the side involved	N	N or hyper- resonant during acute attack	Hyper- resonant
9. Breath sounds	High-pitched bronchial over the area involved	Diminished or absent over the area involved	Low-pitched bronchial over the area involved	Amphoric bronchial over the area involved	Absent or diminished over the area involved	Absent or diminished on the side involved	B/L vesicular with prolonged expiration	B/L vesicular with prolonged expiration	B/L vesi- cular with prolonged expiration
10. Intensity of breath sounds (vocal resonance)	Increased over the area involved. Bronchophony and whispering pectoriloquy present	Decreased over the area involved	Increased over the area involved	Increased over the area involved whisphering pectoriloquy present	Decreased over the area involved	Decreased on the side involved	N	N	N or diminished
11. Added sounds	Fine crepitations early coarse crepitations later on the area involved	None	Coarse crepitations on the area involved	Coarse crepitations on the area involved	Pleural rub in some cases over the area involved	None	Rhonchi with some coarse crepitations on both the sides	Rhonchi, mainly expiratory and high-pitched	Expiratory rhonchi

Abbreviation: N = normal; B/L = bilateral; P = present; A = absent; AP = anteroposterior

Q. Which clinical signs indicate airflow obstruction?

Ans. *Measurement of forced expiratory time (FET).* Ask the patient to exhale forcefully after full inspiration while you are listening over the trachea. Calculate the time taken by the patient (FET >6 sec indicates (COPD)

Q. Name the accessory muscles of respiration.

Ans. *Alae nasi, sternomastoid, trapezius, serratus anterior, scaleni, lattissmus dorsi, pectoralis* and *abdominal muscles* are accessory muscles of respiration seen working in a patient with severe COPD.

Q. How COPD differs from bronchial asthma?

Ans. The differences between COPD and bronchial asthma are given in Table 1.2.

Q. How do you classify severity of COPD?

Ans. Severity of COPD is discussed in Table 1.3.

Q. How do you decide about which component of COPD is predominant, i.e. chronic bronchitis or emphysema?

Ans. Though COPD encompasses both chronic bronchitis and emphysema but one may predominate over the other. Clinically, patients with predominant bronchitis are referred as *"blue-bloaters"* (blue refers to cyanosis, bloater-edema) and with predominant emphysema as pink puffers (pink refers to absence of cyanosis, puffers-pursed-lip breathing). The difference between the two is enlisted in Table 1.4.

Q. What are the signs of advanced airflow obstruction?

Ans. Main signs are as follows:
- Dyspnea and even orthopnea with purse lip breathing (a physiologic response to decreased air entry).
- Excavation of the suprasternal notch, supraclavicular fossae during inspiration, together with indrawing (recession) of intercostal spaces.
- Barrel-shaped chest (AP diameter ≥ transverse diameter) with horizontality of the ribs.
- A reduction in the length of trachea palpable above the suprasternal notch.
- Contractions of extrarespiratory (accessory) muscles (sternomastoid and scalene muscles) on inspiration
- Central cyanosis
- Expiratory filling of neck veins
- Flapping tremors and bounding pulses (due to hypercapnia)
- Wheeze (rhonchi) especially on forced expiration.

Q. What do you understand by the term emphysema? What are its bedside diagnostic signs?

Ans. Emphysema is defined as hyperinflation or overdistention of air spaces (e.g. alveoli) distal to terminal bronchioles as well as destruction of the alveolar septae.

Bedside diagnostic signs are:
- Pursed-lip breathing
- Barrel-shaped chest
- Apex beat is not visible
- Diminished movements of chest with reduced expansion
- Diminished vocal fremitus and vocal resonance
- Hyperresonant percussion note on both sides
- Cardiac and liver dullness masked
- Heart sounds may get muffled
- Usually wheeze or crackles are absent
- Liver may become palpable due to descent of diaphragm.

Q. Why does a patient of COPD has purse lip breathing?

Ans. Purse lip breathing can occur both in COPD and bronchial asthma. A patient purses, her/his lips to maintain high intrabronchial pressure over and above that exists with surrounding alveoli so as to prevent the collapse of bronchial wall by these surrounding distented alveoli.

Q. What are complications of COPD?

Ans. Common complications are as follows:
- *Pneumothorax* due to rupture of bullae into pleural space
- *Recurrent pulmonary infections*
- *Cor pulmonale* (right ventricular hypertrophy with pulmonary arterial hypertension)
- *Congestive cardiac failure* (raised JVP, hepatomegaly, cyanosis, ascites, peripheral edema with RVH).
- *Type 2 respiratory failure* (CO_2 narcosis) with flapping tremors, bounding pulses, worsening hypoxia and hypercapnia
- *Secondary polycythemia* due to hypoxia.

Clinical tips
1. A sudden worsening of dyspnea after prolonged coughing indicate pneumothorax due to rupture of bullae.
2. Oedema of the legs in COPD indicates CHF
3. Flaps on outstretched hands indicate type 2 respiratory failure.

Q. How will you investigate the patient?

Ans. The following investigations are usually performed;
1. *Hemoglobin*, TLC, DLC and PCV for anemia or polycythemia (PCV is increased) and for evidence of infection.

Table 1.2: Differentiating features between bronchial asthma and COPD

Bronchial asthma	COPD (see Fig. 1.1B)
• Occurs in young age, seen in children and adults who are atopic	Occurs in middle or old aged persons
• Allergo-inflammatory disorder, characterised by reversible airflow obstruction, airway inflammation and bronchial hypersensitivity	Inflammatory disorder characterised by progressive airway obstruction
• Short duration of symptoms (weeks or months)	Long duration of symptoms, e.g. at least 2 years
• Episodic disease with recurrent attacks	Nonepisodic usually but acute exacerbations may occur which worsen the symptoms and disease further
• Variable nature of symptoms is a characteristic feature	Symptoms are fixed and persistent, may be progressive
• Family history of asthma, hay fever or eczema may be positive	No positive family history
• A broad dynamic syndrome rather than static disease	A chronic progressive disorder
• Wheezing is more pronounced than cough	Cough is more pronounced and wheezing may or may not be present
• Shape of the chest remains normal because of dynamic airway obstruction but AP diameter may increase with severe asthma	Barrel-shaped chest (AP diameter $\geq$ transverse) in patients with predominant emphysema
• Pursed-lip breathing is uncommon	Pursed-lip breathing common
• Respiratory movement may be normal or decreased, tracheal tug absent. Accessory muscles of respiration may be active and intercostal recession may be present.	Respiratory movement are usually decreased with: • Reduced palpable length of trachea with tracheal tug • Reduced expansion • Excavation of suprasternal notch, supraclavicular and infraclavicular fossae • Widening of subcostal angle • Intercostal recession • Accessory muscles of respiration hyperactive.

Table 1.3: Gold criteria for severity of COPD

Gold stage	Severity	Symptoms	Spirometry
0	At risk	Chronic cough, sputum	Normal
I	Mild	With or without chronic cough or sputum production	FEV_1/FVC <70% FEV_1=80% predicted
II	Moderate	With or without chronic cough or sputum production	FEV_1/FVC <70% FEV_1=50 to 80% predicted
III	Severe	–do–	FEV_1/FVC <70% FEV_1=30-50%
IV	Very severe	–do–	FEV_1/FVC <70% FEV_1 <30% Or FEV_1 <50% predicted with respiratory failure or signs of right heart failure

GOLD: Global Initiative for Obstructive Lung Disease

Table 1.4: Differences between chronic bronchitis and emphysema

Features	Predominant chronic bronchitis (blue bloaters)	Predominant emphysema (pink puffers)
Age at the time of diagnosis (years)	60 $\pm$	50 $\pm$
Major symptoms	Cough > dyspnea, cough starts before dyspnea	Dyspnea > cough; cough starts after dyspnea
Sputum	Copious, purulent	Scanty and mucoid
Cynosis	Common	Usually absent
Episodes of respiratory infection	Frequent	Infrequent
Episodes of respiratory insufficiency	Frequent	Occurs terminally
Hyperinflation of lungs	Absent	Present
Breath sounds	Vesicular beathing with prolonged expiration	Vesicular breathing with diminished intensity
Chest X-ray	Enlarged cardiac shadow with increased bronchovascular markings	Increased translucency of lungs (hyperinflation), central tubular heart, low flat diaphragm
Compliance of lung	Normal	Decreased
Airway resistance	High	Normal or slightly increased
Diffusing capacity	Normal to slight decrease	Decreased
Arterial blood gas	Abnormal in the beginning	Normal until late
Chronic cor pulmonale (raised JVP and edema)	Common	Rare except terminally
Cardiac failure	Common	Rare except terminally

2. *Sputum examination*. It is unnecessary in case of COPD but during acute exacerbation, the organisms *(Strep. pneumoniae or H. influenzae)* may be cultured). Sensitivity to be done, if organisms cultured.

3. *Chest X-ray* (See Fig. 1.1C) will show:
   - Increased translucency with large voluminous lungs
   - Prominent bronchovascular markings at the hilum with sudden pruning/truncation in peripheral fields
   - Bullae formation
   - Low flat diaphragm. Sometimes, the diaphragm shows undulations due to irregular pressure of bullae
   - Heart is tubular and centrally located.
   Tip. An enlarged cardiac shadow with all of the above radiological findings suggests cor pulmonale.

4. *Electrocardiogram (ECG)*. It may show:
   - Low voltage graph due to hyperinflated lungs
   - P-pulmonale may be present due to right atrial hypertrophy.
   - Clockwise rotation of heart
   - Right ventricular hypertrophy (R>S in V1)

5. *Pulmonary function tests*. These show **obstructive ventilatory defect** (e.g. FEV1, FEV1/FVC and PEF- all are reduced, **lung volumes** – total lung capacity and residual volume increased and **transfer factor CO** is reduced). The difference between obstructive and restrictive lung defect are summarised in Table 1.5.

6. *Arterial blood gas analysis* may show reduced PaO_2 and increased $PaCO_2$ (hypercapnia).

7. *Alpha-1 antitrypsin levels:* Reduced level may occur in emphysema (normal range is 24 to 48 mmol/L).

Q. **What is the role of high resolution CT scan in the diagnosis of emphysema?**

Ans. It is most sensitive technique for diagnosis of emphysema. It is useful in evaluating symptomatic patients with normal pulmonary function except for a low CO diffusing capacity.

Q. **What do you understand by the term chronic cor pulmonale? What are its causes?**

Ans. *Chronic cor pulmonale* is defined as right ventricular hypertrophy/dilatation secondary to chronic disease of the lung parenchyma, vasculature and/or bony cage (Read case discussion on cor pulmonale)

Table 1.5: Pulmonary function tests in obstructive and restrictive lung defect

Test	Obstructive defect (COPD)	Restrictive defect (Interstitial lung disease)
Forced expiratory volume during one second (FEV$_1$)	Markedly reduced	Slightly reduced
Vital capacity (VC)	Reduced or normal	Markedly reduced
FEV1/VC	Reduced	Increased or normal
Functional residual capacity (FRC)	Increased	Reduced
Peak expiratory flow (PEF)	Reduced	Normal
Residual volume (RV)	Increased	Reduced
Total lung capacity	Increased	Reduced
Transfer or diffusion factor for CO (T$_{co}$ and D$_{co}$)	Normal	Low
PaO$_2$	Decreased	Decreased
PaCO$_2$	Increased	Low or normal

Acute cor pulmonale refers to acute thromboembolism where pulmonary hypertension develops due to increased vascular resistance leading to right ventricular dilatation with or without right ventricular failure.

Q. **What do you understand by term obstructive sleep-apnea syndrome?**

Ans. Obstructive sleep-apnea syndrome is characterised by spells of apnea with snoring due to occlusion of upper airway at the level of oropharynx during sleep.

Apneas occur when airway at the back of throat is sucked closed during sleep. When awake, this tendency is overcome by the action of the muscles meant for opening the oropharynx which become hypotonic during sleep. Partial narrowing results in snoring, complete occlusion in apnea and critical narrowing in hyperventilation. The major features include, loud snoring, daytime somnolence, unfreshed or restless sleep, morning headache, nocturnal choking, reduced libido and poor performance at work, morning drunkenness and ankle edema. The patient's family report the pattern of sleep as "snore-silence-snore" cycle. The diagnosis is made if there are more than 15 apneas/hyperpneas in any one hour of sleep with fall in arterial O$_2$ saturation on ear or finger oximetry.

Q. **What is Pickwickian syndrome?**

Ans. It is obesity-related alveolar hypoventilation syndrome in which obesity serves to reduce compliance of chest wall and functional residual capacity in the recumbent position.

In these patients obstructive sleep apnea is prominent feature and in some there may be sleep-induced hypoventilation. These patients present with daytime somnolence, unrefreshing sleep, daytime fatigue, snoring, breathlessness, headache, poor concentration, systemic hypertension. They may develop pulmonary hypertension and right heart failure. Arterial blood gas analysis shows hypoxemia and hypercapnia.

Q. **What is treatment of COPD?**

Ans. Stable phase of COPD is treated by:
- **Cessation of smoking** and avoidance of precipitating factors.
- **Bronchodilators**—Inhaled route of bronchodilatation is preferred than oral and parenteral route due to low side effects. Beta-agonists are commonly used. Tremors and trachycardia are common side effects.
- **Anticholinergics**, e.g. ipatropium bromide is not useful in chronic stable phase, is used in acute exacerbation for symptomatic relief.
- **Corticosteroids**—They are not useful in chronic phase, to be used for short-term in tapering doses in acute exacerbations.
- **O$_2$ therapy**—Both the Medical Research Council Trial and Nocturnal O$_2$ therapy trial have documented the benefits of intermittent O$_2$ therapy for long hours in reducing the mortality in COPD.
- **Other agents**
  i. N-Acetylecysteine is used as both mucolytic and antioxidant agent.
  ii. IV alpha-antitrypsin therapy is available for severe deficiency of alpha 1-trypsin. Hepatitis vaccination is must prior to this therapy.
  iii. Lung transplantation is the last resort for end-stage lung disease, e.g. emphysema due to alpha 1-antitrypsin deficiency.

Q. **What do you understand by the term acute exacerbation of COPD?**

Ans. Acute exacerbation implies, an episode of increased dypnea and cough, and change in the amount and character of sputum. There may or may not be associated signs of illness such as fever, myalgia, sore throat.

Exacerbations are a prominent feature in the natural history of COPD.

Q. **What are common precipitants of acute exacerbation?**

Ans. Bacterial and viral respiratory infections.

Q. What are the organisms commonly associated with acute exacerbation?

Ans. *H.influenzae* and *S. pneumoniae* are the most common organisms

- *Moraxella catarrhalis, Chlamydia pneumoniae* and *Pseudomonas* are less common.

Q. What is role of molecular genetics in COPD?

Ans. α_1-antitrypsin deficiency, increased production of tumor necrosis factor-alpha (TNF-α), increased generation of microsomal epoxide hydrolase during smoking are associated with increased risk of COPD.

Q. What is treatment of acute exacerbation?

Ans. 1. *Antibiotics:* Repeated courses of antibiotics are better than rotating antibiotics. Choice of an antibiotic depends on sputum culture and sensitivity report. Most physicians treat acute exacerbation with an antibiotic on empirical basis without an evidence of infection, i.e. fever, leucocytosis.

2. *Bronchodilators and anticholinergics:* These patients are initially nebulised with beta-agonist and anticholinergic, followed by inhalation therapy. This therapy improves most of the patients. If response is not adequate, addition of theophylline I.V. may be considered.

3. *Glucocorticoids:* The Gold guidelines recommend 30-40 mg oral predisolone or its equivalent in tapering doses for 10-14 days. Steroids have been demonstrated to reduce the hospital stay, hasten the recovery and reduce the chances of further exacerbations for a period of 6 months.

4. *Oxygen:* Supplemental O_2 therapy is given to keep arterial saturation above 90%.

5. *Noninvasive positive pressure ventilation (NIPPV):* It is considered if respiratory failure present.

Q. What do you know about noninvasive ventilation?

Ans. Noninvasive ventilation is an alternative approach to endotracheal intubation to treat hypercapnic ventilatory failure which occurs in COPD. Noninvasive positive pressure ventilation (NIPPV) delivered with a face mask and a piece of white foam placed in the face mask to reduce the amount of internal dead space. Recently it has been shown that NIPPV reduces the hospital stay, need for endotracheal intubation and in hospital mortality in patients with acute exacerbation of COPD.

Q. How will you treat acute respiratory failure?

Ans. If PaO_2 is <8KPa, administer 24% O_2 through mask. There is no need of O_2 when PaO_2 >8KPa. Monitor blood gases every one hourly. If PaO_2 continues to rise, administer doxapram; if inspite of this patient deteriorates, artificial respiration may be attempted.

Q. What are uses of long-term domiciliary O_2 therapy?

Ans. 1. COPD with FEV <1.5L and FVC<2L with stable respiratory failure.

2. Terminal ill patients with hypoxia.

Q. What is congenital lobar emphysema?

Ans. Infants rarely develop a check-valve mechanism in a lobar bronchus, which leads to rapid and life-threatening unilateral overdistension of alveoli, called *congenital lobar emphysema.*

Q. What is unilateral emphysema? What are its causes?

Ans. Overdistension of one lung is called *unilateral emphysema.* It can be congenital or acquired (compensatory emphysema). Unilateral compensatory emphysema develops due to collapse or destruction of the whole lung or removal of one lung.

Macleod's or Swyer-James syndrome is characterised by unilateral emphysema developing before the age of 8 years when the alveoli are increasing in number. This is an incidental radiological finding. In this condition, neither there is any obstruction nor there is destruction and overdistension of alveoli, hence, the term emphysema is not true to this condition. In this condition, the number of alveoli are reduced which appear as larger airspaces with increased translucency on X-ray.

Q. What do you understand by the term bullous emphysema?

Ans. Confluent air spaces with dimension > 1 cm are called *bullae,* may occasionally be congenital but when occur in association with generalised emphysema or progressive fibrotic process, the condition is known as *bullous emphysema.* These bullae may further enlarge and rupture into pleural space leading to pneumothorax.

CASE 2: CONSOLIDATION OF THE LUNG (FIG. 1.2)

The patient (Fig. 1.2A) presented with fever, cough, hemoptysis with rusty sputum and pain chest increasing during respiration of 2 weeks duration.

Clinical Presentations

- Short history of fever with chills and rigors, cough, often pleuritic chest pain which is occasionally referred to shoulder or anterior abdominal wall is a classic presentation of a patient with pneumonic consolidation in young age. In children, there may be associated vomiting and febrile convulsions.
- A patient may present with symptoms of complications, i.e. pleural effusion

Figs 1.2A and B: Pneumonic consolidation: A. A patient with pneumonia having hemoptysis; B. Chest X-ray showing right lower lobe consolidation (→)

(dyspnea, intractable cough, heaviness of chest), meningitis (fever, neck pain, early confusion or disorientation, headache, violent behavior, convulsions, etc.)
- A patient with malignant consolidation presents with symptoms of cough, pain chest, dyspnea, hemoptysis, weight loss, etc. Associated symptoms may include hoarseness of voice, dysphagia, fever, weight loss, and loss of appetite. These patients are old and usually smokers.

Points to be Noted in History and Their Relevance

- Recent travel, local epidemics around point source suggest *Legionella* as the cause in middle to old age.
- Large scale epidemics, associated sinusitis, pharyngitis, laryngitis suggest *Chlamydia* infection.
- A patient with underlying lung disease (bronchiectasis, fibrosis) with purulent sputum suggest secondary pneumonia (bronchopneumonia).
- History of past epilepsy, recent surgery on throat suggest aspiration pneumonia.
- Co-existent debilitating illness, osteomyelitis or abscesses in other organs may lead to staphylococcal consolidation.
- Contact with sick birds, farm animals suggest *Chlamydia psittaci* and *Coxiella burnetti* pneumonia.
- History of smoking suggest malignancy
- Recurrent episodes suggest secondary pneumonia
- History of diabetes, intake of steroids or antimitotic drugs, AIDS suggest pneumonia in immunocompromised host.

Physical Signs

General Physical

- Toxic look
- Fever present
- Tachypnea present
- Tachycardia present
- Cyanosis absent
- Herpes labialis may be present
- Neck stiffness absent, if present suggests meningitis as a complication

Systemic Examination

Inspection

- Shape of chest is normal
- Movements of the chest reduced on the side involved due to pain
- In this case (Fig. 1.2), movements of right side of the chest will be reduced.
- Trachea central
- Apex beat normal
- No indrawing of intercostal spaces; and accessory muscles of respiration are not working (active).

Palpation

- Restricted movement on the side involved (right side in this case)
- Reduced expansion of the chest (right side in this case)
- Trachea and apex beat normal in position
- Tactile vocal fremitus is *increased* on the side and over the part involved (in this case, apparent in right axilla and front of central part of right chest).
- *Friction rub* may be palpable over the part of the chest involved.

Percussion

- Dull percussion note on the side and over the part of the chest involved (right axilla and right lower anterior chest in this case).

Auscultation

The following findings will be present on the side and part involved (right axilla and right lower anterior chest in this case).
- Bronchial breath sounds
- Increased vocal resonance with *bronchophony* and *whispering pectoriloquy*.
- Aegophony
- Pleural rub

Note: As the lung is solidified, no crackles or wheeze will be heard at present, but during resolution, crackles will appear due to liquefaction of the contents.

Q. What is the provisional diagnosis and why?

Ans. The provisional clinical diagnosis in this case is right pneumonic consolidation because of short duration of classic triad of symptoms (fever, cough, pleuritic chest pain) with all signs of consolidation on right side (read Table 1.1 for signs of consolidation). Tuberculosis can also be the cause, hence, to be ruled out.

Q. What is differential diagnosis?

Ans. All the conditions that produce consolidation come into differential diagnosis. Read causes of consolidation. Pleural effusion and collapse of lung also produce some signs that resemble consolidation, hence, come in differential diagnosis (Table 1.6).

Q. What is clinical triad of pneumonia?

Ans. Cough and fever, chest pain and hemoptysis is a clinical triad of pneumonia.

Q. What is the site of involvement in your case?

Ans. Because all the signs are present in the right axilla and right lower anterior chest, hence, it is likely due to involvement of right middle and lower lobe.

Table 1.6: Differential diagnosis of consolidation

I. **Bronchogenic carcinoma**
   - Common in male, smokers, middle aged persons
   - Hemoptysis is common
   - Cachexia/emaciation is present.
   - Patient is not toxic
   - Clubbing may be present. There may be cervical lymphadenopathy.
   - No shift of trachea or mediastinum unless there is associated pleural effusion.
   - Crackles are heard over the mass.

II. **Collapse of lung**
   - There is depression of the chest on the side involved. Movements are diminished on the involved side.
   - Intercostal spaces are crowded. Trachea and mediastinum are shifted to same side.
   - Impaired percussion note and decreased intensity of breath sounds.
   - Patient is not toxic
   - History may be suggestive, e.g. aspiration, foreign body, trauma, postoperative condition.

III. **Pleural effusion**
   - Gradual onset of cough and dyspnea
   - Chest may be prominent on the side involved.
   - Trachea and mediastinum are shifted to opposite side.
   - Stony dull percussion note with rising dullness in axilla.
   - Vocal fremitus and vocal resonance are diminished over the area involved.
   - There may a bronchial breathing (amphoric) or aegophony (increased vocal resonance) at the top of effusion posteriorly.

IV. **Pulmonary infarct**
   - Sudden onset of chest pain, fever, hemoptysis.
   - DVT may be present in leg(s).
   - Patient is not toxic
   - Pleural rub may be present, P2 may become loud.
   - ECG shows RVH or S1, QIII, T III syndrome

Q. What is the cause of chest pain in pneumonia?

Ans. Chest pain in pneumonia is acute, occurs due to involvement of overlying pleura leading to friction between two layers of pleura. The pain is pleuritic in origin, increases during respiration. A pleural rub may be heard.

Q. What is pleural rub? What are its causes? How would you differentiate it from crackles?

Ans. For all these questions, read Clinical Methods in Medicine by Prof SN Chugh.

Q. What do you understand by the term consolidation? What are stages of pneumonia and their clinical characteristics?

Ans. Consolidation means solidification of the lung due to filling of the alveoli with inflammatory exudate. It represents second stage (red hepatisation) and third stage (gray hepatization) of pneumonia (Table 1.7).

Table 1.7: Stages of pneumonia

Stage	Signs
I. *Stage of congestion*	Diminished vesicular breath sounds with fine inspiratory crackles due to alveolitis
II. *Stage of red hepatization*	All signs of consolidation present as mentioned (Table 1.1).
III. *Stage of gray hepatization*	— do—
IV. *Stage of resolution*	• Bronchial breathing during consolidation is replaced either by bronchovesicular or vesicular breathing. • Mid-inspiratory and expiratory crackles (coarse crepitations) appear • All other signs of consolidation disappear.

Q. Patient has consolidation on X-ray but is asymptomatic. How do you explain?

Ans. Respiratory symptoms and signs in consolidation are often absent in elderly, alcoholics, immunocompromised and neutropenic patients.

Note: Children and young adults suffering from *Mycoplasma* pneumonia may have consolidation with few symptoms and signs in the chest, i.e. there is discrepancy between symptoms and signs with radiological appearance of consolidation. Deep seated consolidation or consolidation with non-patent bronchus may not produce physical signs on chest examination.

Q. What are the common sites of aspiration pneumonia?

Ans. The site of aspiration depends on the position of patient (Table 1.8).

Table 1.8: Aspiration during supine and upright position

Aspiration during supine position	Aspiration in upright position
• Posterior segment of the upper lobe and superior segment of the lower lobe on the right side (right is more involved than left side)	• Basilar segments of both lower lobes

Q. What are the causes of consolidation?

Ans. Main causes of consolidation are as follows:

1. Pneumonic (lobar consolidation), may be bacterial, viral, fungal, allergic, chemical and radiation induced.
2. Tuberculosis causes apical consolidation.
3. Malignant (bronchogenic carcinoma)
4. Following massive pulmonary infarct (pulmonary embolism – may cause collapse consolidation).
5. Collagen vascular disorders.

Q. How pneumonia in young differs from pneumonia in old persons?

Ans. Pneumonia in young and old persons are compared in Table 1.9.

Q. How do you classify pneumonias?

Ans. Pneumonias can be classified in various ways;

   I. *Depending on the immunity and host resistance*
   • Primary (normal healthy individuals)
   • Secondary (host defence is lowered). It further includes:
      — Acute bronchopneumonia (lobar, lobular, or hypostatic)
      — Aspiration pneumonia

Table 1.9: Differentiating features of pneumonia in younger and older persons

Pneumonia in young	Pneumonia in old
• Primary (occurs in previously healthy individuals)	Secondary (previous lung disease or immunocompromised state)
• Common organisms are; *pneumococci, Mycoplasma, Chlamydia, Coxiella*	Common organisms are; *pneumococci, H. influenzae, Legionella*
• Florid symptoms and signs	Few or no symptoms and signs
• Systemic manifestations are less pronounced	More pronounced systemic features
• Complications are less frequent	Complications are frequent
• Resolution is early	Resolution may be delayed
• Response to treatment is good and dramatic	Response to treatment is slow

   — Hospital–acquired pneumonia (nosocomial)
   — Pneumonias in immunocompromised host
   — Suppurative pneumonia including lung abscess.

   II. *Anatomical classification*
   • Lobar
   • Lobular (bronchopneumonia, bilateral)
   • Segmental (hypostatic pneumonia).

   III. *Aetiological classification*
   • Infective, e.g. bacterial, viral, *Mycoplasma*, fungi, protozoal, *Pneumocystis carinii*
   • Chemical – induced (lipoid pneumonia, fumes, gases, aspiration of vomitus)
   • Radiation
   • Hypersensitivity/allergic reactions.

   IV. *Empiricist's classification (commonly used)*
   • *Community–acquired pneumonia (S. pneumoniae, Mycoplasma, Chlamydia, Legionella, H. influenzae, virus, fungi, anaerobes, Mycobacterium)*
   • *Hospital–acquired pneumonia (Pseudomonas, B. proteus, Klebsiella, Staphycoccus, oral anaerobes)*
   • *Pneumonia in immunocompromised host (Pneumocystis carinii, Mycobacterium, S. pneumoniae, H. influenzae).*

Q. What are the characteristics of viral pneumonia?

Ans. Characteristics of viral pneumonia are as follows:

   • Constitutional symptoms, e.g. headache, malaise, myalgia, anorexia are predominant (commonly due to *influenza, parainfluenza, measles* and *respiratory syncytial virus*).
   • There may be no respiratory symptoms or signs and consolidation may just be discovered on chest X-ray
   • Cough, at times, with mucoid expectoration.
   • Hemoptysis, chest pain (pleuritic) and pleural effusion are rare
   • Paucity of physical signs in the chest
   • Chest X-ray shows reticulonodular pattern instead of lobar consolidation
   • Spontaneous resolution with no response to antibiotics
   • WBC count is normal.

Q. What do you understand about *Mycoplasma pneumonia*?

Ans. *Mycoplasma pneumonia* is an important cause of community-acquired pneumonia and epidemics of this pneumonia are common. Its incubation period is 1-3 weeks and it affects usually children and young adults. It is also common in winter months.

Q. What are the extrapulmonary manifestations of *Mycoplasma pneumonia*?

Ans.
  i. *Articular*, e.g. arthritis, arthralgia
  ii. *Cardiac*, e.g. pericarditis, myocarditis
  iii. *Blood*, e.g. autoimmune hemolytic anemia, DIC
  iv. *Skin*, e.g. erythema multiforme, Stevens-Johnson syndrome
  v. *Hepatitis and glomerulonephritis*

Q. What are the characteristics of various bacterial pneumonias?

Ans. Characteristics of bacterial pneumonias are enlisted in Table 1.10.

Q. What are the complications of pneumonia?

Ans. Common complications of pneumonia are:

- Pleural effusion and empyema thoracis
- Lung abscess
- Adult respiratory distress syndrome
- Meningitis, brain abscess
- Circulatory failure (Waterhouse – Friedrichson's syndrome)
- Septic arthritis, septicemia
- Pericarditis, congestive heart failure (myocarditis)
- Multiorgan failure, renal failure
- Peripheral thrombophlebitis
- Herpes labialis (secondary infection).

Table 1.10: Clinical and radiological features of bacterial pneumonias

Pathogens	Clinical features	Radiological features
Common organisms		
Pneumococcal pneumonia	Young to middle aged, rapid onset, high fever, chills, and rigors, pleuritic chest pain, herpes simplex labialis, *rusty* sputum. Toxic look, tachypnea and tachycardia. All signs of consolidation present	Lobar consolidation (dense uniform opacity), one or more lobes
Mycoplasma pneumoniae	• Children and young adults (5-15 years), insidious onset, headache, systemic features. Often few signs in the chest. IgM cold agglutinins detected by ELISA • Arthralgia or arthritis erythema nodosum, myocarditis, pericarditis, hepatitis, glomerulonephritis, rash, meningoencephalitis, hemolytic anemia, DIC are extrapulmonary manifestations.	Patchy or lobar consolidation. Hilar lymphadenopathy present
Legionella	• Middle to old age, history of recent travel, local epidemics around point source, e.g. cooling tower, air conditioner • Headache, malaise, myalgia, high fever, dry cough, GI symptoms • Confusion, hepatitis, hyponatremia, hypoalbuminemia	Shadowing continues to spread despite antibiotics and often slow to resolve
Uncommon organisms		
H. influenzae	• Old age, often underlying lung disease (COPD), purulent sputum, pleural effusion common	Bronchopneumonia Signs of underlying disease present and are more pronounced
Staphylococcal pneumonia	• Occurs at extremes of ages, coexisting debilitating illness, often complicates viral infection • Can arise from, or cause abscesses in other organs, e.g. osteomyelitis • Presents as bilateral pneumonia, cavitation is frequent	Lobar or segmental thin walled abscesses formation (pneumatoceles)
Klebsiella	Systemic disturbances marked, widespread consolidation often in upper lobes. Red-currant jelly sputum, lung abscess and cavitation frequent	Consolidation with expansion of the affected lobes, bulging of interlobar fissure

Q. What are the causes of recurrent pneumonia?

Ans. Recurrent pneumonias mean two or more attacks within a few weeks. It is due to either reduced/lowered resistance or there is a local predisposing factor, i.e.
- Chronic bronchitis
- Hypogammaglobulinemia
- Pharyngeal pouch
- Bronchial tumor

Q. What is normal resolution? What is delayed resolution and nonresolution? What are the causes of delayed or non-resolution of pneumonia?

Ans. Normal resolution in a patient with pneumonia means disappearance of symptoms and signs within two weeks of onset and radiological clearance within four weeks. Delayed resolution means when physical signs persist for more than two weeks and radiological findings persist beyond four weeks after proper antibiotic therapy. **Causes** are:
- Inappropriate antibiotic therapy
- Presence of a complication (pleural effusion, empyema)
- Depressed immunity, e.g. diabetes, alcoholism, steroids therapy, neutropenia, AIDS, hypogammaglobulinemia
- Partial obstruction of a bronchus by a foreign body like denture or malignant tumor
- Fungal or atypical pneumonia
- Pneumonia due to SLE and pulmonary infarction or due to recurrent aspirations in GERD or cardia achalasia.

Non-resolution means radiological findings persisting beyond eight weeks after proper antibiotic therapy. **Causes** are:
- Neoplasm
- Underlying lung disease, e.g. bronchiectasis
- Virulent organisms, e.g. *Staphylococcus, Klebsiella*
- Underlying diabetes
- Old age.

Q. How will you investigate a patient with community acquired pneumonia (CAP)

Ans. 1. **Radiology:** Chest X-ray is most useful investigation, detects consolidation in most of the cases (see Fig. 1.2B). If pneumonia is suspected on clinical grounds and no opacity is seen on initial chest X-ray, it is useful to repeat either X-ray after 24-48 hours or perform CT scan. High resolution CT scan detects opacities in patients with symptoms and signs suggestive of pneumonia but chest X-ray is normal.

2. **Blood culture:** All patients who are admitted to the hospital should have two sets of blood cultures done before initiation of antibiotic therapy. The most common isolates, in ascending order are; *S. pneumonia, S. aureus and E. coli.*

3. **Sputum stains and culture:** Gram's staining of sputum is used for persumptive etiologic diagnosis. Other types of sputum stainings are also useful for determining the cause of CAP. A variety of stains for acid-fast bacilli are used to diagnose tuberculosis. *Pneumocystis pneumonia* common in HIV patients can be diagnosed with monoclonal antibody staining. Special stains are also available for fungi, etc.

    Sputum should be sent for culture and sensitivity. Bronchoscopy and bronchoalveolar lavage may be attempted in case there is no sputum.

4. **Detection of antigens in urine:** Urine antigen test by ELISA is used to diagnose *Legionnaires disease*. Similarly S. pneumonia urinary antigen detection by ELISA is also useful.

5. **Serology:** The detection of IgM antibody or demonstration of 4-fold rise in titre of antibody in blood to a particular agent between acute and convalescent phase is considered a good evidence that this agent is the cause of pneumonia. The various serological tests used include complement fixation, indirect immunofluorescence and ELISA. The following etiological agents are often diagnosed serologically i.e. *Mycoplasma, C. pneumoniae, Chlamydia, Legionella spp. C. burnetti*, viruses (adeno, influenza, parainfluenza).

6. **Polymerase chain reaction (PCR)**
   A multiplex PCR allows detection of DNA of *Legionella spp, M. pneumoniae* and *C. pneumoniae*.

7. **Blood counts:** Leukocytosis with polymorpho-nuclear response indicate bacterial infection.

Q. How would you treat CAP?

Ans.
- First of all, assess pneumonia severity and pay attention to vital signs.
- Ensure adequate O_2 therapy and support to circulation.
- Perform etiological work-up as described above. Never forget tuberculosis as etiological agent.
- **Antibiotic therapy:** Institute empirical antibiotic therapy followed by antibiotics based on the isolation of organism. The duration of antibiotics therapy is 10-14 days.
- **Monitor and treat comorbid illnesses:** Consider measures such as counseling for cessation of smoking and prevention of pneumococcal and influenza infection by vaccination.
- Follow up chest X-rays.

Q. What are the causes of failure of improvement of CAP?

Ans. Causes are:
- *Incorrect diagnosis*: Reconsider the diagnosis as there may be some illness such as collagen vascular disease presenting as pneumonia

- Incorrect choice of antibiotic
- *Virulent pathogens or antibiotics* are being used for wrong etiology, for example, for tubercular or viral or fungal pneumonia
- *Mechanical reasons* such as underlying lung cancer or sequestrated lung segment
- *Immunocompromised* state or hypogamma-globulinemia.

Q. What do you know about bronchopulmonary sequestration?

Ans. It is a congenital condition in which a portion of non-functioning lung tissue is detached from the normal lung and is supplied by an anomalous systemic artery which arises from the aorta or one of its branches; the segment/tissue has no bronchopulmonary connection/communication. The sequestration may be extralobar (sequestrated segment has separate pleural lining which separates it from the lung) or intralobar (portion or segment shares its pleura with the adjacent normal lung). The patients with lung sequestration present with cough, recurrent pneumonia and occasional hemoptysis.

Q. What are poor prognostic indicators in CAP?

Ans.
- Old age (>65 yr).
- Coexisting conditions such as heart failure, renal failure, COPD, malignancy, lung abscess.
- Immunocompromised state, e.g. diabetes, alcoholism, HIV, immunosupression, etc.
- Severe pneumonia, i.e. respiratory rate >30/min hypotension, high fever, impaired mental status, septicemia
- Multilobar pneumonia
- Hypoxemia, Pa_2 <60 mm Hg while breathing room air or O_2 saturation <90%.
- Virulent organism and presence of pleural effusion.

Q. How would you investigate a patient with suspected malignant consolidation?

Ans.
- *Sputum cytology*; It provides high yield for endobronchial tumors such as squamous cell and small cell carcinoma.
- *Chest X-ray*
- *Pleural fluid* for biochemistry and cytology
- *Bronchoscopy* gives a higher yield when tumor is accessible endobronchially.
- *CT scan* of the chest and upper abdomen for liver metastases.
- *Bone scan* for metastases
- *PET scanning* is highly sensitive and specific for mediastinal staging.
- *Pulmonary function tests* so as to evaluate the patient for treatment.

Q. What is the aim of staging bronchogenic carcinoma?

Ans. The main aim of staging is to identify candidates for surgery, since this approach offers highest potential cure for lung cancer. The staging assessment covers 3 major issues; distant metastases, state of the chest and mediastinum and the condition of the patient.

Q. What is role of surgery in lung cancer?

Ans. Surgery is beneficial in peripheral non-small cell carcinoma. Its role is limited in small cell carcinoma.

Q. Which tumors respond to chemotherapy?

Ans. Small cell carcinoma. The drugs used include cyclophosphamide, doxorubicin, cisplatin, etoposide and vincristine. The combination of etoposide and cisplatin appears to have the best therapeutic index of any regimen.

Q. What are indications of radiotherapy in bronchogenic carcinoma?

Ans.
- Pain either local or metastatic
- Breathlessness due to bronchial obstruction
- Dysphagia
- Hemoptysis
- Pancoast tumor
- Mediastinal compression/superior vena cava obstruction
- Before and after surgery

Q. How do you diagnose pleural effusion in a patient with consolidation?

Ans. The clues to the diagnosis are:
- History suggestive of pneumnoia (fever, pain chest, hemoptysis, cough) and persistence of these symptoms beyond 2-4 weeks
- Signs of pleural effusion, e.g. stony dull percussion note, shifting of trachea and mediastinum.
- The obliteration of costophrenic angle in presence of consolidation on chest X-ray.

Q. What is the mechanism of trachea being shifted to same side in consolidation?

Ans. Usually, trachea remains central in a case of consolidation but may be shifted to the same side if;
- Consolidation is associated with collapse on the same side (Collapse consolidation due to malignancy)
- Consolidation is associated with underlying old fibrosis on the same side.

Q. What is typical or atypical pneumonia syndrome?

Ans. The *typical pneumonia syndrome* is characterised by sudden onset of fever, productive cough, pleuritic chest pain, signs of consolidation in the area of radiological abnormality. This is caused by *S. pneumoniae, H. influenzae, oral anaerobes* and *aerboes* (mixed flora).

The *atypical pneumonia syndrome* is characterised by insidious onset, a dry cough, predominant extrapulmonary symptoms such as headache, myalgia, malaise, fatigue, sore throat, nausea, vomiting and diarrhea, and abnormalities on the chest X-day despite minimal or no physical signs of pulmonary involvement. It is produced by *M. pneumoniae,*

L. pneumophilia, P. carinii, S. pneumoniae, C. psittaci, Coxiella burnetii and *some fungi (H. capsulatum).*

Q. What will be the features in malignant consolidation?

Ans. Common features in malignant consolidation are:
- Patient will be old and usually smoker
- History of dry persistent hacking cough, dyspnea, hemoptysis, pleuritic chest pain.
- There will be weight loss, emaciation due to malignant cachexia.
- Cervical lymphadenopathy may be present.
- Trachea will be central, i.e. but is shifted to same side if there is associated collapse or to the opposite if associated with pleural effusion.
- All signs of consolidation, i.e. diminished movements, reduced expansion, dull percussion note, bronchial breathing may be present if bronchus is occluded. The bronchial breathing is from the adjoining patent bronchi. The bronchial breathing will, however, be absent if there is partial bronchial obstruction.
- Signs and symptoms of local spread, i.e. pleura (pleural effusion), to hilar lymph nodes (dysphagia due to esophageal compression, dysphonia due to recurrent laryngeal nerve involvement, diaphragmatic paralysis due to phrenic nerve involvement, superior vena cava compression), brachial plexus involvement (i.e. pancoast tumor producing monoplegia), cervical lymphadenopathy (Horner's syndrome—cervical sympathetic compression) may be evident.
- Sometimes, signs of distant metastases, e.g. hepatomegaly, spinal deformities, fracture of rib(s) are present.

Q. What are the pulmonary manifestations of bronchogenic carcinoma?

Ans. It may present as;
- Localised *collapse* of the lung due to partial bronchial obstruction.
- *Consolidation*—a solid mass lesion
- *Cavitation* Secondary degeneration and necrosis in a malignant tumor leads to a cavity formation.
- *Mediastinal syndrome* It will present with features of compression of structures present in various compartments of mediastinum (superior, anterior, middle and posterior). These include:
- *Superior vena cava obstruction* with oedema of face, suffused eyes with chemosis, distended nonpulsatile neck veins, and prominent veins over the upper part of the chest as well as forehead. (Read case discussion on Superior Mediastinal Compression).

- Dysphonia and bovine cough due to compression of recurrent laryngeal nerve, stridor due to tracheal obstruction
- Dysphagia due to esophageal compression
- Diaphragmatic paralysis—phrenic nerve compression
- Intercostal neuralgia due to infiltration of intercostal nerves
- Pericardial effusion due to infiltration of pericardium, myocarditis (arrhythmias, heart failure).
- Thoracic duct compression leading to chylous pleural effusion
- Brachial plexus compression (pancoast tumor) producing monoplegia

Q. What are the extrapulmonary nonmetastatic manifestations of carcinoma lung?

Ans. The paraneoplastic/nonmetastatic extrapulmonary manifestations occur in patients with oat cell carcinoma and are not due to local or distant metastatic spread. These are;
a. **Endocrinal** (hormones produced by the tumour)
   ACTH—Cushing's syndrome
   PTH—Hypercalcemia
   ADH—Hyponatremia
   Insulin–like peptide—Hypoglycemia
   Serotonin—Carcinoid syndrome
   Erythropoietin—Polycythemia
   Sex hormone—Gynecomastia
b. **Skeletal** – Digital clubbing
c. **Skin**, e.g. Acanthosis nigricans, pruritus
d. Neurological
   - Encephalopathy
   - Myelopathy
   - Myopathy
   - Amyotrophy
   - Neuropathy
e. Muscular
   - Polymyositis, dermatomyositis
   - Myasthenia –myopathic syndrome *(Lambert-Eaton syndrome)*
f. Vascular
   - Migratory thrombophlebitis
g. Hematological
   - Hemolytic anemia   • Thrombocytopenia

Q. Where do the distant metastases occur in bronchogenic carcinoma

Ans. It spreads to distant organs in three ways:
- Lymphatic spread involves mediastinal, cervical and axillary lymph nodes
- Hematogenous spread involves liver, brain, skin, bone and subcutaneous tissue
- Transbronchial spread leads to involvement of other side.

CASE 3: PLEURAL EFFUSION AND EMPYEMA THORACIS

The patient (Fig. 1.3A) presented with fever, pain chest, dyspnea for the last 6 months. No associated cough or hemoptysis.

Pleural effusion

Figs 1.3A and B: Pleural effusion left side: A. Fluid drainage; B. Chest X-ray

Clinical Presentation

- Fever, non-productive cough and pleuritic chest pain
- Heaviness/tightness of chest in massive effusion
- Dyspnea due to compression collapse of the lung by large amount of fluid and shift of the mediastinum to opposite side leading to reduction of vital capacity
- Presence of signs and symptoms of toxemia in case of empyema thoracis.

History

Points to be Noted in History

- History of breathlessness and pleural pain.
- History of fever, cough, rigors, removal of fluid in the past
- History of trauma
- Past/present history of tuberculosis, malignancy
- Occupational history (exposure to asbestos)
- Any skin rash, swelling of joints, lymphadenopathy
- Any history of dysentery in the past
- Hemoptysis
- Is there history of edema, pain abdomen, distension of abdomen (ascites), edema legs ?
- Any menstrual irregularity in female

Treatment History—Drug taken or being taken.

Examination

Proceed as follows:

I. General Physical Examination (GPE)

- Any puffiness of face or malar flush or rash
- Fever
- Tachypnea
- Tachycardia
- Patient prefers to lie in lateral position on uninvolved side
- Emaciation, clubing of fingers tar stain
- Cervical lymph nodes may be palpable if effusion is tubercular
- Neck veins may be full due to kinking of superior vena cava or raised JVP
- Signs of underlying cause, e.g. rheumatoid hands or butterfly rash.
- Edema may be present if pleural effusion is due to a systemic disorder
- Look for any rash, arthritis/arthralgia
- Note the vitals, pulse, BP, temperature and respiration.
- Comment on aspiration mark, mastectomy scar or radiation mark.

II. Systemic Examination

Inspection
- Increased respiratory rate
- Restricted respiratory movement on affected side (left side in this case)
- Intercostal spaces are full and appear widened on the affected side (left side in this case)

Palpation
- Diminished movement on the side involved (left side in this case)
- Chest expansion on measurement is reduced
- Trachea and apex beat (mediastinum) shifted to opposite side (right side in this case)
- Vocal fremitus reduced or absent on affected side (left side in this case)
- No tenderness
- Occasionally, in early effusion, pleural rub may be palpable

Percussion
- Stony dull note over the area of effusion on the affected side (left side in this case)
- Rising dullness in axilla (S-shaped Ellis' curve) due to capillary action
- Skodiac band of resonance at the upper level of effusion because of compen-satory emphysema
- Traube's area is dull on percussion
- No shifting dullness
- No tenderness

Auscultation
- Breath sounds are absent over the fluid (left side in this case)
- Vocal resonance is reduced over the area of effusion (left side in this case)
- Sometimes, bronchial breathing (tubular – high pitched, bronchophony and whispering pectoriloquy and egophony present at the upper border (apex) of pleural effusion (left interscapular region in this case)
- Pleural rub can be heard in some cases

Q. What is your clinical diagnosis and why?

Ans. The diagnosis is pleural effusion left side probably due to tuberculosis. The positive features in support of diagnosis are:

   i. Diminished movements on the involved side.

   ii. Trachea and mediastinum shifted to opposite side

   iii. Stony dull percussion note with rising dullness in left axilla

   iv. Vocal fremitus reduced on the side involved

   v. Breath sound absent over the effusion but there is bronchial breath sound with egophony at the top of effusion on the back.

Q. What are the causes of dullness at lung base?

Ans. • Pleural effusion

   • Thickened pleura

   • Collapse of lung

   • Raised hemidiaphragm due to amebic liver abscess or ascites

Q. What do you understand by pleural effusion?

Ans. Normal pleural space on each side contains 50 to 150 ml of fluid but excessive collection of fluid above the normal value is called *pleural effusion* which may or may not be detected clinically. Fluid between 150 to 300 ml can be detected radiologically by chest X-ray (obliteration of costophrenic angle). More than 500 ml fluid can be detected clinically.

   Note: USG of the chest is the earliest means of detecting the small amount of fluid.

Q. What are the causes of pleural effusion? What is transudative or exudative fluid?

Ans. Pleural fluid may be clear (hydrothorax) or turbid (pyothorax), may be blood stained (hemorrhagic) or milky white (chylous).

   Biochemically, the fluid may be transudate or exudate; the differences between the two are summarised in Table 1.11. The diagnosis of various types of fluid are given in Table 1.12.

   Various types of effusions and their causes are given in Table 1.13.

Table 1.11: Characteristics of pleural fluid

	Fluid	Transudate (SFAG > 1.1)	Exudate (SFAG < 1.1)
1.	Appearance	Clear, light yellow	Straw-colored, turbid or purulent, milky or hemorrhagic
2.	Protein	< 3 g% or <50% of serum proteins	>3 g% or >50% of serum proteins
3.	Serum/fluid albumin gradient	>1.1	<1.1

Contd...

Contd...

	Fluid	Transudate (SFAG > 1.1)	Exudate (SFAG < 1.1)
4.	Glucose	Normal	Low
5.	pH	>7.3	<7.3
6.	Cells (WBCs)	<1000/mm^3	Usually >1000/mm^3
7.	Fluid LDH	<2/3rd of serum LDH	>2/3rd of serum LDH
8.	Fluid/serum LDH ratio	<0.6	>0.6
9.	Fluid adenosine deaminase (ADA) levels	Low	High
10.	Fluid cholesterol	Low (<60 mg/dl)	High (>60 mg/dl)
11.	Culture	Sterile	May yield organisms

SFAG: Serum fluid albumin gradient.

Table 1.12: Causes of pleural effusion depending on the fluid characteristic

Common	Uncommon
I. Transudate (SFAG > 1.1)	
• Congestive heart failure	• Superior vena cava obstruction
• Cirrhosis of liver	
• Nephrotic syndrome	• Myxedema
• Hypoproteinemia due to any cause	
• Pericardial effusion	• Peritoneal dialysis
II. Exudate (SFAG < 1.1)	
• Infections e.g. tubercular, bacterial (pneumonia), viral	• Chylothorax
	• Pancreatitis
• Malignancy, e.g. broncho-genic (common), mesothe-lioma (rare), lymphoma rare	• Esophageal perforation
	• Subphrenic abscess
	• Post-cardiac injury syndrome
• Collagen vascular disorders e.g. SLE, rheumatoid arthritis, Wegener's granulomatosis	• Uremia
	• Radiation injury
	• Iatrogenic
• Pulmonary emboli	*Drug-induced effusion, e.g*
• Meig's syndrome	Nitrofurantoin
• Sarcoidosis	Dantrolene
• Asbestosis	Methysergide
• Ruptured liver abscess into pleural space	Bromocriptine
	Procarbazine
	Amiodarone

Q. What does raised fluid ADA level indicate?

Ans. Tubercular effusion or effusion due to rheumatoid arthritis

Q. Name the drugs causing pleural effusion?

Ans. Read Table 1.12.

Table 1.13: Various types of fluids and their causes

Chylous (milky) effusion (Triglyceride > 1000 mg% with many large fat globules)
- Nephrotic syndrome
- Tubercular
- Malignancy
- Lymphoma
- Filariasis
- Myxoedema
- Trauma to chest wall

Ether extraction dissolves fat and leads to clearing; confirms true chylous nature of fluid.

Chyliform (fat present is not derived from thoracic duct but from degenerated leukocytes and tumor cells). The fat globules are small. Causes are:
- Tubercular
- Carcinoma of lung and pleura

Pseudochylous. Milky appearance is not due to fat but due to albumin, calcium, phosphate and lecithin. Causes are:
- Tuberculosis
- Nephrosis
- Heart disease
- Malignancy

Alkalinisation dissolves cellular protein and clears the fluid thus differentiates it from true chylous

Cholesterol effusion (Glistening opalescent appearances of fluid due to cholesterol crystals). Causes are:
- Long standing effusion, e.g. tuberculosis, carcinoma, nephrotic syndrome, myxoedema and post-myocardial infarction.

Hemorrhagic effusion (Hemothorax, e.g. blood stained fluid or fluid containing RBCs)
- Neoplasm, e.g. primary or secondary pleural mesothelioma
- Chest trauma (during paracentesis)
- Tubercular effusion
- Leukemias and lymphoma
- Pulmonary infarction
- Bleeding diathesis
  - Anticoagulant therapy
  - Acute hemorrhagic pancreatitis

Q. What are causes of unilateral, bilateral and recurrent pleural effusion?

Ans. **I. Bilateral pleural effusion.** The causes are:
- Congestive heart failure
- Collagen vascular diseases, e.g. SLE, rheumatoid arthritis
- Lymphoma and leukemias
- Bilateral tubercular effusion (rare)
- Pulmonary infarction

II. Unilateral pleural effusion. The causes are:
Right-sided effusion
- Rupture of acute amebic liver abscess into pleura
- Cirrhosis of the liver
- Congestive cardiac failure
- Meig's syndrome—fibroma of ovary with pleural effusion and ascites

III. Causes of recurrent pleural effusion
- Malignancy lung (e.g. bronchogenic, mesothelioma)
- Pulmonary tuberculosis
- Congestive heart failure
- Collagen vascular disorder

Q. What is empyema thoracis? What are its causes?

Ans. Collection of pus or purulent material in the pleural cavity is called *empyema thoracic*.
The causes are:
1. *Diseases of the lung* (Infection travels from the lung to the pleura either by contiguity or by rupture)
   - Lung abscess
   - Pneumonia
   - Tuberculosis
   - Infection
   - Bronchiectasis
   - Bronchopleural fistula
2. *Diseases of the abdominal viscera* (spread of infection from abdominal viscera to pleura)
   - Liver abscess (ruptured or unruptured)
   - Subphrenic abscess
   - Perforated peptic ulcer
3. *Diseases of the mediastinum* There may be infective focus in the mediastinum from which it spreads to the pleura.
   - Cold abscess
   - Esophageal perforation
   - Osteomyelitis
4. *Trauma with superadded infection*
   - Chest wall injuries (gun-shot wound, stab wound)
   - Postoperative
5. *Iatrogenic* Infection introduced during procedure.
   - Chest aspiration
   - Liver biopsy
6. *Blood-borne infection*, e.g. septicemia.

Q. What are physical signs of empyema thoracis?

Ans.
- Patient has a toxic look and prostration
- Signs of toxemia (fever, tachypnea and tachycardia). There is hectic rise of temperature with chills and rigors.
- Digital clubbing may be evident
- Intercostal spaces are full and may be tender
- All signs of pleural effusion will be present except rising dullness in axilla. This is due to collection of thick pus rather than clear fluid which does not obey the law of capillary action.
- The skin is red, edematous and glossy overlying empyema of recent onset. There may be a scar mark of an intercostal drainage (tube aspiration).
- Rarely, a subcutaneous swelling on the chest wall may be seen called *empyema necessitans*. The swelling increases with coughing.

Tip: The presence of signs of toxemia (toxic look, fever, tachypnea, tachycardia, sweating) in a patient with pleural effusion indicates *empyema thoracis*

Q. What is massive pleural effusion?

Ans. It refers to a large collection of fluid causing gross shifting of the mediastinum to the opposite side with stony dull note extending upto 2nd intercostal space or above on front of the chest.

Q. What is Meig's syndrome?

Ans. It comprises right sided transudative pleural effusion associated with an ovarian tumor usually benign (e.g. fibroma).

Q. What is phantom tumor (pseudotumor)?

Ans. This is nothing but an interlobar effusion (effusion in interlobar fissure) producing a rounded homogenous opacity on chest X-ray. This mimics a tumor due to its dense opacity but disappears with resolution of effusion, hence, called *phantom tumor*. This is occasionally seen in patients with congestive heart failure and disappears with diuretic therapy.

Q. What is subpulmonic effusion? When would you suspect it?

Ans. A collection of fluid below the lung and above the diaphragm is called *subpulmonic effusion*. This is suspected when diaphragm is unduly elevated on one side on chest X-ray. Chest X-ray taken in lateral decubitus position shows pleural effusion (layering out of the opacity along the lateral chest wall) which confirms the diagnosis.

Q. How do you explain the position of trachea either as central or to the same side in a case with pleural effusion?

Ans. Remember that negative intrapleural pressure on both sides keeps the trachea central, but, it is shifted to opposite side when a positive pressure develops in one of the interpleural space, therefore, midline trachea despite pleural effusion on one side could be due to?
- Mild pleural effusion (insignificant positive pressure develops)
- Loculated or encysted pleural effusion (positive pressure develops but not transmitted to opposite side—no pushing effect).
- Bilateral pleural effusion (both pleural cavities have positive pressure that neutralise each other's effect)
- Pleural effusion associated with apical fibrosis (fibrosis pulls the trachea to same side and neutralises the pushing effect of pleural effusion on the same side)
- Malignant pleural effusion with absorption collapse due to endobronchial obstruction. Due to collapse, trachea tries to shift towards the same side but pushing effect of effusion keeps it central in position.
- Collapse consolidation due to any cause (Isolated collapse and isolated consolidation has opposing effects).

Trachea can be shifted to same side in a case of effusion, if an underlying lung disease (e.g. collapse or fibrosis on the same side) exerts a pulling effect on the trachea and overcomes the pushing effect of effusion.

Q. What are signs at the apex (upper level) of pleural effusion?

Ans. The following signs develops only and occasionally in moderate (500-1000 ml) pleural effusion.
- Rising dullness; S-shaped Ellis curve in axilla
- Skodiac resonance—a band of hyper-resonance due to compensatory emphysema
- Bronchial breathing—high pitched tubular with bronchophony, whispering pectoriloquy and aegophony
- Pleural rub—rarely

Q. What are the causes of recurrent filling of pleural effusion after paracentesis?

Ans. Recurrent filling of the pleural effusion means appearance of the fluid to same level or above it on X-ray chest within few days (rapid filling) to weeks (slow filling) after removal of the fluid. That is the reason, a chest X-ray is taken before and after removal of the fluid to know the result of the procedure, its complications and later on its refilling. The causes are:
1. *Rapid refilling of pleural effusion*
   - Malignancy
   - Acute tuberculosis
2. *Slow refilling*
   - Tubercular effusion on treatment
   - Congestive cardiac failure – slow response or no response to conventional diuretics
   - Collagen vascular disorders
   - Meig's syndrome

Q. What are the pathogenic mechanisms of pleural effusion?

Ans. 1. Involvement of pleura by malignant infiltration, primary tumor or inflammatory process resulting in increased permeability.
2. Disruption of fluid containing structure in pleural cavity such as thoracic duct, esophagus, blood vessels with leakage of contents into pleural space.
3. Rupture of subpleural lung abscess or amoebic liver abscess into pleura.
4. Abnormal hydrostatic or lower osmotic pressure on an otherwise healthy pleura leading to transudation into pleural cavity.

Q. What are the complications of pleural effusion?

Ans. Common complications of pleural effusion are:
- *Thickened pleura* (indicates healed pleural effusion)
- *Empyema thoracis*—spontaneous or iatrogenic (during tapping of effusion with introduction of infection with improperly sterilized needle)
- *Nonexpansion of the lung.* Usually, after removal of pleural fluid, there is re-expansion of the

compressed lung immediately, but sometimes in long standing cases, it may not occur due to underlying fibrosis.

- *Acute pulmonary edema* is a procedural complication, develops with sudden withdrawl of a large amount of fluid. It is uncommon.
- *Hydropneumothorax* is again iatrogenic (procedural complication) due to lung injury and leakage of air into pleural space during pleural aspiration. To know this complication, a repeat X-ray chest is necessary after aspiration.
- *Cachexia* may develop in long-standing and malignant pleural effusion.

Q. What are clinical differences between thickened pleura and pleural effusion.

Ans. The differences are:

Thickened pleura	Pleural effusion
• Chest is normal or retracted on the side involved	• Chest is normal or prominent on side involved
• Movements are diminished	• Movement of chest are markedly diminished
• No shift of trachea or mediastinum	• Trachea and mediastinum is shifted to opposite side
• Percussion note is impaired with no rising dullness	• Percussion note is stony dull and there is rising dullness.
• Breath sounds are just diminished over the site involved	• Breath sounds are absent over the area of effusion.

88. What are causes of lymphadenopathy with pleural effusion?

Ans. Common causes are:

- Tubercular lymphadenitis with pleural effusion (lymph node in cervical, axillary, mediastinal regions may be enlarged)
- Lymphomas (effusion with generalised lymphadenopathy and splenomegaly)
- Acute lymphoblastic leukemia (cervical and axillary lymph nodes enlargement)
- Malignancy lung (scalene node, Virchow's gland, mediastinal lymph node)
- Collagen vascular disorder (generalised lymphadenopathy)
- Sarcoidosis (cervical, bilateral hilar lymphadenopathy).

Q. What do you know about pleural involvement in rheumatoid arthritis (RA)?

Ans. Pleural involvement in RA is associated with male gender, positive rheumatoid factor in serum (seropositive disease), presence of nodules and other systemic manifestations. The effusion is usually left sided, may be bilateral, develops as an inflammatory response to the presence of multiple subpleural

nodules. The pleural fluid is an exudate with low glucose concentration. Low glucose content is due to consumption of glucose by the inflammatory cells.

Q. What are differences between tubercular and malignant pleural effusion?

Ans. Tubercular and malignant pleural effusions are differentiated in Table 1.14.

Table 1.14: Differentiating features between tubercular and malignant pleural effusion

Tubercular	Malignant
A. *Clinical characteristics*	
• Commonest cause of effusion in all age groups	Common cause in old age
• Slow, insidious onset, can be acute or sudden	• Acute sudden onset
• Slow filling	• Rapid filling
• Cough, fever (evening rise), hemoptysis, night sweats are common complaints	• Cough, hemoptysis, dyspnea, tightness of chest, hoarseness of voice are presenting symptoms
• Cervical, axillary lymph nodes may be enlarged	• Scalene nodes or Virchow's gland enlarged
• Weakness, loss of weight present	• Marked cachexia and prostration
• Clubbing uncommon	• Clubbing common
• No signs of local compression	• Signs of local compression e.g. superior vena cava (prominent neck vein and chest veins), trachea (dysphonia), esophagus (dysphagia), and phrenic nerve (diaphragmatic paralysis) may be accompanying symptoms
• Localized crackles or rhonchi may be present depending on the site and type of lung involvement	• Localized wheeze or rhonchi common than crackles
B. *Fluid characteristics*	
• Straw-coloured exudate	• Hemorrhagic, exudate
• Lymphocytes present	• Malignant cells may be present along with RBCs
• Cob-web coagulum on standing	• RBCs may settle down on standing if hemorrhagic

Q. How will you investigate a case of pleural effusion?

Ans. A pleural effusion being of varied etiology, needs investigations for confirmation of the diagnosis as well as to find out the cause.

1. *Routine blood tests* (TLC, DLC and ESR). High ESR and lymphocytosis go in favor of tubercular effusion.
2. *Blood biochemistry*
   - Serum amylase for pancreatitis
   - Autoantibodies for collagen vascular disorders
   - Rheumatoid factor for rheumatoid arthritis

3. *Chest X-ray* (PA view, Fig. 1.3B) shows:
   - A lower homogenous opacity with a curved upper border which is concave medially but rising laterally towards the axilla.
   - Obliteration of costophrenic angle. It is the earliest sign hence, present in all cases of pleural effusion irrespective of its cause except loculated or encysted effusion.
   - Shift of trachea and mediastinum to opposite side
   - Lateral view is done to differentiate it from lobar consolidation
   - Lateral decubitus view is taken in case of subpulmonic effusion
   - Repeat X-ray chest after therapeutic aspiration of fluid
4. *Sputum examination*
   - For AFB and malignant cells
5. *Mantoux test.* It is not much of diagnostic value, may be positive in tuberculosis, negative in sarcoidosis, lymphoma and disseminated (miliary) tuberculosis or tubercular effusion in patients with AIDS.
6. *FNAC of lymph node,* if found enlarged
7. *Ultrasonography* is done to confirm the diagnosis and to mark the site for aspiration, and to find out the cause
8. *CT scan and MRI* are usually not required for diagnosis, but can be carried out to find out the cause wherever appropriate, and to differentiate localised effusion from pleural tumor.
9. *Aspiration of pleural fluid for;*
   Confirmation of diagnosis. At least 50 ml of fluid is to be removed and subjected to:
   - biochemistry (transudate/exudate), LDH, ADA, cholesterol and pH of fluid if empyema is suspected
   - cytology (for malignant cells, RBCs, WBCs and pus cells)
   - smear examination (e.g. Gram' stain, Ziehl-Neelsen stain, special stains for malignant cells)
   - culture for AFB. Recently introduced BACTEC system gives result within 7 days. Amylase level when malignancy or pancreatitis is suspected
     N.B. For indications of pleural aspiration, read bed side procedures and instruments used.

10. *Bronchoscopy* in a suspected case of bronchogenic carcinoma
11. *Pleural biopsy* for histopathological examination and mycobacterial culture or to find out the cause
12. *Thoracoscopy* to inspect the pleura so as to find out the cause. It is done raely.

Q. What are the uses of ultrasonography in pleural effusion?

Ans. Uses other than described above are:
1. For diagnosis of loculated effusions
2. For guided thoracocentesis, closed pleural biopsy or insertion of a chest drain.
3. To differentiate pleural fluid from pleural thickening.

Q. What investigations would you carry out to find out the cause?

Ans. Pleural Biopsy
CT chest
MRI chest

Q. Name the conditions in which fluid pH and glucose concentration are low?

Ans.
- Empyema thoracis
- Malignancy lungs
- Tuberculosis of lung
- Rheumatoid pleural effusion
- SLE with effusion

Q. What is the role of pleural fluid cytology in diagnosis of pleural effusion?

Ans.
- *Pleural fluid cell count:* Pleural fluid contains 1500 cells/HPF (predominently mononuclear cells). Counts >50,000 are seen in parapneumonic effusion or empyema, where as low count <1000 cells/HPF indicates transudate.
- Pleural fluid lymphocytosis indicates tuberculosis, malignancy, collagen vascular disease, lymphoma and sarcoidosis.
- Computerized interactive morphometry (analyses the size and nuclei of cells in a centrifuged specimen of fluid) differentiates between malignant cells and reactive lymphocytosis.

Q. What does a pleural fluid total neutral fat level > 400 mg/dl and triglyceride levels >1000 mg/dl indicate?

Ans. It indicates chylous pleural effusion. Read the causes in Table 1.13.

The patient whose X-ray is depicted in Figure 1.4A presented with acute severe dyspnea, tachypnea and tachycardia of few days duration. The patient was cyanosed and was admitted as an emergency.

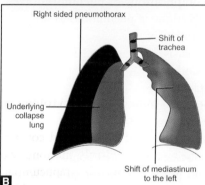

Figs 1.4A and B: Pneumothorax: A. Chest X-ray showing right sided pneumothorax. The collapsed lung is indicated by arrows; B. Diagrammatic illustration of pneumothorax

Clinical Presentations

- Acute onset of dyspnea at rest
- Associated pain chest or tightness of chest
- Symptoms non-progressive
- Palpitation and tachypnea common
- Increasing breathlessness, cyanosis, tachycardia, tachypnea, and hypotension suggest spontaneous tension pneumothorax
- Patient may have wheezing or other symptoms of COPD if it is the cause

- Cough aggravates breathlessness which is not relieved by any means except sitting posture

History

Points to be Noted in History

- Ipsilateral acute pleuritic pain
- Past/present history of COPD, asthma, tuberculosis, hemoptysis or trauma
- History of similar episodes in the past
- History of recent pleural aspiration or insertion of subclavian line or recent surgery on head and neck
- History of Marfan's syndrome
- History of HIV (sexual contact)
- History of positive pressure ventilation
- Any history of IHD (chest pain in the present or past)
- Any history of prolonged immobilisation or calf pain (pulmonary thromboembolism)

Examination

Proceed as follows:

I. General Physical Examination

- *Posture:* Patients prefer to lie on the uninvolved side in lateral decubitus position or propped up position.
- Restlessness.
- Tachypnea (respiratory rate is increased), dyspnea at rest
- Tachycardia
- Central cyanosis, indicates tension pneumothorax
- Lymph nodes may or may not be palpable
- Trachea may be shifted to opposite side (sternomastoid sign or Trail's sign may be positive)
- Accessory muscles of respiration may be actively working
- Ear, nose, throat may be examined
- Note the vitals, i.e. pulse, BP, temperature and respiration. Presence of hypotension or shock indicates tension pneumothorax, creates an emergency situation and warrants removal of the air.

- Look for clues regarding etiology, e.g.
  - Pleural aspiration site
  - Infraclavicular region for a bruise from the central line.
  - Marfanoid features
  - Inhalor or peak flowmeter by bedside to ascertain asthma or COPD.

II. Systemic Examination

Inspection
- Diminished movements on the side involved (right side in this case)
- Intercostal spaces widened and full on the side involved (right side in this case)
- Apex beat displaced to opposite side (left side in this case)
- Accessory muscles of respiration are hyperactive and stand out prominently in tension pneumothorax

Palpation
- Shift of trachea and apex beat (mediastinum) to the opposite side (e.g. left side in this case)
- Diminished movements on the side involved (e.g. right side)
- Expansion of chest decreased (on manual or tape measurement)
- Tactile vocal fremitus is reduced on the side involved (right side)

Percussion
- Hyperresonant percussion note on the side involved (right side). It is a diagnostic sign and differentiates it from pleural effusion
- Obliteration of liver dullness if right side is involved (obliterated in this case), splenic dullness if left side is involved (not applicable in this case)

Auscultation
- Diminished vesicular breathing or absent breath sounds on the side involved (right side in this case). Bronchial breathing indicates bronchopleural fistula (open pneumothorax)
- Vocal resonance diminished over the area involved (right side)
- No adventitous sound

Tip. Silent hyperresonant chest is characteristic of pneumothorax

Q. What is your diagnosis and why?

Ans. Sir, my provisional diagnosis is right sided pneumothorax. The points in favor of diagnosis are;

  i. Prominent chest on the side involved with diminished movements.

  ii. Shifting of trachea and mediastinum to opposite side (left side in this case)

  iii. Reduced vocal fremitus and vocal resonance on the side involved (right side)

  iv. Hyperresonant percussion note with diminished/absent breath sounds on the side involved (right side in this case)

Q. What is pneumothorax?

Ans. Presence of air in the pleural cavity is called *pneumothorax.*

Q. What is your differential diagnosis?

Ans. It has to be differentiated from large air cyst or a large bulla.

Table 1.15 differentiates between bulla and pneumothorax.

Q. What type of pneumothorax does your patient has?

Ans. Table 1.16 discusses various types of pneumothorax and their clinical features.

Q. Does the patient has tension pneumothorax?

Ans. No, patient does not have signs of cardiorespiratory embarrassment, i.e. tachypnea, tachycardia, hypotension), pulsus paradoxsus and cyanosis.

Q. What emergency measure would you adopt on bedside if it develops?

Ans. I will put a large bore needle in second intercostal space in sitting position on the side involved to relieve tension pneumothorax followed by appropriate drainage

Q. How do you classify pneumothorax?

Ans. The pneumothorax is divided into two categories; *spontaneous* and *traumatic*. The spontaneous pneumothorax may be primary (underlying lung is healthy) or secondary (occurs as a complication of some lung disease). The traumatic pneumothorax results from trauma (e.g. chest injury or procedural

trauma). The causes of pneumothorax are given in Table 1.17.

Q. What is recurrent spontaneous pneumothorax?

Ans. This refers to occurrence of second episode of pneumothorax within few weeks following the first episode. It occurs due to rupture of subpleural blebs or bullae in patients suffering from COPD. It is serious condition, needs chemical pleurodhesis (instillation of kaolin, talcom, minocycline or 10% glucose into pleural space) or by surgical pleurodhesis (achieved by pleural abrasions or parietal pleurectomy at thoracotomy or thoracoscopy). The causes of recurrent pneumothorax are given in Table 1.18.

Caution: Patient who are at increased risk of developing recurrent pneumothorax after the first episode (e.g. flying or diving personnel) should undergo preventive treatment (respiratory exercises) after first episode. The respiratory exercises include to inflate air pillows, balloons or football bladder. It will also help to achieve expansion of the collapsed lung.

Q. What are the complications of pneumothorax?

Ans. Common complications of pneumothorax are:

  • Hydropneumothorax
  • Empyema thoracis, pyopneumothorax
  • Hemopneumothorax
  • Thickened pleura
  • Acute circulatory failure—cardiac tamponade in tension pneumothorax
  • Atelectasis of the lung
  • Surgical emphysema and pneumomediastinum.

Q. How would you grade the degree of collapse in pneumothorax?

Ans. British thoracic society grading is:

  • Small; where there is small rim of air (translucent area) around the lung.
  • Moderate; when the lung is compressed towards the hilum (See Fig 1.4A) by a large translucent area containing air.
  • Complete; Airless lung, separate from diaphragm (aspiration is necessary)
  • Tension; Any pneumothorax with signs of cardiorespiratory distress.

Q. When would you suspect tension pneumothorax?

Ans. Tension pneumothorax should be suspected in patients with signs of pneumothorax with any of the following:

  • Severe progressive dyspnea
  • Tachypnea (RR > 30 min) tachycardia (HR > 130/min), cyanosis
  • Hypotension, pulsus paradoxus
  • Marked mediastinal shift

Table 1.15: Differentiating features of bulla from pneumothorax

Large air cyst or bulla	Pneumothorax
May be congenital or acquired	Acquired usually
Mediastinum not shifted (trachea central)	Mediastinum shifted to opposite side (trachea shifted to opposite side)
No underlying collapse of the lung on chest X-ray	Collapse of the lung is demarcated from the pneumothorax by a thin line on chest X-ray

Table 1.16: Types of pneumothorax and their clinical features

Feature	Closed (Fig. 1.4A)	Open	Tension (valvular)
Pathogenesis	The rupture site (opening) gets closed and underlying lung is collapsed (deflated). There is no communication between bronchus and the pleural space	The opening between the bronchus and pleural space does not close, remains patent, hence, called *bronchopleural fistula*	The communication between bronchus and pleural space persists and acts as a check valve (air can get in but cannot get out)
Mean pleural pressure	Negative (less than atmospheric pressure) hence, air can get absorbed and lung re-expands	Mean pleural pressure is atmospheric, hence, lung cannot re-expand. Secondly, due to patent communication, pneumothorax is likely to be infected leading to *pyopneumothorax*—a common complication	Mean pleural pressure is positive, hence, there is compression collapse of the underlying lung. It is an emergency situation because mean pleural pressure goes on building due to constant air entry during inspiration resulting in mediastinal shift and impaired venous return leading to cardiac tamponade requiring urgent drainage.
Causes	• Rupture of subpleural bleb or emphysematous bullae • COPD • Spontaneous due to congenital bleb rupture • Rupture of pulmonary end of pleural adhesion • Secondary to lung disease • Chest injury	• Tubercular cavity • Lung abscess • Necrotizing pneumonia • Chest trauma • Barotrauma • Empyema thoracic • Lung resection	• It can occur due to any cause • Catamenial pneumothorax (endometriosis in female)
Symptoms	• Mild cases may be asymptomatic and only chest X-ray may show pneumothorax • Some patients may present with breathlessness, pain chest/tightness of chest • Onset of dyspnea may be acute or subacute	• Majority of patients with bronchopleural fistula present with cough, fever, mucopurulent or purulent expectoration. Dyspnea is minimal. • Some complain of sensation of splash of fluid in the chest during jumping (e.g. hydropneumothorax)	• The presenting symptoms includes acute onset of dyspnea, cough, tachypnea, tachycardia • Cough worsens dyspnea. No relieving factor known except sitting position • Hypotension or shock and central cyanosis may be present due to cardiac tamponade.
Signs on the side involved	• Reduced chest movement • Shift of trachea and mediastinum to opposite side • Hyperresonant note • Markedly diminished or absent breath sounds • Vocal fremitus and resonance are also reduced • *Coin test* is positive	• All signs of closed pneumothorax present *plus* • Crack-pot sounds on percussion • Amphoric breath sounds with increased vocal resonance • Succussion splash indicates hydropneumothorax • Shifting dullness present if hydropneumothorax develops • *Coin test* may be positive	• All signs of closed pneumothorax present *plus* • Dyspnea, tachypnea, tachycardia, cyanosis • Pulsus paradoxus • Neck veins full, markedly raised JVP • Hypotension • Obtunded consciousness • Progressive mediastinal shift to opposite side with labored respiration
Plan of treatment	• Observation till air is automatically absorbed • Water-seal drainage, if necessary	• Water seal drainage • Treat hydro or pyopneumothorax with proper antibiotic • Thoracic surgeon consultation should be sought	• Immediate relief can be given by putting a wide bore needle (No. 20) in second intercostal space in sitting position in mid-clavicular line on the side involved followed by water-seal drainage system. • Antitubercular drugs/antibiotic therapy as considered appropriate • O_2 inhalation and propped up position • Resuscitation of shock • Morphine 5-10 mg subcutaneous

Table 1.17: Causes of pneumothorax

1. **Spontaneous**
   A. *Primary*
   - Rupture of apical subpleural bleb or bulla in young patients
   - Subpleural emphysematous bullae in old patients
   - Rupture of the pulmonary end of pleuropulmonary adhesion. The risk factors for it include:
     - Tall body habitus
     - Smoking
     - Marfan's syndrome
     - Mitral valve prolapse
     - Going to high altitude
     - Bronchial anatomical abnormalities
   B. *Secondary*
   - COPD
   - Pulmonary tuberculosis (subpleural focus) usually results in hydropneumothorax
   - Infections, e.g. necrotising pneumonia, staphylococcal lung abscess, usually result in hydropneumothorax or pyopneumothorax
   - Occupational lung disease, e.g. silicosis, coal-worker's pneumoconiosis
   - Malignancy lung
   - Interstitial lung disease
   - Catamenial (endometriosis in females)
   - Miscellaneous, e.g. esophageal rupture, cystic fibrosis, Caisson's disease, asthma, pulmonary infarct, post radiation, etc.
2. **Traumatic**

Injury	*Iatrogenic (procedural)*
• Blunt injury to the chest or abdomen	• Pleural tap
	• Pleural biopsy, lung biopsy
• Penetrating chest injury	• Bronchoscopy, endoscopy and sclerotherapy

3. **Induced (artificial)**
   - It was induced in the past to obliterate a tubercular cavity but is now obsolete term.

Table 1.18: Causes of recurrent pneumothorax

- Rupture of apical subpleural bleb or emphysematous bullae.
- Cystic fibrosis
- Rupture of lung cysts
- Rupture of bronchogenic carcinoma or esophageal carcinoma
- Catamenial pneumothorax
- AIDS
- Interstitial lung disease

Q. What do you understand by the term subcutaneous emphysema? What are its causes?

Ans. Subcutaneous emphysema (or surgical emphysema – an older term) refers to presence of air in the subcutaneous space either formed by necrotizing inflammation of the tissue by gas-forming organisms (gas gangrene) or by leakage of air from the lungs or neighboring hollow structures. The causes are:
- Pneumothorax
- Rib fracture or flail chest with leakage of air
- Fractures of paranasal sinuses
- Perforation of a hollow viscus, e.g. esophagus or larynx (spontaneous or procedural)
- Gas gangrene

Always look for subcutaneous emphysema in a case of pneumothroax by palpation with pressure of fingers over the side involved. There will be palpable crepitus on finger pressure.

Q. How will you investigate a patient with pneumothorax?

Ans. Investigations are done for sake of diagnosis and to find out the cause.
1. *Chest X-ray (PA view,* Fig. 1.4A) should be done first of all before any other investigation in case of suspected pneumothorax. It is done in erect position, sometimes expiratory film is taken especially in small pneumothorax. The radiological features are:
   - Increased translucency of the lung on the side involved with absence of peripheral lung markings.
   - The underlying lung is collapsed which is separated from airless peripheral translucent shadow (pneumothorax) by a pencil – sharp border.
   - Mediastinum is shifted to opposite side
   - Costophrenic angle is clear
   - Underlying lung disease may be apparent such as a tubercular cavity.
2. *Routine blood tests,* e.g. TLC, DLC, ESR, (raised ESR with relative mononuclear leukocytosis suggest tubercular etiology).
3. *Mantoux test* may be positive in tuberculosis
4. *Sputum for AFB* (3 consecutive specimens)
5. *Pulmonary function tests* (FEV1, FEV1/VC ratio, PFR etc. for COPD).

Q. What are similarities and dissimilarities between pleural effusion and pneumothorax?

Ans. Similarities and dissimilarities are as follows:
- Some clinical features on chest examination whether there is air or fluid in the pleural space are similar due to shift of the mediastinum to opposite side and collapse of the underlying lung as a result of positive intrapleural pressure (normally there is negative pressure in the pleural

space on both sides which keeps the mediastinum in the center). The similarity of signs include diminished movements and expansion, fullness of intercostal spaces on the side involved, shift of mediastinum to opposite side, hyperactivity of extrarespiratory muscles, diminished or bronchial breath sounds and decreased or increased vocal resonance with no added sounds.

- The dissimilarities include hyperresonant note on percussion in pneumothorax with obliteration or masking of liver dullness in right-sided pneumothorax and splenic dullness on left side pneumothorax. In pleural effusion, the percussion note is stony-dull on the side and over the part involved. The dullness is continuous with liver dullness on right side and cardiac dullness on left side with obliteration of resonance of Traube's area.

Tip. Absolute similarity is silent chest, i.e. no added sounds in both the conditions.

Absolute dissimilarity is hyperresonant note in pneumothorax and stony dull in pleural effusion

Note: Bronchial breath sounds with increased vocal resonance can occur both in pleural effusion (at the upper level or apex) and bronchopleural fistula (open pneumothorax).

N.B. Questions regarding water-seal intercostal tube drainage, its indications, complications and reasons for non-expansion of the lungs after drainage have been discussed in instruments and procedures (Chapter 2).

Q. **How would you manage this patient?**

Ans. As this patient has a large pneumothorax, hence aspiration is needed. Large pneumothorax with normal lungs are managed by simple aspiration rather than an intercostal tube drainage, aspiration is less painful than intercostal drainage, leads to shorter admission and reduces the need for pleurectomy with no increase in recurrence rate.

When there is rapid re-expansion following simple aspiration an intercostal tube with underwater seal drainage is used. The tube should be left for 24 hr. When the lung re-expands, clamp the tube for 24 hr. If repeat chest X-ray shows that lung remains expanded, the tube can be removed. If not, suction should be applied to the tube.

If fails to resolve within one week, surgical pleurodhesis should be considered.

Note: Small pneumothorax (<20% in size) spontaneously resolve within weeks.

Q. **How would you perform a pleurodhesis?**

Ans. By injecting talc into pleural cavity via intercostal tube.

Q. **In which patient, pleurodhesis is not performed?**

Ans. In patients with fibrosis, pleurodhesis is not attempted as they need lung transplantation in future and pleurodhesis would make it technically not feasible.

Q. **What are indications of open thoracotomy?**

Ans. It is considered when one of the following is present.

- A third episode of spontaneous pneumothorax
- An occurrence of bilateral pneumothorax
- Failure of the lung to expand after tube thoracotomy.

CASE 5: HYDROPNEUMOTHORAX

The patient whose X-ray is depicted as Figure 1.5A presented with fever, cough with expectoration, mucopurulent foul smelling without hemoptysis. The patient gave history of some abnormal sounds (crack-pots) on running or walking.

Clinical Presentation

- Dyspnea at rest, cough
- Pain chest or heaviness in chest
- Splashing sound during jumping
- Fever, high grade with chills and rigors if pyopneumothorax

Points to be Noted in the History

- History of fever or injury in the past.
- History of tuberculosis in the past
- Any history of pain chest, hemoptysis or a cardiac disorder.
- Any history of drainage of fluid in the past.

General Physical Examination

- Patient is orthopneic, sitting in the bed

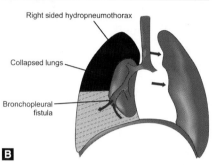

Figs 1.5A and B: Hydropneumothorax: A. Chest X-ray (PA view) shows hydro-pneumothorax (left side); B. Diagrammatic illustration of bronchopleural fistula with hydropneumothorax (right side)

- Fever
- Tachypnea, tachycardia
- Cyanosis
- Clubbing of fingers present in pyopneumothorax
- Accessory muscles of respiration may be active

- Shift of trachea and mediastinum to opposite side – *Sternomastoid sign or Trail sign* may be positive.

Systemic Examination

Inspection

- Signs similar to open pneumothorax

Palpation

- Signs similar to open pneumothorax

Percussion

- A horizontal fluid level, above which percussion note is hyperresonant and below which it is stony dull – hence, there is a clear cut transition between a hyperresonant to stony dull note
- Shifting dullness present because fluid has space (occupied by air) to shift
- Coin test may be positive.

Auscultation

- Succession splash present
- Amphoric bronchial breathing present in bronchopleural fistula—a common cause of hydropneumothorax
- Tingling sounds heard

Q. What is your provisional diagnosis and why?

Ans. Patient has left-sided hydropneumothorax (bronchopleural fistula). The presence of clear cut horizontal fluid level defined on percussion with hyperresonant note above it and presence of shifting dullness, succussion splash and amphoric bronchial sounds support my diagnosis.

Q. What is hydropneumothorax?

Ans. The presence of both air (above) and fluid (below) in pleural cavity is called *hydropneumothorax*. If instead of fluid, pus collects along with air, then it is called *pyopneumothorax*. Similarly collection of air and blood is called *hemopneumothorax*.

Q. What is your differential diagnosis?

Ans. Following conditions may mimic hydropneumothorax:

1. **Pyopneumothorax** (there will be fever, signs of toxemia in addition to hydropneumothorax)
2. **Pleural effusion** (shifting dullness, succussion splash and classical horizontal fluid level will be absent)

3. **Eventration of diaphragm** with herniation of stomach into chest (this will produce succussion splash with resonant percussion note. Borborgymi sounds may be heard over the chest).
4. A **large lung abscess** partially filled with exudate will produce signs of cavity and coarse crackles are characteristics.

Q. What are causes of succussion splash?

Ans. Read clinical methods in medicine by Prof SN Chugh.

Q. What is bronchopleural fistula?

Ans. Actually it is a communication between atmosphere and pleura via the bronchus. It is open type of pneumothorax in which repeated infections are common and result in hydro or pyopneumothorax. All signs of hydropneumothorax are present. Amphoric bronchial sounds indicate a patent communication and confirm the diagnosis.

Q. What are the differences between hydropneumothorax and pleural effusion?

Ans. Table 1.19 differentiates between hydropneumothorax and pleural effusion.

Table 1.19: Differentiating features of hydropneumothorax and pleural effusion

Hydropneumothorax (Fig. 1.5B)	Pleural effusion
• Shifting dullness on percussion present	Shifting dullness absent (the rising dullness – Ellis S-shaped curve is nowadays obsolete term)
• Horizontal fluid level, i.e. there is transition between hyperresonant note (above) and stony dull note (below)	No such level
• Succussion splash present	No succussion splash
• Tingling sounds especially after cough may be audible	No such sound
• Coin-test sound in upper part of hydropneumothorax may occasionally be positive	Coin – test negative
• Diminished breath sounds and vocal resonance except in bronchopleural fistula where amphoric breath sounds may be heard	Sometimes, a tubular bronchial breathing with increased vocal resonance (bronchophony, whispering pectoriloquy and egophony) present over the top of effusion

Q. What are the causes of hydropneumothorax?

Ans. Common causes of hydropneumothorax are:
- Rupture of subpleural tubercular cavity (the most common cause)
- Rupture of lung abscess—actually, it causes pyopneumothorax
- Penetrating chest injury with infection—again a cause of hemopneumothorax
- Acute pulmonary infarction (embolism)
- Following cardiac surgery
- *Iatrogenic*, i.e. introduction of the air during aspiration of pleural effusion
- *Pneumothorax.* Actually bronchopleural fistula (open pneumothorax) of tubercular etiology is the most common cause, but sympathetic collection of fluid in closed and tension pneumothorax may also lead to hydropneumothorax.

Q. What are the causes of bronchopleural fistula?

Ans. Common causes include:
- Rupture of tubercular cavity into pleural space
- Rupture of lung abscess into pleura with patent bronchus.
- Trauma to chest or barotrauma
- Necrotizing pneumonia leading to empyema thoracis.
- Following lung resection.

Q. How would you explain absent shifting dullness in a case of hydropneumothorax?

Ans. Hydropneumothorax contains air above (occupying a large space) and fluid below (occupying smaller space), both in moderate amount and are separated by a horizontal level (a line seen in peripheral lung field on chest X-ray, Fig. 1.5A)). Shifting dullness is present because

fluid has space to shift by displacing air. Therefore, shifting dullness in hydropneumothorax will be absent if above mentioned conditions are not fulfilled.
- Loculated or encysted hydropneumothorax (both air and fluid are tightly packed)
- Too little air in hydropneumothorax
- Too much fluid in hydropneumothorax
- Thick viscid pus (sometime in pyopneumothorax).

Q. What are the characteristic features of pyopneumothorax?

Ans. The patient will have all the clinical features of hydropneumothorax *plus*
- Presence of toxic look and prostration
- Hectic fever with chills and rigors
- Tachycardia, tachypnoea and clubbing of fingers
- Intercostal tenderness and tenderness during percussion (patient winces during percussion).

Q. What are the differences between empyema thoracis and pyopneumothorax?

Ans. Clinical features of both empyema thoracis and pyopneumothorax are similar (hectic fever, signs of toxemia, intercostal tenderness, diminished movements and diminished or absent breath sounds).
The differentiating features between the two are same as in case of pleural effusion versus hydropneumothorax such as presence of a horizontal level (transition between hyperresonant and stony dull percussion note), shifting dullness, succussion splash in pyopneumothorax but not in case of empyema thoracis. However, it will be difficult to differentiate a loculated pyopneumothorax from empyema thoracis because of absence of above mentioned features.

Q. How will you differentiate between a lung abscess and pyopneumothorax?

Ans. Table 1.20 differentiates between lung abscess and pyopneumothorax.

Table 1.20: Differentiating features between pyopneumothorax and lung abscess

Pyopneumothorax	Lung abscess
• Cough and expectoration minimal	Copious purulent expectoration is a predominant feature
• Shift of the mediastinum and trachea to opposite side	No shift of trachea or mediastinum
• Added sounds are absent	Added sounds such as crackles will be present
• Chest X-ray will show horizontal level starting from the periphery	A horizontal fluid level does not touch the periphery of the lung
• Vocal fremitus, breath sounds and vocal resonance diminished or absent	Vocal fremitus and vocal resonance may be decreased (cavity full of pus) or increased if lung abscess is empty and superficially placed. There can be a bronchial breathing as heard over a cavity

Q. How will you investigate a patient with pyopneumothorax?

Ans. Investigations are as follows:
1. *Routine blood tests* such as TLC, DLC and ESR for leukocytosis as an evidence of infection
2. *Sputum examination* for culture and sensitivity
3. *Chest X-ray (PA view)* will show:
   - A horizontal fluid level
   - Increased radiolucency above the horizontal level without lung markings with a homogeneous opacity below the horizontal level (Fig. 1.5A)
   - Shifting of trachea and mediastinum to the opposite side

N.B. X-ray should be taken in upright position to show a fluid level

   - The collapsed lung due to compression from outside is usually hidden within homogeneous opacity of fluid and may not be visible on X-ray.
4. *Aspiration of fluid* or the thick exudate (pus) will be done which is sent for culture and sensitivity.

Q. Name the diagnostic signs of hydropneumothorax/pyopneumothorax. How will you elicit them?

Ans. Diagnostic signs are as follows:
1. A horizontal level, i.e. upper part of hydropneumothorax is hyper-resonant due to presence of air and lower part is dull due to presence of fluid/pus
2. Shifting dullness
3. Succussion splash
4. Tingling sounds on auscultation.
5. Coin test may sometimes be present

Q. What is coin test and how would you elicit it.

Ans. Read Clinical Methods in Medicine by Prof SN Chugh.

Q. How will you treat a patient with hydropneumothorax/bronchopleural fistula?

Ans.
1. Water-seal intercostal tube drainage by putting a Foley's catheter in pleural space and connecting it with water-seal. The fluid will be drained and the air is also expelled with it while remaining air will get absorbed automatically.
2. Antibiotics depending on the cause. If cause is tubercular, institute ATT.
3. Surgery is done in resistant cases especially with pyo or hemopneumothorax.

CASE 6: COLLAPSE OF THE LUNG

The patient whose X-ray (Fig. 1.6A) is depicted and presented with cough, dry hacking without haemoptysis and acute breathlessness.

Clinical Presentations

- Pain on the affected side
- Breathlessness
- Dry cough and fever

Presence of Symptoms Depends on:

- Rapidity with which they develop
- Amount of the lung involved
- Presence or absence of infection

Points to be Noted in the History

- Past history of tuberculosis or malignancy or asthma.
- Any history of swelling in the neck, axilla or groin
- Past history of mumps, measles and whooping cough during childhood
- Past history of rheumatic heart disease or pericardial disease (fever, chest pain).

General Physical Examination

Look for the followings:
- Patient may dyspneic, orthopneic if major bronchus is involved
- Central cyanosis
- Tachypnea, tachycardia

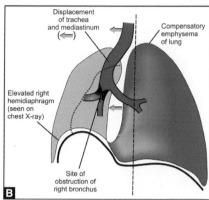

Figs 1.6A and B: A. Chest X-ray showing collapse of right upper lobe; B. Diagrammatic illustration of collapse lung

- Fever (develops in fibrosing alveolitis or in bronchogenic carcinoma)

Systemic Examination

Inspection

- Flattening or depression of the chest on affected side
- Crowding of the ribs and narrowing of intercostal spaces

- Diminished movements on the side involved
- Shifting of trachea, apex beat towards the side involved (pulling effect) – Trail's sign
- Kyphoscoliosis may result in long-standing collapsed lung with fibrosis
- Drooping of shoulder if apex of the lung is collapsed

Palpation

- *Shifting of trachea and mediastinum to the same side*
- Reduced movements of the chest on involved side
- Reduced expansion of the chest on side involved
- Vocal fremitus on the affected side may be;
  — Diminished or absent if bronchus is totally occluded
  — Increased if bronchus is patent.

Percussion

- Impaired or dull note on the side affected

Auscultation

Collapse with obstructed bronchus
- Diminished or absent breath sounds
- Diminished/absent vocal resonance
- No added sounds

Collapse with patent bronchus
- Tubular bronchial breath sounds
- Increased vocal resonance with bronchophony and whispering pectoriloquy
- Coarse crackles may be heard occasionally

Q. What is your diagnosis and why?

Ans. The provisional diagnosis is collapse of right upper lobe. *Points in favour of diagnosis are:*
- Depressed chest and decreased movements on the side involved.
- Shift of trachea and mediastinum to the side involved
- Dull percussion note on the site involved
- Breath sounds are diminished on the affected part of lung

Q. What is the probable cause?

Ans. Could be tubercular due to following reasons;
- Gradual onset of weight loss, anorexia, fever with evening rise and night sweats

- Physical signs are localized to apical region of upper lobe
- No signs of toxaemia or cachexia

Q. What is your alternate diagnosis?

Ans. The only condition from which collapse is to be differentiated is pulmonary fibrosis. Table 1.21 differentiates between collapse and fibrosis.

Table 1.21: Differentiating features of lung collapse and fibrosis

Feature	Collapse	Fibrosis
Onset	Acute	Chronic
Chest wall	Flattened	Retracted
Breath sounds	Absent	Feeble but never absent

Q. What do you understand by the term collapse of the lung?

Ans. Pulmonary collapse or atelectasis is defined as *"airlessness with shrinkage"* of a part or the whole lung. Atelectasis may be present since birth *(atelectasis neonatorum)* due to failure of the lung to expand, or may occur anytime during life (acquired atelectasis) due to absorption of air secondary to obstruction, compression, contraction or surfactant loss.

Q. What are various types of collapse?

Ans. Localised/hemithoracic loss of lung volume (collapse of the lung) can occur with patent bronchus or with occluded bronchus (obstructive collapse) or there is compression of the lung from outside (intrapleural positive pressure), hence, it is of two main types:

1. *Obstructive collapse (absorption or resorption collapse, Fig. 1.6B).* It occurs due to absorption of air distal to obstruction in the alveoli. The site of obstruction can be central or peripheral.
   i. Central obstructive collapse is with obstructed major bronchus.
   ii. Peripheral obstructive (absorption) collapse is always with patent surrounding bronchus.
2. *Compression collapse (Relaxation collapse).* It occurs from relaxation of the lung due to pleural disease (e.g. pleural effusion, pneumothorax and hydropneumothorax).

Q. What are the causes of collapse of the lung?

Ans. 1. *Obstructive (absorption collapse)*
   A. *Central (major bronchus):* The causes are:

Common	Rare
• Bronchial adenoma or carcinoma	• Aortic aneurysm
• Enlarged tracheobronchial lymph nodes (malignant, tubercular)	• Giant left atrium
	• Congenital bronchial atresia
• Inhaled foreign body, misplaced endotracheal tube	• Stricture/stenosis
• Mucus plugging	• Pericardial effusion

   B. *Peripheral (divisions of bronchus/bronchi)*
   • Pneumonias
   • Mucus plugging (sputum retention)
   • Asthma
   • Pulmonary eosinophilia
2. *Compression collapse (relaxation collapse)*
   • Pleural effusion
   • Pneumothorax
   • Hydropneumothorax, pyopneumothorax, hemopneumothorax.

Q. What are the clinical differences between central obstructive and peripheral obstructive collapse?

Ans. Remember that peripheral collapse does not involve the major bronchus, involves divisions of bronchus or bronchi with the result the collapse occurs with patent bronchus (i.e. surrounding bronchi are patent) while, central obstruction of a major bronchus leads to collapse of all its divisions, hence, the whole lobe is airless with no patent bronchus. The differentiating features are summarised in Table 1.22. The causes of both types of obstructive bronchus are given above. Signs of compression collapse means signs of pleural effusion/pneumothorax. The underlying collapsed lung is silent (relaxed hence called relaxation collapse). In this type of collapse, trachea and mediastinum is shifted to the opposite side due to pushing effect of fluid/air.

Q. What are the clinical pulmonary presentations of bronchogenic carcinoma?

Ans. Clinical pulmonary presentations of bronchogenic carcinoma are:
   • Collapse
   • Collapse consolidation
   • Cavitation
   • Mediastinal compression/obstruction-superior vena cava syndrome
   • Pancoast's tumor—Apical carcinoma may involve brachial plexus producing monoplegia
   • Consolidation—a solid tumor
   • Pleural effusion—rapid filling, hemorrhagic.

Q. How will you investigate a patient with lobar collapse?

Ans. Investigations of lobar collapse are:
   • *Routine blood examination*
   • *Sputum examination*—cytology, microbiology and culture
   • *Chest X-ray (PA and lateral view).* It will show:
      • Homogeneous opacity of the collapsed lung
      • Displacement of trachea and cardiac shadow (mediastinum) to the diseased (involved) side
      • Crowding of the ribs with reduction of intercosal spaces due to loss of volume of the lung on the side involved
      • Elevation of hemidiaphragm on the side involved
      • Pleural effusion on the side involved if collapse is due to malignancy of lung
      • Sometimes, the radiological features of underlying cause (hilar lymphadenopathy), foreign body may be evident

Table 1.22: Differentiative features of central obstructive and peripheral obstruction collapse of lung

Feature	Central obstructive collapse (occluded bronchus)	Peripheral obstructive collapse (patent bronchus)
• Shift of trachea and mediastinum	To the same side	To the same side
• Elevated dome of the diaphragm	On the same side	On the same side
• Breath sounds	Absent on the side involved	Tubular (bronchial) breath sounds
• Vocal resonance	Decreased/absent on the side involved	Increased vocal resonance with whispering pectoriloquy
• Common cause	• Tumor or lymph node or a foreign body	• Mucus plugging, ipsilateral bronchial cast or clot
• CT scan or chest X-ray	Collapse with loss of open bronchus sign— Golden's "S" sign	Collapse with open bronchus
• Signs on the other side	Signs of compensatory emphysema i.e. hyperresonant note, vesicular breathing with prolonged expiration	No signs of compensatory emphysema on the other side

- *CT scan* to find out the cause
- *Bronchoscopy* to find out the cause and to take biopsy
- *Scalene node biopsy,* if lymph node enlarged or malignancy lung suspected
- *Pleural fluid examination* if pleural effusion present.

Note: Investigations of compression collapse are same as that of pleural effusion.

Q. What are the complications of collapse?
Ans. Common complications of collapse are:
- Secondary infection
- Spontaneous pneumothorax from ruptured bullae of compensatory emphysema on the uninvolved side of the lung.

CASE 7: DIFFUSE FIBROSING ALVEOLITIS

The patient (i.e. a coal-mine worker) whose CT scan is depicted as Figure 1.7A presented with progressive dyspnea and cough for the last 2 years. The dyspnea was exertional in the begining, increased to occur now at rest. There was history of associated fever, weight loss, malaise and fatigue.

Clinical Presentation

- Progressive exertional dyspnea
- Persistent dry cough

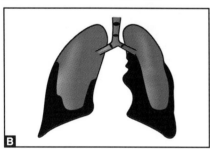

Figs 1.7A and B: A. CT scan chest showing honey-comb appearance in a patient with diffuse fibrosing alveolitis, B. Diagrammatic illustration

- Fever, weight loss, fatigue
- At the late stages, patient may complain of symptoms of cor pulmonale (abdominal pain due to hepatomegaly, ascites, swelling legs)

Points to be Noted in the History

- Past history of tuberculosis or lung suppuration
- Any history of radiation exposure
- Any history of joint pain, arthralgia, rash
- Drug history
- Occupational history, e.g. coal miner, stone cutter, farmer or industrial worker
- Past history of rheumatic heart disease or any other cardiac disorders.

General Physical Examination

- Dyspnea, orthopnea
- Tachypnea
- Central cyanosis (if severe)
- Clubbing of the fingers
- Signs of occupation
- Raised JVP and ankle edema if severe disease
- Examine hands for rheumatoid arthritis, systemic sclerosis
- *Face:* Look for heliotropic rash for dermatomyositis, typical rash of SLE, pinched faces of systemic sclerosis and lupus pernio of sarcoidosis.
- *Mouth:* Look for aphthous ulcers of Crohn's disease, dry mouth of Sjogren's syndrome.

Systemic Examination

Inspection

- Increased respiratory rate

- Bilateral symmetrical reduction in chest movements
- Accessory muscles of respiration may be hyperactive

Palpation

- Reduced bilateral chest movements
- Reduced expansion of the chest
- Bilateral reduction of vocal fremitus

Percussion

- Dullness on percussion at lung bases on both sides

Auscultation

- Bilateral crackles (end-inspiratory) at both the bases (lower zones) of the lungs which may disappear or become quieter on leaning forward but do not disappear on coughing unlike those of pulmonary edema.
- Vesicular breathing diminished in intensity
- Vocal resonance bilaterally diminished

Other System Examination

- Signs of right heart failure (raised JVP, loud P2, hepatomegaly, central cyanosis and pitting oedema) may or may not be present, if present indicates chronic cor pulmonale.

Q. What is your clinical diagnosis?

Ans. The patient being an occupational workers (coal-miner), developed symptoms of progressive dyspnea, cough, fever and weight loss, the probable diagnosis will be occupational lung disease, e.g. coal-miner pneumoconiosis.

Q. Summarize your findings in favor of your diagnosis?

Ans. A middle aged coal miner presented with progressive dyspnea, cough, fever, malaise and weight loss. There is tachypnea, tachycardia, central cyanosis and clubbing of fingers. Chest shows reduced bilateral

chest movements, expansion and vocal fremitus. The lung bases are dull on percussion. On auscultation, there is vesicular breathing with fine, basal end-inspiratory crackles.

Q. What is your differential diagnosis?

Ans. Differential diagnosis lies between the causes of bilateral interstitial fibrosis. (Read the cause of fibrosis). The common conditions to be differentiated are:

- Idiopathic Interstitial fibrosis
- Farmer's lung
- Respiratory bronchiolitis

- Silicosis
- Asbestosis

Q. What are the causes of crackles at the lung bases with clubbing?

Ans. All the following conditions constitute the differential diagnosis:
1. Bronchogenic carcinoma
2. Bronchiectasis
3. Asbestosis
4. Pulmonary edema

Q. What do you understand by fibrosis of the lung? What are its causes?

Ans. Fibrosis of the lung means replacement of lung parenchyma by fibrous tissue. It occurs usually as a reactive process or a healing /reparative process.

Causes
1. *Focal fibrosis*
   - Pneumoconiosis
2. *Reparative fibrosis /replacement fibrosis*
   - Tuberculosis
   - Following bronchiectasis, lung abscess, pulmonary infarction
   - Following radiation
3. *Interstitial fibrosis (it is bilateral fibrosis of alveolar walls and septa)*
   A. *Pulmonary origin*
      - *Hypersensitivity*
        - Diffuse fibrosing alveolitis (Fig. 1.7A)
        - Farmer's lung
      - *Collagen vascular disorders*
        - SLE
        - Systemic sclerosis
        - Rheumatoid arthritis (rheumatoid lung)
      - Lymphangitis carcinomatosis
      - Drug-induced, e.g. busulphan, bleomycin, nitrofurantoin, methysergide, hydralazine, hexamethonium, amiodarone
      - *Miscellaneous*
        - Sarcoidosis
        - Aspiration pneumonitis
        - Histiocytosis
        - Tuberous sclerosis
        - Xanthomatosis
   B. *Cardiac origin*
      - Multiple pulmonary infarcts
      - Mitral stenosis
   C. *Idiopathic*
      - Hamman-Rich disease.

Q. What is Hamman-Rich syndrome? What are its clinical features?

Ans. Diffuse interstitial fibrosis or fibrosing alveolitis of acute onset, progressive course of unknown etiology is called *Hamman-Rich syndrome*. It is characterised by progressive dyspnea, dry cough, fever, weight loss and signs of bilateral fibrosis of the lung.

The clinical characteristics (physical signs) have already been described in the beginning.

Q. What are causes of end-inspiratory crackles?

Ans. Read respiratory system in clinical methods in medicine by Prof SN Chugh.

Q. How will you investigate a patient with cryptogenic fibrosing alveolitis?

Ans. The common investigations are as follows:
1. *Routine blood tests.* ESR in high
2. *Blood* for *rheumatoid factor* and *antinuclear antibodies.* Immunoglubulins are raised
3. *Chest X-ray (PA view) shows:*
   - Diffuse pulmonary opacities in the lower zones peripherally
   - The hemidiaphragm are high and the lungs appear small
   - In advanced disease, there may be "honey-comb" appearance of the lungs in which diffuse pulmonary shadowing is interspersed with small cystic translucencies.
4. *High resolution CT* scan may show honey-combing (Fig. 1.7A) and scarring, most marked peripherally in both the lungs or there may be ground glass appearance. CT scan is useful in early diagnosis when chest X-ray may not show the radiological changes. MRI is useful to determine disease activity.
5. *Pulmonary function tests.* There is restrictive ventilatory defect with reduction in FEV1 and vital capacity (VC). The carbon monoxide transfer factor is low and lung volumes are reduced (Read pulmonary function tests in the beginning of this chapter – Table 1.5).
6. *Bronchoalveolar lavage* may show a large number of lymphocytes and *transbronchial biopsy* may sometimes be helpful.
7. *Open lung biopsy* for histological patterns of idiopathic cases of interstitial lung disease. In early stages, there is mononuclear cell infiltration in alveolar wall with interstitial fibrosis; in late stages, honey combing, bronchial dilatation and cysts are seen.

Q. What is respiratory bronchiolitis?

Ans. Respiratory bronchiolitis is an interstitial lung disease of smokers in which there is accumulation of pigment-laden macrophages in the respiratory bronchioles and adjacent alveoli leading to mononuclear cell infiltration and fibrosis. It may reverse on cessation of smoking.

Clinical picture is similar to cryptogenic fibrosing alveolitis.

Q. What is farmer's lung?

Ans. It is an occupational lung disease caused by an inhalation of organic dust (mouldy hay, straw, grain), characterised by features of extrinsic allergic alveolitis (e.g. headache, muscle pains, malaise, pyrexia, dry cough and breathlessness without wheeze) which may progress to irreversible pulmonary fibrosis.

The pathogenic mechanism is local immune response to fungal antigen, e.g. *Micropolyspora faenae or Aspergillus fumigatus.* The **diagnosis** is based on; (i) clinical features, (ii) characteristic radiological features as described above, (iii) high-resolution CT scan and (iv) identification of potential antigen by ELISA or precipitin antibody test.

The **treatment** is removal of the source of antigen wherever possible and a course of 3-4 week of prednisolone (40 mg/day) may arrest the process.

Q. What is coal-worker's pneumoconiosis?

Ans. The disease follows prolonged inhalation of coal dust hence, is an occupational lung disease seen in coal-workers. The condition is subdivided into *simple pneumoconiosis* and *progressive massive fibrosis* for both clinical purposes and certification.

The simple coal miner's pneumoconiosis is reversible (it does not progress if miner leaves the industry), non-progressive and radiologically characterised by nodulation without cavitation. On the other hand, progressive massive fibrosis—a variety of coal miner's pneumoconiosis is irreversible, progressive and radiologically characterised by large dense masses, single or multiple, occur mainly in upper lobes associated with cavitation. Tuberculosis may be a complication. It carries poor prognosis.

Q. What is Caplan's syndrome?

Ans. It consists of association of rheumatoid arthritis (positive rheumatoid factor) in patients with coal worker's pneumoconiosis with rounded fibrotic nodules (nodular shadowing) 0.5 to 5 cm in diameter distributed mainly in the periphery of the lung field.

Q. What is silicosis?

Ans. This disease is caused by inhalation of silica dust or quartz particles, characterised by progressive development of hard nodules which coalesce as the disease progresses followed by fibrosis. The clinical and radiological features are similar to coal worker's pneumoconiosis though changes tend to be more marked in the upper lobe. The hilar shadow may be enlarged; *egg-shell* calcification in the hilar lymph node is a distinct feature. Tuberculosis may be a complication and may modify the silicotic process with ensuring caseation and calcification. The disease progresses even when the exposure to dust ceases.

Q. What is asbestosis? What are its possible effects on respiratory tract?

Ans. Table 1.23 explains features of asbestosis and its effects on respiratory tract presented diagrammatically.

Table 1.23: Features of asbestosis

Asbestosis is an occupational lung disorder, occurs due to exposure to fibrous mineral asbestos in certain occupations such as in the mining and milling of the mineral. The main types of mineral asbestos involved in asbestosis are:

- *Chrysolite* (white asbestos—a common factor)
- *Crocidolite* (blue asbestos—uncommon factor)
- *A mosite (brown) asbestos*—a rare factor)

The possible effects of asbestosis are depicted in Figure 1.7C.

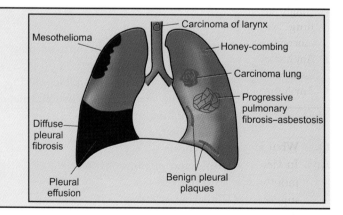

CASE 8: CAVITY WITH FIBROSIS

The young patient whose X-ray is depicted (Fig. 1.8A) presented with cough, fever, hemoptysis and weight loss for the last 6 months. There was history of weakness and decreased appetite and night sweats.

Clinical Presentations

- Cough, fever and night sweats, weakness may be initial manifestations of *tubercular cavity*
- Cough, massive expectoration, fever, purulent sputum with postural and diurnal variation suggest lung *abscess* or *bronchiectasis*
- Cough, hemoptysis, breathlessness, fever, weight loss, anorexia suggest *malignancy* as the cause of cavity.

Points to be Noted in the History

- Onset and progression of the symptoms
- Past history of tuberculosis or malignancy, ankylosing spondylitis.
- Past history of pneumonia (e.g. fever, cough, hemoptysis and pain chest) or lung suppuration (cough with mucopurulent or purulent sputum)
- Any history of headache, vomiting, visual disturbance or neurological deficit.
- Any history of radiation.

Fig. 1.8A: Chest X-ray (PA view) showing a cavity with fibrosis

General Physical Examination

- Patient may be ill-looking, emaciated
- Repeated coughing and bringing out a large amount of sputum
- Tachypnea and tachycardia
- Fever
- Clubbing of fingers and toes
- Weight loss
- Oedema feet if secondary amyloidosis develops and involves the kidneys

Systemic Examination

Inspection

- Diminished movement on the side involved (right side in this case)

Palpation

- Movements of the chest reduced on the side involved (right side in this case)

- Expansion of the chest is reduced if cavity is large
- Shift of trachea and mediastinum to the same side if there is a large cavity with fibrosis (right side in this case)

Percussion

- Dull percussion note over the cavity. Rest of the lung is normally resonant

Auscultation

- Amphoric or cavernous bronchial breathing over the cavity
- Increased vocal resonance over the area of cavity with bronchophony
- Mid-inspiratory and expiratory crackles
- Post-tussive crackles
- Crackpot sounds

Note: All the above mentioned signs will be present only if the cavity is large, superficial and communicates with bronchus. Deep seated cavity may not produce any physical sign.

Q. **What is your clinical diagnosis?**
Ans. In view of history of cough, fever, hemoptysis of 6 months duration and signs of cavitation in this patient suggest either a tubercular or a malignant cavity in the right lung.

Q. **What is your differential diagnosis?**
Ans. 1. **Bronchiectesis,** (could be tubercular). Read clinical case discussion on bronchiectasis
2. **Resolving consolidation** will produce massive expectoration and bronchial breath sounds.
3. **Lung abscess.** Read symptoms and signs of lung abscess in this case discussion
4. **Malignancy lung.** Cough, hemoptysis, weakness, weight loss, cachexia along with signs of a cavity and hilar lymphadenopathy are pointers to its diagnosis.

Q. **What do you understand by the term "cavity"?**
Ans. Pulmonary cavity is an area of liquefaction necrosis within the lung parenchyma in communication with a patent bronchus. The cavity may be empty or may be filled with secretions and infected material. *Pseudocavity* means appearance of a cavity on chest X-ray which may be obtained with summation of shadows of vessels, ribs and calcification.

Q. **What are causes of cavitation in the lung?**
Ans. Common causes are:
1. *Infection*
   - Tuberculosis
   - Bronchiectasis
   - Ruptured hydatid cyst with infection
   - Lung abscess
   - Fungal infection
2. *Congenital*
   - Infected bronchogenic cyst

- Sequestration
- Polycystic lungs

3. Neoplasm
   - Bronchogenic carcinoma • Metastasis
   - Lymphoma
4. *Trauma*
   - Resolving hematoma
5. Immunological
   - Rheumatoid arthritis
   - Wegener's granulomatosis
6. Vascular
   - Pulmonary infarction
7. Infected emphysematous bullae.

Five common causes of cavity in the lung
- Tubercular cavity
- Lung abscess, bronchiectasis
- Malignancy lung
- Pulmonary infarction
- Wegener's granulomatosis

Q. What are the various types of cavity seen in the lung?

Ans. Types of cavities are as follows:
1. *Thin-walled:* A cavity is surrounded by a thin walled margin of lung tissue. The margin may be irregular, shaggy in lung abscess *(staphylococcal)* and bronchogenic carcinoma while it is smooth and regular in tuberculosis, lung cyst, emphysematous bullae, hydatid cyst and fungal infection.
2. *Thicked walled:* A thick wall is formed by thick exudative material or heaps of cells such as in lung abscess, tuberculosis and bronchogenic carcinoma.

Q. What are the physical signs of a cavity?

Ans. Typically, a superficial large cavity communicating with the bronchus produces signs which depend on whether the cavity is empty or filled with fluid at the time of examination. The signs of cavity are given in Table 1.24.

Table 1.24: Physical signs over a cavity

Sign	Empty	Filled
• Movement of chest on the side and area involved	Diminished	Diminished
• Retraction/flattening of chest	Present	Present
• Tactile vocal fremitus and vocal resonance	Increased	Decreased
• Percussion note	Crackpot sound	Diminished
• Breath sounds	Amphoric/ cavernous	Diminished
• Whispering pectoriloquy	Present	Absent
• Post-tussive crackles/ rales	Absent	Present

Q. What is post-tussive crackles?

Ans. These are crackles which are heard after coughing due to dislodgement of secretions in a cavity. They are characterstic of a tubercular cavity.

Q. What is amphoric breath sounds? What are its causes?

Ans. Read Clinical Methods by Prof SN Chugh.

Q. Which type of breathing occurs over a cavity?

Ans. • Thin walled cavity with narrow bronchus produces **amphoric bronchial breathing**
- Thick walled cavity with patent (narrow or wide) bronchus produces **cavernous breathing.**

Q. What are complications of a tubercular cavity?

Ans. • A source of intercurrent infections
- Meningitis (tubercular) or miliary tuberculosis
- Secondary amyloidosis in case of long-standing cavity
- Hydropneumothorax
- Chronic cavity may lead to malnutrition or hypoproteinemia

Q. What do you understand by the term lung abscess? What are its causes?

Ans. *Definition:* It is defined as collection of purulent material in a localized necrotic area of the lung parenchyma. It is a suppurative lung disease.
Causes: Most of the lung abscesses are pyogenic in origin, but, sometimes it may be nonpyogenic such as necrosis in a tumor followed by cavitation and collection of material. This is called *malignant lung abscess.* The causes of the abscesses are given in Table 1.25.

Table 1.25: Causes of lung abscess

1. **Necrotising infection**
   a. *Pyogenic,* e.g. *Staph. aureus, Klebsiella, group A streptococci, Bacteroides, anaerobes, Nocardia*
   b. *Tubercular*—a tubercular cavity with collection of purulent material
   c. *Fungi,* e.g. *Aspergillus, Histoplasma*
   d. *Amebic lung abscess* secondary to liver abscess
2. **Embolic infarction with cavity formation**
   - Thromboembolism of the lung
   - Metastatic lung abscess
3. **Malignancy of the lung with cavitation**
   - Bronchogenic carcinoma with secondary degeneration and cavitation
   - Metastatic lung abscess
4. **Miscellaneous**
   - Infected congenital cysts
   - Coal miner's pneumoconiosis

Q. What are its clinical features?

Ans. Clinical presentations and examinations of lung abscess are given in Table 1.26.

General physical examination	Systemic examination
• Toxic look • Fever, sweating, tachycardia, tachypnea • Poor nutrition • ± Cyanosis • Clubbing of the fingers present • Edema of legs if secondary renal amyloidosis or hypoproteinemia due to massive expectoration develops • Foul smelling (fetid) sputum and breath (halitosis) • Source of infection in upper respiratory tract, e.g. tonsillar or parapharyngeal abscess or throat sepsis may be evident • Cervical lymphadenopathy may be present	• All the signs present in a cavity filled with secretion/necrotic material will be present as discussed above • In case of rupture lung abscess, either the signs of empyema thoracis, or pyopneumothorax as discussed earlier will be present • In case of rupture amoebic liver abscess, there will be h__um w__expectoration of anchovy sauce spu__malignancy.__er hepatomegaly • In case of __cachex__there will be marked weight los__r conso__a, hemoptysis with signs of collapse __lidation. In addition, there may be feat__metastatic spread to the mediastinal __h nodes or evidence of compression of neighboring structures

Fig. 1.8B: Chest X-ray PA view showing lung abscess on right side (↑)

Clinical presentations
- Fever, sweating, palpitations, tachypnea
- Copious purulent or mucopurulent sputum with diurnal (more in the morning) and postural (more in lying down than sitting position) relation
- Hemoptysis
- Pain chest due to pleuritis if pleura involved
- May present with symptoms of underlying disease, e.g. tuberculosis, amebic liver abscess, malignancy lung
- May present with complication, e.g. meningitis, empyema thoracis

Q. How will you investigate a case with lung abscess?
Ans. The tests done are:
- *Blood examination* for anemia and leukocytosis. Raised ESR that suggests infection especially tuberculosis (markedly elevated).
- *Sputum examination* for isolation of the organisms (Gram's staining, Ziehl-Neelsen stain), for cytology including malignant cell; and culture and sensitivity.
- *Blood culture* to isolate the organism. It is mostly sterile.
- *Urine examination* for proteinuria, pus cells and casts. Albuminuria indicates secondary renal amyloidosis.
- *Chest X-ray* (PA view—Fig. 1.8B and lateral view) will show:
  - An area of consolidation with breakdown and translucency. The walls of the abscess may be outlined
  - The presence of a fluid level inside the translucent area confirms the diagnosis

- Empyema, if develops, will be detected by radiological appearance of a pleural effusion (read radiological appearance of pleural effusion)

Lateral film will show the site of an abscess depending on the position of patient at the time of abscess formation (Table 1.27).

Table 1.27: Localization of lung abscess

1. **Patient in lying down position**
   - Right lung (commonest site)
     - Posterior segment of upper and superior segment of lower lobe
2. **Patient in upright position**
   - Basal segments of both the lobes

Note: The lung abscess is more common on right side due to less obliquity of right bronchus

- *Bronchoscopic aspiration* for diagnosis. The aspirate is subjected to cytology, microbiology and culture

- *Aspiration of empyema* – if develops.
- *MRI* of upper lobe.

Q. **What is common site for lung abscess?**

Ans. Right middle lobe.

Q. **What are pathogens of lung abscess?**

Ans. Read causes of lung abscess

Q. **What are the complications of a lung abscess?**

Ans. Common complications are:
- Involvement of other lung (transbronchial spread)
- Septicemia, brain abscess
- Meningitis, pyopneu
- Empyema and amyloi nothorax
- Secondary rena dosis
- Massive hemopty
- Emaciation and poproteinemia in long-standing cases.

Q. **What does edema indicate in a patient with lung abscess?**

Ans. 1. *Hypoproteinemia* due to loss of protein through massive expectration
2. *Malnutrition/malabsorption*
3. *Renal amyloidosis* leading to albuminuria and nephrotic syndrome.

4. *Cor pulmonale* and *congestive cardiac failure*, through rare, may develop in some cases when the disease is extensive or bilateral.

Q. **How does a lung abscess lead to brain abscess? What is the common site?**

Ans. Lung abscess leads to meningitis and brain abscess by hematogenous spread. These abscesses are common in the posterior frontal region or parietal lobes and are usually multiple.

Q. **Which is the imaging procedure for upper lobe lesions?**

Ans. MRI is better for upper lobe lesions than CT scan of the chest, otherwise MRI is less useful than CT scan because of poorer imaging of lungs parenchyma and inferior spatial resolution.

Q. **How would you treat such a case?**

Ans. 1. *Postural drainage of the cavity*, sitting position is best for upper lobe cavity.
2. *Antibiotics* for pyogenic lung abscess and ATT for tubercular cavity.
3. *Expectorants and mucolytic agents*
4. *Surgery* in localised lung cavity which is nidus for recurrent pulmonary infection or haemoptysis.
5. *Chest physiotherapy*

CASE 9: PULMONARY TUBERCULOSIS

The patient whose X-ray is depicted (Fig. 1.9A) presented with cough, fever, hemoptysis, pain chest and weakness for the last 8 months. There was history of loss of weight, appetite and night sweats. There were crackles in the right infraclavicular region without bronchial breathing.

Clinical Presentations (Fig. 1.9B)

Major manifestations
1. A cavity
2. Consolidation or collapse
3. Pleural effusion/empyema
4. Miliary tuberculosis
5. Hydropneumothorax or bronchopleural fistula
6. Hilar lymphadenopathy
7. Bronchiectasis.

History

Point to be Noted

- Write chief complaints in chronological order
- Note the onset and progression of the symptoms
- History of fever, cough, hemoptysis, breathlessness, pain chest/discomfort, any neurological deficit
- Any history of weight loss, decreased appetite, night sweats or evening rise in temperature
- Ask complaints pertaining to other systems.

Examination

Proceed as follows:

I. General Physical Examination

- Ill-look
- Phlyectenular conjunctivitis
- Cervical or axillary lymphadenopathy

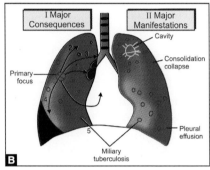

Figs 1.9A and B: Primary pulmonary tuberculosis. Consequences if left untreated are (Fig. 1.9B):
1. The primary focus may spread to hilar or mediastinal lymph node to form primary or Ghon's focus
2. Direct extension of primary focus into other part of lung
3. Extension of primary focus to bronchus
4. Extension of primary focus to pleura
5. Dissemination into blood stream leading to miliary tuberculosis

- Look for anaemia, jaundice, cyanosis and edema feet
- Look for JVP, trachea, etc.
- Note any clubbing of the fingers
- Any joint involvement.

II. Systemic Examination

Inspection
- Shape and symmetry of chest, Note any bulging or retraction.
- Look at the movements of chest at every quadrant of chest. Compare both sides with each other.
- Look at the apex beat e.g. location.
- Look for any distended veins or scar mark or mark for aspiration over the chest.
- Count the respiratory rate and note the type of breathing.
- Look for pulsations in supraclavicular fossa, epigastrium or other sites.

Palpation
- Palpate the apex beat to confirm its position.
- Palpate the trachea for any deviation.
- Note the expansion of the chest and measure it.
- Compare the vocal fremitus on both the sides.
- Palpate the intercostal space for any widening or narrowing.
- Palpate the crepitus or crackles or rub if any.

Percussion
- Percuss the lungs for resonance.
- Define cardiac and liver dullness.
- Percuss 2nd left and right intercostal spaces for dullness or resonance.
- Percuss directly the clavicles and supraclavicular areas for resonance.

Auscultation
- Hear the breath sounds and note the character and intensity and compare them on both the sides.
- Hear for any added sounds e.g. crackles, wheezes rub, etc.
- Vocal resonance to be compared on both sides for increase or decreases.
- Elicit other specific signs depending on the underlying disease, e.g. succussion splash, coin test, etc.

Other Systems
- Examine the spine for deformity and tenderness
- Examine abdomen for fluid or any organ enlargement
- Examine eyes for phlyctenular conjunctivitis or choroid tubercles.
- Elicit the signs of meningitis if suspected.

Q. What is your clinical diagnosis?

Ans. Postprimary pulmonary tuberculosis (Fibroexudative apical tuberculosis).

Q. What is fibroexudative apical tuberculosis?

Ans. It is a local infiltrative lesion of tuberculosis involving the apex of the lung. The features are:
- Depressed chest in the infraclavicular region.
- Trachea may/may not be shifted to the same side.
- No mediastinal shift
- Percussion note over the area involved is impaired.
- Coarse/medium/fine crackles are heard at the apex.
- No bronchial breath sounds.

Q. What do you understand by the term primary pulmonary tuberculosis? How does it differ from postprimary tuberculosis?

Ans. Infection with *M tuberculosis* occurring most frequently through inhalation of infected droplets with the primary involvement of the lung is called primary *pulmonary tuberculosis*. Following inhalation, of *M tuberculosis*, a subpleural lesion (*Ghon focus*) develops that causes a rapid transport of bacilli to the regional (hilar) lymph nodes leading to development of primary complex (Table 1.28). The fate of the primary complex is as follows:
1. It may heal spontaneously within 1-2 months and *tuberculin skin test* becomes positive.
2. Spread of the primary focus to hilar and mediastinal lymph nodes to form primary complex which in most cases heals spontaneously.
3. It may remain dormant, becomes reactivated when the body defenses are lowered.
4. Direct extension of primary focus – called *progressive pulmonary tuberculosis* merging with post primary TB.
5. Hematogenous spread leading to *miliary tuberculosis*, or *tubercular meningitis*.

Table 1.28: Primary tuberculosis

- Subpleural lesion (*Ghon focus*)
- Draining lymphatics from this focus to hilar lymph nodes
- Hilar lymphadenopathy

Clinical Features of Primary Tuberculosis

I. *Symptoms and signs of infection*, i.e. fever, influenza like illness , primary complex, skin test conversion.

II. *Symptoms and signs of the disease*, i.e. lymphadenopathy (hilar, paratracheal, mediastinal), collapse or consolidation (right middle lobe), obstructive emphysema, pleural effusion, endobronchial tuberculosis, miliary tuberculosis or, meningitis and pericarditis.

III. *Symptoms and signs of hypersensitivity*, e.g. erythema nodosum, phlyctenular conjunctivitis, dactylitis.

Clinical Features of Postprimary Pulmonary Tuberculosis

However, 85-90% of patients develop latent infection (positive tuberculin test or radiographic evidence of self-healed tuberculosis); and within this group 5-10% reactivate during their life-time resulting in post-primary disease, predominantly pulmonary (50% smear positive). Re-exposure to these smear – positive pulmonary tuberculosis may result in post-primary disease/tuberculosis. The difference between progressive primary complex and post-primary tuberculosis are enlisted in Table 1.29.

Table 1.29: Differences between progressive primary and postprimary tuberculosis

Progressive primary complex	Postprimary tuberculosis
Common in children	*Common in adults*
1. Hilar lymphadenopathy	Absence of lymph node enlargement
2. Subpleural focus or focus in any part of the lung	Usually apical fibrosis
3. Cavitation rare	Cavitation common
4. Fibrosis uncommon	Fibrosis common
5. Miliary tuberculosis common	Miliary tuberculosis uncommon
6. Direct extension of primary focus	Re-exposure to smear positive pulmonary disease

Q. What are clinical presentations of postprimary pulmonary tuberculosis?

Ans. Clinical presentations are as follows:
- Chronic cough, hemoptysis with signs and symptoms of exudative/infiltration or a cavity or collapse/fibrosis
- Pyrexia of unknown origin (PUO)
- Unresolved pneumonia (consolidation)
- Pleural effusion
- Asymptomatic (diagnosed on chest X-ray)
- Weight loss, night sweats, evening rise of temperature, general debility (cryptic tuberculosis)
- Spontaneous pneumothorax.

Q. What is time table of tuberculosis?

Ans. As already described, in 85-90% cases the primary complex heals spontaneous with or without calcification. In 10-15% cases, multiplication of tubercular bacilli is not contained and lymph nodes enlargement results in either local pressure effects or lymphatic spread to the pleura or pericardium or rupture into adjacent bronchus or pulmonary blood vessel. The time table of tuberculosis is given in Table 1.30.

Q. Who are at high risk of tuberculosis?

Ans. • Asian immigrants
- Older persons
- Alcoholic and debilitated persons or destitutes
- Immunocompromised individuals, i.e. AIDS and diabetic patients

Table 1.30: Time table of tuberculosis

Time from infection	Manifestations
3-8 weeks	• Primary complex, positive tuberculin skin test, erythema nodosum
3-6 months	• Collapse and bronchiectasis, adult pulmonary tuberculosis, miliary tuberculosis
Within 1 year	• Pneumonia, pleural effusion
Within 3 years	• Tuberculosis affecting bones, lymph node, joints, GI tract and genitourinary
From 3 years onwards	• Post-primary disease due to reactivation or reinfection
Around 8 years	• Urinary tract disease

- Professional, e.g. doctor, nurses, physiotherapists.
- Close contacts, i.e. family members of a case with tuberculosis

Q. What is cryptic tuberculosis? What is its presentation?

Ans. The term 'cryptic' means 'hidden'. A patient of tuberculosis with normal chest radiograph is called *cryptic tuberculosis*. Its presentation is as follows;
- Age over 60 years
- Intermittent low grade fever (PUO) with night sweats and evening rise
- Unexplained weight loss, general debility
- Hepatosplenomegaly (seen in 25% cases only)
- Normal chest X-ray
- Negative tuberculin skin test
- Leukemoid reaction or pancytopenia
- Confirmation is done by biopsy (liver or bone marrow).

Q. What are the stigmata of tuberculosis (evidence of present or past infection or disease)?

Ans. Stigmata attached with the tuberculosis are as follows:
- Phlyctenular conjunctivitis
- Erythema nodosum
- Tubercular lymphadenopathy with or without scars and sinuses
- Thickened, beaded spermatic cord
- Scrofuloderma
- Positive Mantoux test
- Localized gibbus, spinal deformity, paravertebral soft tissue swelling.

Q. What are the chronic complications of pulmonary tuberculosis?

Ans. Common complications of pulmonary TB include;
1. *Pulmonary complications*
   - Massive hemoptysis
   - Cor pulmonale
   - Fibrosis/emphysema (compensatory)
   - Recurrent infections
   - Tubercular empyema
   - Lung/pleural calcification
   - Obstructive airway disease (endobronchial)
   - Bronchiectasis
   - Bronchopleural fistula
2. *Non-pulmonary complications*
   - Empyema necessitans
   - Laryngitis
   - Enteritis following ingestion of infected sputum
   - Anorectal disease following ingestion of infected sputum
   - Amyloidosis (secondary)
   - Poncet's polyarthritis

Q. How will you investigate a case of pulmonary tuberculosis?

Ans. Investigations are as follows:
1. *Routine blood examination,* i.e. TLC, DLC, ESR for anemia, leucocytosis. Raised ESR and C-reactive protein suggest tuberculosis.
2. *Montoux test* is non-specific (low sensitivity and specificity)
3. *Sputum* (induced by nebulized hypertonic saline, if not expectorated), or *gastric lavage* (mainly used for children) or *bronchoalveolar lavage* for acid-fast bacilli isolation (Ziehl-Neelsen stain) and culture.
4. *Chest X-ray* (AP, PA and lateral and lordotic views) for radiological manifestations of tuberculosis in the lungs. The varied manifestations are;
   - Soft fluffy shadow (confluent)
   - Apical infiltration
   - Dense nodular opacities.
   - Miliary mottling shadows (miliary tuberculosis)
   - A cavity or multiple cavities (irregular, thin walled)
   - Fibrocaseous lesions
   - Tuberculoma
   - Calcification – lung and/or pleura
   - Bronchiectasis especially in the upper zones
   - Mediastinal (unilateral) lymphadenopathy (enlarged hilar lymph nodes)
   - Primary complex (Ghon focus) in children

5. *CT scan* for diagnosis and differential diagnosis
6. *PCR (polymerase chain reaction)* with blood or any other fluid
7. *ADA (adenosine deaminase)* levels increase in tuberculosis
8. *Transbronchial biopsy.*

Q. Which test gives an early diagnosis of tuberculosis?

Ans. Polymerase chain reaction (PCR) gives rapid diagnosis.

Q. How would you investigate close contacts of a patient with tuberculosis?

Ans. Close contacts are investigated as follows:
- First confirm the history of close contacts with the patient having open tuberculosis
- Enquire about BCG vaccination.
- Perform Mantoux or Heaf testing.
- Advise chest X-ray examination.

Q. How would you treat newly diagnosed sputum positive tuberculosis?

Ans.
1. Isolation of the patient in a single room for 2 weeks if smear positive.
2. Barrier nursing care
3. For new smear-positive or new cases of pulmonary tuberculosis are put on WHO DOTS regimen category I which comprises of
   - HRZE daily/thrice a week for 2 months
   - Assess sputum for AFB. If negative use two drugs (HR) for 4 months.
   - If sputum remain positive, extend four drugs regimen for one month more, then use 2 drugs (HR) for 2 months and if sputum is negative continue it for 2 months more or if positive, shift to category II.

Q. What are various categories of WHO DOTS regimen

Ans. Read Textbook of Medicine.

Q. What are the toxic effects of antitubercular drugs.

Ans. Read Commonly used Drugs Unit 3 of this book.

Q. Name second-line antitubercular drugs.

Ans. Paraminosalicylic acid, ethionamide, capreomycin, cycloserine, ciprofloxacin.

Q. What are indications of BCG vaccination?

Ans.
- Previous unvaccinated contacts.
- Persistently Mantoux test negative contacts below 35 years of age.

Q. What are indications of chemoprophylaxis?

Ans.
1. Mantoux test positive persons with no clinical or radiological evidence of tuberculosis
2. Children under 5 years of age who are close contacts of smear positive adult patient.
3. Immunocompromised contacts irrespective of immune status

Q. Which drug is used for chemoprophylaxis?

Ans. Isoniazid is used in usual dosage for one year.

Q. What is miliary tuberculosis? What is the status of immunity in this disease?

Ans. It is defined as dessemination of tuberculosis through the blood stream producing miliary tubercles in various organs. Immunity is lowered in it, hence, dissemination occur. Mantoux test is negative which confirms lowered immunity.

Q. What is treatment of multidrug resistant tuberculosis?

Ans. Drug resistant tuberculosis may be primary or acquired during treatment with inappropriate regimen or due to irregular treatment. MDR (multidrug resistant) tuberculosis is a big problem in Asia. Although 6 month regimen of RZE (excluding H) is effective for patients with initial isoniazid resistance, all the 3 drugs to be continued for 6 months.

For patients resistant to isoniazid (H) and rifampicin (R), combinations of a fluoroquinolones, ethambutol (E), pyrazinamide (Z) and streptomycin (S) is given for 18-24 months and for at least a months after sputum culture conversion. For those resistant to streptomycin, injectable amikacin can be used in its place.

For patients resistant to all first line drugs, cure may be obtained with combination of 4 second line drugs, (ethionamide, cycloserine, quinolone and PAS) including one injectable agent for full 24 months.

Q. Name new antitubercular drugs.

Ans. Following drugs are being evaluated.
- Rifapentine—a rifamycin antibiotic, is bacteriostatic similar to rifampicin. Other drugs include gatifloxacin, moxifloxacin, clarithromycin, linezolid and oxazolidinones.

CASE 10: BRONCHIAL ASTHMA

The patient (Fig. 1.10) presented with acute attack of breathlessness and cough. There was no history of pain chest or hemoptysis. There was history of such attacks in the past. On examination, wheezes were heard all over on both sides of the chest.

Fig. 1.10: A patient of acute severe asthma being nebulized

Clinical Presentations

- Typical symptoms include wheeze, breathlessness, cough and tightness of chest. These symptoms may occur for the first time at any age and may be episodic or persistent.
- Episodic asthma presents with intermittent acute attacks, remains asymptomatic between attacks. The precipitating factor is either respiratory viral infection or exposure to allergens. This type of asthma occurs in children or young adults who are atopic.
- Persistent asthma presents with chronic wheezing and breathlessness, has to be differentiated from left heart failure (cardiac asthma). This is called adult onset asthma seen in older non-atopic individuals. Typically there is diurnal pattern in symptoms and PEF shows morning diping. Cough and wheezing are nocturnal and disturb the sleep-hence called *nocturnal asthma*.

History

Important Points to be Noted in History

- Present history should cover the present symptoms in details. Note seasonal or nocturnal attacks of asthma. Is there worsening of symptoms in the morning (morning diping) ?
- Past history should include any history of cough and cold in the childhood, chronic exposure to dust and smoke. Any history of recurrent attacks of nasal discharge, sneezing and angioneurotic oedema.
- *Personal history* .e.g. smoking, alcohol, occupation, habits, diet (food allergy)
- *Family history* of bronchial asthma, hay fever and eczema
- Ask about any precipitant.

Examination

Proceed as follows:

I. General Physical Examination

- *Resting position:* Patient is dyspneic and tachypneic during acute attack, sits in prop up position and uses extrarespiratory muscles for respiration
- *Pulse:* Tachycardia is usually present in acute attack. Marked tachycardia and bounding pulses indicate CO_2 narcosis (retention). Presence of *pulsus* paradoxus indicates severe acute asthma
- BP and temperature normal
- *Cyanosis* is present in severe acute asthma
- *Level of consciousness:* Patients with mild attacks are fully conscious but anxious looking. Marked anxiety, drowsiness and restlessness indicate increasing severity of airway obstruction
- *Respiration:* Rate is more, respiration is rapid and shallow
- *Speech:* If the patient can speak easily and in full sentences, the dyspnea is mild. Monosyllabic speech suggests moderate dyspnea. Inability to speak sentences without stopping to take a breath indicate severe asthma

- *Flapping tremors (asterixis)* on outstretched hands, papilledema, and bounding pulses indicate CO_2 narcosis
- *Nasal examination* for polyp or allergic rhinitis. Throat examination for septic focus
- *Skin examination* for allergy

II. Systemic Examination

Inspection
- Patient is dyspneic at rest
- Accessory muscles of respiration and alae nasi are working
- Respiratory rate is increased
- Audible wheezing
- Excavation of suprasternal notch and supraclavicular fossae may be present with recession of intercostal spaces during inspiration
- Shape of the chest normal, but there may be pigeon-shape chest in long standing childhood asthma
- Tracheal tug absent

Palpation
- Trachea is central
- Apex beat may not be palpable due to overinflated lungs
- Movements of the chest are bilaterally and symmetrically decreased.
- Expansion of the chest on the *measurement* is reduced
- Vocal fremitus is reduced uniformly on both the sides
- Wheeze/rhonchi may be palpable

Percussion
- Resonant note all over the chest
- Liver dullness intact at normal 5th intercostal space in right mid-clavicular line
- Normal cardiac dullness

Auscultation
- Vesicular breathing with prolonged expiration present all over the chest
- Vocal resonance reduced uniformly all over the chest
- Polyphonic expiratory and inspiratory wheezes (rhonchi) are heard over the chest
- Coarse crackles at both the bases
- No pleural rub

Q. What is your clinical diagnosis and why?

Ans. Sir, my clinical diagnosis is bronchial asthma. *The points in favor of diagnosis are:*

 i. Episodic nature of cough, wheeze, breathlessness and tightness in chest

 ii. Exacerbation of cough or wheeze at night or after exercise

 iii. Precipitation of attacks during summer, dusty and rainy seasons (seasonal attacks)

 iv. History of atopy (eczema, hay fever) or rhinitis (seasonal) present

 v. Examintion of chest shows tachypnea, excavation of suprasternal and supraclavicular, fossa; reduced movements and expansion of chest, indrawing of intercostal spaces. Resonant percussion note on both sides, and bilateral scattered wheezes and rhonchi.

Q. What is your differential diagnosis?

Ans. The differentiation of asthma from other diseases associated with dyspnoea and wheezing is not difficult, following conditions have to be kept in mind during an attack of asthma.

1. **Chronic bronchitis/COPD.** The differences between asthma and chronic bronchitis have been discussed as a separate question (Read the differences)

2. **Upper airway obstruction by tumor or laryngeal edema.** In this condition, there is usually stridor and there are harsh respiratory sounds limited to the area of trachea not all over the chest as heard in bronchial asthma. Diffuse wheezing is absent. Indirect laryngoscopy and bronchoscopy confirms the diagnosis.

3. **Endobronchial disease** due to tumor, tuberculosis, foreign body or bronchostenosis produces paroxysms of coughing with persistent wheezing limited to one area of the chest.

4. **Left ventricular failure** (cardiac asthma) produces cough, dyspnea, PND with moist basal rales, gallop rhythm, blood stained sputum and other signs of heart failure.

5. **Carcinoid syndrome,** episodic flushing, diarrhea, pruritus, salivation along with diffuse wheezing in the chest are characteristics. Cardiac lesions may also occur. The diagnosis is confirmed by measurement of urinary or plasma serotonin or its metabolites in urine.

6. **Recurrent pulmonary thromboembolism:** Recurrent episodes of dyspnea, particularly on exertion with or without hemoptysis can occur in pulmonary embolism. Sometimes, wide spread wheezing simulating asthma may occur causing confusion with it, lung scans and pulmonary angiography may be necessary to confirm the diagnosis.

7. **Eosinophilic pneumonia.** Acute eosinophilic pneumonia is characterized by episodes of cough, fever, chills, dyspnea and wheezing following an exposure to an antigen. Neutrophila, eosinophilia and lymphopenia can occur. Chest X-ray shows nodular infiltrates or reticulonodular opacities. Pulmonary function tests reveal restrictive defect. High resolution CT scan is diagnostic.

Q. What do you understand by the term bronchial asthma?

Ans. *Bronchial asthma* is defined as a disorder characterized by chronic airway inflammation and increased responsiveness of tracheobronchial tree to a variety of stimuli resulting in temporary narrowing of the air passages leading to symptoms of cough, wheeze, tightness of chest and dyspnea. Airflow obstruction is transient and reversible with treatment. It is not a uniform disease but rather a dynamic clinical syndrome comprising of two common distinct pattern; (i) episodic asthma in which acute attacks are precipitated by allergens or infection by respiratory virus. These attacks are short-lived and patient in between attacks is symptom free. These attacks are common in children who are atopic hence, called *extrinsic asthma.* The other pattern (ii) is persistent form in which there is chronic wheeze and breathlessness, these cases resemble patients of COPD. These individuals are nonatopic, and asthma develops in old age – called *intrinsic asthma.*

Q. What are causes of wheezes?

Ans. 1. Bronchial asthma

2. COPD, predominently chronic bronchitis

3. Left ventricular failure (cardiac asthma)

4. Bronchial tumor

5. Eosinophilic lung disease (pulmonary eosinophilia)

6. Carcinoid syndrome

7. Recurrent thromboembolism

8. Anaphylaxis

9. Systemic vasculitis with pulmonary involvement

10. Mastocytosis

Q. What are the difference between extrinsic and intrinsic asthma?

Ans. Table 1.31 differentiates atopic (extrinsic) and non-atopic instrinsic asthma.

Q. What is acute severe asthma?

Ans. This term has replaced the previous horrifying term *status asthmaticus.* It is defined as either an acute attack of prolonged asthma or paroxysmal attacks of

Table 1.31: Differentiating features of extrinsic and intrinsic asthma

Extrinsic asthma (atopic)	Intrinsic asthma (non-atopic)
• Episodic, sudden onset	Non-episodic, chronic or persistent
• Early onset or childhood asthma	Late onset or adult asthma
• More wheeze, less cough	More cough, less wheeze
• Mostly seasonal	Mostly non-seasonal
• Attacks may occur at any time of the day or night	Mostly attacks occur at night (nocturnal)
• Diurnal pattern, e.g. symptoms and peak expiratory flow show morning dipping with subsequent recovery	Non-diurnal pattern
• Non-exercise induced attacks	Exercise-induced attacks
• Positive family history of an allergic disorder	No family history
• Skin hypersensitivity tests positive	Skin tests negative
• Sodium cromoglycate is most effective	Not effective

acute asthma where there is no remission of attacks in between and they are not controlled by conventional bronchodilators. It is a life-threatening emergency, needs proper diagnosis and urgent treatment. The diagnosis is suggested by:

- Acute dyspnea, orthopnea with wheeze, tachycardia, tachypnea and perspiration.
- Central cyanosis
- Dry (unproductive) cough with mucoid expectoration
- Respiratory distress with hyperactivity of extra-respiratory muscles (accessory muscles of respiration)
- Pulsus paradoxus
- Diminished breath sounds due to reduced air entry and minimal or absence of high-pitched polyphonic rhonchi (wheezes)

Silent chest is a characteristic feature of acute severe asthma and is an ominous sign

- PEFR (peak expiratory flow rate) is <50% of predicted or patient's best.

Q. What are the parameters of assessment of severity of asthma?

Ans. The parameters of life-threatening asthma are;
1. *Bed side parameters*
   - Pulse rate >110/min, respiratory rate >25 min.
   - Pulsus paradoxus
   - Tachypnea (rapid shallow respiration)

- Unable to speak in sentences (i.e. one sentences in one breath)
- PEF <50% of predicted or <100 L/min

2. *Clinical parameters*
   - Cannot speak
   - Central cyanosis
   - Exhaustion, confusion, obtunded consciousness
   - Bradycadia, hypotension
   - *"Silent chest", feeble respiratory effort.*
   - Uncontrolled PEF or PEF <33% of predicted or best

3. *Investigative parameters of life-threatening asthma*
   - Arterial blood gas analysis
     A normal (5-6 kPa) or high CO_2 tension
   - Severe hypoxemia (< 8 kPA) especially if being treated with O_2
   - A low pH or acidosis

Q. What are various allergens for asthma and how to avoid them?

Ans. It is a hard fact that certain allergens/drugs can precipitate asthma in sensitised individual, their knowledge is essential so as to prevent the development of life-threatening situation. The allergens encountered at home or at work place are listed along with preventive measures (Table 1.32).

Q. What is persistent rhonchi/wheeze? What are its causes?

Ans. A localized wheeze persisting in a localized area could be due to
- Bronchostenosis
- Foreign body obstruction
- Bronchial adenoma.

Q. What are the causes of pulsus paradoxus?

Ans. Read clinical methods in medicine by prof. S. N. Chugh.

Q. What are precipitating factors for acute attack of asthma?

Ans. 1. **Allergens** (Read Table 1.32)
2. **Pharmacological stimuli** e.g. drugs such as;
   - Aspirin and NSAIDs
   - Beta blockers
   - Coloring agents e.g. tartrazine
   - Sulfiting agents e.g. potassium metabisulfite, potassium and sodium bisulfite, sodium sulfite and SO_2 which are used in food industries. Exposure usually follows ingestion of these compouds in food and beverages e.g. Salads, fresh fruit, potatoes, shellfish and wine.
3. **Environmental and air pollutions.**
   - Ozone, nitrous dioxide and SO_2
   - Dust, fumes, pollens

47

Table 1.32: Various allergens and other substances likely to provoke an attack of asthma

Allergen	Efficacy/propensity	Preventive measures
1. More common		
• Pollens	Low	• Try to avoid exposure to flowering vegetation • Keep bed room windows closed
• House dust	Low/doubtful	• Vacuum cleaning of the matress daily • Shake out the blankets and bed sheets daily • Dust bed room thoroughly
• Animal dander	High	Avoid contact with animal pets, e.g. dogs, cats, horses, etc
• Feathers in pillows or quilts	High	Substitute foam pillows and terylene quilts
• Drugs	High	Avoid all preparations of relevant drugs
• Insect web	High	Do not allow the insect web to collect
2. Less Common		
• Food/food items	Low	Identify and eliminate them from diet
• Chemicals/pollutants	High	Avoid exposure to chemicals/pollutants and/or change of an occupation

4. **Occupational factors**
   • Metal salts e.g. platinum, chromium, nickle
   • Wood and vegetable dusts e.g. grain, flour, cast or bean, coffee beans, gum acacia, etc.
   • Drugs e.g. antibiotics, piperazine.
   • Industrial chemicals and plastics e.g. dyes
   • Biological enzymes e.g. laundry detergents and pancreatic enzymes
   • Animal and insect dusts and secretions
5. **Infections** e.g. viral, bacterial
6. **Exercise** (exercise-induced asthma)
7. **Emotional stress**

Q. What is wheeze? What are its types? What are its causes?

Ans. Read Clinical methods of Prof. S.N. Chugh.

Q. What are the causes of recurrent bronchospasm?

Ans. • Bronchial asthma
   • Carcinoid tumor
   • Recurrent pulmonary emboli
   • Chronic bronchitis with acute exacerbation
   • Recurrent LVF (cardiac asthma)

Q. What are the complications of asthma?

Ans. • Severe acute asthma (status asthmaticus)
   • Recurrent pulmonary infection leading to superadded bronchitis and pneumonia.
   • Sputum retention syndrome leading to atelectasis of lung
   • Pneumothorax
   • Emphysema, can occur in long-standing asthma
   • Respiratory failure (type II common)
   • Chronic cor pulmonale
   • Precipitation of syncope, hernias, prolapse, sub conjunctival hemorrhage due to repeated coughing

Q. How does bronchial asthma differ from chronic bronchitis?

Ans. See the Table 1.33.

Q. What are indications of steroids in asthma?

Ans. 1. Nocturnal asthma (sleep is disturbed by wheeze)
   2. Persistence of morning tightness until mid-day.
   3. Symptoms and peak expiratory flow deteriorates progressively each day.
   4. Maximum treatment with bronchodilators
   5. When there is need of emergency nebulisers

Q. Name the inhalational steroids.

Ans. Beclomethasone
   Budesonide
   Ciclesonide
   Fluticasone
   Triamcinolone

Q. What are the indications for mechanical ventilation with intermittent positive-pressure ventilation?

Ans. • Worsening hypoxia ($PaO_2 < 8kPa$) despite 60% inspired O_2
   • Hypercapnia ($PaO_2 > 6$ kPa)
   • Drowsiness
   • Coma

Q. How will you manage a case of severe acute asthma?

Ans. • Nebulized beta-agonists e.g. terbutaline or salbutamol
   • High concentration of O_2
   • High doses steroids e.g. IV hydrocortisone or oral prednisolone or both
   • Order immediately blood gases and X-ray chest to rule out pneumothorax
   • When life-threatening features are present;
     – Add ipratropium bromide to nebulized beta-agonist
     – IV aminophylline or salbutamol or terbutaline

Table 1.33: Differences between bronchial asthma and chronical bronchitis

Feature	Asthma	Chronic bronchitis
Onset	Acute	Slow, insidious
Age	Childhood, adolescents and middle age	Usually middle age or old patients
Pathogenesis	Allergic	Allergic-inflammatory
H/o Smoking	Absent	Present
Family history	May be positive	Negative
H/o Allergy e.g. rhinitis, hay fever eczema	Present	Absent
Duration of symptoms	No fixed duration	At least of 2 years duration
Nature of symptoms and signs	Intermittent episodic	Persistent, acute exacerbation can occur
Seasonal variation	Present	Absent
Symptoms	Dyspnea > cough	Cough > dyspnea
Signs	Wheezes/rhonchi are more pronunced than crackles	Both wheezes and crackles are present
Sputum and blood eosinophilia	Common	Uncommon
Pulmonary function tests	Usually normal	Usually abnormal

Q. **What is step-care regimen for management of chronic asthma in adults?**

Ans. British thoracic society regimen is depicted in Figure 1.10 B.

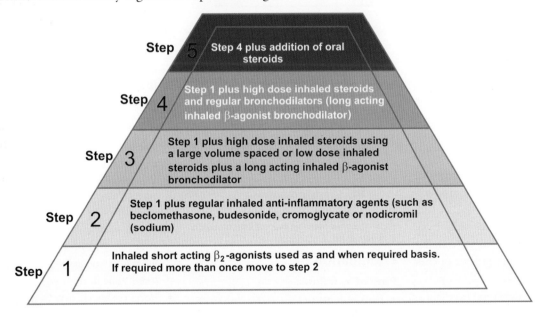

Fig. 1.10B: Pyramid of step care treatment of chronic bronchial asthma

49

The patient (Fig. 1.11A) presented with history of cough with massive purulent (foul smelling) expectoration more than 250 ml a day with frequent streaking of the sputum with blood. The cough and expectoration was more in the morning in left lateral position. Chest examination revealed coarse crackles in right infra-axillary and infrascapular region.

Clinical Presentations

- Chronic cough, massive expectoration related to diurnal variation and posture
- Recurrent hemoptysis
- Recurrent pneumonias (fever, cough, pain chest due to pleurisy)
- Dyspnea and wheezing
- Associated systemic symptoms, e.g. fever, weight loss, anemia, weakness
- Edema feet due to development of either cor pulmonale or involvement of kidneys by secondary amyloidosis

History

Points to be Noted in the History

- Write the complaints in chronological order and detail them.
- Ask specifically about the amount of sputum, color, consistency, smell, etc.
- Is there any relationship between posture and cough?
- Past history of tuberculosis or childhood measles, mumps or whooping cough.
- Past history of recurrent fever or chest infection or asthma.
- Any history of edema feet, swelling of the abdomen, etc.
- Any history of fever, headache, vomiting, or neurological deficit.

Bilateral bronchiectasis

Figs 1.11A to C: A. A patient with bronchiectasis bringing out massive mucoid expectoration; B. X-ray chest; C. Diagram

Examination

Proceed as follows:

I. General Physical Examination

- Patient may be dyspneic and has lots of coughing (coughing-coughing-coughing)

- Toxic look and fever if patient develops severe infection
- Pulse rate increased
- Respiratory rate may be high
- Nutrition may be poor due to hypoproteinemia as a result of massive expectoration
- Cyanosis may be present, if disease is bilateral and severe or patient develops respiratory failure or cor pulmonale
- Clubbing of fingers and toes common; may be grade I to IV
- Edema feet if there is cor pulmonale or hypoproteinemia

II. Systemic Examination

Inspection

- The affected side of the chest may be retracted (right side in this case)
- There may be diminished movement on the side involved
- There is wasting of muscles of thorax
- Look for the apex beat for dextrocardia.

Palpation

- Chest may be retracted with diminished movements and crowding of the ribs in the lower parts (s). There may be palpable wheeze or rhonchi and coarse mid-inspiratory and expiratory crackles.

Percussion

The percussion note is impaired over the area involved.

Auscultation

- Breath sounds may be bronchial, with coarse, bubbling leathery mid inspiratory and expiratory crackles (right lower zone in this case)
- Vocal resonance may be increased

N.B. All the signs will be seen on both sides in bilateral disease.

Q. What is your clinical diagnosis and why?

Ans. In view of long history of cough with massive purulent expectoration, more in the morning and in left lateral position; with retraction of chest on right side and diminished movements and presence of coarse, mid and late inspiratory crackles, bubbling in nature, rhonchi and wheezes in right infra-axillary and infrascapular region, my provisional diagnosis is right sided bronchiectasis.

Q. What are your other possibilities?

Ans. 1. *Lung abscess*-Read case discussion in lung abscess
2. *Tubercular cavity filled with exudate* (Read case discussion)
3. *Resolving pneumonia*
4. *Empyema thoracis* with bronchopleural fistula.

Q. What are causes of massive expectoration?

Ans. 1. Bronchiectasis
2. Lung abscess
3. Necrotising pneumonia, or
4. A tubercular cavity filled with exudates
5. Empyema thoracis or ruptured amebic liver abscess with communication to exterior through patent bronchus
6. Cystic fibrosis and
7. Chronic bronchitis

Q. What do you understand by the term bronchiectasis?

Ans. *Bronchiectasis* is a localized irreversible dilatation and distortion of bronchi. Although the definition is based on histopathological changes, yet clinical diagnosis is applied when chronic and recurrent infections occur in the dilated airways resulting in collection of secretions within them leading to massive expectoration, more so in the morning. It may be focal and unilateral (involvement of airway within limited region of the lung parenchyma) or diffuse and bilateral.

Q. What are its pathological types (Reid's classification)?

Ans. Pathological types of bronchiectasis are:
1. *Cylindrical bronchiectasis.* The bronchi are uniformly dilated
2. *Varicose bronchiectasis.* The affected bronchi have irregular or beeded pattern of dilatation.
3. *Saccular (cystic) bronchiectasis.* The bronchi have ballooned or cystic appearance.
   These pathological shapes can only be seen on bronchoscopy and CT scan.

Q. What are the causes of bronchiectasis?

Ans. The causes of bronchiectasis are enlisted in Table 1.34. The most common cause is infection of bronchi with or without obstruction. Impaired pulmonary defense mechanisms such as immuno-globulin deficiency, cystic fibrosis may lead to bronchiectasis by repeated infections without obstruction. Some noninfective causes also lead to bronchiectasis.

Table 1.34: Causes of bronchiectasis

1. Postinfective e.g. postpneumonic, following, measles, whooping cough and post-tubercular (tubercular bronchiectasis common in upper-lobe)
2. Mechanical bronchial obstruction (obstructive bronchiectasis) as in endobronchial tuberculosis, carcinoma, extrinsic lymph node compression
3. Allergic bronchopulmonary aspergillosis
4. γ-globulin deficiency e.g. congenital or acquired.
5. Immobile cilia syndrome (Kartagener's syndrome)
6. Cystic fibrosis
7. Neuropathic disorders (namely Riley-day syndrome, (Chagas' disease)
8. Idiopathic

Q. What are major pathogens in bronchiectasis?

Ans. Major pathogens are
- *S. aureus*
- *H. influenzae*
- *Pseudomonas aeruginosa*

Q. What are common sites for localized disease?

Ans. Left lower lobe and lingula.

Q. What is Kartagener's syndrome?

Ans. It consists of the following:
- Sinusitis
- Dextrocardia
- Bronchiectasis
- *Primary ciliary dyskinesia.* The normal sperm motility also depends on proper ciliary function, males are generally infertile.

Q. Where does bronchiectasis occurs in allergic bronchopulmonary aspergillosis?

Ans. The bronchial dilatation occurs in more proximal bronchi due to type III immune complex reactions.

Q. What other abnormalities may be associated with bronchiectasis?

Ans. 1. Congenital absence of bronchial cartilage (*Camp bell syndrome*)
2. Tracheobronchomegaly
3. Azoospermia
4. Chronic sinopulmonary infection
5. Congenital kyphoscoliosis
6. Situs inversus and paranasal sinusitis (Kartagener's syndrome)

Q. What is dry or wet bronchiectasis?

Ans. Chronic cough with massive purulent sputum, more in the morning and in one of the lateral or lying down position (postural relation depends on the side (s) involved), hemoptysis, and dilated airways on the bronchoscopy or high resolution CT scan are characteristic features of *wet bronchiectasis.*

The term *dry bronchiectasis* refers to either asymptomatic disease or a disease with recurrent nonproductive cough associated with intermittent episodes of hemoptysis and bronchiectasis in an upper lobe. The hemoptysis can be life-threatening as bleeding occurs from the bronchial vessels under systemic pressure. There is usually a past history of tuberculosis or granulomatous infection.

Q. How will you investigate a case of bronchiectasis?

Ans. Following investigations are to be done:

- *Hemoglobin, TLC, DLC, ESR.* Polymorpho-nuclear leucocytosis with raised ESR suggest acute infection. There may be normocytic normochromic anemia due to repeated infections.
- *Sputum for culture and sensitivity.* The sputum volume, color, cellular elements are useful guide for active infection. Sputum for eosinophilia provides a clue to asthma and/or broncho-pulmonary aspergillosis.
- *Urine examination* for proteinuria if amyloidosis is being suspected.
- *Blood culture and sensitivity* if there is evidence of bacteremia or septicemia
- *Chest X-ray (PA view).* The chest X-ray (Fig. 1.11B) may be normal with mild disease or may show prominent (dilated) cystic spaces (saccular bronchiectasis) either with or without airfluid levels, corresponding to the dilated airways. These dilated airways are often crowded together in parallel, when seen longitudinally, appear as "*tram-tracks*", and when seen in cross section appear as, "*ring shadows*". These may be difficult to distinguish from enlarged airspaces due to bullous emphysema or from regions of honeycombing in patients with severe interstitial lung disease. Because these spaces may be filled with secretions, the lumen may appear dense rather than radiolucent, producing opaque tubular or branched tubular structures.
- *Bronchography a gold standard for diagnosis* shows an excellent visualization of bronchiectatic airways, but, now-a-days is not done because of availability of high resolution CT scan.
- *High resolution CT scan* will show dilated airways in one or both of the lower lobes or in an upper lobe. When seen in cross-section, the dilated airways have a ring like appearance.

- *Fiberoptic bronchoscopy.* It is done to find out the cause. When the bronchiectasis is focal, fiberoptic bronchoscopy may show an underlying endobronchial obstruction. Bronchiectasis of upper lobe is common either due to tuberculosis or bronchopulmonary aspergillosis.
- *Pulmonary function tests.* These tests demonstrate airway obstruction as a consequence of diffuse bronchiectasis or associated COPD. Pulmonary function tests are useful to define the extent, severity of the disease, need for bronchodilators and to plan surgery.
- *Specific tests for aspergillosis* i.e. precipitin test and measurement of serum IgE.

Q. What are the complications of bronchiectasis?

Ans. Common complications are as follows:

- Recurrent pneumonias (e.g. repeated infections)
- Bacteremia and septicemia
- Massive hemoptysis (from dilated bronchial vessels) leading to pulmonary apoplexy
- Right ventricular failure or cor pulmonale
- Secondary amyloidosis
- Meningitis or brain abscess
- Aspergilloma (fungal ball) in a bronchiectatic cavity.

Q. What is difference between standard and high resolution CT?

Ans. In standard CT, the resolution (the slice thickness) is 10 mm thick where as in high resolution CT the slice thickness is 1-2 mm and high spatial resolution algorithms are used to reconstruct images.

Q. What do you know about spiral CT?

Ans. This is a rapidly evolving technique to image the chest which has the advantage of imaging truly contiguous sections; with the result completely seamless reconstructions are possible. This may allow virtual-reality bronchoscopy imaging.

Q. How would you treat bronchiectasis?

Ans.
- Postural drainage
- Antibiotics
- Bronchodilators and mucolytics
- Surgery in selected cases
- Treat the complication when they arise

Q. What is indication of surgery in bronchiectasis?

Ans.
- Localized disease involving a segment or a lobe without involvement of other parts of the lung on bronchographic or CT evidence.
- Recurrent hemoptysis

Gastrointestinal and Hepatobiliary Diseases

CASE 12: JAUNDICE

The patient (Fig. 1.12A) presented with fever for few days followed by jaundice and dark coloration of urine. There was history of pain abdomen, and distaste to food.

Clinical Presentations

The clinical presentation of a case with jaundice varies according to the cause.
1. Patients with hepatitis present with fever, abdominal pain, jaundice, tender hepatomegaly, anorexia, distaste to food and smoking.
2. Patients with hemolytic jaundice complain of insidious onset and long duration of jaundice with dark colored urine and stools.
3. Patients with obstructive jaundice present with abdominal pain, pruritus and acholic stools in case the bile duct stone is the cause; while carcinoma of the pancreas produces painless progressive jaundice with palpable gallbladder.
4. Patient with cirrhosis of liver present with features of portal hypertension (ascites, hematemesis, melena, splenom-

Fig. 1.12A: A patient with jaundice

Fig. 1.12B: Infected needle—a common cause of hepatitis B

egaly) and jaundice develops during decompensation of liver disease, i.e. hepatic encephalopathy (mental features will be present)
5. Jaundice may present during each pregnancy in a patient with benign intrahepatic cholestatic jaundice of pregnancy.
6. A young patient with recurrent jaundice of long duration usually suffer from congenital hyperbilirubinemia.

History

Points to be Noted in History

A complete medical history is perhaps the most important part of evaluation. Ask for the followings:
- Duration of jaundice
- Sore throat and rash (infectious mononucleosis)
- Occupation (Weil's disease in sewerage workers and farmers)
- Abdominal pain (cholecystitis, gallstones, cholangitis, carcinoma of pancreas)
- Pruritus (cholestatic hepatitis, primary biliary cirrhosis)
- Triad of fever, rigors and upper abdominal pain (cholangitis)
- Any change in appetite, taste, weight and bowel habits (hepatitis)
- Any history of blood transfusions, I.V. injections (Fig. 1.12B), tattooing, unprotected sexual activity (Hepatitis B)
- Recent travel history
- Exposure to people with jaundice either in the family, or locality or outside (hepatitis)
- Exposure to possibly contaminated food
- Occupational exposure to hepatotoxins or chemicals
- Detailed drug history, (especially oral contraceptive and phenothiazines) i.e. taken in the past or are being taken. History of taking herbal or indigenous medicine
- History of alcohol intake
- History of pregnancy (Pregnancy induced or pregnancy associated jaundice)
- History of epistaxis, hematemesis or bleeding tendency (pale stool in obstructive jaundice)
- Family history for congenital hyperbilirubinemia, i.e. Gilbert's, Crigler-Najjar and Dubin-Johnson and Rotor syndromes

- Presence of any accompanying symptoms such as arthralgias, myalgias, weight loss, fever, pain in abdomen, pruritus and change in color of stool or urine
- Symptoms of encephalopathy, i.e. mental features.

Examination

Proceed as follows:

I. General Physical Examination

- Assess the patient's nutritional status
- Look for stigmatas of chronic liver disease. These are commonly seen in alcoholic cirrhosis.
  - Spider nevi
  - Palmar erythema
  - Gynecomastia
  - Caput medusae
  - Dupuytren's contracture
  - Parotid glands enlargement
  - Testicular atrophy, axillary and pubic hair loss
- Look for enlarged lymph nodes
  - An enlarged left supraclavicular node (*Virchow's node*) or periumbilical nodule (*Sister Mary Joseph's nodule*) suggests an abdominal malignancy
- JVP and other signs of right heart failure
- Look for pulse rate (bradycardia in obstructive jaundice), anemia and scratch marks, xanthelasma/xanthomatosis occur due to hypercholesteremia in obstructive jaundice.

II. Systemic Examination

Abdominal Examination for
- Hepatomegaly, e.g. note, size, shape, surface, movement with respiration, consistency and whether pulsatile or not. Elicit tenderness
- Splenomegaly—define its characteristics
- Ascites. Elicit all the signs for detection of fluid
- Prominent venous collaterals or veins must be looked for determine the flow of blood
- Look at the hernial sites
- Look for scratch marks.

Other Systems Examination
- Cardiovascular, i.e. valvular heart disease, pericardial effusion

Respiratory System for
- Pleural effusion especially right-sided

Examination of excreta
- Urine
- Stool.

53

Q. What is your provisional diagnosis and why?

Ans. The provisional diagnosis of this case is acute hepatitis probably viral. The *points in favor of diagnosis are;*

i. Presence of prodromal symptoms i.e. fever, malaise, distaste for food, anorexia

ii. Acute onset of jaundice with dark colored urine and stool with no pruritus

iii. Tender moderate hepatomegaly which is soft, smooth.

Q. How do you define jaundice? Where will you look for jaundice?

Ans. Jaundice or icterus refers to yellow disoloration of sclera, conjunctiva, mucous membrane of the tongue and skin due to raised serum bilirubin. Normal serum bilirubin is 0.3 to 1.5 mg%. Scleral staining or jaundice becomes clinically evident when serum bilirubin is at least 3.0 mg/dl. Raised bilirubin in between 1.5 and 3 mg/dl indicates subclinical jaundice.

Sites to be seen for Jaundice

Jaundice should be seen in sclera in broad day light because icterus is difficult to examine in the presence of tube light or fluorescent light because of yellow reflection. The sclera provides white background.

Jaundice first appears in sclera due to affinity of bilirubin to stain elastin in sclera. A second place to examine the jaundice is underneath tongue.

Q. What is differential diagnosis in your case?

Ans. A large number of conditions that produce fever, jaundice and tender hepatomegaly come into differential diagnosis of viral hepatitis such as;

1. *Infectious mononucleosis:* Fever, lymphadenopathy, jaundice and hepatomegaly constitute clinical hallmark. Peripheral blood film will show atypical lymphocytosis. Serology (*Paul-bunnel test*) helps in the diagnosis.

2. *Nonviral hepatitis* such as toxoplasmosis and nocardiosis can produce similar picture. Serology can differentiate the non-viral conditions from viral hepatitis.

3. *Autoimmune hepatitis*—Read Table 1.34

4. *Alcoholic and drug induced/hepatitis*—Read Table 1.34.

5. *Amoebic liver abscess.* Acute amoebic liver abscess produces, fever, large tender hepatomegaly. Jaundice can occur occasionally. There may or may not be past history of dysentery. USG is diagnostic which reveals an abscess.

6. *Congestive hepatomegaly.* Signs of right ventricular failure. e.g. raised JVP, cyanosis, oedema feet and signs of pulmonary hypertension (loud P2, narrow split of S2 and Grahm-steel murmur) separates congestive hepatomegaly from viral hepatitis.

7. *Budd-Chiari syndrome* (occlusion of hepaic vein or inferior vena cava) and *veno-occlusive disease* (involvement of small hepatic veins and venules due to consumption of bush tea) also produce massive hepatomegaly, jaundice but presence of ascites and signs of portal hypertension differentiate it from viral hepatitis. The absence of signs of congestive heart failure differentiates it from congestive hepatomegaly.

8. *Malignancy liver* - read Table 1.35.

9. In *pregnant women, acute fatty liver of pregnancy* and cholestasis of pregnancy and eclampsia constitute differential diagnosis of viral hepatitis.

Q. To which group of viral hepatitis your case belong?

Ans. Hepatitis A (short incubation, epidemic form of hepatitis)

Q. Name the types of viral hepatits?

Ans. Viral hepatitis A, B, non A - non B (hepatitis C), hepatitis D and E.

Q. What is the source of infection in your case?

Ans. Contaminated food, milk, water or other food items.

Q. How does hepatitis A spread?

Ans. Feco-oral route, percutaneous and sexual transmission rare.

Q. How would you confirm the diagnosis?

Ans. The diagnosis of hepatitis A is made during an acute illness by demonstrating anti-HAV of IgM class. After acute illness, anti HAV of IgG class remains detectable indefinitely indicating past or previous infections.

Q. What is prophylaxis of hepatitis A?

Ans. Both passive immunization with IG (Immuno-globulin) and active immunization with vaccines are available. All preparations of IG contain anti-HAV concentration sufficient to be protective. It gives immediate protection, formalin-inactivated vaccine used for pre-exposure prophylaxis gives long-lasting protection.

Q. What are the indications of hepatitis A prophylaxis?

Ans. I. *Passive immunization with IG (immunoglobulin)* is indicated in

i. Pre-exposure prophylaxis or early incubation period prophylaxis.

ii. For post-exposure-hepatitis of intimate contact (household, sexual, institutional).
Dose is 0.02 ml/kg intramuscular

II. *Active immunization by vaccine*
   - It is indicated as pre-exposure prophylaxis for travellers to tropical countries, developing countries or other areas outside standard tourist routes.

III. *Both passive and active immunization*
   Passive immunization with IG at different site and active immunization with vaccine at another site are indicated during imminent travel or immediate travel.

   Two doses of vaccine are given at 0 month and at 6-12 months.

Q. Which hepatitis spread by blood transfusion?
Ans. Hepatitis B, C, D.

Q. Which hepatitis is most dangerous?
Ans. Hepatitis B

Q. What would be the color of other fluids in jaundice?
Ans. Body fluids (CSF, tears, joint fluid) become yellow colored if there is predominant conjugated hyperbilirubinemia as conjugated bilirubin being water soluble gets excreted into these secretions.

Q. What are other causes of yellow discoloration of tissue?
Ans. Besides jaundice, other causes are;
   - Carotenoderma (hypercarotenemia) due to excessive consumption of fruits and vegetables rich in carotene (e.g. carrots, oranges, squash, peeches)
   - Use of antimalarial drug, e.g. mepacrine, quinacrine. They are not used nowadays.
   - Excessive exposure to phenols

Carotenoderma can be distinguished from jaundice by sparing of the sclera and normal colored urine while it stains all other tissues. On the other hand, quinacrine stains the sclera and produces yellow discolouration of urine.

Q. What are the causes of jaundice?
Ans. Jaundice reflects hyperbilirubinemia, indicates an imbalance between bilirubin production and clearance. Increased production and decreased clearance are the underlying mechanisms for production of jaundice. Hyperbilirubinemia may result from (i) overproduction of bilirubin, (ii) impaired uptake, conjugation or excretion of bilirubin, or (iii) regurgitation of unconjugated or conjugated bilirubin from damaged hepatocytes or bile ducts. *Unconjugated hyperbilirubinemia* results from either overproduction or impaired uptake or

conjugation of bilirubin. On the other hand, *conjugated hyperbilirubinemia* is due to decreased excretion into the bile ductules or backward leakage of the pigment. The causes of jaundice are tabulated (Table 1.35).

Q. How do you classify jaundice?
Ans. Jaundice is classified in different ways;
   1. *Based on coloration of sclera*
      - *Medical jaundice* (yellow coloration)
      - Surgical jaundice (greenish yellow coloration). The green color is produced by oxidation of bilirubin to biliverdin in long-standing cases of jaundice.
   2. *Based on the etiology*
      - Hemolytic or prehepatic (excessive destruction of RBCs)
      - Hepatic (cause lies inside the liver)
      - *Obstructive or posthepatic* (cause lies outside the liver in extrahepatic biliary system)
   3. *Based on chemical nature of bilirubin*
      - Unconjugated hyperbilirubinemia
      - Conjugated hyperbilirubinemia (conjugated bilirubin is $\geq$ 50% of total bilirubin. The normal conjugated bilirubin is just 15-20%)

Table 1.35: Causes of jaundice depending on the type of hyperbilirubinemia

Jaundice with predominantly unconjugated hyperbilirubinemia
1. *Hemolysis* (excessive destruction of RBCs and/or ineffective erythropoiesis)
   - Intracorpuscular or extracorpuscular defects
   - Drug-induced especially in patients with G6PD deficiency
   - Infections, e.g. malaria, viral
   - Immune hemolysis
   - Microangiopathic hemolytic anemia
   - Paroxysmal nocturnal hemoglobinuria
   - Ineffective erythropoiesis due to folate, vitamin B_{12} and iron deficiency and thalassemia
2. *Decreased uptake of bilirubin*
   - Drugs, sepsis
   - Hepatitis (acute or chronic), decompensated cirrhosis
   - Gilbert's syndrome (congenital defect)
3. *Decreased conjugation of bilirubin*
   - Neonatal jaundice
   - Gilbert's and Crigler-Najjar syndrome – type I (complete absence) type-II (partial deficiency of enzyme glucuronyl transferase)

Jaundice with predominantly conjugated hyperbilirubinemia
1. Cholestasis
   A. *Intrahepatic*
      - Congenital (Dubin-Johnson and Rotor syndrome)

Contd...

- Benign intrahepatic cholestasis
- Cholestatic jaundice of pregnancy
- Drugs and alcohol
- Hepatitis (acute and chronic)
- Primary biliary cirrhosis
- Hodgkin's lymphoma
- Postoperative

B. *Extrahepatic*
- Bile duct stone, stricture, cholangitis
- Parasite (round worm)
- Trauma to bile duct
- Bile duct obstruction due to tumor (bile duct, pancreas, duodenum)
- Secondaries in liver or at porta-hepatis
- Pancreatitis
- Choledochal cyst

Q. What are characteristic features of hemolytic jaundice?

Ans. These are as follows:

- Anemia with mild jaundice

- Freshly voided urine is not yellow, becomes yellow on standing due to conversion of excessive urobilinogen in the urine to urobilin on oxidation
- Preceding history of fever (malaria, viral), or intake of drugs if patient is G6PD deficient or intake of heavy metals.
- Typical facies, e.g. chipmunk facies seen in thalassemia due to excessive marrow expansion leading to frontal bossing and maxillary marrow hyperplasia
- Mild hepatosplenomegaly. The liver is nontender
- No pruritus or itching. No xanthelasma/ xanthomatosis
- Peripheral blood film examination and other tests for hemolysis will confirm the diagnosis.

Q. What is differential diagnosis of hepatocellular jaundice?

Ans. Common causes of hepatocellular jaundice are differentiated in Table 1.36.

Table 1.36: Differential diagnosis of hepatocellular jaundice

Viral hepatitis	Autoimmune hepatitis	Alcoholic hepatitis	Carcinoma of liver	Drug induced
• Fever followed by jaundice. As the jaundice appears, fever disappears • Anorexia, nausea and vomiting, distaste to food and smoking • Arthralgia, myalgia, headache, pharyngitis, cough, fatigue, malaise • Dark colored urine and clay-colored or normal colored stool • History of exposure to a patient with jaundice or use of contaminated food or I.V. injection/ blood transfusion or sexual contact, etc. • *Hepatomegaly.* Liver is moderately enlarged, soft, tender, smooth	• Splenomegaly in 20% cases only • Insidious onset. Chronic course • Common in females • Fever with jaundice, anorexia, fatigue, arthralgia, vitiligo, epistaxis. Amenorrhea is the rule • Sometimes a *"cushingoid"* face with acne, hirsutism, pink cutaneous striae • Bruises may be seen • Hepatosplenomegaly, spider telangiectasis are characteristic • Other autoimmune disorders may be associated • Serological tests for specific auto-antibodies confirm the diagnosis	• History of alcoholism • Anorexia, weight loss • Stigmata of chronic liver disease (spider naevi, palmar erythema, gyneco-mastia, testicular, atrophy, Dupuytren's contractures, parotid enlargement) may be present • Jaundice with enlarged tender liver • May be associated with other manifestations of alcoholism, e.g. cardiomyopathy, peripheral neuropathy	• Common in old age • Progressive jaundice with loss of appetite and weight • Liver enlarged, tender, hard, nodular. Hepatic rub may be heard • Anemia, fever lymphadenopathy in neck and marked cachexia present • Jaundice is deep yellow or greenish • Ascites may be present • Evidence of metastatic spread to lungs, bone, etc • USG and liver biopsy will confirm the diagnosis	• History of intake of hepatotoxic drugs, e.g. INH, rifampicin oral contraceptives • Malaise before the onset of jaundice • Occasionally rash, fever, arthralgia present • Liver is enlarged and tender • Tests for viral hepatitis are negative

Q. List few differences between intrahepatic and extrahepatic obstructive jaundice?

Ans.

Extrahepatic jaundice (Surgical jaundice)	Intrahepatic obstruction (Medical jaundice)
Common in old and middle age	Common in young
Associated history of dyspeptic symptoms (gallbladder dyspepsia)	History of hepatitis (contacts, blood transfusion in Injections) or intake of drugs
Jaundice is slow to develop, intermittent with pain	Transient painless Jaundice of sudden onset
Pruritus is characteristic (scratch marks may be present)	Pruritus is minimal
Hepatomegaly is usually present due to dilated biliary sytem.	No hepatomegaly. Splenomegaly can occur in 5-10% cases of hepatitis
Gallbladder may be palpable due to obstruction below the cystic duct.	Gallbladder is not palpable as obstruction is within liver above the cystic duct.
Signs of infection or inflammation absent	Fever, alteration in WBC count may be present
Serum bilirubin is usually high (>10 mg%)	Varies with the severity.
Serum lipids (triglyceride, cholesterol) and alkaline phosphatase are very high	They are mildy raised
Ultrasonography and CT scan are diagnostic and help to find out the cause	They show just altered echotexture
Stone, tumor, parasite are common causes	Viral infection, autoimmunity and drugs are common causes.

Q. What are clinical characteristic of obstructive jaundice?

Ans. The clinical characteristics are:
- Deep yellow or greenish yellow jaundice – called *surgical jaundice*
- Pruritus or itching present due to retention of bile salts
- Urine is dark colored due to excretion of bile pigments but stools are clay-colored (acholic)
- There may be associated pain abdomen, severe, colicky with intermittent jaundice, if bile duct stone is the cause
- Gallbladder is palpable if bile duct is obstructed either by an impacted stone or by carcinoma of head of pancreas. A palpable gallbladder in obstructive jaundice unlikely due to chronic cholecystitis (Courvosier's law)
- Slowing of pulse rate or bradycardia may occur due to retention of bile salts
- Fever, shaking chills and rigors with jaundice indicate cholangitis and biliary obstruction (Charcot's fever)

- In long-standing obstructive jaundice, xanthomas, weight loss, malabsorption or steatorrhea may occur
- Conjugated hyperbilirubinemia with dilatation of intrahepatic or extrahepatic ducts on USG confirm the diagnosis.

Q. Name the few causes of postoperative jaundice?

Ans.
- Hemolysis and reabsorption of hematoma, hemoperitoneum or blood transfusions.
- Impaired liver functions due to sepsis, anesthesia, shock
- Extrahepatic biliary obstruction due to biliary stones or unsuspected injury to biliary tree.

Q. What are medical causes of extrahepatic obstruction?

Ans. Read causes of extrahepatic obstruction in Table 1.35.

Q. What are characteristics of various viral hepatitis?

Ans. The characteristics of viral hepatitis are enlisted in Table 1.37.

Q. What are causes of acute hepatitis?

Ans. Hepatitis occurs due to a variety of infective and noninfective causes (Table 1.38).

Q. Name the familial congenital hyperbilirubinemia.

Ans.
- *Gilbert's syndrome* (predominantly unconjugated hyperbilirubinemia)
- *Crigler-Najjar syndrome* (type I:complete absence of glucuronyl transferase, type II, partial deficiency of enzyme)
- *Dubin-Johnson* (decreased excretion of bilirubin/ syndrome
- *Rotor*-Excretory defect of bilirubin with pigmentation of liver.

Q. What is Dubin-Johnson syndrome?

Ans. It is familial conjugated hyperbilirubinemia in which there is excretory defect of bilirubin excretion and there is pigmentation of liver due to melanin (rotor syndrome) detected on liver biopsy. It is detected by delayed bromosulphthalein excretion test.

Q. What are causes of prolonged jaundice (i.e. duration > 6 months)?

Ans. Causes of prolonged jaundice are as follows:
- Chronic hepatitis or cholestatic viral hepatitis, chronic autoimmune hepatitis
- Cirrhosis of liver
- Malignancy liver
- Hemolytic jaundice (e.g. thalassemia)
- Congenital hyperbilirubinemia
- Drug-induced
- Alcoholic hepatitis
- Primary biliary cirrhosis
- Wilson's disease
- Obstructive jaundice (extrahepatic biliary obstruction).

Table 1.37: Distinguishing features of main hepatitis viruses

Virus	A	B	C	D	E
Group	Enterovirus	Hepadna	Flavivirus	Delta particle (incomplete virus)	—
Nucleic acid	RNA	DNA	RNA	RNA	RNA
Size	27 nm	40-42 nm	30-35 nm	35 nm	27 nm
Incubation period in weeks	2-6	4-26	2-20	5-9	3-8
Spread					
Faeco-oral	Yes	No	No	No	Yes
Parenteral (blood)	Uncommon	Yes	Yes	Yes	Yes
Saliva (kissing)	Yes	Yes	Yes	—	—
Sexual act	Uncommon	Yes	Uncommon	Yes	Unknown
Vertical transmission	No	Yes	Uncommon	Yes	No
Chronic infection					
Incidence	Not known	5-10%	>50%	—	—
Severity	Mild	Often severe	Moderate	Unknown	Mild to moderate
Prevention					
Active	Vaccine	Vaccine	No	Prevented by hepatitis B	No
Passive	Immune serum globulins	Hyperimmune serum globulins	No	Virus infection	No
Prognosis	Good	Worst with age and debility	Moderate	Same as with hepatitis B	Good

Table 1.38: Causes of acute hepatitis

Infective
- *Viral*, e.g. hepatitis A, B, C, D, E, Epstein-Barr virus, cytomegalovirus, herpes simplex and yellow fever virus
- *Postviral*
  Reye's syndrome in children (aspirin-induced)
- *Nonviral*, e.g. leptospira, toxoplasma, coxiella

Noninfective
- Drugs, e.g. paracetamol, halothane, INH, rifampicin, chlorpromazine, methyldopa, oral contraceptives
- *Poisons*, e.g. carbon tetrachloride, mushrooms, aflatoxin
- Metabolic, e.g. Wilson's disease, pregnancy
- *Vascular*, e.g. CHF, Budd-Chiari syndrome, oral contraceptives

Q. What are complications of acute viral hepatitis?

Ans. Complications are common in type B or type C viral hepatitis; type A hepatitis usually resolves spontaneously. The complications are;
- Fulminant hepatitis – a dreadful complication
- Cholestatic viral hepatitis
- Relapsing hepatitis (transient subclinical infection)
- Chronic carrier state
- Chronic hepatitis
- Post-hepatitis syndrome (symptoms persist but biochemical investigations normal)

- Cirrhosis of the liver
- Hepatocellular carcinoma.

Q. What is carrier state in hepatitis?

Ans. Some asymptomatic patients carrying the HbsAg for more than 6 months after the episode of acute hepatitis B are called *chronic carriers*. Carrier stage does not exist in hepatitis A and E. These carriers are potential source of transmission of infection.

Q. How will you investigate a case with acute viral hepatitis?

Ans. Following are the investigations:
1. *TLC and DLC* may show leucopenia or lymphopenia, atypical lymphocytes may be seen. The ESR may be high.
2. *Hepatic profile*
   - *Serum bilirubin* raised, equally divided between conjugated and unconjugated fractions, or sometimes conjugated fraction may predominate (cholestatic phase).
   - *Serum transaminases (SGOT/SGPT)* are raised more than ten times (400-4000 IU).
   - *Serum alkaline phosphatase* may or may not be raised; if raised, indicates cholestasis
   - *Plasma albumin* is normal, may become low if jaundice is prolonged.

- *Prothrombin time* is normal, if increased, indicates extensive hepatocellular damage and bad prognosis
- *Urine* may show;
  - Urobilinogen in urine, appears during preicteric phase, disappears with onset of jaundice and reappears during recovery.
  - Bilirubinuria occurs during subclinical stage
  - Presence of bile salt and bile pigment indicates cholestasis
  - Stool may be normal colored or clay–colored (obstructive jaundice)

3. *Ultrasound of liver* may reveal hepatomegaly with normal echotexture. CT scan is not superior to USG.
4. *Serological tests* (Table 1.39) These are done in acute hepatitis.
5. *Special investigations* e.g. mitochondrial antibodies, ERCP, CT scan and liver biopsy (if needed)

Table 1.39: Diagnostic serology of acute hepatitis

Hepatitis	Serology			
	Hbs Ag	IgM anti-HAV	IgM anti-HBC	Anti-HCV
Acute hepatitis A	–	+		–
Acute hepatitis B	+	–		+
Acute hepatitis A Super imposed on chronic hepatitis B	+	+		–
	+	-		–
Acute hepatitis A and B	+	+	+	–
Acute hepatitis C	–	–	–	–

Q. Which hepatitis produces extrahepatic manifestations? What are these manifestation?

Ans. Hepatitis B produces extrahepatic manifestations are as follows:
- Serum sickness like syndrome
- Polyarthritis
- Acute glomerulonephritis (immune-complex)
- Atypical pneumonia
- Aplastic anemia or agranulocytosis
- Autoimmune hemolytic anemia
- Guillain-Barre syndrome
- Skin rashes (urticaria).

Q. What is acute fulminant hepatitis? How does it present clinically?

Ans. Acute fulminant hepatitis is said to be present when a previously healthy person develops acute hepatitis and goes into acute hepatic insufficiency/failure within 2 weeks of illness. This is due to acute massive necrosis (acute yellow atrophy) with shrinkage of liver (liver span <10 cm on USG).

The causes are; Type B, C and D viral infection, drugs, pregnancy, Wilson's disease and liver poisons (mushrooms, carbon tetrachloride, phosphorous) and Reye's syndrome in children.

The symptoms and signs of acute fulminant hepatitis are due to acute hepatic encephalopathy without stigmatas of the liver disease and signs of portal hypertension.

Q. What is chronic hepatitis? What are its causes?

Ans. It is defined as an inflammation of the liver (acute viral hepatitis) lasting for ≥ 6 months. The causes are;
- Autoimmune hepatitis
- Hepatitis B, C, D
- Drug-induced hepatitis
- Wilson's disease
- Alcoholic hepatitis
- Alpha-1 antitrypsin deficiency

The diagnosis of chronic hepatitis is made when clinical and biochemical evidence of hepatitis (e.g. jaundice, raised liver enzymes) persist for >6 months. The diagnosis is confirmed by liver biopsy and blood serology.

Q. Whom will you advise prophylaxis against hepatitis B (Table 1.40)

Ans. The indications are given in Table 1.40. Recently there has been mass prophylaxis program for hepatitis B in general population in India.

Table 1.40: Indications for hepatitis B vaccination in endemic areas

- **Parenteral drug abusers**
- *Male homosexuals*
- *Close contacts* (relatives or sexual partners) of infected persons
- *Patients receiving maintenance dialysis*
- *Laboratory staff*
- *Medical personnel*
  - Dentists
  - Surgeons/obstetricians
- *Medical /paramedical staff of:*
  - Intensive care department
  - Accident and emergency department
  - Endoscopy units
  - Oncology units
- *Nursing staff* involved in care of such patients

CASE 13: ASCITES

The patient (Fig. 1.13) presented with progressive distension of abdomen with abdominal discomfort and dyspnea. No history of jaundice or hematemesis. No history of edema feet or puffiness of face. No history of palpitation, PND or orthopnea. No past history of jaundice or rheumatic fever. No history of pain chest, cough with expectoration or hemoptysis. Examination revealed flanks full, positive fluid thrill and shifting dullness.

Clinical Presentations

- Often considerable number of patients with ascites may go unnoticed for weeks or months either because of coexistent obesity or because the ascites formation has been insidious, without pain or localizing symptoms.
- Ascites may first be noticed by the patient as an abdominal swelling with progressive increase in belt or size of clothing.
- Progressive abdominal distension due to ascites produces sensation of stretching or pulling of the flanks or groins and vague low back pain.
- Tense ascites may produce an increase in intra-abdominal pressure resulting in indigestion and heart burn due to gastroesophageal reflux; or dyspnea, orthopnea and tachypnea due to elevated domes of diaphragm and abdominal wall hernias (inguinal or abdominal).
- Patient may complain of respiratory embarrassment due to massive ascites or right sided pleural effusion due to leakage of ascitic fluid through lymphatic

Fig. 1.13: A patient with ascites. Note the distended abdomen with everted umbilicus and a ventral hernia (↓) above the small umbilical hernia

channels in diaphragm. A large pleural effusion obscuring the most of the lung may occasionally develop, is known as *hepatic hydrothorax.*

History

Points to be Noted on History

- Onset and progression of symptoms
- Past history of jaundice, hematemesis and melena, CHF, tuberculosis, rheumatic fever, renal failure, polyarthritis.
- Personal history-alcoholism, diet
- History of malignancy (mesothelioma, secondaries in liver) e.g. loss of appetite and weight.
- Family history, e.g. cirrhosis, Wilson's disease, hemochromatosis.
- History of pain in abdomen (spontaneous bacterial peritonitis, malignancy).

Examination

Proceed as follows:

I. General Physical Examination

Look for the followings:

- *Face:* vacant look, emaciated face and sunken cheeks indicate cirrhosis of the liver (cirrhotic facies)
- *Mental features,* e.g. confusion, disorientation, disturbed sleep pattern, bizarre handwriting, disturbed speech with jaundice indicate hepatic encephalopathy
- *Puffiness of face* with periorbital edema. It occurs in nephrotic syndrome
- Generalized or localized lymph adenopathy (e.g. tubercular, malignancy collagen vascular disorders)
- Raised JVP and cyanosis (congestive heart failure, constrictive pericarditis)
- Cyanosis, clubbing of fingers (e.g. bacterial endocarditis, hepatic encephalopathy)
- *Stigmatas of chronic liver disease,* e.g. muscle wasting, gynecomastia, testicular atrophy, loss of axillary and pubic hair, parotid enlargement and Dupuytren's contractures)
- Palmar erythema or painful fingertips or gangrene or flapping tremors
- Pedal edema, sacral edema, scrotal edema
- Signs of multiple nutrients deficiency e.g. angular stomatitis, cheilosis, anemia, atrophic or bald tongue, muscle

flabbyness, wasting and pigmentation of tongue and mucous membranes.

II. Systemic Examination

Inspection

- Fullness of flanks or tense abdominal distension
- The umbilicus is either transversely slit e.g. smiling umbilicus (moderate ascites) or everted with or without umbilical hernia (massive ascites)
- Prominent distended veins over the abdomen or around umbilicus (*caput medusae*) in a patient with cirrhotic portal hypertension or inferior vena cava obstruction
- Ventral, umbilical or inguinal hernia may or may not be seen
- There may be a mark of tapping of ascites (a mark with staining of tincture)

Palpation

- Increased abdominal girth
- Tenderness of abdomen in peritonitis with ascites
- Flow of blood in distended veins is away from the umbilicus in portal hypertension and from below upwards in IVC obstruction
- Palpable spleen in a patient with ascites (*by dipping method*) indicate portal hypertension
- Hepatomegaly. It indicates *Budd-Chiari syndrome* (malignancy or postnecrotic nodular conolasis)
- Elicit for abdominal wall edema

Percussion

- Percussion note is dull. Dullness is more marked in flanks with central sparing
- *Shifting dullness* is present in moderate ascites but becomes absent in huge ascites
- Fluid thrill is present in huge ascites, moderate ascites and localized ascites but absent in mild ascites
- Puddle's sign (dullness around umbilicus in knee-elbow position) is positive in mild ascites

Auscultation

- A venous hum around umbilicus indicate cirrhotic portal hypertension (*Cruveihlier-Bombgarten's syndrome*)
- A bruit over the liver indicates malignancy or recently done biopsy.

Other system examination

- Cardiovascular
- Urogenital system

Q. What is your provisional diagnosis?

Ans. My provisional diagnosis is ascites. *The points in favor are:*
- Distended abdomen with full flanks and transverse slit (smiling) umbilicus.
- Presence of both fluid thrill and shifting dullness.
- Flanks are dull with central sparing.
- Intestinal sounds are heard in the center of abdomen.

Q. How do you define ascites?

Ans. Normal amount of fluid in the peritoneal cavity is 100-150 ml of lymph, not detected by any means. Abnormal collection of fluid (>300 ml) in the peritoneum is called *ascites*. This amount is detected on USG abdomen. Significant amount of fluid (>500 ml) produces fullness of flanks on lying down position, is detected clinically. Larger amount of fluid (e.g. 1 liter) produces horse-shoe shape of the abdomen. Tense ascites means the peritoneal cavity is filled with free fluid producing cardiorespiratory embarrassment.

Q. What are causes of distended abdomen?

Ans. Five "F" denotes distension such as Fat, Fluid, Flatus, Feces and Fetus.

Q. What important points will you ask in history from a patient with ascites?

Ans. The followings points are to be noted in a case of ascites:
- Onset, e.g. sudden or gradual
- Past history of rheumatic fever, joint pain, jaundice, alcoholism, hematemesis or melena. Low grade fever or past history of tuberculosis or polyarthritis
- History of heart failure, liver disease, malignancy.
- Decrease or loss of appetite
- Diet and nutrition
- Cough and hemoptysis (present or past)
- Loss of weight, malignant cachexia
- Prolonged history of diarrhea >3 months, alteration in bowel habits
- Pain abdomen (acute pancreatitis) spontaneous bacterial peritonitis.
- History of puffiness of face or edema or chronic renal failure.

Q. What are causes of ascites?

Ans. Ascites occurs due to transudation of fluid into peritoneum in hypoproteinemic states or exudation into peritoneum by inflammation or infiltration of peritoneum by malignant process. The common causes are given in Tables 1.41 and 1.42.

Table 1.41: Causes of ascites

Systemic (ascites with edema)	Local (ascites only without edema)
• Nephrotic syndrome • Cirrhosis of the liver • Hypoproteinemia: nutritional or following chronic diarrhea or mal-absorption • Congestive heart failure or constrictive pericarditis • Malignancy liver • Meig's syndrome (ovarian tumor) • Hypothyroidism	• Peritonitis (serous, exudative) • Tuberculosis • Malignancy with secondaries in peritoneum • Spontaneous bacterial peritonitis • Pancreatitis • Portal vein thrombosis • Hepatic vein thrombosis (Budd-Chiari syndrome) • Chylous ascites

Table 1.42: Causes of ascites depending on the nature of fluid

Transudate (serum ascitic fluid albumin gradient > 1.1)
- Non-inflammatory fluid, serous or straw colored
- Fluid protein content <3.0 g/dl (or <50% of serum proteins)
- Specific gravity low or normal
- Occasional cell, mostly mesothelial
- Serum-ascites albumin gradient >1.1 g/dl (serum albumin minus ascitic fluid albumin)

Causes
- Nephrotic syndrome
- Congestive heart failure, pericadial effusion
- Hypoproteinemia, protein-losing states
- Cirrhosis of the liver
- Meig's syndrome

Exudate (serum/ascitic fluid albumin gradient > 1.1)
- Inflammatory thick, turbid or mucinous, hemorrhagic or straw colored fluid
- Protein content >3.0 g/dl (>50% of serum proteins)
- Specific gravity is high
- Cell count (100-1000 cells/mm^3), mostly either mononuclear or neutrophils
- Serum-ascites albumin gradient <1.1 g/dl

Causes
- Peritonitis, e.g. pyogenic, tubercular, malignant, subacute bacterial
- Leukemias, lymphomas
- Chylous ascites
- Budd-Chiari syndrome
- Pancreatitis (pancreatic ascites)

Q. What is differential diagnosis of ascites?

Ans. The differential diagnosis of ascites depends on the cause of ascites and whether ascites is a part of generalised *anasarca* (ascites, edema, fluid in serous cavities) or is localized.

1. *Ascites of nephrotic syndrome:* Puffiness of face in the morning, pitting ankle edema, slowly developing ascites with or without anemia indicate ascites to be of renal origin. The massive albuminuria confirms the diagnosis.

2. *Ascites due to cirrhosis of the liver:* Past history of jaundice or chronic liver disease, with history of recent episode of hematemesis and jaundice in a patient with ascites suggest cirrhosis. The gynecomastia, loss of axillary and pubic hair, weakness, weight loss are stigmata of chronic liver disease. Prominent abdominal veins, splenomegaly suggest portal hypertension due to cirrhosis.

3. *Ascites due to hypoproteinemia:* Anemia, multiple deficiencies, muscle flabbyness and atony of muscles with ascites and edema indicate hypoproteinemia to be its cause. The patient may have history of chronic diarrhea or recurrent diarrhea.

4. *Ascites of congestive heart failure:* Raised JVP, tender hepatomegaly, dyspnea, orthopnea, paroxysmal nocturnal dyspnea (PND), cardiomegaly with or without murmurs, ascites, edema with or without peripheral cyanosis are points in favor of congestive heart failure as the cause of ascites.

5. *Tubercular ascites:* A slow developing ascites with anorexia, low grade fever, common occurrence in females than males, night sweats and evening rise of fever with or without any evidence of tuberculosis elsewhere are points in favor of tubercular ascites if it develops in young age.

6. *Malignant ascites:* Rapid filling tense ascites in old age with decrease or loss of appetite, marked cachexia, hemorrhagic nature of ascites could be due to malignancy anywhere in the abdomen with secondaries in the peritoneum. (e.g. ovary, uterus, stomach pancreas, lung, breast).

7. *Pancreatic ascites* is due to collection of a large amount of pancreatic secretions either due to disruption of pancreatic duct or pseudocyst formation. It is painless, mild to moderate collection seen in patients with chronic pancreatitis. The ascitic fluid is exudate with low SAAG (<1.1) and high, fluid amylase levels (>1000 unit/l).

Q. What is chylous ascites? What are its causes?

Ans. It is the presence of milky fluid containing lymph in the peritoneal cavity. Milky fluid (turbidity) may be due to large number of cells (e.g. leucocytes, degenerated cells or tumor cells) or due to increased amount of protein content called *pseudochylous.*

Causes: Chylous ascites is most commonly due to obstruction to the lymphatics or thoracic duct especially by lymphoma, contains a large amount of triglycerides (>1000 mg/dl), and results from;

1. Trauma or penetrating abdominal injury to the thoracic duct
2. Tumors (malignant tumors of lymph nodes or others infiltrating the lymphatics)
3. Tuberculosis with lymphadenitis
4. Filariasis (filarial worms obstructing the lymphatics).
5. Occasionally cirrhosis and pancreatitis.

Turbidity of fluid disappears after extraction with ether; a diagnostic clue to the presence of fat and differentiates it from pseudochylous ascites.

Pseudochylous ascites refers to increased amount of proteins and calcium in the fluid leading to turbidity which is not dissolved by ether.

Chyliform ascites means a large number of cells (leucocytes, degenerated epithelial cells or tumor cells) as the cause of turbidity which disappears on extraction with alkali.

Q. What would be nature of ascites when both fluid thrill and shifting dullness are absent?

Ans. Mucinous ascites.

Q. What is mucinous ascites?

Ans. Rarely, ascitic fluid may be mucinous (gelatinous) in character, giving lobulated (jelly like mass) appearance to the ascites. The fluid thrill and shifting dullness are absent. It is difficult to aspirate (ascitic tap is dry). It may be either due to *pseudomyxoma peritonei* (rupture of mucocele of appendix or mucinous ovarian cyst) or rarely colloid carcinoma of stomach or colon with peritoneal metastases.

Q. What it serum ascitic albumin gradient (SAAG)?

Ans. It is calculated by substracting the ascitic fluid albumin concentration from serum albumin concentration from samples obtained at the same time. This gradient differentiates transudative from exudative ascites and also correlates directly with portal pressure; those whose gradient is >1.1 g/dl have portal hypertension and those with gradients <1.1g/dl do not. The accuracy of such determination is 97%

Q. What is refractory ascites?

Ans. Ascites is said to be refractory if it persists inspite of the maximum dose of diuretics (400-600 mg of spironolactone and 120-160 mg of furosemide) and salt restriction.

   i. Noncompliance of salt restriction

   ii. Hepatorenal syndrome, e.g. functional renal failure in cirrhosis of the liver

   iii. Low serum sodium or failure of diuretic therapy

   iv. Infections or subacute bacterial peritonitis

v. Superimposition of hepatoma
vi. GI bleeding
vii. Development of hepatic or portal vein thrombosis.

Q. What is genesis of ascites in cirrhosis?

Ans. Increased hydrostatic pressure due to splanchnic vascular dilatation and increased portal venous flow.

- Sodium retention due to hyperaldosteronism as a result of activation of renin-angiotensin aldosterone system.
- Decreased oncotic pressure due to hypoalbuminemia
- Increased formation of lymph due to vascular dilatation and increased portal venous blood flow
- Stimulation of antidiuretic hormone due to hypoperfusion of kidneys.

Q. What are physical signs of ascites?

Ans. Read "Clinical Methods in Medicine" by Dr. SN Chugh.

Q. What does presence of fluid thrill and absence of shifting dullness indicate?

Ans. Fluid thrill is present while shifting dullness is absent in following situations in the abdomen.
1. Mild ascites (≤ 500 ml of fluid)
2. Huge or massive ascites where there is no space for fluid to get shifted
3. Localized ascites
4. Ovarian cyst
5. Distended bladder

Q. How would you differentiate ascites from ovarian cyst?

Ans.

Ascites	Ovarian cyst
• Generalized distention	Localized distention
• Flanks full	Central or aniliac fossa swelling
• Umbilicus is transurgery slit or everted	Vertically slit or everted umbilicus
• Umbilicus to symphysis pubis distance is more than xiphisternum to umbilicus	The distances from umbilicus to pubis is smaller than umbilicus to xiphisternum
• Swelling does not have well defined demarcation	Swelling is rounded with well defined upper border i.e. you can reach above the swelling
• Horse-shoe shape dullness on percussion (flanks dull, center spares)	"Dullness is limited to midline or in one or two quadrants (quardrantic dullness)
• Shifting dullness present and characteristic	Shifting dullness absent
• Vaginal examination is negative	Vaginal examination is diagnosis
• USG is diagnostic, defects free fluid and its cause	USG defects localized fluid and confirms the ovarian cyst

Q. What are physical signs of mild, moderate and massive ascites?

Ans. The signs are given in the Table 1.43.

Table 1.43: Physical signs in various grades of ascites

Grade		Signs
0	Minimal	Puddle's sign
1	Mild	Shifting dullness present fluid thrill absent
2	Moderate	Shifting dullness and fluid thrill present
3	Massive	Fluid thrill present, shifting dullness absent

N.B. Localized ascites will behave like massive ascites, hence, in this also fluid thrill will be present and shifting dullness absent.

Q. What are the causes of rapid filling of ascites?

Ans.
- Malignancy (primary and secondary)
- Tuberculosis
- Chylous
- Spontaneous bacterial peritonitis
- Budd-Chiari syndrome.

Q. What are causes of purulent and hemorrhagic ascites?

Ans. They are depicted in Table 1.44.

Table 1.44: Purulent vs hemorrhagic ascites

Purulent ascites	Hemorrhagic ascites
• Pyogenic peritonitis	• Abdominal trauma or trauma during tapping of ascites
• Septicemia	• Malignancy of peritoneum (primary or secondary)
• Ruptured amebic liver abscess	• Tubercular peritonitis
• Pelvic inflammatory disease	• Bleeding diathesis
• Penetrating abdominal trauma with introduction of infection	• Acute hemorrhagic pancreatitis

Q. What are the causes of ascites disproportionate to edema feet (ascite precoax)?

Ans. These are as follows:
- Constrictive pericarditis
- Restrictive cardiomyopathy
- Hepatic vein thrombosis
- Cirrhosis of liver
- Tubercular peritonitis
- Intra abdominal malignancy
- Meig's syndrome

Q. What are the causes of hepatosplenomegaly with ascites?

Ans. Hepatosplenomegaly with ascites indicates lymphoreticular malignancy, leukemia, malignancy of liver, secondaries in the liver, hepatic vein thrombosis (Budd-Chiari syndrome), postnecrotic cirrhosis, congestive heart failure, pericardial effusion.

Q. How will you investigate a patient with ascites?

Ans. Investigations are done to confirm the diagnosis and to find out its cause. These include:

1. *Blood examination:* Anemia may be present. Presence of neutrophilic leukocytosis indicates infection.

2. *Urine examination:* Massive albuminuria (>3.5 g/day) is present in nephrotic syndrome. Small amount of proteinuria occurs in pericardial effusion and congestive heart failure.

3. *Stool for occult blood:* If present, may indicate gastrointestinal malignancy as the cause of ascites.

4. *Ultrasonography:* It is of proven value in detecting ascites, presence of a masses, evaluation of size of liver and spleen, portal vein diameter and presence of collaterals and enlargement of caudate lobe.

5. *Plain X-ray abdomen* in standing position is useful. It may show ground glass opacity or diffuse haziness with loss of psoas muscle shadow. It may show intestinal obstruction (3-5 fluid levels in step-ladder pattern), raised right dome suggests either amebic liver abscess or hepatoma.

6. *Diagnostic paracentesis:* 50-100 ml of ascitic fluid is withdrawn with the help of a needle and biochemically analysed to establish the etiology of ascites and to plan its treatment. It is also sent for bacteriological examination. The differences between transudative and exudative ascites with their respective causes have already been discussed.

7. *Serum-ascites albumin gradient:* The albumin in serum and ascitic fluid is determined to calculate the gradient. The serum albumin *minus* ascitic fluid albumin determines the gradient. The gradient >1.1 g/dl indicates transudative ascites and <1.1 g/dl indicates exudative ascites. The fluid protein <50% of serum protein also indicates transudate; while ≥ 50% indicates exudate.

8. *Further investigations* are done to find out the cause, e.g. serum proteins, serum cholestrol for nephrotic syndrome, X-ray chest, ECG, echo for congestive heart failure/pericadial effusion, liver function tests and tests for portal hypertension.

Q. What does paracentesis mean? What are its indications?

Ans. Paracentesis means removal of fluid. Paracentesis of ascitic fluid is indicated as follows:

i. *Diagnostic:* A diagnostic tap of ascitic fluid is done by putting the needle in the flank in one of lateral positions. The fluid removed is 50-100 ml for diagnostic purpose, i.e. for biochemical, cytological and bacteriological analysis.

ii. *Therapeutic:* It is done as a part of treatment. Ascitic fluid is rich in proteins, hence should not be routinely tapped. It is removed if patient has cardiorespiratory embarrassment (acute respiratory distress with tachycardia). The amount of fluid removed depends on the relief of symptoms or maximum of 3-5 liters of fluid may be removed in one setting. Repeated tapping should be avoided unless absolutely necessary as this may predispose to secondary infection of peritoneum and also causes protein loss.

iii. *Refractory ascites* (nonresponse to treatment)

iv. *Paracentesis* is attempted before *needle biopsy* of liver, *ultrasonogoraphy* or for *better palpation* of *underlying viscera*.

Q. What would you see on ultrasound in cirrhotic ascites?

Ans.
i. To detect presence of ascites (free or loculated)
ii. To detect splenomegaly
iii. To detect portal vein thrombosis or formation of collaterals
iv. To measure the portal vein diameter.
v. Condition of liver and its echotexture

Q. How does ultrasound help in the diagnosis of tubercular ascites?

Ans. It may reveal:

- Enlargement of mesenteric, pre-aortic and para-aortic lymph nodes
- Thick fibrinous septae may be seen traversing ascites (septate ascites)
- Thickened mesentery or rolled up omentum
- Tuberculosis of the liver, spleen, etc.

Q. What are ultrasound findings in Budd-Chiari syndrome?

Ans.
- Altered echotexture of liver
- Enlargement of caudate lobe
- Presence of ascites
- Reversal of portal blood flow on Doppler study.

Q. What are complications of paracentesis?

Ans. Common complications of paracentesis are as follows:

- Sudden withdrawal of a large amount of fluid may lead to dilatation of splanchnic blood vessels with subsequent *development of shock.*
- *Introduction of infection (peritonitis)* if sterile precautions are not observed.
- *Hypoproteinemia.* Ascitic fluid is rich in proteins, repeated large amount of aspiration may lead to development of hypoproteinemia.
- *Precipitation of hepatic coma.* Sudden withdrawal of ascites in a patient with cirrhotic portal hypertension may precipitate hepatic encephalopathy
- *Constant oozing of the ascites* due to formation of a track (especially in tense ascites).

Q. What are sequele/complications of a ascites?

Ans. These are as follows:

- *Cardiorespiratory embarrassment*
- *Right sided pleural effusion* due to leakage of ascitic fluid through lymphatic channels in the diaphragm.
- *Spontaneous bacterial peritonitis*
- *Abdominal hernia* (umbilical, inguinal) and diverication of recti due to tense ascites as a result of increased intraabdominal pressure
- *Functional renal failure*
- *Mesenteric venous thrombosis.*

Q. How would you manage a case with ascites?

Ans. 1. Rest in bed

2. *Dietary salt restriction.* In severe ascites, sodium should be strictly restricted to less than 10 meqld.

3. *Diuretics*: A combination of frusemide/torsamide with spironolactone is better than either alone.

4. *Fluid restriction* in severe ascites

5. *Paracentesis*: It should be done for therapeutic purpose when there is an evidence of cardiorespiratory embarrassment. Repeated tapping should be avoided as far as possible.

6. *Salt free albumin* infusion.

7. *Treatment of the underlying cause* i.e. ATT for tuberculosis, appropriate treatment of CHF, nephrotic syndrome, pericardial effusion.

8. If cirrhotic portal hypertension is the cause then *peritoneovenous shunting or TIPS* may be employed (Read the case discussion on cirrhotic portal hypertension and ascites)

Q. What is treatment of refractory ascites?

Ans. 1. Dietary sodium restriction plus diuretic.

2. Large volume paracentesis plus albumin.

3. Transjugular intrahepatic portosystemic shunt.

4. Liver transplantation.

CASE 14: HEPATOMEGALY

The patient (Fig. 1.14) presented with pain in the abdomen especially in right hypochondrium with swinging temperature, chills and rigors of 2 weeks duration. There was past history of loose motions and blood. Pain was more marked in left lateral position.

Clinical Presentations

Patients having hepatomegaly present with;
1. No symptoms (asymptomatic), Hepatomegaly is detected during routine examination.
2. Pain in right upper quadrant: It occurs in acute hepatomegaly due to stretching of the capsule of the liver which is pain-sensitive structure.
3. Mass in right hypochondrium.
4. Patients may present with fever, jaundice, distaste for food, dark urine and sometimes pruritus.
5. Patient may present, acute pain with fever and chills. This may occur following an episode of dysentery.
6. Patients with alcoholic liver disease may present with other toxic manifestations of alcoholism e.g. peripheral neuropathy, proximal sympathy, cerebella ataxia,

Fig. 1.14: A patient with hepatomegaly

Wernickes' encephalopathy (ocular nerve palsy) and Korsakoff's psychosis (loss of recent memory and confabulation)

History

Points to be Noted in History

- Present history of dysentery or GI disorder
- Any history of bleeding from any site
- History of fever, pigmentation, neck swelling, jaundice, anorexia, weight loss
- Full drug history
- Past history of tuberculosis, jaundice, diabetes, RHD (congestive heart failure)
- Personal history, e.g. alcoholism
- Nutritional history
- Family history of polycystic disease.

Examination

Proceed as follows:

I. General Physical Examination

- Assess the nutritional status
- Examine neck for lymph nodes, JVP
- Look at the skin for purpuric spots, ecchymosis, bruises, pigmentation
- Note anemia, cyanosis, jaundice, palmer erythema, spider angiomata
- Look for stigmatas of chronic liver disease and hepatic flap.
- Note pedal edema
- Examine vitals, e.g. respiration, pulse, temperature and BP

II. Systemic Examination

Inspection
- A right upper quadrantic fullness due to mass that moves with respiration (present in this case)

- Umbilicus is normal unless ascites present
- Normal abdominal movements
- Hernia sites are usually normal
- Prominent abdominal veins and collateral with flow away from umbilicus suggest portal hypertension

Palpation
- Define the mass and study its characteristics, e.g. solid or cystic, smooth or irregular, soft, firm or hard, tender or nontender, etc. Note whether it is pulsatile or not
- Elicit intercostal tenderness (thumbing sign). It was positive in this case.
- Elicit the signs of ascites if suspected
- Palpable the abdomen for other mass or masses such as spleen or lymph nodes.

Percussion
- Define upper and lower borders of the liver and calculate the liver span. It was 22 cm in this case
- Hydatid sign if hydatid cyst is syspected
- Percuss flanks for ascites.

Auscultation
- A bruit indicates a vascular hepatic tumor or hemangioma
- A rub indicates hepatic infarction or a nodular liver
- A venous hum around umbilicus indicates portal hypertension
- Auscultate for bowel sounds.

III. Systemic Examination

- Cardiovascular system for heart failure
- CNS examination for alcoholism

Q. What is your clinical diagnosis and why?
Ans. In view of painful and tender mass in right hypochondrium with swinging temperature and chills, positive intercostal tenderness with massive hepatomegaly without jaundice and signs of portal hypertension; and past history of dysentery the diagnosis of amebic liver abscess is most likely in this case.

Q. What is differential diagnosis?
Ans. The followings are differential conditions:
Congestive Hepatomegaly: It is due to chronic venous congestion of the liver as a result of congestive heart failure due to any cause, i.e. constrictive pericarditis, pericardial effusion and hepatic vein thrombosis (*Budd-Chiari syndrome*). Symptoms of dyspnea, orthpnea, paroxysmal nocturnal dyspnea and

cough with physical signs such as raised JVP, cyanosis, peripheral edema, crackles at both lung bases, heart murmurs, cardiomegaly and hepatomegaly indicate congestive heart failure. Nonvisible apex, pulsus paradoxus, low pulse pressure, widening of cardiac dullness and dullness of 2nd and 3rd left space, feeble heart sounds with other peripheral signs of congestive heart failure indicates hepatomegaly due to either constrictive pericarditis or pericardial effusion. In hepatic vein thrombosis (*Budd-Chiari syndrome*), there is an intractable ascites, jaundice, prominent abdominal veins and collaterals formation due to development of portal hypertension. Hepatomegaly is a part of the syndrome.

In these congestive states, liver is moderately or massively enlarged, tender, has smooth surface and round well defined edge. Further investigations should be done to confirm the diagnosis.

Inflammatory Hepatomegaly: Inflammation of liver due to hepatitis or typhoid fever produces enlargement of liver. In hepatitis, there is history of fever, distaste for food, nausea, vomiting followed by jaundice and pain in right hypochondrium. Typhoid fever is characterized by moderate to high grade fever, abdominal symptoms (nausea, vomiting, diarrhea with or without blood), tenderness of abdomen, rose spots and slow pulse rate. At about 7 to 10th day of illness, spleen also becomes enlarged.

Liver in inflammatory disorders shows mild to moderate enlargement, is tender and has smooth surface. Further investigations are required to confirm the respective inflammatory cause.

Infiltrative Hepatomegaly: Liver becomes enlarged when it gets infiltrated with leukemic cells or lymphoma cells or with fat and glycogen. Fatty infiltration of liver occurs in pregnancy, malnutrition, diabetes mellitus and alcoholism. Fatty liver is mildly enlarged, non-tender and has smooth surface. In leukemia, there is evidence of anemia, bleeding tendency (purpuric spots, ecchymosis, epistaxis, bruising etc), fever, lymph node enlargement and splenomegaly; while fever with hepatosplenomegaly and lymphadenopathy are characteristics of lymphoma. Peripheral blood film examination will confirm the diagnosis. In these disorders, liver is moderately enlarged, soft to firm in consistency, nontender with smooth surface. Further investigations are needed to confirm the diagnosis.

Hepatomegaly due to Parasitic Infection/Infestations: Malaria, kala-azar, hydatid disease and amebic infection can produce hepatomegaly by various mechanisms. Chronic malaria produces massive enlargement of liver along with other characteristics, such as fever of several days duration with classical bouts on alternate days with shaking chills and rigors. Jaundice is also common due to hepatitis or hemolysis. There is splenomegaly. Hepatomegaly is non-tender. Peripheral blood film will confirm the diagnosis of this condition.

Fever, hyperpigmentation of skin, especially face and hands, hepatosplenomegaly and anemia support the diagnosis of kala-azar in endemic area. The diagnosis can easily be confirmed by demonstrating the parasite in stained smears of aspirate of bone marrow, lymph nodes, spleen or liver or by culture of these aspirates.

Hydatid disease of liver produces cystic enlargement with positive hydatid sign on percussion with peripheral eosinophilia. USG is useful for confirming the diagnosis.

Hematological Disorders: All types of anaemia, especially hemolytic anemia, lead to mild to moderate non-tender hepatomegaly. The presence of mild jaundice, dark colored urine and stools with mild to moderate hepatosplenomegaly support the diagnosis of hemolytic anaemia. The diagnosis is further confirmed by tests for hemolysis and peripheral blood film examination. Malaria can also produce hemolysis, jaundice and hepatomegaly as already discussed.

Tumors of Liver: The tumors (primary or secondary) can enlarge the liver. Liver in malignancy is massively enlarged, tender and has nodular surface and hard consistency. Friction rub may be audible in some cases. Jaundice, pruritus may or may not be present, depending on the presence or absence of cholestasis. USG and biopsy of liver will confirm the diagnosis.

Hepatomegaly due to Diseases of Liver: Posthepatitic or post necrotic cirrhosis can produce non-tender, mild to moderate hepatomegaly with other stigmatas of cirrhosis and portal hypertension (muscle wasting, loss of axillary and pubic hair, gynecomastia, palmar erythema, spider angiomata, ascites, caput medusae and splenomegaly). The diagnosis is confirmed by liver biopsy and by biochemical and radiological tests.

Q. How do you define hepatomegaly?

Ans. Liver is placed just below the right dome of diaphragm and its edge is normally palpable on deep inspiration in right hypochondrium in some people and in children. The palpable liver does not mean hepatomegaly because if liver is displaced downwards due to any cause (emphysema, subphrenic abscess) it becomes palpable. Therefore, before commenting on hepatomegaly, the upper border must be defined by percussion in midclavicular line. Upper border of liver dullness is in 5th intercostal space.

Hepatomegaly refers to actual enlargement of liver (enlarged liver span) without being displaced downwards, i.e. the upper border of liver dullness stays as normal.

N.B. Always tell liver span in a case of hepatomegaly instead of commenting palpable liver by so many centimeters.

Q. What are the causes of palpable liver without its actual enlargement?

Ans. This denotes downwards displacement of normal liver due to:
- Emphysema
- Thin and lean person
- Subphrenic abscess (right side)
- Visceroptosis (Liver descends down during standing due to weak support)
- Any mass or fluid interposed between liver and the diaphragm will push liver downwards e.g. subpulmonic effusion. Massive right sided pleural effusion or pneumothorax.

Q. Where are the points to be noted in hepatic enlargement?

Ans. Following are important points:
1. *Extent of enlargement.* Liver span should be defined. Normal liver span is 10-14 cm. Less than 10 cm is considered as acute fulminant hepatitis (acute yellow atrophy) and >14 cm is taken as hepatomegaly.
2. *Movements with respiration.* Liver always moves with respiration, i.e. descends 1-3 cm downwards with deep inspiration.
3. *Tenderness* (tender or nontender). Tender hepatomegaly suggests acute enlargement or infarction.
4. *Edge* (sharp or blunt)
5. *Surface* (smooth, irregular or nodular)
6. *Consistency* (soft, firm, hard)
7. *Upper border of liver dullness* (normal or shifted)
8. *Whether left lobe* is enlarged or not. Is there any enlargement of caudate lobe?
9. Any *rub, bruit, venous hum.*
10. Any *pulsation* (intrinsic or transmitted).

Q. What are the causes of hepatomegaly?

Ans. Table 1.45 explains the causes of hepatic enlargement.

Table 1.45: Etiology of hepatic enlargement

1. **Vascular**
   - Congestive heart failure (CHF)
   - Pericardial effusion or constrictive pericarditis
   - Hepatic vein thrombosis (Budd-Chiari syndrome)
   - Hemolytic anemia
2. **Bile duct obstruction (Cholestasis)**
   - Bile duct stone
   - Tumor
3. **Infiltrative**
   - Leukemias (acute and chronic leukemia especially chronic myeloid leukemia)
   - Lymphoma
   - Fatty liver (e.g. alcoholism, diabetes, malnutrition)
   - Amyloidosis
   - Fat storage diseases such as Gaucher's disease, Niemann-Pick's disease in children.
   - Granulomatous hepatitis (e.g. typhoid, tuberculosis and sarcoidosis)
4. **Parasitic**
   - Malaria
   - Kala azar
   - Hydatid disease
   - Amebic liver abscess
5. **Infective/inflammatory**
   - Hepatitis
   - Typhoid fever
6. **Tumors**
   - Hepatocellular carcinoma
   - Secondaries or metastatic deposits in liver
7. **Rare**
   - Polycystic disease of the liver
   - Hemangioma of liver
   - A large hepatic cyst

Q. What are the common causes of mild to moderate hepatomegaly?

Ans. They are;
- Typhoid fever, tuberculosis
- Leukemias
- Congestive splenomegaly (e.g. CHF, pericardial effusion)
- Budd-Chiari syndrome
- Hemolytic anemia
- A hemangioma or congenital cyst
- Fatty liver
- Postnecrotic cirrhosis

Q. What are the causes of tender hepatomegaly?

Ans. Causes are as below:
- Acute viral hepatitis
- Amebic liver abscess
- Congestive hepatomegaly (e.g. CHF, constrictive pericarditis, pericardial effusion, Budd-Chiari syndrome)

- Pyogenic liver abscess
- Malignancy of the liver
- Perihepatitis (e.g. after biopsy or hepatic infarct)
- Infected hydatid cyst.

Q. What are the causes of enlargement of left lobe?

Ans. Causes are as below:
- Amebic liver abscess (left lobe abscess)
- Hepatoma
- Metastases in liver.

Q. What are different consistencies of the liver?

Ans. Table 1.46 explains the answer.

Table 1.46: Differential diagnosis of hepatomegaly depending on consistency of liver

Consistency	Causes
Soft	Congestive heart failure, viral hepatitis, fatty liver, acute malaria, visceroptosis (drooping of liver)
Firm	Cirrhosis, chronic malaria and kala-azar, hepatic amebiasis, lymphoma
Hard	Hepatocellular carcinoma, metastases in liver, chronic myeloid leukemia, myelofibrosis

Q. What are the causes of irregular surface of liver?

Ans. Followings are causes:
- Cirrhosis (micronodular or macronodular)
- Secondaries in the liver
- Hepatocellular carcinoma
- Hepatic abscesses (pyogenic, amebic)
- Multiple hepatic cysts.

Q. What are the causes of massive hepatomegaly?

Ans. Massive hepatomegaly means enlargement > 8 cm below the costal margin. The causes are:
1. Malignancy liver (primary or secondary)
2. Amebic liver abscess
3. Chronic malaria and kala-azar
4. Hepatitis (sometimes)
5. Hodgkin's disease
6. Polycystic liver disease

N.B. Acute malaria does not produce hepatomegaly

Q. What are the causes of hepatic bruit and rub?

Ans. Followings are the causes:

Bruit
- Hepatocellular carcinoma
- Hemangioma liver
- Alcoholic hepatitis/liver disease

Rub
- Infections of liver
- Following liver biopsy
- Hepatic infarction (embolic)
- Perihepatitis due to any cause (gonococcal perihepatitis in women)
- Carcinoma of liver

Q. What does the presence of abdominal venous hum medicate?

Ans. It is virtually diagnostic of cirrhotic portal hypertension. When present with hepatic arterial bruit in the same patient, then it suggests cirrhosis with either alcoholic hepatitis or malignancy liver

Q. What is Cruveilhier–Baumgarten syndrome?

Ans. It is the presence of the abdominal venous hum in portal hypertension secondary to cirrhosis.

Q. What does a presence of hepatic rub, bruit and venous hum indicate?

Ans.
i. The presence of hepatic rub with bruit indicates cancer of the liver.
ii. The presence of the hepatic rub, bruit and venous hum indicates that a patient with cirrhosis has developed a hepatoma.

Q. What do you understand by pulsatile liver? How will you demonstrate it?

Ans. Pulsatile liver means pulsations felt over the liver which could be;
1. *Intrinsic pulsations due to:*
   - Tricuspid regurgitation (systolic pulsations) either organic or functional
   - Hemangioma of the liver
2. Transmitted pulsation from right ventricle due to
   - Right ventricular hypertrophy.

Method of Demonstration of Pulsations of Liver: The presystolic or systolic pulsations of the heart can be transmitted to venous circulation in the liver in the presence of tricuspid incompetence, which can be detected as follows:
- Make the patient to sit in a chair, stand on the right side of the patient
- Place your right palm over liver in right hypochondrium and left palm over the back in the same manner as used for bimanual palpation.
- Ask the patient to hold his breath after taking deep inspiration
- Observed the lifting and separation of hands from the side with each heart beat.

In case of pulsatile liver, the hands are lifted and separated to some extent.

Clinical Tip

In case of pulsatile liver, always look for other signs of tricuspid regurgitation (engorged pulsatile neck veins, v and y collapse and a pansystolic murmur) and congestive heart failure (cyanosis, dyspnea, edema).

Q. What do you understand by the term liver span? What is its significance?

Ans. The liver span is the vertical distance between the upper and lower borders of the liver which is defined either clinically (on percussion) or on ultrasound. Normal liver span in an adult is variable (10-14 cm), greater in men than in women, greater in tall people than in short.

Significance

- Liver span is actually reduced when liver is small and shruken (acute fulminant hepatitis) or masked when free air is present below the diaphragm as from a perforated viscus (liver dullness is masked, hence, span appears to be reduced).
- Liver span is increased when liver is enlarged not when liver is displaced.
- Serial observations may show a decreasing span of dullness with resolution of hepatitis, CHF or less commonly with progression of fulminant hepatitis.
- It is used to define actual vs apparent enlargement of liver.
  - Actual or real enlargement means palpable liver with increase in liver span.
  - Apparent enlargement means liver is palpable without being actually enlarged (liver span is normal). It is displaced downwards by right sided pleural effusion, pneumothorax, COPD or low diaphragm.

Q. What is Reidle lobe of the liver?

Ans. *Reidle' lobe of liver* is a tongue like projection of the right lobe of the liver, represents a variation in shape of the normal liver. It is commonly found in females or those with a lanky built. It is usually mistaken for a gallbladder or right kidney, can be differentiated on ultrasound.

CASE 15: PORTAL HYPERTENSION

The patient (Fig. 1.15A) presented with distension of abdomen, weakness, dull abdominal ache and mild exertional dyspnea for the last 3 months. There was history of hematemesis and jaundice in the past.

Clinical Presentations

Patients usually present with;
- Progressive distension of abdomen, swelling of legs, hematemesis and melena (e.g. portal hypertension)
- Fatigue, weight loss, flatulent dyspepsia, anorexia, malnutrition, muscle wasting drowsiness, disturbed sleep pattern (e.g. hepatic encephalopathy)

Points to to Noted in the History

- History of fever, jaundice, bleeding from any site
- History of disturbance in consciousness, sleep or behavior problem
- Past history of alcoholism, drug intake, jaundice, delivery (in female)
- Family history of jaundice or similar illness
- Nutritional history.

General Physical Examination

- Look for hepatic facies, e.g. earthy look, sunken (hollow) cheek and malar prominence—present in this case
- Assess nutritional status—poor in this case
- Look for stigmatas of cirrhosis (wasting of muscles, palmar erythema, spider angiomatas, testicular atrophy, gynecomastia, bilateral parotid enlargement and Dupuytren's contractures). Few stigmatas were present.
- Look for signs of hepatic insufficiency, i.e. mental features, jaundice, bleeding (purpura, ecchymosis and bruising) clubbing of fingers, flapping tremors.
- Look for signs of portal hypertension, e.g. ascites, collaterals formation and fetor hepaticus, splenomegaly. Ascites and splenomegaly present.

Figs 1.15A to C: A. Patient with symptoms and signs of portal hypertension due to cirrhosis of the liver; B. Classification of portal hypertension depending on the site of obstruction C. Cirrhotic liver—a common cause of portal hypertension

- Look for anemia, jaundice, Keyser-Fleischer's rings
- Look for signs of malnutrition and vitamin deficiency
- Look for peripheral pitting edema, which was present.

- Look for signs of CHF or pericardial effusion, e.g. raised JVP, cyanosis, neck pulsations, etc.
- Note the vital signs, e.g. temperature, respiration, BP and pulse.

Systemic Examination

Inspection

- Skin over the abdomen may be thin, shiny due to edema of abdominal wall
- Abdominal distension with increased abdominal girth—present in this case.
- Prominent veins with flow of blood away from umbilicus
- Hernias (umbilical or inguinal) may or may not be present
- Umbilicus may be everted or transversely slit (smiling umbilicus) in presence of ascites (umbilicus was transversely slit in this case).

Palpation

- Liver was palpable, nontender, firm with sharp irregular margins. Left lobe was enlarged. In some cases, liver may not be palpable
- Spleen was also palpable, nontender, soft to firm
- Ascites was detected by fluid thrill
- Flow of blood in dilated veins was away from umbilicus.

Note: Palpate the liver and spleen by dipping method in presence of ascites.

Percussion

- Shifting dullness confirmed the presence of ascites
- Flanks were dull with central sparing
- Liver and splenic areas were dull.

Auscultation

Hear for;
- Bruit over liver. It indicates malignant liver
- Rub. It indicates perihepatitis due to infarction or may be heard over a nodule
- Venus hum around umbilicus. Its presence indicates portal hypertension (*Cruveihlier-Bomgarten's syndrome*)

Q. What is your clinical diagnosis and why?

Ans. The clinical diagnosis is cirrhotic portal hypertension without hepatic encephalopathy. The points in favor are:
- Long history
- Past history of jaundice and hematemesis
- Poor nutritional status e.g. sunken cheeks
- Presence of stigmata of cirrhosis
- Presence of ascites, splenomgaly and collaterals with flow of blood away from umbilicus
- Pitting edema.

Q. What is portal hypertension? How do the patients present with it?

Ans. Normal portal venous pressure is low (5 to 10 mm Hg) because vascular resistance in hepatic sinusoids is minimal. Portal hypertension is defined as elevated portal venous pressure more than 10 mm Hg, results from increased resistance to portal blood flow. As the portal venous system lacks valves, therefore, obstruction at any level between right side of the heart and portal vein will result in retrograde transmission of elevated blood pressure.

Portal hypertension results in congestion of viscera (stomach and intestine), formation of collaterals and subsequent rupture, and precipitation of hepatic failure. Patient commonly present with;
- *Variceal bleeding*, e.g. hematemesis; melena, piles
- *Chronic iron deficiency anemia* due to congestive gastropathy and repeated minor bleeding.
- *Abdominal distension* (ascites), splenomegaly.
- Spontaneous bacterial peritonitis.
- Symptoms and signs of hepatic encephalopathy (discussed below) may be associated with portal hypertension.
- Oliguria/anuria due to hepatorenal syndrome
- Hypersplenism leading to pancytopenia.

Q. How do you classify of portal hypertension?

Ans. Increased portal pressure can occur at three levels relative to hepatic sinusoids (Fig. 1.15B).
1. *Presinusoidal.* It means obstruction in the presinusoidal compartment outside the liver (between sinusoids and portal vein).
2. *Sinusoidal.* Obstruction occurs within the liver itself at the level of sinusoids.
3. *Postsinusoidal.* Obstruction is outside the liver at the level of hepatic veins, inferior vena cava or beyond sinusoids within liver (veno-occlusive disease).

Q. What are the causes of portal hypertension?

Ans. Cirrhosis is the most common cause, accounts for >90% of cases (Table 1.47).

Table 1.47: Causes of portal hypertension depending on the site of obstruction (Fig. 1.15 B)

1. **Postsinusoidal**
   - Extrahepatic postsinusoidal, e.g. Budd-Chiari syndrome
   - Intrahepatic postsinusoidal, e.g. veno-occlusive disease

2. **Sinusoidal**
   - Cirrhosis of the liver (Fig. 1.15 C)
   - Cystic liver disease
   - Metastases in the liver
   - Nodular transformations of the liver

3. **Presinusoidal**
   - *Intrahepatic presinusoidal*, e.g. schistosomiasis, sarcoidosis, congenital hepatic fibrosis, drugs and toxins, lymphoma, leukemic infiltrations, primary biliary cirrhosis.
   - *Extrahepatic presinusoidal*, e.g. portal vein thrombosis, abdominal trauma, compression of portal vein at porta hepatis by malignant nodules or lymph node, pancreatitis.

Q. Define noncirrhotic portal hypertension. What are its causes?

Ans. This is defined as portal hypertension without hepatocellular damage and lack of nodular regeneration activity in the liver. These cases manifest usually with splenomegaly, anemia, recurrent variceal bleed and chances of hepatic encephalopathy are remote.

This disorder is usually associated with either congenital or acquired hepatic fibrosis, which may be localized or generalized. Some causes of noncirrhotic portal fibrosis are given in Table 1.48.

Table 1.48: Causes of noncirrhotic portal fibrosis

1. **Idiopathic portal hypertension (noncirrhotic portal fibrosis, Banti's syndrome)**
   - Intrahepatic fibrosis and phlebosclerosis
   - Portal and splenic vein sclerosis
   - Portal and splenic vein thrombosis
2. **Schistosomiasis** (pipe-stem fibrosis with presinusoidal portal hypertension)
3. **Congenital hepatic fibrosis**
4. **Lymphomatous infiltration** around portal triad
5. **Chronic arsenic poisoning** (deposition of arsenic in liver)

Q. What are difference between cirrhotic and noncirrhotic portal hypertension?

Ans. Differences between cirrhotic and noncirrhotic portal hypertension are given in the Table 1.49.

Table 1.49: Differentiation between cirrhotic and noncirrhotic portal hypertension

Cirrhotic	Noncirrhotic
• Slow insidious onset	• Acute or sudden
• Ascites present	• Ascites absent
• Recurrent haematemesis uncommon	• Recurrent haematemesis is common and presenting feature
• Anaemia moderate	• Anaemia severe
• Hepatic encephalopathy common	• Hepatic encephalopathy uncommon
• Oedema present	• No edema
• Liver biopsy shows cirrhosis	• No evidence of cirrhosis; only portal fibrosis seen

Q. Why does ascites absent in noncirrhotic portal hypertension?

Ans. Ascites is sign of cirrhosis (liver cell dysfunction), hence, absent in noncirrhotic portal hypertension.

Q. What are pathological types of cirrhosis?

Ans. • Micronodular   • Macronodular
• Mixed

Q. What are clinical types of cirrhosis?

Ans. • Post hepatitis   • Alcoholic
• Cardiac   • Biliary
• Cryptogenic

Q. Define cirrhosis of the liver. What are its clinical characteristics?

Ans. Cirrhosis is the pathological term, denotes irreversible destruction of liver cells (necrosis) followed by fibrosis and nodular regeneration of the liver cells in such a way that the normal liver architecture is lost.

Clinical Features of Cirrhosis: Cirrhosis may be totally asymptomatic, and in life time may be found incidentally at surgery or may just be associated with isolated hepatomegaly. The liver in cirrhosis is usually small but may become large due to large transformation. When palpable, it is firm, nodular, nontender with sharp and irregular borders.

It may present with nonspecific complaints such as weakness, fatigue, muscle cramps, weight loss, nausea, vomiting, anorexia and abdominal discomfort.

The common clinical features of the cirrhosis are due to either liver cell failure with or without hepatic encephalopathy or portal hypertension.

Q. What are signs and symptoms of liver cell failure?

Ans. Signs of liver cell failure are:
• *Hepatomegaly* or *small shrunken liver*
• *Jaundice, fever*
• *Circulatory changes,* e.g. palmar erythema, spider angiomata, cyanosis (due to AV shunting in lungs), clubbing of the fingers, tachycardia, bounding pulses, hyperdynamic circulation.

• *Endocrinal changes,* e.g.
  – Loss of libido, hair loss
  – Gynecomastia, testicular atrophy, impotence in males
  – Breast atrophy, irregular menses, amenorrhoea in females
• *Haemorrhagic manifestations,* e.g.
  – Bruises, epistaxis, purpura, menorrhagia
• *Miscellaneous*
  – Diffuse pigmentation
  – White nails
  – Dupuytren's contractures
  – Parotid enlargement.
• *Hepatic Encephalopathy* – read below

Q. What are signs of portal hypertension?

Ans. Signs of portal hypertension
• *Splenomegaly*
• *Collateral vessels* formation at gastroesophageal junction, around the umbilicus, behind the liver and in the rectum.
• *Variceal bleeding* (hematemesis and melena)
• *Fetor hepaticus* due to excretion of mercaptans in breath.

Q. What are signs of hepatic encephalopathy?

Ans. It comprises of features of liver cells failure described above plus mental feature described below:
• Mental features (e.g. reduced alertness, restlessness, behavioral changes, bizarre handwriting, disturbance in sleep rhythm, drowsiness, confusion, disorientation, yawning, and hiccups). In late stages, convulsions may occur and patient lapses into coma.

Q. What are precipitating factors for hepatic encephalopathy?

Ans. There are certain factors that push the patient with compensated cirrhosis liver into decompensation phase (hepatic encephalopathy). These include:
• Drugs-like sedatives, hypnotics
• Gastrointestinal bleeding (e.g. varices, peptic ulcer, congestive gastropathy)
• Excessive protein intake
• Diuretics producing hypokalaemia and alkalosis
• Rapid removal of large amount of ascitic fluid in one setting (>3L)
• Acute alcoholic bout
• Constipation
• Infections and septicemia, surgery
• Azotemia (uremia)
• Portosystemic shunts, e.g. spontaneous or surgical.

Q. What is probable pathogenesis of hepatic encephalopathy?

Ans. Although, hepatic encephalopathy is called *ammonia encephalopathy* but NH_3 is not only the culprit. The possible mechanisms are;

- Increased NH_3 levels in blood
- Increased levels of short-chain fatty acids
- Increase in false neurotransmitters like octopamine and rise in GABA level (true neurotransmitter)
- Rise in methionine levels
- Rise in certain amino acids (ratio of aromatic amino acids to branched chain amino acids is increased) and mercaptans.

All these products described above are retained in blood in higher concentration due to combined effect of liver cell failure (decreased metabolism) and portosystemic shunting (delivery of these substances into circulation by bypassing the liver).

Q. How do you stage/grade the hepatic encephalopathy?

Ans. Clinical staging of hepatic encephalopathy is important in following the course of illness and to plan the treatment as well as to assess the response to therapy (Table 1.50).

Table 1.50: Clinical staging of hepatic encephalopathy

Stage	Mental features	Tremors	EEG change
I	Euphoria or depression, confusion, disorientation, disturbance of speech and sleep pattern	+/–	Normal EEG
II	Lethargy, moderate confusion	+	High voltage triphasic slow waves (abnormal EEG)
III	Marked confusion, incoherent speech, drowsy but arousable	+	High voltage Triphasic waves (2-5/sec) (abnormal EEG)
IV	Coma, initially responsive to noxious stimuli, later unresponsive	–	Delta activity (abnormal EEG)

Q. What are diagnostic criteria for hepatic encephalopathy?

Ans. The four major criteria are:

1. Evidence of acute or chronic hepatocellular disease with extensive portosystemic collaterals
2. Slowly deterioration of consciousness from reduced awareness to confusion, disorientation, drowsiness or stupor and finally into coma.

3. Shifting combination of neurological signs including asterixis (tremors), rigidity, hyper-reflexia, extensor plantar response and rarely seizures.
4. EEG changes. Symmetric high voltage triphasic waves changing to delta slow activity.

Q. What will you look on general physical examination in a patient with alcoholic cirrhosis of the liver?

Ans. Examination of a patient with cirrhosis is as follows: (Read case summary also in the beginning)

General Physical Signs

Look for;

- Malnutrition, vitamin deficiency
- Anemia
- Jaundice (icterus)
- Hepatic facies, e.g. earthy look, shunken shiny eyeballs, muddy facial expression, sunken cheeks with malar prominence, pinched up nose and parched lips, icteric tinge of conjunctiva
- Edema feet
- Obvious swelling of abdomen
- Wasting of muscles
- Foul smell (fetor hepaticus)
- Flapping tremors
- Cyanosis.

Signs of chronic alcoholism (alcoholic stigmata)

- Red tip of nose and redness of cheeks
- Spider naevi
- Pigmentation of skin; may or may not be present
- Gynecomastia and testicular atrophy in males
- Palmar erythema
- Scanty axillary and pubic hair in male, breast atrophy in females
- White nails
- Dupuytren's contracture.

Q. What are alcoholic stigmata?

Ans. These stigmata preceed the development of cirrhosis, hence, are usually present in alcoholic cirrhosis. They have been discussed above.

Q. What are stages of alcoholic cirrhosis?

Ans. 1. Fatty liver
2. Alcoholic hepatitis/steatohepatitis
3. Alcoholic cirrhosis

Q. What are complications of cirrhosis?

Ans. Followings are complications:

- Portal hypertension (fatal variceal bleeding)
- Hepatocellular failure and subsequent hepatic encephalopathy

- Spontaneous bacterial peritonitis (Ascitic fluid leukocytes count >500 cells/µl or >250 polymorphs/µl).
- Septicaemia
- Increased incidence of peptic ulcer and hepatocellular carcinoma
- Nutritional debility (e.g. anemia, hypoproteinemia)
- Hepatorenal and *hepatopulmonary syndromes*. It is functional acute renal failure in a patient with cirrhosis of the liver, develops due to circulatory or hemodynamic changes. The exact etiology is unknown. The kidneys structurally are normal but functionally abnormal, hence called *functional renal failure*. The prognosis is poor. Hepatorenal syndrome rarely can develop in hepatitis also. *Hepatopulmonary syndrome* is development of cyanosis and clubbing of the fingers due to arteriovenous shunting in the lungs.
- Hemorrhagic tendency.

Q. What are the causes of death in cirrhosis?

Ans. Common causes are as follows:
1. Most common cause is fatal septicemia (gram-negative)
2. Hepatic encephalopathy
3. Cerebral edema
4. Fatal bleeding
5. Renal failure (hepatorenal syndrome)
6. Hypoglycemia, hypokalemia etc.

Q. What are causes of upper GI bleed in cirrhosis of liver?

Ans. The causes are:
1. Esophageal varices
2. Gastric varices/erosions
3. Congestive gastropathy
4. Gastroduodenal ulcerations
5. Mallory-Weiss tear
6. Bleeding tendencies

Q. How will you investigate a case with cirrhosis of the liver?

Ans. Investigations of cirrhosis are as follows:
1. *Complete hemogram and ESR:*
   - *Anemia.* Anemia in cirrhosis is due to haematemesis, melena, anorexia with poor intake of nutrients, piles, malabsorprtion and hypersplenism. Anemia is commonly microcytic and hypochromic.
   - Pancytopenia (anemia, leukopenia and thrombocytopenia) is due to hypersplenism.
   - Raised ESR indicates infections.

2. *Stool for occult blood (Guaiac test)* may be positive. Bleeding in cirrhosis is intermittent, hence, test may be performed at least for 3 consecutive days. Vitamin C intake may give false positive result.
3. *Rectal examination* for internal piles
4. *Chest X-ray* for lung pathology or pleural effusion
5. *Hepatic profile*
   - Total serum proteins and albumin may be low. The albumin/ globulin ratio is altered.
   - Serum bilirubin is normal or raised
   - Serum transaminases are normal or mildly elevated
   - Alkaline phosphatase is mildly elevated
   - Serum cholesterol is low
   - Prothrombin time is normal or increased and does not return to normal with vitamin K therapy. Low PT is bad prognostic sign
   - Viral markers (HbsAg) are negative
   - Serum autoantibodies, antinuclear, anti-smooth muscle and antimitochondrial antibodies level increase in autoimmune hepatitis, cryptogenic cirrhosis and biliary cirrhosis.
   - Serum immunoglobulins, e.g. IgG is increased in autoimmune hepatitis, IgA increased in alcoholic cirrhosis and IgM in primary biliary cirrhosis.
6. *Other blood tests,* e.g. serum copper (Wilson's disease), iron (hemochromatosis), serum alpha-1-antitrypsin (cystic fibrosis) and serum alpha-fetoprotein (hepatocellular carcinoma).
7. *Imaging*
   - Ultrasound for liver may reveal change in size, shape and echotexture of the liver. Fatty change and fibrosis produce diffuse increased echogenicity. The presence of ascites, portal vein diameter (>14 mm indicates portal hypertension), presence of varices and splenomegaly can be determined on USG.
   - Barium swallow for esophageal varices (worm-eaten appearance due to multiple filling defects).
   - CT scan is not better than USG in cirrhosis of liver.
8. *Upper GI endoscopy* shows esophageal and gastric varices, peptic ulcer or congestive gastro-pathy (petechial hemorrhages both old and new, seen in gastric mucosa-mosaic pattern of red and yellow mucosa).

9. *Pressure measurement studies*
   - Percutaneous intrasplenic pressure is increased in portal hypertension.
   - Wedged hepatic venous pressure is increased.
10. ***Dynamic flow studies.*** These may show distortion of hepatic vasculature or portal vein thrombosis
   - Doppler ultrasound for visualization of portal venous system and duplex Doppler for measurement of portal blood flow and flow reversal in portal and splenic vein.
   - Portal venography by digital substraction angiography.
11. ***Electroencephalogram (EEG)*** may show triphasic pattern in hepatic encephalopathy.
12. ***Liver biopsy.*** It is a gold standard test to confirm the diagnosis of cirrhosis and helps to find out its cause. Special stains can be done for iron and copper.
13. ***Tapping of the ascites.*** Ascites is transudative (serum albumin/ascites albumin gradient > 1.1). The fluid should be sent for cytology, biochemistry and for culture if bacterial peritonitis is suspected.

Q. How would you manage a patient of cirrhosis and ascites?

Ans. The steps of management would be:
   - *Sodium restriction* to 80-90 mEq/day
   - *Diuretics*: A combination of frusemide and spironolactone is effective, serial monitoring of Na^+ concentration helps to determine the optimal dose of diuretic; doses are increased until a negative sodium balance is achieved.
   - *Paracentesis*: About 3-5 liters of fluid can be removed in a patient with cardiorespiratory embarrassment to relieve symptoms
   - *If ascites is diuretic resistant*, then
     - Therapeutic paracentesis with infusion of salt free albumin
     - Peritoneovenous shunting (Laveen shunt) is of limited use nowaday because of high rate of infection and development of DIC.
     - Transjugular intrahepatic portosystemic shunt (TIPS). It is side to side shunt consisting of stented channel between portal vein and hepatic vein.
     - Extracorporeal ultrafiltration of ascitic fluid with reinfusion
     - Liver transplantation

Q. What are indications of TIPS?

Ans.
   - A huge or tense ascites refractory to treatment
   - Recurrent ascites

CASE 16: CHRONIC DIARRHEA AND MALABSORPTION

The 14 years male adolescent (Fig. 1.16) was brought by the mother with complaints of stunted growth and reduction in weight. There was history of chronic diarrhea since childhood. There was history of intermittent loose motion since then.

Clinical Presentations (Fig. 1.16)

These patients present with;
1. Passage of loose stools >3 per day for the last 3 months.
2. Patients may complain of nonspecific symptoms, e.g. ill health, weakness, fatigue, weight loss with signs and symptoms of malnutrition, anemia, vitamins and mineral deficiency.
3. Specific symptoms and signs depending on the underlying cause;
   - Fever, pain abdomen, diarrhea with or without blood may suggest underlying inflammatory bowel disease.

Fig. 1.16: An adolescent male with stunted growth and chronic diarrhea. There was anemia, edema feet and signs of multiple nutrient deficiency

- Presence of edema face and feet, anemia, muscle wasting and weight loss indicate hypoproteinemia due to protein-losing enteropathy.
- The presence of steatorrhea (large, offensive stools with increased fat content) indicates either pancreatic or hepatic cause of malabsorption.
- Diarrhea with features of vitamin B_{12} deficiency (red tongue-glossitis, macrocytic anemia, peripheral neuropathy and subacute combined degeneration of the cord) indicate chronic gastritis or malabsorption due to involvement of terminal ileum (site of vitamin B_{12} absorption) due to any cause or bacterial proliferation in blind loop syndrome or stricture of bowel.
- Diarrhea following ingestion of milk or milk product indicates milk allergy or milk intolerance.

Points to be Noted in History

- Ask about onset, duration, frequency, nature and any associated symptoms e.g nausea, vomiting or pain in abdomen.
- Whether or not it is nocturnal ? Is there any blood in stool ?
- History of fever, worm expulsion or recurrent episodes of diarrhoea
- Any relation of diarrhoea with food or milk
- History of oedema feet, distension of abdomen, loss of appetite or weight
- Developmental history including milestones
- Nutritional history
- Family history
- Any history of foreign travel.

General Physical Examination

- Record height and weight, and calculate BMI
- General appearance, e.g. facial puffiness, protuberant abdomen
- Look for deficiency signs of nutrients e.g. protein (weakness, muscle wasting, flabbyness, edema, protuberant abdomen, thin-peppary skin), fat (thin extremities, sunken cheeks, flat buttocks and thin chest, etc.)

- Look for signs of vitamin deficiency, e.g. xerosis, Bitot's spots, cheilosis, angular stomatitis, aphthous ulcers, spongy and bleeding gums, bowing of the legs, rickety rosary, purpuric or ecchymotic patches, peripheral neuropathy and anaemia
- Record pulse, BP, temperature and respiration
- Look for lymphadenopathy any where in the body e.g. neck, axilla, groin, etc.

Systemic Examinations

All the major systems have to be examined.

I. Abdomen

- Note abdominal protuberance, flabby abdominal muscle and edema of abdominal wall
- Look for the signs of ascites due to hypoproteinemia
- Look for enlargement of spleen, liver due to anemia or intercurrent infection
- Look for any abdominal lymph nodes.
- Rectal examination

II. CVS Examination

- Examine the heart for any enlargement, murmur, rub or abnormal sound

III. Examination of Nervous System

- Look for evidence of beri-beri, Korsakoff psychosis, Wernicke's encephalopathy, peripheral neuropathy or mental subnormality

IV. Endocrine and Metabolism

- Look for signs of hypopituitarism, hypothyroidism, rickets

V. Other Systems

- Respiratory system for any evidence of tuberculosis or infection
- Skin for any dryness, bleeding, etc.
- Joints
- Hematopoietic system for anemia, bleeding

Q. What is probable diagnosis of the patient in picture?

Ans. In an adolescent child with diarrhea since childhood, reduced weight and height, history of delayed milestones, presence of anemia, protuberant abdomen, muscle wasting, edema feet, signs of multiple nutrients and vitamins deficiency, the clinical diagnosis of malabsorption syndrome is most likely.

Q. How do you define diarrhea?

Ans. Diarrhea is defined as passage of frequent loose stools, i.e. more than 3 in a day. Quantitatively it is defined as fecal output >200 mg/day when dietary fibre content is low.

Acute diarrhea means rapid onset of diarrhea occurring in an otherwise healthy person not lasting for more than 2 weeks. It is usually infective in origin (viral or bacterial).

Chronic diarrhea refers to slow onset of diarrhea persisting for more than 3 months. It is usually a symptom of some underlying disease or malabsorption syndrome.

Malabsorption syndrome refers to defective absorption of one or more essential nutrients through the intestine. The malabsorption may be specific or generalized. The examples of specific malabsorption include lactose intolerance, vitamin B$_{12}$ malabsorption etc.

Q. What are causes of malabsorption?

Ans. Malabsorption may be due to diseases of pancreas, GI tract and the liver. The causes of malabsorption are given in Table 1.51.

Q. What are the common causes of chronic diarrhea?

Ans. The causes are:
- Inflammatory bowel disease, e.g. ulcerative colitis, Crohn's disease
- Celiac disease (gluten-induced) or tropical sprue
- Intestinal diseases, e.g. tuberculosis, stricture, fistula
- Worm infestations, e.g. giardiasis
- Pancreatic disease, e.g. chronic pancreatitis, malignancy
- Endocrinal causes, e.g. diabetes, Addison's disease, thyrotoxicosis, etc.

Q. How will you diagnose malabsorption?

Ans. Diagnosis of malabsorption is based on:
1. *Symptoms and signs suggestive of malabsorption* (diarrhea >3 months with deficiency signs of one or more nutrients).
2. *Biochemical tests* or other investigations documenting the evidence of malabsorption to one or more nutrients.

Table 1.51: Causes of malabsorption syndrome

A. **Pancreatic disorders (disorders of maldigestion)**
   1. Chronic pancreatitis
   2. Cystic fibrosis
   3. Malignancy pancreas
   4. Ulcerogenic tumors of pancreas (Zollinger-Ellison's syndrome)

B. **Disorders causing deficiency of bile acids/bile salts**
   1. **Interruption of enterohepatic circulation of bile acids/salts or reduced bile salt concentration.**
      a. Ileal resection or inflammatory bowel disease
      b. Parenchymal liver disease or cholestasis (intra or extrahepatic)
   2. **Abnormal bacterial proliferation in small intestine leading to bile salt deconjugation**
      a. Blind loop (stagnant loop) syndrome
      b. Strictures or fistulas of small intestine
      c. Hypomotility of small intestine due to diabetes
   3. **Drugs causing sequestration or precipitation of bile salts,** e.g. neomycin and cholestyramine
   4. **Inadequate absorptive surface**
      a. Intestinal resection or bypass surgery of intestine.
   5. **Mucosal defects of absorption (inflammatory, infiltrative or infective disorders)**
      a. Tropical sprue .
      b. Lymphoma
      c. Whipple's disease
      d. Radiation enteritis
      e. Amyloidosis
      f. Giardiasis
      g. Scleroderma
      h. Eosinophilic enteritis
      i. Dermatitis herpetiformis

C. **Biochemical or genetic abnormalities**
   1. Celiac disease (gluten-induced enteropathy)
   2. Disaccharidase deficiency
   3. Hypogammaglobulinemia
   4. Abetalipoproteinemia

D. **Endocrinal or metabolic defects**
   a. Diabetes mellitus
   b. Addison's disease
   c. Carcinoid syndrome
   d. Hyperthyroidism

E. **Specific malabsorption (mucosa is histologically normal)**
   a. Lactase deficiency
   b. Vitamin B$_{12}$ malabsorption

3. *Radiology of small intestine* may show either gastrointestinal motility disorder, fistula, stricture, Zollinger-Ellison's syndrome or characteristic intestinal changes of malabsorption, i.e. breaking up of barium column with segmentation, clumping and coarsening of mucosal folds (*Moulage's sign*).

4. *Biopsy and histopathology of small intestine* shows partial villous atrophy with lymphocytic infiltration.

Q. How will you investigate a case of malabsorption?

Ans. The various tests of malabsorption of different nutrients are enlisted in Table 1.52.

Q. What are diagnostic criteria for nontropical sprue?

Ans. Diagnostic clues to nontropical sprue (celiac disease) are given in Table 1.53.

Table 1.52: Investigations for malabsorption

Test	Normal values	Malabsorption (non-tropical sprue)	Maldigestion (pancreatic insufficiency)
I. Fat absorption			
1. Fecal fat (24 hours excretion)	< 6.0 g/day	> 6.0 g/day	>6.0 g/day
2. Fat in stools (%)	< 6	< 9.5 and > 6	>9.5 (steatorrhea)
II. Carbohydrate absorption			
1. D-xylose absorption (25.0 g oral dose)	5 hours urinary excretion >4.5 g	Decreased	Normal
2. Hydrogen breath test (oral 50.0 gm lactose and breath H_2 measured every hour for 4 hours)	Less than 10 ppm above baseline in any sample	Increased	Normal
III. Protein absorption			
1. Fecal clearance of endogenous alpha-1 antitrypsin measured in three days collection of stools	Absent in stools	Increased	Increased
2. Nitrogen excretion (3-5 days collection of stools)	< 2.5 g/day	>2.5 g/day	>2.5 g/day
IV. Vitamins absorption			
1. Radioactive B_{12} absorption test (0.5 mg of labelled vitamin B_{12} is given orally followed 2 hours later by 1000 µg of non-labelled B_{12} given by IM injection. Radioactivity in the urine is seen after 24 hours)	>16% radioactivity in urine	Frequently decreased	Frequently decreased
V. Other tests			
1. *Breath tests*			
a. Breath $^{14}CO_2$ (^{14}C xylose)	Minimal amount	Decreased	Normal
b. Bile salt breath test (radioactive)	< 1% dose excreted $^{14}CO_2$ in 4 hrs	Normal	Normal
2. *Blood tests*			
a. Serum calcium	9-11 µg/dl	Frequently decreased	Normal
b. Serum albumin	3.5-5.5 g/dl	Frequently decreased	Normal
c. Serum iron	80-150 µg/dl	Decreased	Normal
d. Serum vitamin A	>100 IU/dl	Decreased	Decreased
VI. Miscellaneous			
1. Bacterial (culture)	<10^5 organisms/ml	Normal but abnormal in blind loop syndrome	Normal
2. Secretin test	Volume (1.8 ml/kg/hr) and bicarbonate (>80 mmol/L) Concentration in duodenal aspirate	Normal	Abnormal
3. Barium study (follow through)	Normal pattern	Flocculations and segmentations of barium column (malabsorption pattern –see text)	Normal pattern
4. Small intestine biopsy	Normal mucosa	Abnormal	Normal

Table 1.53: Diagnostic criteria for nontropical sprue

1. Clinical	Symptoms and signs of long duration suggestive of malabsorption (Table 1.54)
2. Biochemical	Positive evidence of fat, carbohydrate, protein, vitamin B_{12}, folate malabsorption (Table 1.52)
3. Immunological	Antigliadin, antireticulin and antiendomysial antibodies are seen in high titres in majority of patients
4. Histopathology of small intestine	Villous or subvillous atrophy with mononuclear cells infiltration of lamina propria and submucosa
5. Therapeutic response	Clinical, biochemical and histopathological improvement on gluten-free diet

Table 1.54: Deficiency signs in malabsorption syndrome

Deficiency	Signs and symptoms
Vitamin A	• Night blindness, xerosis, Bitot's spots, keratomalacia, dryness of eyes and follicular hyperkeratosis of skin
Vitamin C	• Scurvy
Vitamin D	• Rickets in children and osteomalacia in adults
Vitamin K	• Bleeding tendencies
Vitamin B complex	• Bald tongue, angular cheilosis, stomatitis, glossitis, peripheral neuropathy, subacute combined degeneration, megaloblastic anemia, dermatitis and dementia (pellagra)
Deficiency of nutrients (carbohydrate, proteins, loss fats)	• Vague ill health, fatigue, weight • Muscle wasting and edema
Iron deficiency	• Anaemia
Calcium deficiency	• Bone pain, tetany, paresthesias, muscle wasting
Potassium deficiency	• Distension of abdomen, diminished bowel sounds, vomiting, muscle weakness and EKG changes
Sodium and water depletion	• Nocturia, hypotension

Q. What are symptoms and signs of malabsorption syndrome?

Ans. Due to fecal loss of certain nutrients, vitamins and minerals, their deficiency symptoms and signs appear (Table 1.54).

Q. What are symptoms and signs of various vitamins deficiency?

Ans. Read Table 1.54

Q. What are signs of iron deficiency?

Ans. Read Table 1.54

Q. What are signs of vitamin B complex deficiency?

Ans. Read Table 1.54

Q. What are deficiency signs of vitamin B_1?

Ans. Beri-Beri e.g. wet beri-beri (high cardiac output state) and dry beri-beri (peripheral neuropathy).

Q. What are deficiency signs of vitamin B_2?

Ans. Cheilosis and angular stomatitis

Q. What are signs of pellagra?

Ans. It is due to niacin deficiency. It produces diarrhea, dermatitis, dementia and rarely death can occur.

Q. What is Traveller's diarrhea?

Ans. It is an acute infective diarrhea frequently seen in tourists caused by the following pathogenic organisms;
- *Enterotoxigenic E. coli*
- *Shigella*
- *Salmonella*
- *Campylobacter*
- *Rota virus*
- *Giardia intestinalis*
- *Entamoeba histolytica.*

It is characterized by sudden onset of diarrhea with watery stools, fever, nausea, vomiting, abdominal pain which lasts for 2-3 days. On examination, there may be diffuse tenderness of abdomen. Treatment is tetracycline or ciprofloxacin *plus* metronidazole combination with correction of dehydration.

Q. What is pseudomembranous colitis?

Ans. It is an antibiotic-induced diarrhea caused by an opportunistic commensal *clostridium difficile*. It can occur in immunocompromised state also. The antibiotics incriminated are: ampicillin, clindamycin and cephalosporins.

Q. What is spurious diarrhea?

Ans. It occurs following fecal impaction in constipated patients, seen in old persons, characterized by sense of incomplete evacuation and gaseous distension with diarrhea. It is relieved by enema.

Q. What do you know about blind-loop syndrome? What are its causes?

Ans. The term refers to small intestinal abnormality associated with outgrowth of bacteria (bacterial count is >108 /ml) causing steatorrhea, and vitamin B_{12} malabsorption, both of which improve dramatically after oral antibiotic therapy. This also called *"contaminated bowel syndrome"*, or "small *intestinal stasis syndrome"*.

N.B. Normally the small intestine is either sterile or contain < 10^4 organism/ml.

The **causes** are:
- Gastric surgery
- Diverticulosis
- Fistulae
- Bowel resection
- Diabetic autonomic neuropathy
- Hypogammaglobulinemia.

All these structural abnormalities lead to delivery of the coliform bacteria from colon to small intestine and predispose to their proliferation.

The triphasic malabsorption test for vitamin B_{12} as detailed below is diagnostic.

Stage 1. Malabsorption without replacement of intrinsic factor

Stage 2. Malabsorption persists with replacement of intrinsic factor

Stage 3. Malabsorption to B_{12} improves after a 5-7 days course of antibiotic therapy.

Q. What is lactose intolerance?

Ans. It occurs due to deficiency of an enzyme *lactase* – a disaccharidase which normally hydrolyses lactose to glucose and galactose. The deficiency may be primary (inherited) or secondary (acquired), is characterized by abdominal colic, distension of abdomen and increased flatus followed by diarrhea on ingestion of milk; withdrawal or substitution therapy with enzyme *lactase* improves the condition.

Q. What do you understand by the term protein-losing enteropathy?

Ans. The term implies excessive loss of proteins through the GI tract leading to hypoproteinemia and its clinical manifestations such as edema face and feet, muscle wasting (flabbiness of muscles) and weight loss.

A variety of disorders lead to it (Table 1.55).

The diagnosis of protein-losing enteropathy is confirmed by measurement of fecal nitrogen content (increased) and fecal clearance of alpha-1-antitrypsin or ^{51}Cr labelled albumin after IV injection. Excessive intestinal clearance of alpha-1-antitrypsin >13 ml/day (normal <13 ml/day) confirms the diagnosis.

Q. What is the difference between food intolerance and food allergy?

Ans. *Food intolerance* is an adverse reaction to food. It is not immune-mediated and results from a wide range

Table 1.55: Disorders producing protein-losing enteropathy

1. ***Disorders of stomach***
a. Hypertrophic gastritis (Menetrier's disease)
b. Gastric tumors
2. ***Disorders of intestine***
a. Intestinal lymphangiectasia
b. Whipple's disease
c. Tropical sprue
d. Coeliac disease (nontropical sprue)
e. Intestinal tuberculosis
f. Parasitic infections
g. Lymphoma
h. Allergic gastroenteropathy
i. Inflammatory bowel disease, e.g. regional enteritis
3. ***Cardiac disorders***
a. Congestive heart failure
b. Constrictive pericarditis

of mechanisms such as contaminants in food, preservatives and lactase deficiency etc.

Food allergy is an immune-mediated disorder due to IgE antibodies and type I hypersensitivity reaction to food. The most common food associated with allergy are; milk, egg, soya bean and shellfish. Food allergy may manifest as:

- *Oral allergy syndrome*—contact with certain fruit juices results in urticaria and angioedema of lips and oropharynx.
- *Allergic gastroenteropathy* leading to diarrhea with discharge of eosinophils in the stools.
- *Gastrointestinal anaphylaxis* leading to nausea, vomiting, diarrhea, and sometimes cardiovascular or respiratory collapse.
- Diagnosis is confirmed by double-blind placebo-controlled food challenges.

Q. What are inflammatory bowel disorders?

Ans. These are nonspecific inflammatory disorders of bowel having similar etiopathogenesis, pathology, investigations, complications and treatment. Exact causes of these disorders are unknown. Two common disorders are:

- Crohn's disease
- Ulcerative colitis

The clinical characteristics of both these disorders are compared in Table 1.56.

Table 1.56: Clinical features of two common inflammatory bowel disorders

Features	Crohn's disease	Ulcerative colitis
Presenting symptoms	Diarrhea and pain abdomen in right lower quadrant with tenderness and guarding	Diarrhea with blood, mucus and pus. Pain in left lower abdomen and fever may be present. Tenderness in left side of abdomen or left iliac fossa
Palpation	A mass may be palpable on abdominal and/or rectal examination. It is an inflammatory mass	No mass palpable
Colics/diffuse pain	Recurrent abdominal colics are common due to obstruction	No colicky pain. Toxic megacolon may produce diffuse pain associated with distension of abdomen and stoppage of loose motions
Signs and symptoms of malabsorption	Moderate diarrhea and fever. Stools are loose or well formed. Features of malabsorption of fat, carbohydrate, protein, vitamin D and vitamin B_{12} are common. These patients have anemia, weight loss, growth retardation (in children)	Patients have severe diarrhea with tenesmus. Anemia, weight loss present. Malabsorptive features are less common but dehydration common
Relapses or remissions	Common	Common
Stricture/anal fissure	Common	Less common
Abscess and fistulas	Common	Less common
Carcinoma in situ	Less common	More common in long-standing disease
Systemic involvement (hepatic, ocular, skin, ankylosing spondylitis, arthritis)	Less common	More common

Note: These distinctions in clinical features are arbitrary and should not be interpreted in absolute sense.

Renal Diseases

CASE 17: ACUTE NEPHRITIC SYNDROME

Renal Diseases

The female patient (Fig.1.17A) presented with pain abdomen, puffiness of face and passed dark colored small amount of urine < 400 ml (Fig. 1.17B) following an episode of fever for 3 weeks.

Clinical Presentations

- The patients usually children or young adults present with the complaints of puffiness of face especially around the eyes in the early hours of the morning on getting out of bed (Fig. 1.17A).
- They may complain of reduced urine output or change in coloration of the urine (Fig. 1.17B).
- They may complain of headache, fatigue, weakness, breathlessness, cough, hemoptysis due to hypertension or left heart failure.
- Sometimes they may present with symptoms and signs of underlying disease.
- Sometimes they may present with features of hypertensive encephalopathy (mental changes, headache seizures) or uremia (GI symptoms or ill health).

Points to be Noted in History

- *Age:* The patient is usually a child or adolescent
  Ask for the following;
- History of fever, sore throat, tonsillitis, pharyngitis, otitis media or cellulitis
- History of collagen vascular disorder or a hematological disorder
- History of vaccination (DPT)
- History of oliguria, puffiness of face, change in color of urine
- H/O drug rash, jaundice breathlessness, headache and edema feet
- History of disturbance in consciousness, lazziness, lethargy, nausea, vomiting, pruritus, palpitation (features of uremia).

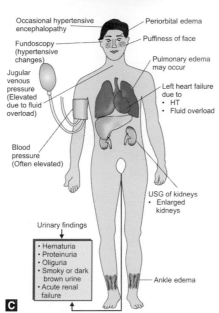

Occasional hypertensive encephalopathy
Fundoscopy (hypertensive changes)
Jugular venous pressure (Elevated due to fluid overload)
Blood pressure (Often elevated)
Periorbital edema
Puffiness of face
Pulmonary edema may occur
Left heart failure due to
• HT
• Fluid overload
USG of kidneys
• Enlarged kidneys
Ankle edema

Urinary findings
• Hematuria
• Proteinuria
• Oliguria
• Smoky or dark brown urine
• Acute renal failure

Figs 1.17A to C: A: A young female patient having puffiness of face. B: 24 hour Urine of the patient which is small in amount, smoky and shows RBCs and proteinuria. C: Clinical manifestations of acute nephritic syndrome (diagram)

General Physical Examination

Look for
- Face (periorbital edema, puffiness present)
- Pulse and BP (BP is high)
- JVP. It is raised
- Edema feet, sacral edema present
- Note the change in color of urine (red, brown, or smoky).

Systemic Examinations

I. Examination of CVS

- Look for the signs of cardiomegaly. Auscultate the heart for any murmur or rub or abnormal sound (3rd heart sound)

II. Examination of Lungs

- Auscultate the lungs for crackles or rales for fluid overload or noncardiogenic pulmonary edema due to LVF

III. Examination of Abdomen

- Inspect the abdomen for distension or ascites
- Elicit the signs for presence of ascites or edema of abdominal wall
- Palpate the abdomen for any organ enlargement

IV. Examination of CNS

- Note the features of hypertensive-encephalopathy
- Fundoscopy

Q. What is the clinical diagnosis of the patient in picture?

Ans. The young female patient presenting with morning puffiness of face, oliguria, smoky urine and hypertension probably has acute nephritic syndrome as the first possibility due to any cause.

Q. What is your differential diagnosis?

Ans. The differential diagnosis lies within the causes of acute nephritic syndrome (Table 1.58).

Q. How do you define acute nephritic syndrome?

Ans. *Acute nephritic syndrome* is characterized by an acute transient inflammatory process involving mainly the glomeruli and to lesser extent the tubules, manifests clinically with oliguria, hypertension, hematuria, edema and rapid renal failure. Acute glomerulonephritis (AGN) is interchangeably used as acute nephritic syndrome.

The term *rapidly proliferative glomerulonephritis* (RPGN) is used for those patients of AGN who do not go into remissions, spontaneously develop acute renal failure over a period of weeks to months. These patients belong to either a primary glomerular disease or a complicating multisystem disease (secondary glomerular disease).

Q. What are clinical hallmark of acute nephritic syndrome and what is their pathogenesis?

Ans. The clinical hallmarks of acute nephritic syndrome are depicted in Figure 1.17C. Their pathogenesis is given in the Table 1.57A.

Table 1.57A: Acute nephritic syndrome

Feature	Mechanism (Cause)
• *Early morning puffiness or periorbital edema*	• Collection of fluid in loose periorbital tissue
• *Hematuria (gross or microscopic)*	• Glomerular inflammation
• *Hypertension*	• Retention of Na and H_2O
• *Edema*	• Retention of salt, H_2O and hypertension
• *Uremia*	• Retention of urea and creatinine
• *Oliguria*	• Reduced GFR

Q. What is its etiopathogenesis?

Ans. It is an immune complex glomerulonephritis characterised by production of antibodies against glomerular antigen, deposition of immune complexes in the walls of glomerular capillaries which modify the immune system leading to inflammation of the glomeruli. The stepwise pathogenesis is given in Table 1.57B.

Table 1.57B: Stepwise pathogenesis of nephritic syndrome

1. *Binding of antibodies* directed against glomerular basement membrane antigen
2. *Trapping* of soluble immune complexes in the glomerular capillary wall (subepithelial or subendothelial).
3. *In situ immune complex formation* between circulating antibody and fixed antigen or antigen planted either in the mesangium and/ or in capillary wall.
4. *Action of circulating primed T cells* with macrophages.

Q. What are causes of acute nephritic syndrome?

Ans. All the causes that lead to acute glomerular injury may lead to acute nephritic syndrome (Table 1.58).

Table 1.58: Causes of AGN (acute nephritic syndrome)

I. **Infectious diseases**
   a. Post-streptococcal glomerulonephritis
   b. Non-streptococcal glomerulonephritis
      i. Bacterial: Infective endocarditis, staphylococcal and pneumococcal infection, typhoid, syphilis and meningococcemia
      ii. Viral: Hepatitis B, infectious mononucleosis, mumps, measles, coxsackie and echoviruses
      iii. Parasitic – malaria
II. **Systemic disorders**
   Systemic lupus erythematosus (SLE), vasculitis, Henoch-Schonlein purpura, Goodpasture's syndrome
III. **Primary glomerular diseases**
   Mesangiocapillary glomerulonephritis, mesangial proliferative glomerulonephritis
IV. **Miscellaneous**
   Guillain-Barre syndrome, serum sickness, DPT vaccination, IgA nephropathy

Q. What are the causes of rapidly proliferative glomerulonephritis (RPGN)?

Ans. It is a complication of acute glomerulonephritis or a manifestation of a multisystem disease (Table 1.59). The clinical features are summarized in Table 1.60.

Table 1.59: Causes of RPGN

I. **Infectious diseases**
   a. Poststreptococcal glomerulonephritis
   b. Infective endocarditis
II. **Multisystem diseases**
   a. Systemic lupus erythematosus (SLE)
   b. Goodpasture's syndrome
   c. Vasculitis
   d. Henoch-Schonlein purpura
III. **Primary glomerular disease**
   a. Idiopathic
   b. Mesangiocapillary glomerulonephritis
   c. Membranous glomerulonephritis (anti-glomerular basement membrane antibodies nephritis)

Table 1.60: Clinical manifestations of rapidly proliferative glomerulonephritis

---

1. **Signs and symptoms of azotemia**
   Nausea, vomiting, weakness. The azotemia develops early and progresses faster.
2. **Signs and symptoms of acute glomerulonephritis**
   It includes oliguria, abdominal flank pain due to large kidneys, hematuria, hypertension and proteinuria

---

Q. **Eneumerate the complications of acute nephritic syndrome.**

Ans. Complications are either due to retention of salt and water (volume overload) or hypertension or capillaritis. These include:
- Fluid overload
- Hypertensive encephalopathy
- Acute left heart failure
- Noncardiogenic pulmonary edema
- Rapidly progressive glomerulonephritis (RPGN)
- Uremia
- Massive hemoptysis

Q. **How will you proceed to investigate a patient with acute nephritic syndrome?**

Ans. The investigations to be done are given in Table 1.61.

Table 1.61: Investigations for acute nephritic syndrome

Investigation	Positive finding
1. Urine microscopy	1. RBCs and red cell casts
2. Urine complete	2. High specific gravity, proteinuria present
3. Blood urea and serum creatinine	3. May be elevated
4. Culture (throat swab, discharge from ear, swab from infected skin)	4. Nephrogenic streptococci – not always
5. ASO titre	5. Elevated in poststreptococcal nephritis
6. C3 level	6. Reduced
7. Antinuclear antibody (ANA)	7. Present in significant titres in lupus (SLE) nephritis
8. X-ray chest	8. Cardiomegaly, pulmonary edema – not always
9. Renal imaging (Ultrasound)	9. Usually normal or large kidneys
10. Renal biopsy	10. Glomerulonephritis

CASE 18: NEPHROTIC SYNDROME

A-18-year male (Fig. 1.18) presented with complaints of puffiness of face in the morning, edema feet and distension of the abdomen for the last 1 year. Patient is passing normal amount of urine of normal color. There is no history of headache, blurring of vision, dizziness, breathlessness or orthopnea nausea, vomiting. There is no history of disturbance in consciousness.

Clinical Presentations

- The patients usually children, adolescents or adults present with puffiness of eyelids or periorbital edema especially in the morning on awakening followed by edema face and feet (Fig. 1.18).
- Patients with progressive disease present with ascites and generalized anasarca.
- Patients may present with complications, e.g. pulmonary infection, pleural effusion, thromboembolism, renal vein thrombosis, protein malnutrition and microcytic hypochromic anemia.
- Patients may present with symptoms and signs of underlying disorder, i.e. infections (malaria, leprosy, syphilis,

Fig. 1.18: A patient with puffiness of face and edema feet. There was ascites and scrotal edema. There was no anemia, jaundice or cyanosis. Blood pressure was normal. CVS examination was normal

streptococcal sore throat), collagen vascular disorders, lymphomas, diabetes mellitus and toxemia of pregnancy or hypertension.

Points to be Noted in the History

Ask the followings on history;
- Symptoms, their duration, progression, relapse or remission, aggravating and relieving factors, diurnal variation

- History of jaundice, sore throat, diabetes hypertension, neck swelling (lymphoma)
- Past history of infections (malaria, leprosy) collagen vascular disorder (SLE), skin rashes
- Drug history and history of alcoholism

General Physical Examination

- General appearance – moon facies or puffiness of face, periorbital edema xanthelasma
- Nutritional status
- Look for jaundice, anemia, cyanosis
- Neck veins for JVP
- Lymph nodes
- Pulse and BP
- Skin for alopecia, rash, xanthomas
- Feet for pitting edema
- External genitalia for edema and hydrocele.

Systemic Examination

1. Abdomen–distended, presence of ascites, edema of abdominal wall, shiny skin, nontender renal angle, scrotal (or vulval) edema, presence of hydrocele
2. Respiratory system. Thoracoabdominal respiration, edema chest wall and legs, pleural effusions. Sometimes evidence of infection may be present.
3. CVS examination–non contributory.

Q. **What is the clinical diagnosis of the patient in picture?**

Ans. Presence of morning puffiness of face follwed by edema feet during day time with ascites without hypertension in a young patient suggests the possibility of nephrotic syndrome.

Q. **What is its differential diagnosis?**

Ans. The differential diagnosis of nephrotic syndrome lies within the causes of ascites with anasarca (read differential diagnosis of ascites). Such as CHF, cirrhosis of liver, hypoproteinemia, constrictive pericarditis etc.

Q. **How do you define nephrotic syndrome?**

Ans. Nephrotic syndrome is defined as a heterogenous clinical complex comprising of following features;
1. Massive proteinuria >3.5 g/day or protein creatinine ratio of >400 mg/mmol
2. Hypoalbuminemia/hypoproteinemia
3. Pitting pedal edema
4. Hyperlipidemia and lipiduria
5. Hypercoagulopathy.

Q. **What are its causes?**

Ans. A wide variety of disease processes including immunological disorders, toxic injuries, metabolic abnormalities, biochemical defects and vascular disorders involving the glomeruli can lead to it (Table 1.62).

Table 1.62: Common causes of nephrotic syndrome

1. **Primary glomerular diseases**
   a. Minimal change disease
   b. Mesangioproliferative glomerulonephritis
   c. Membranous glomerulonephritis
   d. Membranoproliferative glomerulonephritis (crescents formation)
   e. Focal glomerulosclerosis
2. **Secondary to other diseases**
   A. *Infections*
      a. Post-streptococcal glomerulonephritis
      b. Post-streptococcal endocarditis
      c. Secondary syphilis
      d. Malaria (vivax and malariae infection)
      e. Lepromatous leprosy
   B. *Drugs and toxins*
      Gold, mercury, penicillamine, captopril, NSAIDs antitoxins, antivenoms and contrast media
   C. *Neoplasm*
      a. Wilms' tumor in children
      b. Hodgkin and non-Hodgkins lymphoma
      c. Leukemia
   D. *Systemic disorders*
      a. Systemic lupus erythematosus (SLE)
      b. Goodpasture's syndrome
      c. Vasculitis, e.g. polyarteritis nodosa
      d. Amyloidosis
      e. Diabetes mellitus
   E. *Heredo-Familial*
      a. Congenital nephrotic syndrome
      b. Alport's syndrome
   F. *Miscellaneous*
      a. Toxemia of pregnancy
      b. Renovascular hypertension

Q. What is its etiopathogenesis?

Ans. Massive proteinuria >3.5 g/day is an essential criteria for the diagnosis. Other components are its consequences as described in Table 1.63.

Table 1.63: Pathogenesis of components of nephrotic syndrome

Components	Pathogenesis
Proteinuria	Altered permeability of GBM and the podocytes and their slit diaphragms
Hypoalbuminemia	Increased urinary protein loss not compensated by increased hepatic synthesis of albumin
Edema	Decreased oncotic pressure and stimulation of renin-angiotensin system resulting in salt and H_2O retention.
Hyperlipidemia and lipiduria	Increased hepatic lipoprotein synthesis triggered by reduced oncotic pressure
Hypercoagulability	• Increased urinary loss of antithrombin III • Altered levels and/or activity of protein C and S • Hyperfibrinogenemia • Impaired fibrinolysis • Increased platelet aggregation.

Q. How will you investigate such a patient?

Ans. Investigations of nephrotic patient are as follows:
1. *Urine examination* reveals proteinuria and casts (fatty casts). Hematuria is uncommon.
2. *24 hours urine* shows excretion of albumin or proteins > 3.5 g or protein/creatinine ratio > 400 mg/mmol. In early stages of the disease or in patients receiving treatment, the proteinuria may be less.
3. *Serum lipids.* Low density lipoproteins and cholesterol are increased in majority of the patients. Hyperlipidemia is an integral component of the syndrome.
4. *Serum proteins or albumin.* Total serum proteins may be normal or low. Serum albumin is usually low <3 g/dl, also forms an important diagnostic criteria.
5. *Other renal function tests,* e.g. blood urea, creatinine, creatinine clearance and electrolytes are normal in uncomplicated cases, become abnormal if renal failure sets in.
6. *DNA antibody, antinuclear antibody (ANA), complement level.*
7. *Chest X-ray* may show hydrothorax.
8. *Ultrasound of abdomen.* It may show normal, small or large kidneys depending on the cause. Amyloid and diabetic kidneys are large; while kidneys in glomerulonephritis are small.
9. *Renal biopsy.* It is done in adult nephrotic syndrome to show the nature of underlying disease, to predict the prognosis and response to treatment.

Renal biopsy is not required in majority of children with nephrotic syndrome as most of them belong to minimal change disease and respond to steroids.

Q. What is selective and nonselective proteinuria?

Ans. *Selective proteinuria* means filtration of low molecular weight proteins especially the albumin through the glomeruli. It is seen in minimal change glomerulonephritis and early phase of other glomerulonephritis. These cases respond well to steroids.

Nonselective proteinuria means filtration of albumin along with high molecular weight proteins, e.g. globulins, antithrombin III, transferrin, immunoglobulins, thyroxine-binding globulins calciferol-binding globulin, etc. This occurs in advanced glomerular disease and does not respond to steroids. It is a bad prognostic sign. The loss of these proteins constitute the clinical spectrum of the nephrotic syndrome in adults.

Q. What is the differences between glomerular proteinuria and tubular proteinuria?

Ans. Following are the differences:

Glomerular proteinuria. The damage to the glomeruli allows filtration of larger molecular weight proteins especially the albumin. The presence of albumin in the urine is sure sign of glomerular abnormality. The proteinuria in glomerular disease is >1 g/day. The severity of proteinuria is a marker for an increased risk of progressive loss of renal function. The glomerular proteinuria is associated with cellular casts (RBCs, WBCs) which are dysmorphic, i.e. get distorted as they pass through the glomerulus.

Tubular proteinuria is secretion of Tamm-Horsefall proteins or excretion of low molecular weight proteins especially retinol-binding proteins, β-macroglobin. The proteinuria is <1 g/day occurs in tubulointerstitial diseases. Tubulointerstitial diseases are not the cause of either nephritic or nephrotic syndrome. The casts in tubulointestinal diseases are epithelial or granular.

Q. What is orthostatic proteinuria?

Ans. It occurs on standing and disappears on lying down. It is due to compression of inferior vena cava by liver during standing. The prognosis is good. Proteinuria is absent in the morning on rising from the bed.

Q. What are characteristics of minimal change disease (MCD) or lipoid nephrosis, nil disease or foot process disease?

Ans. The characteristic features are:

i. Most common cause of nephrotic syndrome in children (70-80%) and more common in males than females.

ii. It is named so because light microscopy of renal biopsy specimen does not reveal any abnormality of glomeruli. Electron microscopy reveals effacement of the foot processes of epithelial cells

iii. Proteinuria is highly selective.

iv. Hematuria is uncommon.

v. Spontaneous relapses and remissions are common.

vi. Majority of the patients respond promptly to steroids. The disease may disappear after steroid therapy.

vii. Progression to acute renal failure is rare.

viii. Prognosis is good.

Q. What are characteristics of membranous glomerulonephritis?

Ans. The characteristic features are as follows:

i. It is a leading cause of nephrotic syndrome in adults (30-40%) but is a rare cause in children.

ii. It has peak incidence between the ages of 30 and 50 years, more common in males.

iii. It is named so because the light microscopy of renal biopsy specimen shows diffuse thickening of glomerular basement membrane (GBM) which is most apparent on PAS staining

iv. Proteinuria is nonselective

v. Hematuria is common (50%)

vi. Spontaneous remissions may occur in only 30-40% patients

vii. Renal vein thrombosis is a common complication.

viii. Response to steroids therapy is inconsistent, it may reduce proteinuria but does not induce remission.

ix. 10-20% cases progress to end-stage renal disease (ESRD) requiring transplantation of kidney.

Q. What are complications of nephrotic syndrome?

Ans. Common complications are as follows:

1. **Vascular**
   - Accelerated atherogenesis due to hyperlipidemia leading to accelerated hypertension and early coronary artery disease.
   - Peripheral arterial or venous thrombosis, renal vein thrombosis and pulmonary embolism due to hypercoaguable state.

2. **Metabolic**
   - Protein malnutrition
   - Iron-resistant microcytic hypochromic anemia
   - Hypocalcemia and secondary hyperparathyroidism.

3. **Infections**
   - Pneumococcal and staphylococcal infections (respiratory and peritonitis) due to depressed immunity (low levels of IgG).

4. **Chronic renal failure**

Q. What are causes of hypertension in nephrotic syndrome?

Ans. Hypertension is not a feature of nephrotic syndrome, but may be seen in diseases that cause nephrotic syndrome such as;
   - Diabetic nephropathy
   - SLE and polyarteritis nodosa
   - Nephrotic syndrome complicated by CRF
   - Focal glomerulosclerosis is commonly associated with hypertension.

Q. What is indication of renal biopsy in nephrotic syndrome?

Ans. The renal biopsy is done in adults for following reasons:
   - To confirm the diagnosis
   - To know the underlying pathological lesion

- To plan future treatment
- To predict the prognosis and response to treatment.

Q. What is the common pathological lesion in diabetic nephropathy?

Ans. *Kimmelstiel-Wilson syndrome* (diabetic nodular glomerulosclerosis) is the common pathological lesion.

- It occurs commonly in type I diabetes than type 2 diabetes
- Usually develops as a long-term microvascular complication of diabetes (duration of diabetes >10 years)
- Common presentation is moderate to massive proteinuria. Hypertension may develop later on.
- With the onset of this lesion, the requirement of insulin falls due to excretion of insulin antibodies in urine.
- Progresses to end-stage renal disease (ESRD) over a period of few years.
- The characteristic histological lesion is nodular glomerulosclerosis.

Q. How does nephrotic syndrome differ from nephritic syndrome?

Ans. The differences are tabulated (Table 1.64)

Table 1.64: Differences between nephrotic and nephritic syndrome

Feature	Nephrotic syndrome	Nephritic syndrome
Onset	Slow, insidious chronic disorder	Sudden, acute renal disorder
Proteinuria	Massive > 3.5 g/d	Moderate 1-2 g/d
Hyperlipidemia and lipiduria with faulty casts	Present	Absent
Hypertension	Not a feature	An important feature
Volume of urine passed in 24 hr	Normal	Oliguria
Hematuria	Not common	A common and integral component of syndrome
Acute renal failure	Uncommon	Common
Relapse and remission	Commom	Uncommon
Course	Chronic progressive disorder	70-80% cases recover completely while others pass on to RPGN

Blood Disorders

A 19 years female (Fig. 1.19A) presented with pallor, fatigue, malaise, weakness and breathlessness on exertion. There was no history of fever, loose motion, blood loss, any surgery. No history of drug intake. She has generalized pallor with slight puffiness of face. Physical examination revealed pallor and koilonychia.

Clinical Presentations

- Patients with mild anemia are asymptomatic. Anemia is discovered on routine hemoglobin estimation done for some other purposes. On symptomatic enquiry, they may admit history of occasional exertional dyspnea, palpitations and fatigue.
- Patients with severe anemia usually complain of weakness, weight loss, dyspnea, palpitation, throbbing headache, dizziness, tinnitis and menstrual irregularity in females, tingling in extremities and GI symptoms (nausea, anorexia).
- Anemia may be a presenting feature of certain chronic disorders, e.g. malabsorption, chronic renal failure, chronic blood loss (hematemesis, malena, menorrhagia) or malignant disorders.

Note: Anemia is a sign not a complete diagnosis, hence, cause of anemia must be mentioned in the diagnosis, e.g. malabsorption with anemia, CRF with anemia etc.

The patient has pale tongue, conjunctival along with puffiness of face

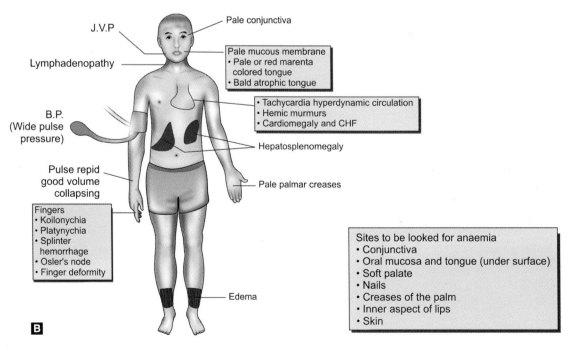

Figs 1.19A and B: A. A patient with severe anemia. B. Clinical features of anemia

History

Points to be Noted

- Symptoms and their analysis
- History of fever, blood loss, drug intake (NSAIDs, chloramphenicol, phenytoin), loose motions, jaundice, dysphagia, vomiting
- Menstrual history, history of recent delivery and blood loss if any
- History of piles or repeated hematemesis, melena
- Nutritional history, e.g. malnutrition
- Past history of tuberculosis, bleeding, any surgery, trauma, repeated abortions/deliveries
- Personal history, e.g. alcoholism
- Family history of jaundice.

General Physical Signs

- Facial appearance or look (e.g. pallor)
- Puffiness of face or periorbital edema
- Look for anemia at different sites, nails for koilonychia, platynychia, and look for bleeding from gums or nose
- See the tongue for glossitis (Magenta colored tongue in Vit B_{12} deficiency, bald atrophic tongue in iron deficiency)
- Mouth for cheilosis, angular stomatitis and ulcerations (agranulocytosis)
- Neck examination for JVP, lymph nodes and thyroid

Systemic Examinations

I. Examination of CVS

Inspection
- Look for apex beat, e.g. location, type
- Any chest deformity
- Chest movements

Palpation
- Trachea—Note any deviation
- Apex beat—confirm the findings of inspection
- Chest movements and expansion

Percussion
- Heart borders, cardiac and liver dullness
- Lung resonance

Auscultation
- Heart, e.g. sounds, murmurs, if any murmur, note its various characteristics
- Lung sounds, e.g. breath sounds, crackles and rales.

II. Examination of Abdomen

Inspection
- Contour, shape of umbilicus, hernial sites, any swelling or mass or distention

Palpation
- Palpate for any mass
- Pulse, BP, temp, respiration
- Skin for any bleeding spots or rash or bruising
- Edema feet, leg ulcers (see in hemoglobinopathies)
- Look for deficiency signs of hypoproteinemia, e.g. flabby muscles, wasting, thin skin.
- Palpate for liver, spleen and kidneys
- Elicit any tenderness

Percussion
- Percussion note. Note over the mass if present. Define upper border of the liver

Auscultation
Hear for sound, bruit or rub

III. Examination of CNS

- Look for signs of neuropathy

IV. Endocrine System

- Look for signs of hyper- or hypothyroidism.

V. Rectal Examination

- Piles, rectal bleeding, fissure, etc.

Q. What is the clinical diagnosis of the patient in picture?

Ans. The young patient presented with exertional breathlessness, fatigue and malaise. She was found to have generalized pallor, paleness of mucous membrane and koilonychia. The clinical diagnosis is anemia the cause of which is nutritional.

Q. How do you define anemia?

Ans. A hemoglobin level $\leq 11.0\%$ g in an adult female and < 12.0 g% in an adult male is taken as anemia.

Q. What are symptoms and signs of anemia?

Ans. For symptoms – read clinical presentations. For sign – see Figure 1.19B.

Q. What are the causes of anemia?

Ans. The common clinical causes of anemia in India are:
- *Nutritional*, e.g. deficient intake of iron, folate and protein in diet
- *Hookworm infestation*
- *Chronic blood loss*, e.g. piles, hematemesis, menorrhagia, melena, etc.
- *Chronic diarrhea and malabsorption*.
- *Pregnancy* associated anemia

- *Hypoproteinemia*, e.g. nephrotic syndrome, cirrhosis liver
- *Hemolytic anemia*, e.g. malarial parasite or drug-induced in G6PD deficiency.
- *Anemia of chronic infection*, e.g. tuberculosis, SLE, rheumatoid arthritis.
- *Anemia associated with malignancies*, e.g. leukemia, lymphoma, carcinoma stomach, colon etc.
- *Hereditary anemia*.

Q. What are common causes of iron deficiency anemia (microcytic hypochromic)?

Ans. Common causes are as follows:
1. *Nutritional deficiency*, e.g. inadequate iron intake
2. *Increased demands*, e.g. pregnancy and lactation
3. *Blood loss*
   - *GI loss*, e.g. bleeding peptic ulcer, piles, cancer of GI tract, hematemesis, hookworm disease, angiodysplasia of colon
   - *Uterine*, e.g. menorrhagia, repeated abortions, dysfunctional uterine bleeding

- *Renal* – hematuria
- *Nose* – epistaxis
- *Lung* – hemoptysis

4. *Malabsorption* due to any cause.

5. *Hereditary hemorrhagic telangiectasia*

Q. What are clinical signs of iron deficiency anemia?

Ans. Clinical signs are:

- Pallor
- Glossitis (bald atrophic tongue), angular stomatitis, cheilosis
- Koilonychia
- Dysphagia (*Plummer-Vinson syndrome*)
- Mild splenomegaly
- History of *pica* (eating of strange items, e.g. coal, earth).

Q. What is Plummer Vinson (Paterson-Kelly) syndrome?

Ans. It comprises of koilonychia, iron deficiency anemia and dysphasia due to esophased webs. It is common in middle aged females and is considered as a precancerous condition.

Q. What is sideroblastic anemia? What are its causes?

Ans. A red cell containing iron is called *siderocyte*. A developing erythroblast with one or two iron granules is called *sideroblast*. Iron granules free in cytoplasm of RBCs are normal, but when they form a ring round the nucleus in red cells, then they are considered abnormal and called *ring sideroblasts*. The anemia in which ring sideroblasts are present is called *sideroblastic anemia*. It is due to nonutilization of the iron in the bone marrow resulting in accumulation of iron as granules in developing red cells. Sideroblastic anemia may be primary (hereditary or congenital) or secondary (acquired). The **causes** are:

1. *Hereditary (congenital)*
2. *Acquired*
   - Inflammatory conditions
   - Malignancies
   - Megaloblastic anemias
   - Hypothyroidism
   - Drug induced
   - Lead poisoning
   - Pyridoxine deficiency.

Q. What are causes of megaloblastic anemia?

Ans. It occurs due either to folate or Vit. B$_{12}$ deficiency or both. The causes are:

1. *Nutritional*, e.g. inadequate intake, alcoholism.
2. *Increased demands of folic acid*, e.g. pregnancy, lactation.
3. *Following hemolysis*

4. *Malabsorption syndrome;*
   - Ileal disease
   - Gastrectomy
   - Blind – loop syndrome

5. *Drug induced*, e.g. anticonvulsants, methotrexate, oral contraceptive, pyrimethamine.

6. *Parasitic infestation*, e.g. Diphylobothrium latum.

Q. What are causes of haemolytic anaemia?

Ans. (Read haemolytic jaundice).

Q. What are causes of aplastic anemia?

Ans. Followings are the causes:

1. **Primary** – red cell aplasia.
2. **Secondary**
   i. *Drugs*
      - Dose related, e.g. methotrexate, busulfan, nitrosourea
      - Idiosyncratic, e.g. chloramphenicol, sulpha drugs, phenylbutazone, gold salts.
   ii. *Toxic chemicals*, e.g. insecticides, arsenicals, benezene derivatives
   iii. *Infections*, e.g. viral hepatitis, AIDS, other viral infections
   iv. *Miscellaneous*, e.g. irradiation, pregnancy, paroxysmal nocturnal hemoglobinuria.

Q. What are causes of reticulocytosis and reticulopenia?

Ans. *Reticulocyte* is a young red cell with basophilic cytoplasm (polychromasia). It matures into an adult RBC within 3 days. The normal reticulocyte count is 0.5-2% in adults and 2-6% in infants. An absolute increase in reticulocyte count is called *reticulocytosis*. The causes are:

- Hemolytic anemia
- Accelerated erythropoiesis
- Polycythemia rubra vera

Reticulocytopenia means low reticulocyte count ($\leq 0.5\%$), is seen in aplastic anaemia and *megaloblastic anemia*.

Q. What is corrected reticulocyte count? What is reticulocyte production index ?

Ans. Reticulocyte count corrected for anemia is called corrected reticulocyte count. It is calculated as reticulocyte count multiplied by hemoglobin of patient divided by normal hemoglobin; for example if reticulocyte count is 9% and Hb is 7.5 g/dl then Corrected reticulocyte count= $9 \times 7.5 \div 15 = 4.5$

Reticulocyte production index is calculated by dividing corrected reticulocyte count by reticulocyte maturation time which varies from 1-3 depending on severity of anemia. For moderate anemia, a correction of 2 is used as follows:

Reticulocyte production index

$$\frac{\text{corrected reticulocyte count}}{2} = \frac{4.5}{2} = 2.25$$

Q. What is significance of reticulocyte production index?

Ans. It implies bone marrow response to anemia. It is calculated by correcting the reticulocyte count first for degree of anemia (see above) secondly for maturation time. A normal cut off limit is 2.5. Index ≤ 2.5 indicates hypoproliferative anemia due to maturation defect. Index > 2.5 indicates invariably hemolytic anemia.

Q. Name the chronic systemic diseases associated with anemia

Ans. Following are the systemic diseases:
- Chronic infections, e.g. tuberculosis, SABE, osteomyelitis, lung suppuration
- Collagen vascular disorders, e.g. SLE
- Rheumatoid arthritis
- Malignancy anywhere in the body
- Chronic renal failure
- Endocrinal disorders, e.g. Addison's disease, myxedema, thyrotoxicosis, panhypopituitarism
- Cirrhosis of the liver especially alcoholic.

Q. What is morphological classification of anemia?

Ans. Morphological classification refers to average size and hemoglobin concentration of RBCs.
1. *Microcytic hypochromic* (reduced MCV, MCH and MCHC)
   - Iron deficiency anemia
   - Sideroblastic anemia
   - Thalassemia
   - Anemia of chronic infection
2. *Normocytic normochromic* (MCV, MCH and MCHC normal)
   - Hemolytic anemia
   - Aplastic anemia
3. *Macrocytic* (MCV is high. MCH and MCHC relative low)
   - Folate and Vit. B12 deficiency (read the causes of megaloblastic anemia)
4. *Dimorphic anemia* (microcytic as well as macrocytic)
   - Nutritional deficiency
   - Pregnancy
   - Malabsorption syndrome
   - Hookworm infestation.

Q. What is functional classification of anemia?

Ans. Functional classification: Anemia is classified (Fig. 1.19 C) into functional defect in RBC

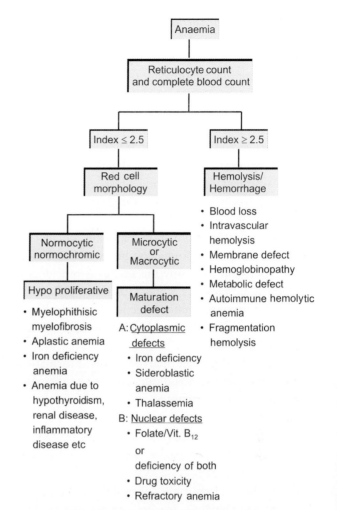

Fig. 1.19C: Classification of anemia based on reticulocyte production index

production (low reticulocyte production index ≤ 2.5) and decreased red cell survival (high reticulocyte index ≥ 2.5)

Q. What are diagnostic clues to hookworm infestation?

Ans. The clues are:
- Occupation (e.g. workers in tea - garden, farmers, coal-miners)
- History of walking bare-footed
- Presence of ground itch in interdigital spaces
- Pain abdomen (epigastrium simulating peptic ulcer)
- History of pica
- Diarrhea or steatorrhea
- Iron deficiency or dimorphic anemia
- Prevalence of hookworm disease in that area.

Q. How will you investigate a patient with anemia?

Ans. Investigations are done to confirm anemia and to find out the cause of anemia:

Test to Confirm Anemia

- Hemoglobin and red cell count
- *Peripheral blood film* for type of anemia and to find out any abnormality of the shape of RBCs and presence of malarial parasite or any other abnormal cells. Reticulocytosis indicates accelerated erythropoiesis.
- *Bone marrow examination.* It provides assessment of cellularity, details of developing RBCs, assessment of iron store, presence of marrow infiltration by parasites, fungi and secondary carcinoma.

It gives valuable information regarding reticulocyte count, reticulocyte production index and myeloid/erythroid ratio to classify the anemia A reticulocyte production index < 2.5 and M:E ratio of 2 or 3:1 indicates hypoproliferative anemia while reticulocyte production index > 2.5 and M:E ratio 1:1 indicates hemolytic disease.

In addition, bone marrow gives information regarding iron stores and can demonstrate the cause of anemia such as parasites

Specific Tests

Anemia with low reticulocyte count index (≤ 2.5)

I. *For iron deficiency anemia (microcytic hypochromic)*
- Serum iron is low (normal 50-150 mg/dl)
- Iron binding capacity is raised (normal 300-360 mg/dl)
- Serum ferritin low. (normal about 100 µg/dl in males and about 30 µg/dl in females)

  Transferrin saturation low (normal 25–50%)
- Stool for occult blood
- Upper GI endoscopy
- Colonoscopy, Barium Studies
- Prothrombin time and INR
- Hemoglobin for electrophoresis

II. *For megaloblastic anemia*
- Plasma LDH markedly elevated
- Serum iron elevated
- Serum ferratin elevated
- Serum bilirubin—unconjugated hyperbilirubinemia
- Antiparietal cell antibodies and an abnormal Vit. B_{12} absorption studies (Schilling test) may be observed in Vit B_{12} deficiency anemia or pernicious anemia.
- Serum folate levels/ Red cell folate levels.
- Upper GI endoscopy

Anemia with high reticulocyte count index (> 2.5)

Hemolytic anemias
- PBF for morphology of the RBCs (spherocytes, ovalocytes, elliptocytes, sickle cells) and for malarial parasite
- Hemoglobin electrophoresis for thalassemia (HbF > 2%)
- Coombs' test (direct and indirect)—may be abnormal
- Osmotic fragility test may be positive
- Serum bilirubin shows unconjugated hyperbilirubinemia
- Red cell survival studies may reveal decreased survival
- Sickling test positive in sickle cell anemia.

Q. What are causes of refractory anemia?

Ans. The anemia that does not respond to appropriate treatment given for optimal period is called *refractory anemia*. The **causes** are:
- Aplastic anemia
- Thalassemia
- Sideroblastic anemia (pyridoxine responsive)
- Refractory anemia due to myelodysplastic syndrome
- Anemia due to leukemia, e.g. erythroleukemia or aleukemic leukemia.

CASE 20: LEUKEMIA

A patient (Fig. 1.20A) presented with fever, dyspnea and bleeding from the nose. There was history of a big mass in the left hypochondrium with dragging pain. Another patient (Fig. 1.20B) presenting with bleeding from the gums, excoriation of mouth, fever, breathlessness and pallor. There was also history of mass abdomen and pain abdomen.

Clinical Presentations

- Patients with acute leukemia usually children or adolescents present with acute onset of symptoms and signs of bone marrow failure, i.e. anemia (pallor, lethargy, dyspnea, palpitations, etc.), thrombocytopenia (bleeding from gums, epistaxis, petechiae and spontaneous bruising) and neutropenia (infections leading to fever, excoriation of mouth and respiratory infection). They may also present with hepatosplenomegaly and/ or lymphadenopathy.
- Patients with chronic leukemia usually middle aged or old persons present with insidious onset of symptoms of anemia, bone pain, infections (fever) and bleeding tendencies. These cases especially with chronic myeloid leukemia present with mass abdomen while that of chronic lymphoid leukemia with lymphadenopathy and spleno-megaly. A significant number of cases are discovered incidentally.

N.B. Hepatosplenomegaly with anemia is classic feature of CML. A mass abdomen with dragging pain is a presenting feature.

Points to be Noted in History

- Onset and progression of symptoms
- History of fever, sore throat, ulceration in the mouth
- History of bleeding from any site, e.g. gum, nose, urine, sputum, skin
- History of weakness of any part of the body, convulsions
- History of visual impairment or loss

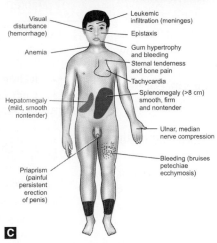

Figs 1.20A to C: Chronic myeloid leukemia. A. Patient presented with epistaxis. B. Patient presented with gum bleeding. C. Clinical manifestation of CML (diagram)

- History of breathlessness, fatigue or pain abdomen.

General Physical Examination

- *Face:* expression, puffiness
- *Oral cavity*, e.g. gum bleeding, anemia or excoriation or aphthous ulceration
- *Neck* examination for JVP, lymphaden-opathy, thyroid enlargement

- *Pulse, BP, temperature* and *respiration*
- *Hands* for koilonychia or platynychia, clubbing, sublingual hematoma or bleeding
- *Skin* for bleeding spots or ecchymotic patches
- Elicit *sternal tenderness*
- *Edema* feet

Systemic Examination
Examination of abdomen

Inspection

- A mass in the left hypochondrium. Describe all its characteristics
- Shape and position of the umbilicus may be normal or disorted by the mass if it is huge
- Hernial sites normal.

Palpation

- A palpable mass in left and right hypochondrium. Described its characteristics
- Any tenderness of abdomen.

Percussion

- Percuss over the mass. There will be dullness over splenic and liver mass
- Normal abdominal resonance
- Define the upper border of liver to confirm liver enlargement.

Auscultation

- Auscultate the bowel sounds
- Auscultate over the mass for any bruit, rub etc.

Other Systems

CVS Examination

- Look for anemia
- Auscultate for sounds, murmurs or rubs
- Looks for signs of CHF.

Nervous System

- Look for entrapment neuropathy, e.g. carpel tunnel syndrome or peripheral neuropathy.

Q. What is the clinical diagnosis of the patients in picture?

Ans. Both the patients are adults and presented with bleeding from nose (A) and gums (B) with a mass in left abdomen (both patients), the diagnosis of chronic myeloid leukemia is most likely.

Q. What is your differential diagnosis?

Ans. Read the differential diagnosis of hepatosplenomegaly with anemia (case 23)

Q. What are points in favor of your diagnosis?

Ans. 1. Adult patient with insidious onset of symptoms and signs
2. Presence of anemia.
3. Sternal tenderness
4. Massive splenomegaly and mild hepatomegaly

Q. How do you define leukemia? What is subleukemic or aleukemic leukemia?

Ans. The leukemias are a group of white cell disorders characterized by malignant transformation of blood white cells primarily in the bone marrow resulting in increased number of primitive white cells (blasts cells) in the bone marrow which ultimately spill into peripheral blood raising the total leukocyte count in peripheral blood.

Subleukemic or aleukemic leukemia is defined as the presence of immature cells in the bone marrow with little or no spilling into peripheral blood, hence, the WBC count is not high; may be normal or even reduced. The diagnosis is confirmed on bone marrow examination.

Q. What is difference between acute and chronic leukemia?

Ans. Depending on the clinical behavior of leukemia, it has been classified into acute and chronic. In **acute** leukemia, the history is short and life expectancy without treatment is short while in **chronic** leukemias, the patient is unwell for months and survives for years. The difference between acute and chronic leukemia are summarized in Table 1.65.

Q. How do you classify leukemias?

Ans. The leukemia on the basis of cell types are classified into *myeloid* and *lymphoid* and on the basis of natural history into acute and chronic as described above. The subclassification of leukemia is depicted in Table 1.66.

Q. What are symptoms and signs of leukemia?

Ans. Clinical symptoms (see Fig. 1.20C)are:
1. **Symptoms due to anemia**
   - Weakness
   - Pallor
   - Dyspnea
   - Tachycardia
2. **Symptoms due to hypermetabolism**
   - Weight loss
   - Anorexia
   - Lassitude
   - Night sweats

Table 1.65: Differentiation between acute and chronic leukemias

Acute	Chronic
Common in children and adolescents	Common in adults and old age
Acute onset	Slow insidious onset
Presentation is bone marrow failure, i.e. anemia, thrombocytopenia and leukopenia with their systemic effects	Presentation is extramedullary hematopoiesis, e.g. hepatosplenomegaly
Cell count varies in thousands, usually does not cross a lac	Cell count varies in lacs
Predominant cell type is blast cells	Predominant cell type is cytic cells (myelocytic, premyelocytic, metamyelocytic)
Blast cells usually exceed 30% in the marrow	Blast cells are usually less than 10%
Prognosis is bad, usually months to a year	Prognosis is good usually few years

Table 1.66: Subclassification of leukemia

1. **Acute lymphoblastic**
   - Common type (Pre B)
   - T cell
   - B cell
   - Undifferentiated
2. **Acute myeloid (FAB* classification)**
   M0 = Undifferentiated
   M1 = Minimal differentiation
   M2 = Differentiated
   M3 = Promyelocytic
   M4 = Myelomonocytic
   M5 = Monocytic
   M6 = Erythrocytic
   M7 = Megakaryocytic
3. **Chronic lymphocytic/lymphoid**
   - B cell – common
   - T cell – rare
4. **Chronic myeloid**
   - Ph' positive
   - Ph' negative, BCR – ABL positive
   - Ph' negative
   - Eosinophilic leukemia

FAB = French, American, British
Ph' = Philadelphia chromosome
BCR = Break point cluster region abl; Abelson oncogene

3. **Symptoms due to hyperplasia of bone marrow or infiltration of marrow by leukemic cells**
   - Bone pain
   - Sternal or iliac tenderness

4. **Symptoms due to infection**
   - Fever
   - Perspiration
5. **Bleeding tendencies**
   - Easy bruising, ecchymosis
   - Epistaxis
   - Menorrhagia
   - Hematomas
6. **Symptoms of hyperuricemia produced by drug treatment**
   - Asymptomatic
   - Uric acid stones
   - Precipitation of an attack of gout
   - Uric acid nephropathy

Q. How will you arrive at the diagnosis of CML?

Ans. CML is diagnosed on the clinical findings and confirmed on investigations.

Clinical findings in CML
- Adult patient
- Gradual onset of dragging pain and mass in the left hypochondrium
- Progressive anemia; anorexia, abdominal fullness, marked weight loss
- Moderate hepatomegaly with huge splenomegaly (> 8 cm below the costal margin)
- Sternal tenderness

Confirmation of CML
- Peripheral blood and bone marrow examination
- Ph' chromosome, if present, clinches the diagnosis
- Low leukocyte alkaline phosphatase score
- RNA analysis for presence of BCR-abl oncogene

Q. What are causes of bleeding gums?

Ans. Leukemias, e.g. acute (myelomonocytic common) and chronic (CML)
- Bleeding disorders, e.g. thrombocytopenia scurvy
- Dilantin toxicity (hypertrophy cum gum bleeding)
- Gingival disorders
- Local trauma

Q. What are causes of sternal tenderness?

Ans. Sternal tenderness is usually due to expansion of the bone marrow due to its proliferation, hence, can be present in all those conditions which cause bone marrow proliferation, i.e.
- Acute leukemia (AML and ALL)
- CML
- Severe anemia especially acute hemolytic anemia or crisis
- Multiple myeloma
- Following sternal puncture. This is easily diagnosed by the presence of either sternal puncture mark or attached cotton seal or benzene stain over sternum.

Q. What is genetics of CML?

Ans. The fusion of C-ABL (normally present on chromosome 9) with BCR sequences on chromosome 22 is pathognomonic of chronic phase of CML called the philadelphia chromosome

The p53 gene is the culprit in CML with blast transformation and there are structural alterations of RBI of N-ras in few case (<10%) of myeloid blast crisis.

Q. What do you understand by the term "myeloid metaplasia"?

Ans. Myeloid metaplasia also called extramedullary hematopoiesis means formation of blood at sites other than bone marrow, i.e. in the liver and spleen. It is commonly associated with bone marrow fibrosis (angogenic myeloid metaplasia).

Q. What is myelodysplastic syndrome (MDS)? What are conditions included in it?

Ans. Myelodysplasia (MDS) describes a group of acquired bone marrow disorders that are due to defect in the stem cells. They are characterized by increasing bone marrow failure with qualitative or quantitative abnormalities of all three myeloid cell lines (red cells, WBCs and platelets).

WHO and FAB classified myelodysplasia into 3 categories.

Category	Pheripheled blast (1%)	Bone marrow (1%)
1a (Reflactory anemia)	<1	Blasts <5, rings, sideroblast <15
2a (Reflactory anemia with sideroblasts)	<1	Blast <5, ring sideroblasts >15
3a (Reflactory anemia with excess blasts-I	1-4	Blasts 5-10
3b Reflactory anemia with excess blasts II	5-19	Blasts 11-19

Q. What are complications of CML?

Ans. Common complications of CML are as follows:
- Blastic crisis or blastic transformation of CML
- Hemorrhage or bleeding
- Recurrent infections (respiratory infection common)
- Hyperuricemia (due to disease as well as treatment)
- Leukemic infiltration in cranial nerves (compression neuropathy), pleura (pleural effusion), bones (paraplegia)
- Priaprism – persistent painful erection of penis

- Infarction or rupture of the spleen. Presence of splenic rub indicates infarction; while tender spleen can occur both in infarction and rupture.

Conversion of CML to acute leukemia indicates blastic crisis.

Q. What is blastic crisis?

Ans. It refers to transformation of chronic stable phase of chronic leukemia into acute unstable phase characterized by progressive anemia, onset of severe bleeding (e.g. petechiae, bruises, epistaxis, GI bleed) and on examination one would find;
- Sternal tenderness
- Appearance of lymphadenopathy (due to transformation to ALL).

The diagnosis is confirmed by peripheral blood examination which shows >30% blast cells (usually in CML, blast cells are <10%).

N.B.: Blastic crisis in CML is seen in patients with long duration of disease being treated with myelosuppressive drugs.

Q. What are differences between acute myeloid and acute lymphoid leukemia?

Ans. The ALL is common in children while AML is common in adults. The contrasting features of two types of leukemia are summarized in Table 1.67.

Q. What are similarities between CML and CLL? How they differ from each other?

Ans. Table 1.68 differentiates between CML and CLL.

Q. Which lymphomas can convert to leukemias?

Ans.
- Small cell lymphoma to CLL
- Burkitt's lymphoma to B cell ALL
- Lymphoblastic lymphoma to T cell ALL

Q. What is significance of Philadelphia Chromosome?

Ans. The significances are:
- The philadelphia chromosome (Ph') results from reciprocal translocation between the parts of long arms of chromosomes 9 and 22.
- Found in 90% cases of CML. Rest 10% are philadelphia chromosome negative. It is considered as diagnostic tool for CML.
- Ph'-chromosome positive cases have better prognosis than Ph'- chromosome negative cases.
- It is found in myeloid and erythroid series of blood cells in bone marrow. It is never seen in lymphocytes.
- It can differentiate AML from blastic crisis in CML
- Philadelphia chromosome is positive throughout the course of the disease during treatment, however, philadelphia positive cells decrease with alpha-interferon and Imatinib mesylate therapy.

Table 1.67: Two common types of acute leukemia—similarities and dissimilarities

Features	AML	ALL
Age	Adults (15-40 years)	Children (<15 years)
Incidence	Constitutes 20% of childhood leukemia	Constitute 80% of childhood leukemia
Symptoms	Fever, tiredness, bleeding manifestations, mouth ulceration and recurrent infections	Same as AML. Bone pain and tenderness common
Physical findings	Hepatosplenomegaly (+)	Hepatosplenomegaly (+++)
	Lymphadenopathy (+)	Lymphadenopathy (++)
	Gum hypertrophy (+)	Gum hypertrophy (++)
	Bone tenderness (+)	Bone tenderness (++)
	Chloroma (common) i.e. localized tumor masses in orbit, skin and other tissue	Chloroma – rare
	Anemia (++)	Anemia (+++)
	Leukemic meningitis (uncommon)	Leukemic meningitis (common)
	Sternal tenderness (++)	Sternal tenderness (++)
Laboratory findings	Low to high WBC count with predominant myeloblasts (>30%)	Low to high WBC count with predominant lymphoblasts
Cytochemical	Myeloperoxidase positive	PAS positive
Stain	Sudan black positive	—
Remissions	Remission rate is low, duration of remission short	Remission rate high and duration of remission prolonged

Signs used (+) means present (++) to (+++) means a marked feature

Table 1.68: Similarities and dissimilarities between CML and CLL

Features	CML	CLL
Age	Peak age 55 years	Peak age 65 years
Onset	Insidious	Very insidious
Symptoms and signs	Hepatosplenomegaly marked	Hepatosplenomegaly mild
	Anemia early	Anemia develops late
	Lymphadenopathy uncommon	Lymphadenopathy is common presentation
	Sternal tenderness present	Sternal tenderness absent
	Blast crisis (common)	Blast crisis (uncommon)
Laboratory findings	Very high WBC count with predominant myelocytes and metamyelocytes	WBC count high, predominant cells are lymphocytes
	Philadelphia chromosome positive	Philadelphia chromosome negative
Response to treatment	Good	Excellent
Prognosis	Good	Excellent

Q. How will you investigate a case with CML?

Ans. Investigations are as follows:

1. *Blood examination*
   - Hemoglobin and RBC count. They are low
   - WBC count high (1-5 lac/mm^3). Differential count shows 20-30% myelocytes, 20-25% metamyelocytes, 2-3% promyelocytes and rest are polymorphs. Myeloblasts (< 10%) may be seen. There may be increase in basophils and eosinophils in early disease.
   - Platelet count – normal to increased in early stages but decreased in late stages.

2. *Bone marrow examination.* It is not must for diagnosis as presence of immature cells (>30%) in the peripheral blood are sufficient for diagnosis. It shows increased myelocyte series of cells with increased myeloid and erythroid ratio (20:1). Bone marrow is hypercellular. Myeloblasts >30% in the bone marrow in CML indicates blastic crisis.

3. *Chromosomal study for philadelphia* chromosome. It is positive in 90% cases

4. *RNA analysis* for BCR-abl oncogene

5. *Leukocyte alkaline phosphatase* score is diminished

6. *Other tests*
   - High uric acid and LDH level
   - High serum Vit. B$_{12}$ level

Q. What is busulphan lung?

Ans. Interstitial lung fibrosis seen during therapy with busulphan is called *busulphan lung.*

CASE 21: LYMPHADENOPATHY

The patient 30 years male (Fig. 1.21) presented with multiple swelling in the neck with low grade fever, fatigue and malaise for the last 8 months. On examination, there was lobulated mass in the cervical region.

Clinical Presentations

1. *Asymptomatic*. Lymphadenopathy may be an incidental finding in patients being examined for various reasons.
2. *When symptomatic*, the symptoms may vary according to size, site and cause of involvement. They may present with:
   - Multiple swellings at one site or at different sites, e.g. neck, axillae and groins.
   - Mediastinal lymph node enlargement may present as superior mediastinal compression syndrome or superior vena caval obstruction syndrome
   - Intra-aortic abdominal lymph node enlargement produce pain abdomen and mass abdomen.
3. Patients may present with P.U.O. (fever), night sweats, weight loss or pain in the nodes.
4. Patients may present with the symptoms and signs of basic disease, e.g. leukemia, lymphoma, acute infections etc. and lymphadenopathy is a part and parcel of the clinical spectrum.

History

Points to be Noted in History

- Site(s), duration and extent
- Any history of swelling in the axilla or groin

Fig. 1.21: A patient with cervical lymphadenopathy presented with mass in the neck which has irregular surface, is firm in consistency, adherent to overlying skin with a sinus and skin discoloration

- Any history of pain abdomen or mass abdomen (e.g. spleen and/or liver)
- Any history of fever, night sweats, fatigue, malaise and weight loss
- Any history of cough, dyspnea or hoarseness of voice (for hilar lymphadenopathy)
- Any history of injury or infection of neck or extremity
- Past history of fever, tuberculosis, malignancy or injury/infection (HIV)
- Personal history including occupation.

General Physical Examination

- *Face* for puffiness or edema
- *Mouth* for anemia or evidence of infection, petechiae and pharyngitis (glandular fever)
  Skin for evidence of bleeding or infection.
- *Neck*. Examine the various groups of cervical lymph nodes and describe the number, consistency, tenderness, matting, adherence to underlying structures or overlying skin. Note the temperature over the mass. Look for JVP and thyroid. Examine the neck for

preauricular, post-auricular, submental, etc (see Fig. 1.21B).
Examine axilla and inguinal region in addition to all other sites of lymph node.
- Look for *engorgement of neck/chest veins, suffusion of the face* and *cyanosis* (e.g. superior mediastinal compression).
- Pulse, BP respiration and temperature
- Look for *anemia, jaundice, edema,* etc.

Systemic Examinations

I. Examination of Abdomen

- Inspect the abdomen for any swelling or protuberance
- Palpate the abdomen for liver, spleen or lymph node enlargement
- Look for the presence of ascites.

II. Examination of Respiratory System

- Inspect the chest for any retraction or deformity
- Palpate the trachea for any deviation
- Look for any evidence of mediastinal shift due to lung collapse
- Look for signs of superior mediastinal compression, e.g. periorbital edema, chemosis, conjunctival suffusion, prominence of neck veins and veins over the chest, absent venous pulsation in the neck.

III. Examination of Hematopoietic System

- Look for any evidence of purpuric or ecchymotic patches
- Elicit sternal tenderness
- Any evidence of infection
- Ocular fundus examination.

Q. What the clinical diagnosis of the patient in picture?

Ans. The presence of a lobulated irregular mass in cervical region with irregular surface, firm in consistency, not mobile, fixed to the skin with formation of a sinus and skin pigmentation indicate a lymph node mass due to tuberculosis, e.g. tubercular lymphadenitis with sacrofuloderma.

Q. What is differential diagnosis?

Ans. The following conditions come into differential diagnosis of cervical lymphadenopathy:

- Tubercular lymphadenitis, HIV infections
- Infectious mononucleosis
- Hodgkin's and non-Hodgkin's lymphoma, leukemia (ALL)
- Lung carcinoma
- Infection in the draining area, i.e. face, neck
- Sarcoidosis

Q. How do you define lymphadenopathy? What is meant by significant lymphadenopathy?

Ans. Lymphadenopathy literally means enlargement of lymph nodes which may be significant or insignificant.

Significant lymphadenopathy means enlargement that needs further evaluation. Lymph nodes enlargement ≥ 1 cm in size anywhere in the body is considered as significant except the groin where ≥ 2 cm size of the lymph node is considered significant. Insignificant enlargement means nonspecific, small lymph nodes usually <0.5 cm in diameter, may be palpable due to past infection.

Q. What are the causes of lymphadenopathy?

Ans. Localized or regional lymphadenopathy implies involvement of a single anatomical area. A generalized adenopathy has been defined as involvement of three or more noncontiguous lymph node areas. Many of the causes of lymphadenopathy (Table 1.69) can produce localized or generalized adenopathy, so this distinction is of limited utility in differential diagnosis.

Table 1.69: Diseases associated with lymphadenopathy

1. **Infectious diseases**
   a. *Viral infections,* e.g infectious mononucleosis syndromes (EBV, CMV), infectious hepatitis, HIV, herpes infections.
   b. *Bacterial infections,* e.g. streptococcal, staphylococcal, salmonella, brucella, pasteurella pestis.
   c. *Fungal infections,* e.g. histoplasmosis, coccidioidomycosis
   d. *Mycobacterial infections,* e.g. tuberculosis, leprosy.
   e. *Spirochetal,* e.g. syphilis, leptospirosis
   f. *Parasitic,* e.g. toxoplasmosis
2. **Immunological disease**
   - Rheumatoid arthritis, juvenile rheumatoid arthritis
   - Mixed connective tissue disorders
   - SLE, dermatomyositis
   - Sjogren's syndrome
   - Serum sickness
   - Drug hypersensitivity, e.g. diphenylhydantoin, gold, hydralazine, carbamazepine, allopurinol, etc.
   - Graft vs host disease
   - Silicone - associated
   - Primary biliary cirrhosis
3. **Neoplastic disorders**
   - Primary, e.g. leukemia, lymphomas
   - Metastatic or secondary, e.g. breast, lung, thyroid, stomach
4. **Lipid storage diseases,** e.g. Gaucher's disease, Niemann–Pick's disease, Tangier disease.
5. **Miscellaneous**
   - Amyloidosis
   - Sarcoidosis
   - Histiocytosis X
   - Inflammatory pseudotumor of lymph node
   - Mucocutaneous lymph node syndrome (Kawasaki's disease)
   - Castlemen's disease (giant lymph node hyperplasia)
   - Familial mediterranean fever

Q. What are common causes of generalized lymphadenopathy?

Ans. Nevertheless, generalised lymphadenopathy is frequently associated with nonmalignant disorders rather than malignant disorders. The common causes are:
- Tuberculosis
- Infectious mononucleosis
- Toxoplasmosis
- AIDS and other viral infections
- Collagen vascular disorders, e.g. SLE, mixed connective tissue disorders
- Leukemias, e.g. acute and chronic lymphocytic leukemias
- Lymphomas (Hodgkin's and non-Hodgkin's).

Q. What is differential diagnosis of a case with regional adenopathy?

Ans. The site of regional lymphadenopathy may provide a useful clue to the cause (Table 1.70).

Q. How will you proceed to examine a case of lymphadenopathy?

Ans. Points to be noted in lymphadenopathy are:
- Site
- Size and shape
- Consistency or texture (soft, firm, hard, rubbery)
- Tenderness (present or absent)
- Fixation (mobile or fixed to the underlying or overlying structures)
- Matted or discrete
- Local temperature is raised or not (hot or cold)
- Change in color of the skin – *sacrofuloderma*
- Margins – defined or ill-defined
- Associated features
- Associated splenomegaly or hepatosplenomegaly.

Q. What are the causes of painful tender lymph nodes?

Ans. The causes are:
1. *Acute inflammation or infection*
   - Viral – infectious mononucleosis
   - Bacterial – pyogenic infections, tuberculosis, brucellosis, plague, diphtheria, leprosy
   - Parasitic – toxoplasmosis
   - Fungal infections
2. *Immunological causes*
   - SLE and other collagen vascular disorders
   - Rheumatoid arthritis
3. *Neoplastic*
   - Acute leukemia (lymphoblastic)
   - Metastases in the lymph node

Note: Tenderness or pain in lymphadenopathy is due to stretching of the capsule as a result of rapid or sudden enlargement of lymph node due to any cause

Table 1.70: Site of involvement of lymph node as a clue to the diagnosis

Site	Cause(s)
Occipital adenopathy	Scalp infection
Preauricular adenopathy	Conjunctival infection
Left supraclavicular lymph node (Virchow's gland)	Metastasis from gastric or gastrointestinal cancer
Supraclavicular nodes enlargement	• Tuberculosis, sarcoidosis, toxoplasmosis • Metastases from lung, breast, testis or ovary
Axillary lymphadenopathy	• Injuries of upper limb • Localized infection of ipsilateral upper extremity • Malignancies, e.g. melanoma, lymphoma and breast carcinoma
Inguinal lymphadenopathy	• Infections or trauma of lower extremity, plague • Sexually transmitted diseases, e.g. lymphogranuloma venereum, primary syphilis, genital herpes or chancroid • Lymphomas and metastases from rectum and genitalia
Thoracic lymph nodes (hilar lymphadenopathy)	• Tuberculosis, sarcoidosis, fungal infection • Lymphoma, malignancy lung with metastases in lymph node
Abdominal lymphadenopathy (retroperitoneal, para-aortic)	• Tuberculosis (mesenteric lymphadenitis) • Lymphoma • Metastases from the abdominal viscera

Q. What is the cause of egg-shelled calcification in hilar lymph nodes?

Ans. Silicosis

Q. What do you know of Sister Joseph's nodule?

Ans. It refers to a nodule around umbilicus seen in gastric adenocarcinoma, represents either a metastatic deposit or an enlarged anterior abdominal wall lymph node.

Q. What are the causes of fixation of the lymph nodes to surrounding structures?

Ans. The causes are:
- Tuberculosis
- Malignancy or metastases in the lymph nodes

Q. What are the causes of lymphadenopathy with splenomegaly?

Ans. The causes are:
- Infectious mononucleosis
- Lymphoma
- Acute or chronic leukemia especially lymphatic
- Sarcoidosis
- Collagen vascular disorders, e.g. SLE, RA
- Toxoplasmosis
- Cat-scratch disease
- Disseminated or miliary tuberculosis.

Q. What is non-Hodgkin's lymphoma?

Ans. They are heterogenous group of malignant disorder of lymphoid tissue involving chiefly the B cells and to some extent T cells. They vary in their presentation and natural history varying from slow indolent course to a rapidly progessive disease.

Q. How do you classify non-Hodgkin's lymphoma

Ans. Previous classification of non-Hodgkin's lymphoma into low grade (slow, indolent and favorable prognosis) and high grade (aggressive, unfavorable) has been replaced by WHO (2001) as follows

   I. B. Cell lymphoma
   - Precursor B cell lymphoma
   - Mature B cell lymphoma

   II. T/NK cell lymphoma
   - Precursor T cell lymphoma
   - Mature T/NK cell lymphoma

The main two groups are further subdivided to include aggressive forms also.

Q. What is mode of presentation of Hodgkin's disease?

Ans.
- Usually as a painless lymph node enlargement in young age
- Other presenting symptoms include systemic features such as pyrexia, drenching night sweats, weight loss, pain in the affected lymph nodes after ingestion of alcohol and generalized itching.

Q. How do you stage Hodgkin's disease?

Ans. Stage I : One lymph node site involved

Stage II : More than 2 lymph nodes sites involved on one side of the diaphragm

Stage III : Lymph nodes involved on both sides of diaphragm

Stage IV : Disseminated disease with extranodal involvement (e.g. bone marrow, liver)

A means absence of systemic symptoms and B means presence of systemic symptoms e.g. fever, sweating, weakness and weight loss.

Q. What do you understand by the term Hodgkin's disease?

Ans. It is abnormal proliferation of lymphoid tissue (neoplasm of lymphoid tissue), characterized by development of lymphadenopathy at single or multiple sites. The pathological hallmark is Reed-Sternberg cells derived from germinal center B cells, rarely peripheral T cells.

Q. What are histological subtypes of Hodgkin's disease?

Ans. The 4 subtypes are:
- Lymphocyte predominance
- Nodular sclerosis
- Mixed cellularity
- Lymphocyte depletion

Q. How would you treat Hodgkin's lymphoma?

Ans.
- Localized disease (stage IA, IIA) is treated by radiotherapy.
- Disseminated disease (IIIB and IV stages) is treated with combination chemotherapy (e.g. A B V D and M O P P regimen).
- Stages II B & III A are now a days treated with combination chemotherapy

Q. How will you investigate a case with lymphadenopathy?

Ans. The investigations are done to find out the cause. They are planned depending on the site and type of involvement.

1. *Complete hemogram.* Presence of anemia (low hemoglobin) with lymphadenopathy indicates chronic infections, chronic disorders (e.g. rheumatoid arthritis, or Felty syndrome, SLE) or malignant disease (e.g. leukemias, lymphomas, metastasis). Anemia in these conditions is normocytic and normochromic.

   Complete blood count can provide useful data for diagnosis of acute or chronic leukemia (leukocytosis with immature cells), infectious mononucleosis (leukopenia), lymphoma, pyogenic infections (leukocytosis) or immune cytopenias in illness like SLE.

   Raised ESR suggests tuberculosis, rheumatoid arthritis, SLE, acute infections.

2. *Serological tests*
   - To demonstrate antibodies specific to components of EBV, CMV, HIV and other viruses, toxoplasma gondii, brucella
   - VDRL test for syphilis
   - Antinuclear antibodies, LE cell phenomenon and anti-DNA antibodies for SLE and other collagen vascular disorders
   - Rheumatoid factor for rheumatoid arthritis

3. *Blood culture* for causative organism in acute infections

4. *Chest X-ray.* It will reveal hilar or mediastinal lymph node enlargement, if any. Unilateral hilar lymph node enlargement usually suggests malignancy lung or tuberculosis; bilateral enlargement indicates sarcoidosis, histoplasmosis or lymphoma.

The chest X-ray will also confirm the involvement of lung in acute infections, tuberculosis, and primary or metastatic lung tumours.

5. *Imaging techniques* (ultrasound, color Doppler ultrasonography, CT scan, MRI) have been employed to differentiate benign from malignant lymph nodes especially in head and neck cancer. These techniques especially USG have been used to demonstrate the ratio of long (L) axis to short (S) axis in cervical nodes. An L/S ratio of <2.0 is used to distinguish between benign and malignant lymph nodes in head and neck cancer and has sensitivity and specificity of 95%. This ratio has greater sensitivity and specificity than palpation or measurement of either the long or short axis alone.

   Ultrasonography or CT scan abdomen will also reveal lymph node enlargement in the chest and abdomen (mesenteric, para-aortic) which are not palpable on per abdomen examination. These imaging techniques are used for staging lymphomas and to detect enlargement of spleen before it becomes palpable.

6. *Lymph node biopsy.* The indications for lymph node biopsy are imprecise inspite of so many studies done in this regard, yet it remains a valuable diagnostic tool. It is useful to carry out lymph node biopsy;
   - If history and physical findings suggest a malignancy, i.e. a solitary, hard, nontender cervical node in an older patient who is chronic smoker.
   - Supraclavicular lymphadenopathy
   - Generalized or solitary lymphadenopathy with splenomegaly suggestive of lymphoma.

Fine needle aspiration should not be performed as the first diagnostic procedure. Most diagnoses require more tissue than obtained on FNAC.

- A young patient with peripheral lymphadenopathy (lymph node size >2 cm in diameter with abnormal chest X-ray.

Generally, any lymph node >2 cm in diameter should be biopsied for etiological diagnosis.

CASE 22: SPLENOMEGALY

A female patient (Fig. 1.22A) presented with a mass in the left hypochondrium and associated dragging pain. There was no history of fever, hematemesis or bleeding from any site. She gave history of weakness and exertional dyspnea. No history of jaundice or drug intake or prolonged cough in the past. A mass was palpable in the left hypochondrium.

Clinical Presentations

- Splenomegaly may be asymptomatic and without any disease
- Pain and dragging sensation in the left upper quadrant is a common presentation with chronic splenomegaly. Massive splenomegaly can produce early satiety.
- Acute pain in left upper quadrant may result due to acute splenomegaly with stretching of the capsule or infarction (vascular occlusion of splenic vessels in subacute bacterial endocarditis, sickle cell crisis in children) or inflammation (perisplenitis) of the spleen.
- Rupture of the spleen either from trauma or infiltrative disease means rupture of the capsule with intraperitoneal bleeding, may result in shock, hypotension and death. The rupture itself may be painless. The disease associated with rupture of spleen include; *chronic leukemias, myelofibrosis, congestive splenomegaly.*

History

Points to be Noted

- History of abdominal distention.
- History of fever, sore throat bleeding from nose, mouth, rectum, etc.
- History of piles and/or hematemesis, jaundice
- History of palpitation, dyspnea, orthopnea and PND
- Any history of weight loss, fatigue, bone pain, night sweats (CML)
- Is the area endemic for malaria or Kala-azar?
- Family history of Gaucher's disease.

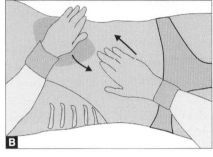

Figs 1.22A and B: A. A patient with massive (> 8 cm) splenomegaly producing left hypochondriac protrusion; B. Method of palpation for splenomegaly (diagram)

- Past history of jaundice hematemesis, RHD, tuberculosis, malignancy.

General Physical Examination

- Face for puffiness or edema
- Mouth for any evidence of infection, ulceration or excoriation or thrush
- Tongue and mucous membranes—look for anemia
- *Neck* for lymphadenopathy, JVP, thyroid enlargement
- Pulse, BP, respiration and temperature
- Hands for clubbing, splinter hemorrhage, Roth's spots, gangrene
- Feet for edema.
- Normally the spleen is neither palpable nor becomes palpable unless enlarged by two and half times, hence, spleen may be enlarged but not palpable. Therefore, percussion of 9th, 10th and 11th space (*Traube's area*) is a useful diagnostic technique.

Systemic Examinations

I. Examination of Abdomen

- Look for any swelling or protuberance of abdomen especially in left hypochondriac region

- Palpate the abdomen for enlargement of spleen, liver and lymph nodes. In case spleen or liver is enlarged, note the details of characteristics of liver or splenic mass
- *Rule of palpation for spleen (Fig. 1.22B):* Start low while examining the spleen and be gentle during palpation. Even if you are certain it is spleen, you must follow the rules of palpation of spleen to rule out renal mass. Do not forget to do a bimanual palpation (spleen is bimanually palpable and kidney is ballottable). Feel for the splenic notch and auscultate for the splenic rub.
- Percussion over the mass. In a case with splenomegaly percuss for Traube's area for dullness. In case of hepatomegaly, define the upper border of liver dullness on percussion and record the liver span by measurement
- Auscultate over the mass for any rub, bruit etc.

II. Examination of Respiratory System

- Examine for signs of hilar lymphadenopathy (e.g. superior mediastinal syndrome—read short case discussion on it)
- Look for signs of LHF.

III. Examination of CVS

- Inspect the precordium for any precordial bulge or cardiac enlargement
- Palpate the apex for any evidence of derivation/shift or thrill
- Ausculate the heart for sounds, murmurs or rub and for evidence of LVF or pericardial disease especially pericardial effusion or rheumatic valvular disease.

IV. Examination of Blood

- Look for signs of hemorrhage or bleeding into the skin or organ
- Elicit sternal tenderness.

Q. What is your clinical diagnosis?

Ans. Massive splenomegaly due to chronic myeloid leukemia.

Q. What are the points in favor of your diagnosis?

Ans. 1. History of fever, bone pains, night sweats, dyspnea
2. Presence of anemia and sternal tenderness
3. Massive non-tender splenomegaly

Q. How do you define splenomegaly?

Ans. Splenomegaly literally means enlargement of spleen. Palpable spleen means its enlargement 2 to 3 times than normal. Normal spleen measures 12 × 7 cm on ultrasonography, radionuclide scan and CT scan. Spleen is palpable in 1-3% normal individuals without any cause. Its incidence in normal population in New Guinea has been reported to be very high (up to 60%). Spleen is said to be enlarged if its span on USG is > 14 cm.

Q. What is differential diagnosis of massive splenomegaly (>8 cm)?

Ans. The following conditions must be considered;
- Chronic malaria
- Kala-azar
- Chronic myeloid leukemia/Hairy cell leukaemia
- myelofibrosis/myelosclerosis
- Gaucher's disease.

N.B.: Read the characteristics of these disorders as well as that of spleen in case discussion of hepatosplenomegaly.

Q. Which bed side investigation would you carry out to confirm the diagnosis?

Ans. Peripheral blood film examination for total leucocyte count and immature cells. Immature cells >30% will clinch the diagnosis.

Q. Name the conditions producing moderate splenomegaly.

Ans. Read Table 1.71.

Q. What are causes of mild splenomegaly (e.g. spleen is just palpable)?

Ans. Read the Table 1.71.

Q. What are the causes of palpable spleen without enlargement?

Ans. Normally spleen may be palpable without being enlarged in;
- Some children below 10 years of age
- Thin lean persons
- COPD (spleen is pushed down by hyperinflated lung
- Visceroptosis (drooping of viscera including spleen)

Q. What are causes of splenomegaly with fever?

Ans. Spleen enlarges within few days to few weeks of fever. Causes are:
- Bacterial endocarditis
- Acute malaria
- Kala-azar
- Tuberculosis
- Infectious mononucleosis
- Histoplasmosis
- Typhoid fever
- Acute leukemia
- Lymphoma
- SLE
- Hemolytic crisis

Q. What are the causes of splenomegaly with anemia?

Ans. The causes are:
- Bacterial endocarditis
- Hemolytic anemia

Table 1.71: Causes of various grades of splenomegaly

Mild (<3 cm)	Moderate (3-8 cm)	Massive (78 cm)
• Congestive heart failure	• Cirrhosis of liver with portal hypertension	• Chronic malaria and kala-azar
• Bacterial endocarditis	• Lymphomas	• Chronic myeloid leukemia (CML)
• Typhoid fever	• Hemolytic anemia	• Myelofibrosis/myelosclerosis
• SLE	• Infectious mononucleosis	• Chronic lymphatic leukemia (CLL)
• Acute malaria (chronic malaria produces massive splenomegaly)	• Amyloidosis	• Hairy cell leukemia
	• Chronic lymphatic leukemia	• Gaucher's disease in children
• Rheumatoid arthritis, sarcoidosis	• Hairy cell leukemia	• Diffuse splenic hemangiomatosis
• Glandular fever (infectious mononucleosis)	• Splenic abscess or cyst	
	• Idiopathic thrombocytopenic purpura	
• Idiopathic thrombocytopenia purpura		
• Polycythemia		

- Cirrhotic portal hypertension with repeated hematemesis
- Myeloproliferative syndromes
- Malaria
- Felty's syndrome
- SLE
- Rheumatoid arthritis.

Q. What are causes of splenomegaly with jaundice?

Ans. Jaundice may be hemolytic or hepatic. Causes are;
- Cirrhosis of liver
- Acute viral hepatitis (uncommon)
- Acute malaria (*P. falciparum*) due to hemolysis
- Hepatic vein thrombosis (Budd-Chiari syndrome)
- Hemolytic anemia
- Lymphoma
- Miliary tuberculosis

Q. What are the common causes of fever, lymphadenopathy, splenomegaly with or without rash?

Ans. The conditions are:
- Infectious mononucleosis
- Sarcoidosis
- Acute leukemia or blast crisis in chronic leukemia
- SLE
- Lymphoma
- Felty's syndrome

Q. What are the causes of splenomegaly with ascites?

Ans. The causes are:
- Portal hypertension
- Budd-Chiari syndrome
- Lymphoma
- CML
- Viral hepatitis with hepatocellular failure

Q. What are the causes of splenic rub? Where do you hear it? What does it indicate?

Ans. Splenic rub can be heard over the enlarged spleen with stethoscope in conditions associated with splenic infarction (perisplenitis) due to vascular occlusion of spleen. The patient complains of acute left upper quadrantic pain abdomen which may radiate to tip of left shoulder. The spleen is enlarged and tender. The causes are:
- Subacute bacterial endocarditis
- Chronic myeloid leukemia
- Sickle cell anemia
- Following splenic puncture for diagnosis of kala-azar

Splenic rub is heard over the spleen or left lower chest during respiration

Q. What is hypersplenism? What are its causes?

Ans. Hypersplenism refers to overactivity of the splenic function, has nothing to do with the size of the spleen. It is characterized by a tetrad consisting of;
- Splenomegaly of any size
- Cytopenias/pancytopenias (anemia, leukopenia and/or thrombocytopenia)
- Normal or hypercellular marrow
- Reversibility following splenectomy

Causes of Hypersplenisms are:
- Lymphoma
- Cirrhosis of the liver
- Myeloproliferative disorders
- Connective tissue disorders

Pancytopenia of hypersplenism differs from pancytopenia due to aplastic anemia by hypercellular or normal bone marrow. It is due to the fact that in hypersplenism, all the formed elements of blood (RBCs, WBCs and platelets) are being destroyed in the spleen which stimulates the bone marrow and makes it hypercellular. On the other hand, in aplastic anemia, bone marrow is hypocellular due to aplasia or hypoplasia of the marrow elements.

Q. What are causes of hyposplenism or asplenia?

Ans. It refers to virtual absence of spleen (asplenia) or malfunctioning spleen (hyposplenism). It is usually associated with;
- Dextrocardia
- Sickle cell disease leading to multiple infarcts
- Coeliac disease
- Fanconi's anemia (aplastic anemia with hypoplasia of spleen, kidney, thymus, etc.)
- Surgical removal of the spleen.
- Splenic irradiation for autoimmune or neoplastic disease.

Q. How will you investigate a patient with splenomegaly?

Ans. The investigations to be done are:
- *Hemoglobin and RBCs count.* Hemoglobin is *low* in thalassemia major, SLE, cirrhotic portal hypertension and *increased* in polycythemia rubra vera.
- *WBC count.* Granulocyte counts may be *normal, decreased* (Felty's syndrome, congestive splenomegaly, aleukemic leukemia) or *increased* (infections, or inflammatory disease, myeloproliferative disorders).
- *Other investigations* are same as discussed under hepatosplenomegaly (read them there).

Q. What are indications of splenectomy (removal of spleen)?

Ans. Indications are:

1. For correction of cytopenia in immune-mediated destruction of one or more cellular blood elements, for example, in immune thrombocytopenia
2. For sickle cell crises (splenic sequestration) in young children
3. Hereditary spherocytosis
4. For correlation (reversibility) of cytopenias in patients with hypersplenism
5. For disease control in patients with splenic rupture.
6. More often splenectomy is performed in stage III and IV of Hodgkin's disease. Splenectomy is necessary for routine staging of Hodgkin's disease (stage I and II in whom radiation therapy is done)
7. For symptom control in patients with painful massive splenomegaly in CML unresponsive to chemotherapy.

Q. What are the clinical manifestations of splenectomy?

Ans. These will be:

The immediate manifestation within 2-3 weeks is leukocytosis and thrombocytosis.

- *Marked variations in size and shape of RBCs* (anisocytosis, poikilocytosis)
- *Presence of Howell-Jolly bodies* (nuclear remnants), *Heinz bodies* (denatured Hb), *basophilic stippling* and an occasional *nucleated RBC* in the peripheral blood.

Q. What will be the consequences of splenectomy?

Ans. The consequences will be:

1. The most serious consequence of splenectomy is predisposition to bacterial infections, particularly with *S. pneumoniae, H. influenzae* and some gram-negative enteric organisms. They should be immunized against these organisms. The vaccination recommended are given in the box.
2. The splenectomized patients are more susceptible to a parasitic disease – *babesiosis*, hence, they should avoid visit to areas where the parasite – Babesia is endemic.

Vaccination before and after splenectomy

The Advisory Committee on Immunization Practices recommends that pneumococcal vaccine should be administered to all patients before elective splenectomy and a repeat dose of vaccination 5 years later.

The vaccination against N. meningitidis should also be given to patients in whom elective splenectomy is planned.

Q. What is abscopal effect?

Ans. Tumor regression or regression of systemic illness following splenectomy or splenic irradiation in patients with CML and prolymphocytic leukemia is known as abscopal effect.

Q. What is Traube's area? What is its significance?

Ans. Normal Traube's area is bounded above by the lung resonance, below by the costal margins; on the right by left border of the liver and on the left by the normal splenic dullness. It lies in left lower chest behind 9th, 10th and 11th rib.

- Normally it is resonant because it is occupied by stomach (tympanic note)
- It becomes dull in:
  — Left side pleural effusion
  — Splenomegaly
  — Distended stomach with fluid or solid growth.

Q. What are differences between a splenic and left renal mass?

Ans. Read clinical method by Prof. SN Chugh.

Q. How will you palpate spleen in the presence of ascites?

Ans. For method of palpation of spleen (Fig. 1.22B), read clinical methods. However, in the presence of ascites, spleen is palpated by dipping method.

Q. What are characteristics of a splenic mass?

Ans. Read Clinical Method in Medicine.

Q. What are other causes of mass in left hypochondrium?

Ans. Read Clinical Method in Medicine.

CASE 23: HEPATOSPLENOMEGALY

The patient (not in picture) presented with gradual onset of fever, malaise, weakness. There was history of masses in the abdomen with dyspnea, pallor. Patient gave history of taking anti-malarial drug following which the fever subsided.

Clinical Presentation of Hepatosplenomegaly

These patients usually present either with dull ache or pain in right and left hypochondrium, but most of the time they may complain of masses in the abdomen (Fig. 1.23).

History

Points to be Noted

- History of fever or sore throat, jaundice, bleeding from any site
- History of palpitation, breathlessness, orthopnea, PND

- Any history of infection, mouth ulcerations, mouth thrush, excoriation, etc.

General Physical Examination

Look at
- Face for puffiness, edema
- Mouth for ulceration, excoriation or thrush
- Tongue for anemia. Look other sites for anemia
- Neck for lymph node enlargement, JVP and thyroid enlargement
- Pulse, BP, temperature and respiration
- Hands for koilonychia, platynychia, splinter hemorrhage, clubbing
- Feet for edema

Systemic Examination

I. Abdomen

- Look for any swelling or bulge
- Palpate the masses in the abdomen and describe their characteristics
- Percuss for Traube's area for splenic dullness and define the upper border of the liver for its enlargement and liver span measurement

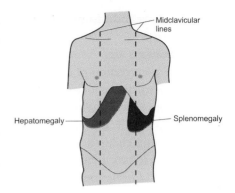

Fig. 1.23: Hepatosplenomegaly—a diagram

- Auscultate over the mass(es) for any bruit or rub

II. CVS Examination

- Examine the heart for any enlargement, murmur, sounds or rub
- Look for the signs of valvular heart disease, LVF, SABE and pericardial disease especially pericardial effusion.

III. Examination of Blood

- Look for any hemorrhage into the skin or joint or organ
- Examine ocular fundi for hemorrhage

Q. What is your clinical diagnosis?
Ans. Hepatosplenomegaly
Q. What are the causes of hepatosplenomegaly?
Ans. The causes are:
1. *Infections,* e.g. malaria, kala azar, typhoid, acute miliary or disseminated tuberculosis, viral hepatitis (occasional) and brucellosis.
2. *Blood disorders,* e.g. hemolytic anemia, chronic myeloid leukemia, lymphoma, polycythemia rubra vera, chronic lymphatic leukemia, acute leukemias.
3. *Extramedullary erythropoiesis,* e.g. myelofibrosis, myelosclerosis.
4. *Diseases of liver,* e.g. cirrhosis, Budd-Chiari syndrome.
5. *Congestive hepatosplenomegaly,* e.g. pericardial effusion, constrictive pericarditis and congestive cardiac failure (cardiomyopathy)
6. *Infiltrative disorders,* e.g. amyloidosis
7. *Miscellaneous,* e.g. sarcoidosis.

Q. What is the differential diagnosis of hepatosplenomegaly in an adult?
Ans. The conditions that come into differential diagnosis are discussed below.

Chronic Malaria: The characteristic features are;
- Patient belongs to an endemic zone
- Fever with chills and rigors. Fever may come on alternate days periodically
- Anemia and mild jaundice may be present if hemolysis occurs
- Massive splenomegaly with moderate hepatomegaly, firm to hard and nontender
- Diagnosis is confirmed by demonstration of the parasite in the peripheral blood.

Chronic Kala-azar
- Patient belongs to an endemic area
- Double rise or peak in temperature (biphasic pattern) in 24 hours may be present
- Patient is well despite symptoms and signs
- The skin is dry and pigmented
- Hepatosplenomegaly in which spleen is massively enlarged while liver enlargement is moderate. Both are firm and nontender.
- The diagnosis is confirmed by demonstration of LD bodies in buffy coat preparations of blood or in the bone marrow smear or lymph node, liver, or spleen aspirates (splenic puncture).

Thalassemia (Cooley's Anemia)

- A heredofamilial disorder of hemoglobin (hemoglobinopathy) hence, the patient is usually a child or young person with positive family history.
- Stunded growth and mongoloid facies
- Moderate hepatosplenomegaly, nontender, soft to firm
- Severe anemia and mild jaundice (hemolysis)
- Anemia is microcytic and hypochromic
- Leg ulcers
- Diagnosis is confirmed by radiological study of skull and presence of abnormal hemoglobin (HbF >2%) on electrophoresis.

Hemolytic Anemia

- Granual onset of anemia
- Mild jaundice
- Dark colored urine and stool during an episode of hemolysis
- Moderate nontender hepatosplenomegaly
- Positive tests for hemolysis will confirm the diagnosis.

Chronic Myeloid Leukemia

- Patient is middle aged or old aged person with slow onset of symptoms
- The presenting symptoms are dragging pain in left hypochondrium due to massive splenomegaly and profound weakness, weight loss and sweating.
- Moderate anemia
- Hepatosplenomegaly due to extramedullary erythropoiesis. The spleen is massively enlarged (>8 cm), firm to hard and occasionally a splenic rub may be present if a splenic infarct occurs. The liver is moderately enlarged.
- Sternal tenderness is present
- Diagnosis is confirmed by presence of anemia, high WBC count (in lacs) with immature WBCs (myelocytes, metamyelocytes and promyelocytes with few myeloblasts (<10%).

Lymphoma

- Painless progressive enlargement of cervical, axillary and inguinal lymph nodes, discrete, firm, but rubbery in consistency in Hodgkin's lymphoma.
- Fever, weight loss, weakness, pruritus with drenching night sweats may occur
- Moderate hepatosplenomegaly
- Moderate anemia
- Eosinophilia present
- Lymph node biopsy is diagnostic.

Cirrhosis (Postnecrotic) of Liver

- Symptoms and signs of chronic liver disease, e.g. weakness, malaise, muscle wasting.
- Past history of jaundice, e.g. viral hepatitis
- Features of portal hypertension, e.g. hematemesis, melena, splenomegaly, fetor hepaticus, caput medusae or distended veins on the abdomen with ascites.
- Moderate hepatosplenomegaly, firm, nontender
- Diagnosis is made by esophageal varices, splenoportal venography and liver biopsy
- Presence of other stigmatas of cirrhosis (Read case discussion on Cirrhosis of Liver).

Budd-Chiari Syndrome (Hepatic Vein Thrombosis)

- Gradual onset of symptoms
- The triad of signs and symptoms includes; gross intractable ascites, jaundice and massive tender hepatomegaly.
- Splenomegaly will occur along with hepatomegaly in patients who develop portal hypertension. Other signs of portal hypertension will also appear.
- Peripheral edema is present if there is inferior vena cava obstruction
- The diagnosis is confirmed on (i) *Doppler ultrasound* (obliteration of hepatic veins, reversed flow or associated portal vein thrombosis), (ii) *CT scan* showing enlargement of caudate lobe, (iii) *hepatic venography* showing obstruction of hepatic veins and (iv) *liver biopsy* demonstrates centrilobular congestion with fibrosis.

Enteric Fever

- History of fever which rises in step-ladder pattern, headache, diarrhea or constipation, epistaxis, cough, rose spots over skin and relative bradycardia.
- The tongue is red (angry-looking)
- Mild to moderate hepatosplenomegaly which is soft and tender, appears on 7th to 10th of fever
- Diagnosis is confirmed by blood culture and rising titers of antibodies on widal test.

Myelofibrosis/Myelosclerosis

- It may be primary or secondary to toxins, malignant infiltration of bone marrow, lymphoma or irradiation.
- Massive splenomegaly with moderate hepatomegaly due to extramedullary hematopoiesis. Splenic rub may be present occasionally.
- Leucoerythroblastic blood picture with high platelet count
- Ground glass appearance of bones on X-ray

- Bone marrow examination may yield a *"dry tap"*, hence, trephine biopsy is needed to confirm the diagnosis.

Miliary Tuberculosis

- Gradual onset of symptoms with fever, anorexia, weight loss and night sweats
- Cough, breathlessness, headache, hemoptysis may be present
- Tachycardia, tachypnea with few chest signs such as fine crackles.
- Mild to moderate hepatosplenomegaly
- Signs of meningitis may be present. CSF shows changes of meningitis
- Fundus examination may reveal choroid tubercles (25% cases)
- Leukocytosis is absent
- Montoux test is negative
- Chest X-ray shows miliary mottling shadows widely distributed in both the lungs
- Sputum examination may or may not be positive.

Amyloidosis

- It is secondary to suppurative lung disease (lung abscess, bronchiectasis), Crohn's disease, multiple myeloma, rheumatoid arthritis, leprosy
- Macroglossia may be present
- Mild to moderate hepatosplenomegaly
- Evidence of renal involvement, i.e. massive proteinuria (nephrotic syndrome)
- Other associated involvement include malabsorption, lymphadenopathy, peripheral neuropathy, cardiomyopathy
- The diagnosis is confirmed on liver, gingival or rectal biopsy.

Q. What are the causes of fever with hepatosplenomegaly?

Ans. The presence of fever indicates infection or inflammation, hence, may be associated with leukocytosis or leukopenia. The causes are:
- Parasitic infections, e.g. malaria, kala-azar
- Bacterial infection, e.g. enteric fever, brucellosis, miliary tuberculosis
- Viral infection, e.g. acute lupoid hepatitis
- Acute leukemia and lymphoma
- Hemolytic crisis.

Q. What are the causes of hepatosplenomegaly with lymphadenopathy?

Ans. The liver, spleen and lymph nodes constitute the lymphoreticular system, hence, the disorders involving this system will produce their enlargement such as;
- Acute leukemia especially ALL in children

- Lymphoma (Hodgkin's and non-Hodgkin's)
- Miliary tuberculosis
- Sarcoidosis
- AIDS
- Infectious mononucleosis
- Collagen vascular disorder, e.g. SLE.

Q. What are the causes of hepatosplenomegaly with jaundice?

Ans. Jaundice in presence of hepatosplenomegaly occurs either due to decompensation of liver or infection of the liver or due to hemolysis. The causes are:
- Cirrhosis of liver with decompensation
- Budd-Chiari syndrome (hepatic vein thrombosis)
- Lupoid hepatitis
- Malaria (falciparum infection producing hemolysis)
- Lymphoma (especially non-Hodgkin's)
- Miliary tuberculosis.

Q. What are conditions that produce hepatosplenomegaly with ascites?

Ans. Ascites in the presence of hepatosplenomegaly may be a sign of portal hypertension or hepatocellular failure or may be due to malignant infiltration of the peritoneum. The causes are:
- Malignancy liver with portal hypertension
- Cirrhosis of liver with portal hypertension
- Budd-Chiari syndrome with portal hypertension
- Chronic myeloid leukemia
- Lymphoma (non-Hodgkin's)
- Subacute or lupoid hepatitis with or without hepatocellular failure.

Q. What are the causes of congestive hepatosplenomegaly?

Ans. The conditions are:
- Congestive heart failure
- Pericardial effusion/Constrictive pericarditis
- Budd-Chiari syndrome
- Extramedullary erythropoiesis, e.g. chronic myeloid leukemia, myeloid metaplasia.

Q. How will you investigate a case of hepatosplenomegaly?

Ans. The investigations to be done are:
1. *TLC and DLC.* Leukocytosis indicates pyogenic infections, polycythemia and leukemia while leukopenia occurs in malaria, enteric fever, kala-azar. Pancytopenia indicates hypersplenism.
2. *Peripheral blood film* for MP, kala-azar (LD bodies) and hemolytic anemia (abnormal type of cells) or other types of anemia. Reticulocytosis indicates hemolytic anemia. Presence of premature WBCs indicate leukemia (acute or chronic).

3. **Blood culture** for enteric
4. **Special tests**
   - Paul-Bunnell test for infectious mononucleosis
   - Widal test for typhoid and brucella
   - Serum bilirubin for jaundice
   - Aldehyde test for kala azar
   - Tests for hemolysis, e.g. osmotic fragility, Coombs' test
5. **Radiology**
   - Chest X-ray for:
     - miliary tuberculosis (miliary mottling)
     - lymphoma and sarcoidosis (mediastinal widening due to mediastinal lymphadeno-pathy)
   - X-ray bones
     - Skull ('Hair on end' appearance in thalassemia)
     - Long bones, e.g. expansion of lower ends of the bone in Gaucher's disease. Increased density of the bones in myelofibrosis or myelosclerosis
6. **USG of abdomen**
   - To confirm hepatosplenomegaly

   - To detect the presence of ascites, portal hypertension (portal vein diameter >14 mm) and dilated venous collaterals.
   - To detect echogenic pattern of the liver (heterogenous pattern indicates cirrhosis)
7. **Biopsy**
   - Lymph node biopsy for tuberculosis, sarcoidosis and lymphoma
   - Liver biopsy for cirrhosis of the liver and amyloidosis
   - Bone marrow biopsy (trephine) for myelofi-brosis
   - Bone marrow aspiration for leukemia, lymphoma, Gaucher's disease and, hypersplenism (pancytopenia with hypercellular marrow), splenic aspirate for kala-azar.
8. **Skin tests**
   - Mantoux test for tuberculosis
   - Kveim test for sarcoidosis (not done now-a-days)
9. **CT scan abdomen**
   - To detect lymph node enlargement
   - To confirm the findings on USG
   - To stage the lymphoma.

Endocrine Disorders

CASE 24: THYROTOXICOSIS

The young female (Fig. 1.24) presented with palpitation, drenching sweats and a neck swelling. There was history of off and on loose motions and she had lost 3 kg weight past 1 month.

Examination of the patient revealed-tachycardia, rapid collapsing pulse, exophthalmose, staring look, lid log and lid retraction. The thyroid was enlarged with smooth texture. A bruit was heard over the thyroid.

Clinical Presentations

- Patients usually present with goiter (swelling in the neck) and symptoms of thyrotoxicosis. These are cases of Graves' disease and nodular goiter (Fig. 1.24).
- Patients may present with unexplained weight loss inspite of good appetite, without any diarrhea or malabsorption.

Fig. 1.24: Graves' disease

These are usually cases of occult thyro-toxicosis.

- Patients may present with arrhythmias (atrial fibrillation) especially old patients
- The young patients present with symptoms of sympathetic overactivity, i.e. palpitations, nervousness, sweating, insomnia, tremulousness, weakness, menstrual irregularity (in females)
- Patients may present with psychiatric manifestations, e.g. irritability, anger, hyperactivity, depression.

Note: Patients present in variety of ways because thyrotoxicosis disturbs the general metabolism in such a way that every system is affected and patient may present with symptoms related to any system.

History

Points to be Noted

- Record the chief complaints in chronological order and describe their details
- Ask for any restlessness, irritability, behavior change, hyperexcitability
- Ask for weight loss, increased appetite, nausea, vomiting, diarrhea
- Ask for palpitation, breathlessness, heat intolerance
- Ask for menstrual irregularity, loss of libido, gynecomastia, etc
  Ask for proximal muscle weakness or periodic paralysis.

General Physical Examination

- Look at the face for perspiration, staring look, exophthalmos, loss of frowning or wrinkling

- Look for eye signs of thyrotoxicosis, e.g. lid lag, lid retraction, exophthalmos, ophthalmoplegia, loss of accommodation
- Examine neck for thyroid enlargement. Describe the size, shape, measurement, palpate thyroid for smooth texture or nodularity and auscultate for bruit. Examine the neck veins for JVP
- Record the pulse (AF), BP (wide pulse pressure), temperature and respiration
- Look at the hands for tremors, clubbing, moistness, perspiration, warmth, palmar erythema. Shake hands with the patient to note sweaty palms.
- Examine feet for edema and legs for pretibial myxoedema.

Systemic Examination

I. CVS Examination

- Inspect the apex beat and look for cardiac enlargement
- Palpate the apex beat, define its location and other characters
- Percuss the heart for cardiomegaly
- Ausculate the heart for third heart sound, murmurs(s) or any other abnormal sound or rub.

II. Respiratory System

- Examine for crackles and rales for LVF.

III. Nervous System

- Higher function testing for psychosis
- Abnormal movements, e.g. tremors, choreoathetosis
- Examine for peripheral neuropathy, proximal myopathy, etc.

Q. What is the clinical diagnosis of the patient in picture?

Ans. The young female has symptoms and signs suggestive of thyrotoxicosis with diffuse thyroid enlargement. The probable diagnosis is Graves' disease.

Q. How do you define thyrotoxicosis?

Ans. Thyrotoxicosis implies a state of hyperthyroidism in which the thyroid hormone is toxic to the tissues producing clinical features; while hyperthyroidism

simply implies excessive thyroid function. However, both are not synonymous, yet are used interchangeably.

Q. What is Graves' disease?

Ans. It is an autoimmune disorder characterized by hyperthyroidism, diffuse goiter, ophthalmopathy and dermopathy (pretibial myxedema) and thyroid acropachy (clubbing of fingers). A thyroid scan and antithyroid antibodies (TPO, TRAb) are diagnostic.

Q. What is the differential diagnosis of thyrotoxicosis?

Ans. The two common conditions causing thyrotoxicosis are compared in the Table 1.72.

Q. What are the causes of thyrotoxicosis?

Ans. Causes of thyrotoxicosis are described in Table 1.73.

Q. What are symptoms and signs of thyrotoxicosis?

Ans. See the Table 1.74. The symptoms and signs are due to sympathetic stimulation induced by excess of thyroid hormones.

Q. How do you classify the eye changes in Graves' disease?

Ans. Many scoring systems have been used to gauge the extent and severity of orbital changes in Graves' disease. As a mnemonic, the NOSPECS scheme is used to class the eye signs as follows;

- o = **N**o sign or symptom
- 1 = **O**nly sign (lid lag or retraction), no symptoms
- 2 = **S**oft tissue involvement (pretibial myxoedema)
- 3 = **P**roptosis (>22 mm)
- 4 = **E**xtraocular muscle involvement (diplopia)
- 5 = **C**orneal involvement
- 6 = **S**ight loss

Q. How would you assess proptosis?

Ans. It is assessed by Hertel's exophthalmometer (>20 mm is considered as an exophthalmos)

Q. What is pretibial myxoedema?

Ans. Pretibial myxoedema is a late manifestation of Graves' disease.

The name justifies the site of skin changes, i.e. over the anterior and lateral aspects of the lower leg in front of tibia. The typical skin change is noninflamed, indurated, pink or purple color plaque giving an "orange-skin" appearance. Nodular involvement can uncommonly occur.

Q. What are various types of pretibial myxedema?

Ans.
1. Nonpitting edema accompanied by hyperkeratosis pigmentation and pinkish, brownish red or yellow discoloration.
2. Plaque form consisting of raised, discrete or confluent plaques.
3. Nodular form characterized by formation of nodules.

Table 1.72: Differential diagnosis of thyrotoxicosis

Feature	Graves' disease	Toxic multinodular goiter
• *Age*	Young age	Old age
• *Sex*	Common in females	Common in females
• *Goiter*	Diffuse, firm, smooth. Bruit is heard commonly	Nodular, firm to hard, irregular surface. No bruit
• *Eye signs*	Common	Uncommon
• *Dermopathy (pertibial myxoedema)*	May occur	Does not occur
• *Thyroid bruit*	*Common*	*Uncommon*
• *Severity of thyrotoxicosis*	Moderate to severe	Mild to moderate
• *Atrial fibrillation*	Uncommon	Common
• *Compressive symptoms*	Uncommon	Common
• *Cause*	Autoimmune, may be associated with other autoimmune diseases	Autonomous
• *Treatment of choice*	Drug therapy	Surgery or radioactive iodine

Q. How will you investigate a case of thyrotoxicosis?

Ans. The investigations to be performed are:
1. *Measurement of radioactive iodine uptake.* It is increased.
2. *Thyroid hormones.* The total or free T3 and T4 are increased while TSH is decreased in primary thyrotoxicosis (Graves' disease or MNG); while all the three are increased in secondary (pituitary or ectopic) thyrotoxicosis
3. *Ultrasound of thyroid* will demonstrate either the diffuse (Graves' disease) or multinodular goitre.
4. *Thyroid scan.* A radionuclide scan of thyroid either by ^{131}I or ^{99m}Tc will demonstrate functioning thyroid tissue. It will show diffuse increased uptake in Graves' disease but increased or decreased uptake in multinodular goiter. A **hot nodule** means increased uptake while **cold**

Table 1.73: Causes of thyrotoxicosis

Common (>95%)	Less common (3-5%)	Rare (<1%)
• Graves' disease	• Thyroiditis, e.g. subacute (de Quervain's and postpartum)	• Pituitary or ectopic TSH by a tumor
• Multinodular goiter	• Drug-induced (e.g. amiodarone, radioactive contrast media or iodine prophylaxis program)	• Thyroid carcinoma
• Autonomously functioning solitary thyroid nodule	• Factitious (self-induced)	
	• Struma ovarii	

Table 1.74: Symptoms and signs of Graves' disease or hyperthyroidism

1. **Goiter** (e.g. diffuse or rarely nodular)
2. **Gastrointestinal**
   - Weight loss in spite of good appetite, Vomiting, Diarrhea or steatorrhea
3. **Cardiovascular**
   - High resting pulse rate or tachycardia, Good volume pulse with wide pulse pressure (> 60 mm Hg)
   - Exertional dyspnea, Systolic hypertension
   - Arrhythmias (atrial fibrillation is common)
   - Precipitation of angina in a patient, With ischemic heart disease or cardiac failure
4. **Neuromuscular**
   - Nervousness, irritability, Restlessness, psychosis
   - Tremors of hands
   - Proximal myopathy, Exaggerated tendon reflexes
5. **Dermatological**
   - Perspiration (moist hands, increased sweating or hyperhydrosis). Warm and vasodilated peripheries
   - Clubbing of fingers (rare), Loss of hair
   - Pre-tibial myxoedema, Thyroid acropathy
   - Redness of palms (palmar erythema)
6. **Reproductive**
   - Menstrual irregularity (amenorrhea is common)
   - Abortions, Infertility, Loss of libido or impotence
7. **Ophthalmological**
   - Lid lag or lid retraction, Staring look
   - Wide palpebral fissure, Exophthalmos
   - Diplopia or ophthalmoplegia, Excessive watering of eyes
8. **Miscellaneous**
   - Heat intolerance, Excessive thirst
   - Outburst of anger, Fatiguability or apathy

nodule indicates decreased uptake. Thyroid scan will also detect an ectopic thyroid tissue in the neck or chest.

5. *Antithyroid antibodies.* Antithyroid antibodies are detected in Graves' disease and Hashimoto's thyroiditis. TRAb antibodies and TPO antibodies are raised in Graves' disease.

6. *Needle biopsy* of the thyroid is done in MNG to detect underlying malignancy.

7. *Other tests* such as ECG for tachycardias and arrhythmias.
   - CT scan or MRI, TSH suppression tests for pituitary origin of thyrotoxicosis.

8. *Other biochemical abnormalities* are; (i) raised bilirubin and transferases, (ii) raised calcium and glycosuria or impaired glucose tolerance. These are due to other autoimmune diseases associated with it.

Q. What are the causes low TSH?

Ans.
- Subclinical hyperthyroidism
- Overt hyperthyroidism
- First trimester of pregnancy
- Medications e.g. dopamine, steroids
- Non-thyroidal illness with low free T4.

Q. Name the other autoimmune diseases associated with thyrotoxicosis.

Ans. These are:
- Diabetes mellitus
- Hyperparathyroidism
- Chronic active hepatitis
- Autoimmune hemolytic anemia

Q. What is subclinical hyperthyroidism?

Ans. In this condition, the serum T3 and T4 are either normal or lie in the upper limit of their respective reference range and the serum TSH is undetectable. This combination is found in patients with nodular goiter. These patients are at increased risk of atrial fibrillation and osteoporosis, hence, the consensus view is to treat such cases with ^{131}I. As these cases can transform to overt hyperthyroidism, therefore, annual review is mandatory.

Q. What is thyroiditis (hyperthyroidism with reduced iodine uptake)?

Ans. In patients with hyperthyroidism, the RAIU is usually high but a low or negligible uptake of iodine occurs in some rare causes of hyperthyroidism such as thyroiditis (subacute or postpartum). If a radioactive iodine uptake (RAIU) test is not routinely performed in patients with hyperthyroidism, such cases are likely to be missed and inappropriate treatment may be given.

1. *Subacute (de Quervain's) thyroiditis.* It is a viral – induced (*coxsackie, mumps, adenovirus*) thyroiditis in which there is release of colloid and thyroid hormones into circulation leading to hyperthyroidism.

   It is characterized by fever, pain in the region of thyroid gland which may radiate to angle of the jaw and the ears, made worse by swallowing, coughing and movements of neck. The thyroid gland is enlarged and tender. It is seen in young females 20-40 years.

   The thyroid hormones levels are high for 4-6 weeks but RAIU is low indicating transient hyperthyroidism which is followed by asymptomatic hypothyroidism and finally erythyroid state is achieved with full recovery within 3-6 months. No treatment is required except steroids and betablockers for initial period of hyperthyroidism.

2. *Postpartum thyroiditis.* It is subacute autoimmune thyroiditis occurring during postpartum period or within 6 month of delivery. These women exhibit biochemical disturbances of thyroid function reflecting hyperthyroidism, hypothyroidism and hyperthyroidism followed by hypothyroidism lasting for few weeks. These patients have antithyroid peroxidase (TPO) antibodies in the serum in early pregnancy. Thyroid biopsy shows lymphocytic thyroiditis. These patients are asymptomatic. Thyroid scan shows low iodine uptake.

Postpartum thyroiditis tends to recur after subsequent pregnancies, hence may ultimately lead to permanent hypothyroidism.No treatment is needed except beta blockers during early period of hyperthyroidism.

Q. **What are the causes of hyperthyroidism with reduced iodine uptake?**

Ans. • Thyroiditis (de Quervain's and postpartum)
• Malignancy thyroid
• Struma ovarii

Q. **What are the complications of hyperthyroidism?**

Ans. They are:
1. Precipitation of angina in a patient with IHD and CHF and digitalis toxicity in patients with valvular heart disease receiving digitalis.
2. Cardiac arrhythmias (atrial fibrillation is the most common)
3. Thyrotoxic myopathy (proximal muscle weakness)
4. Thyrotoxic hypokalemic periodic paralysis
5. Thyrotoxic crisis/thyroid storm
6. Malabsorption syndrome.

Q. **What are the eye signs of thyrotoxicosis?**

Ans. The various eye signs are:

von Graefe's: Upper lid lag

Joffroy's: Absence of wrinkling on forehead when asked to look upwards with face inclined downward.

Gilford's: Non-retraction of upper lid manually.

Loclur's: Stare look.

Naffziger's: Protrusion from superciliary phase

Dalrymple's: Visible upper sclera.

Moebius: Failure to converge eyeballs.

Stellwags': Stare look, infrequent blinking, widening of palpebral fissure.

N.B.: Read the signs and their method of demonstration in clinical methods in medicine by Dr SN Chugh.

Q. **Name the treatment modalities available for Graves' disease**

Ans. • Drug treatment
• Subtotal thyroidectomy
• Radioactive iodine therapy

Q. **Which drugs are used in thyrotoxicosis?**

Ans. • Carbimazole
• Methimazole
• Propylthiouracil

Q. **Which drug is safest in pregnancy?**

Ans. Propylthiouracil

Q. **What are disadvantages of drug treatment in thyrotoxicosis?**

Ans. • High rate of relapse once treatment is withdrawn
• Troublesome hypersensitivity reaction
• Rarely life threatening agranulocytosis and hepatitis may occur

Q. **What are indications of radioiodine therapy in thyrotoxicosis?**

Ans. • Graves' disease with large goiter and relapse on treatment
• Multinodular goiter
• Toxic adenoma
• Ablation therapy in those with severe manifestations such as heart failure, AF or psychosis.

Q. **What are contraindications of radioiodine in thyrotoxicosis?**

Ans. • Breastfeeding and pregnancy
• Allergy to iodine

Q. **Does thyrotoxicosis affect bone?**

Ans. Yes, it causes osteoporosis

Q. **What is the effect of iodine on thyroid status?**

Ans. It may cause transient hypothyroidism (*Wolff-Chaikoff effect*) or hyperthyroidism (*Jod-Basedow effect*)

Q. **What are indications of subtotal thyroidectomy?**

Ans. • Large goiter
• Patient's preference
• Drug noncompliance
• Disease relapse on drug withdrawl

CASE 25: HYPOTHYROIDISM

The young girl (12 yr) (Fig. 1.25A) presented with puffiness of face, weight gain, hoarseness of voice, protuberent abdomen, laziness, and lethargy. She has dropped schooling at the age of 10. She has delayed milestones and has mental insufficiency according to the parents. The another patient 35 yr F (Fig. 1.25B) presented with recent weight gain, constipation, cold intolerance and puffiness of face with hoarseness of voice.

Examination revealed mental insufficiency (IQ 50%) in patient (Fig. 1.25A), otherwise both the patients have coarse facial features, thick lips, puffiness of face, thick dry rough skin, bradycardia, hoarseness and nonpitting pedal edema. The patient (Fig. 1.25B) has hypertension (BP 150/100 mmHg).

Clinical Presentations

1. Infants (<1 year) present with mental retardation, pot belly, large protruding tongue (macroglossia), flat nose, dry skin, sparse hair and delayed milestones of development. Other features of hypothyroidism are present. The condition is called *Cretinism*. This may persist in childhood.
2. The adolescents with hypothyroidism (juvenile hypothyroidism) present with short stature, retarded growth, poor performance at school, delayed puberty and sexual maturation. Other features of adult hypothyroidism are present.
3. The adult patients present usually with myxedema in which features of hypothyroidism are associated with myxomatous changes in skin (dry, toad-like skin, puffiness of face, hands and feet), larynx (hoarseness of voice or slurred speech), and ear (leading to deafness). They may complain of carpal tunnel syndrome (entrapment neuropathy).
4. Majority of the women with mild hypothyroidism present with increase in weight, menstrual irregularity, mental feature (depression) or slowness of activity and generalized ache and pains.

History

Points to be Noted

- Onset of symptoms and their progression
- History of recent weight gain, change in appearance and voice, malaise, tiredness and slowness of activity
- History of cold intolerance, change in mood or behavior disturbance, deafness
- History of arthralgia, myalgia, dryness of skin, decreased sweating
- History of menstrual irregularity, poor libido, sterlity
- History of anorexia, constipation
- History of delayed milestones, slow mentation or mental insufficiency in a child
- History of infertility, depression, muscle cramps, dementia
- History of radioiodine therapy for Graves disease or medications (e.g. lithium, amiodarone, contrast agents, iodine containing expectorant's
- Family history of thyroid disorder, DM, Addison's disease etc.

General Physical Examination (GPE)

- *Face.* Note puffiness or periorbital edema, coarse thick facial appearance, rounded face, peaches and cream complexion (Fig. 1.25)
- *Eyes* for xanthelasma, loss of outer third of eyebrows
- *Tongue.* Large protruding (macroglossia)
- *Lips* thick
- Neck examination for JVP, thyroid enlargement and lymph node, scar of thyroidecomy
- Pulse, BP, temp. and respiration
- *Skin.* Note the texture, dryness, coarse (toad-like)
- *Hair.* The hair are sparse, thin, brittle in hypothyroidism
- *Hands.* Dry cold hands, thick skin, creases of palm prominent, carpal tunnel syndrome
- *Feet.* Note dryness and nonpitting edema.

Systemic Examination

I. CVS Examination

- Examine the heart for evidence of CHF and pericardial effusion.

II. Examination of Abdomen

- For adynamic ileus and any organ enlargement.

III. Nervous System

- Higher function for mental insufficiency
- VIII nerve exam. For deafness
- Motor system for myopathy (proximal), myotonia and for delayed reflexes
- Sensory system for peripheral neuropathy, carpal tunnel syndrome

IV. Respiratory System

- Chest wall is thick with decreased and slow movements

Figs 1.25A and B: Hypothyroidism. A. Cretinism (infantile onset of hypothyroidism); B. Adult hypothyroidism

Q. What is your clinical diagnosis?

Ans. The patient 1 (12-yr F) has features suggestive of juvenile hypothyroidism (cretinism). Read the features in next question. The patient 2, adult female has all features suggestive of myxoedema (adult hypothyroidism).

Q. What are the clinical features of hypothyroidism in these cases?

Ans. The clinical features of hypothyroidism are tabulated (Table 1.75). Most of the clinical features were present.

Q. What are cardiovascular manifestations in hypothyroidism?

Ans. Read Table 1.75

Q. What are neurological manifestations in hypothyroidism?

Ans. Read Table 1.75

Q. What is hypothyroidism?

Ans. Hypothyroidism is a clinical condition reflecting hypofunctioning of thyroid gland, characterized by low levels of circulating thyroid hormones. It is called *primary* when the cause of it lies in the thyroid gland itself. It becomes *secondary* when hypothyroidism occurs due to disease of anterior pituitary or hypothalamus.

Goitrous hypothyroidism means enlargement of thyroid gland associated with hypothyroidism.

Subclinical hypothyroidism means biochemical evidence of hypothyroidism (low to normal T3 and T4 but raised TSH) without any symptoms of hypothyroidism (asymptomatic hypothyroidism). The cause of subclinical hypothyroidism are same as described under transient hypothyroidism. It may persist for many years. Treatment with replacement therapy with small dose of thyroxine is indicated.

Transient hypothyroidism refers to a state of reversible thyroid function, often observed during the first 6 months of:

1. Subtotal thyroidectomy or I^{131} treatment of Graves' disease
2. Post-thyrotoxic phase of subacute thyroiditis
3. Postpartum thyroiditis
4. In some neonates, transplacental passage of TSH receptors-binding antibodies (TRAbs) from the mother with Graves' disease or autoimmune thyroid disease may cause transient hypothyroidism.

Congenital hypothyroidism is asymptomatic state detected during routine screening of TSH levels in spot blood samples obtained 5-7 days after birth. It results either from thyroid agenesis, ectopic hypoplastic glands or from dyshormogenesis. Early detection and early treatment with replacement thyroxine therapy is mandatory to prevent irreversible brain damage.

Q. What are the causes of hypothyroidism?

Ans. These are:

1. *Spontaneous atrophic or idiopathic hypothyroidism*
2. *Goitrous hypothyroidism*
   - Hashimoto's thyroiditis
   - Iodine deficiency
   - Drug-induced (PAS, phenylbutazone, lithium, iodides)
   - Dyshormogenesis
3. *Postablative*
   - Following surgery
   - Following ^{131}I
4. *Transient during thyroiditis*
   - Subacute
   - Postpartum
5. *Maternally transmitted* (iodides, antithyroid drugs, TRABs antibodies)

Table 1.75: Symptoms and signs of adult hypothyroidism

General features	Tiredness, weight gain, cold intolerance, hoarseness of voice and lethargy are common. Somnolence and goiter are less common. Non-pitting edema over feet and legs common. "Peaches and cream" complexion may occur
Cardiovascular	Slow pulse rate or bradycardia, hypertension and xanthelasma are common
	Pericardial effusion, precipitation of angina and cardiac failure less common
Neuromuscular	Aches and pains, delayed relaxation of ankle jerks, muscle stiffness are common
	Carpal tunnel syndrome, deafness, psychosis, depression, myotonia and proximal myopathy are less common, myxoedema madness and myxoedema coma are rare. Hoffmann's syndrome (muscle aches with myotomia) is also rare.
Hematological	Anemia may be present
Dermatological	Dry thick skin (toad skin), sparse hair including loss of hair on lateral third of eyebrow, nonpitting edema are common. Hypothermia is common. Vitiligo and alopecia are rare
Reproductive	Menorrhagia, infertility (common), galactorrhoea and impotence (less common)
Gastrointestinal	Constipation (common) and adynamic ileus (less common)

Q. What is thyroid status in Hashimoto's thyroiditis?

Ans. Read Table 1.76. Usually there is hypothyroidism in Hashimoto's thyroiditis

Q. What is best clinical parameter of hypothyroidism?

Ans. Delayed ankle jerks

Q. How would you record delayed ankle jerks?

Ans. Photomotogram

Q. What is the cause of delayed relaxation of jerks in hypothyroidism?

Ans. The exact cause is unknown. It is probably due to decreased muscle metabolism

Q. What is Pendred's syndrome?

Ans. It is a genetically determind syndrome (autosomal inheritance) consisting of a combination of dyshormonogenetic goitre, mental retardation and nerve deafness. The dyshormogenesis is due to deficiency of intrathyroidial peroxidase enzyme.

Q. What is the relation between iodine and hypothyroidism?

Ans. Both iodine deficiency and iodine excess can produce hypothyroidism.

Iodine when taken for prolonged period (iodine excess) in the form of expectorants containing potassium iodide or use of amiodarone (contains a significant amount of iodine) may cause goitrous hypothyroidism by inhibiting the release of thyroid hormones. This is common in patients with underlying autoimmune thyroiditis.

Iodine deficiency in certain parts of the world especially Himalayas, produces endemic goiter (>70% of the population is affected). Most of the patients usually are euthyroid and have normal or raised TSH levels. In general, more severe is the iodine deficiency, the greater is the incidence of hypothyroidism.

Q. How will you diagnose hypothyroidism?

Ans. The diagnosis is made on the basis of:

1. Clinical manifestations
2. Investigations

The investigations are done to confirm the diagnosis, to differentiate between primary and secondary hypothyroidism, for follow-up of treatment and to monitor the response. The TSH levels are used to monitor the response to treatment (Table 1.77).

Q. What are other laboratory changes in hypothyroidism?

Ans. • *Serum cholesterol* is high (hypercholestrolemia)
• *ECG* may show bradycardia, low voltage graph and ST-T changes
• *Blood examination* may reveal anemia (usually normocytic or macrocytic)
• *Thyroid peroxidase antibodies (TPO)* help to find out the cause of hypothyroidism. Their presence indicate autoimmune thyroiditis as the cause of hypothyroidism.
• *X-ray chest*. It may be normal or may show cardiomegaly due to pericardial effusion – common in primary rather than secondary hypothyroidism.

Table 1.77: Thyroid hormone levels in various forms of hypothyroidism

Hormone	Primary	Secondary	Subclinical
T3	Low	Low	Normal (lower limit of normal)
T4	Low	Low	Normal (lower limit of normal)
TSH	High	Low	Slightly high

Table 1.76: Differentiation between two common diffuse goiter

Features	Simple diffuse goiter	Goiter due to Hashimoto thyroiditis
Age	Common in young girls (15-25 years) or during pregnancy	Common in young females (20-50 years)
Thyroid enlargement	Mild, tends to be noticed by friends and relatives	Large, visible from distance
Goiter	Soft, nontender	Firm, tender
Prevalence	Endemic or sporadic	Sporadic
Symptoms	Asymptomatic or there is a tight sensation in neck Patient seeks medical attention from asthetic point of view	Pain radiating to jaw or neck, increased during swallowing, coughing and neck movements
Cause	Suboptimal dietary iodine intake and minor degrees of dyshormogenesis	Autoimmune disease, may be associated with other autoimmune conditions
Thyroid status	Normal	25% cases are hypothyroid at presentation, others become later on. Initially, there may be transient thyrotoxicosis
Thyroid antibodies (TPO antibodies)	Negative	Positive (95% cases)

118

- Hyperprolactinemia
- Hyponatremia

Q. What is best laboratory indicator in hypothyroidism?

Ans. Elevated TSH level

Q. What are causes of raised TSH?

Ans.
- Subclinical hypothyroidism
- Overt hypothyroidism
- Medications such as lithium and amiodarone.
- Recovery from hypothyroxinemia of non thyroidal disorders.

Q. What do you understand by subclinical hypothyroidism?

Ans. This is a condition characterized by low normal serum thyroxine levels with elevated serum TSH > 10 mIU.

Q. How would you treat hypothyroidism?

Ans. Oral thyroxine replacement is given for life long. Therapeutic dose varies from 100 to 200 μg/day taken as single dose empty stomach and adjustments are made once in 3 weeks. The dose is adjusted depending on the clinical response and suppression of TSH levels.

Lack of response indicates poor compliance, an underlying psychiatric abnormalities or an associated autoimmune disease (e.g. Addison's disease)

Q. What precaution would you take while prescribing thyroxine in elderly?

Ans. Rapid T4 replacement in elderly may precipitate angina and myocardial infarction, hence, starting dose of thyroxine in elderly should be low (50 μg/day)

Q. How does simple goiter differ from goitrous hypothyroidism?

Ans. The difference between simple diffuse goiter and Hashimoto's thyroiditis are given in Table 1.76.

Q. What are the complications of myxedema?

Ans. Complications arise as a result of infiltration of myxomatous tissue in various other structures, especially in primary myxedema.

1. *CVS*, e.g. pericardial effusion, restrictive cardiomyopathy, conduction disturbances
2. *Respiratory*. Cor pulmonale, type 2 respiratory failure
3. *Myxedematous* madness and myxedema coma
4. *Entrapement neuropathy* (Carpal-Tunnel syndrome).

CASE 26: DIABETES MELLITUS

I. An 18 years male (Fig. 1.26A) presented with diabetic ketoacidosis as an emergency. On recovery he gave history of polyuria, polydipsia, polyphagia and weakness.

II. A 45 years female (Fig. 1.26B) presented with history of polyuria, polydipsia and puffiness of face and edema feet. She admitted a past history of diabetes for the last 5 yrs taking antidiabetic medication. Her BP was 160/100 mm Hg in right arm in lying down position.

Clinical Presentations

1. Asymptomatic diabetes. The diabetes is detected on investigations.
2. Type 1 diabetics (acute presentation)
   - Type I diabetics present with a symptom triad of polyuria, polydipsia and polyphagia along with weakness and marked weight loss.
3. Subacute presentation: The clinical onset may be over several months; occurs commonly in older patients who complain of thirst, polyuria, weight loss, lack of energy, visual disturbance, changes in eye-refraction and pruritus vulvae (in females).
4. Type 1 diabetics may also present with complications such as ketoacidosis, diabetic neuropathy and/or nephropathy.
5. Type 2 diabetics present in different speciality with different complaints (Table 1.78).

Fig. 1.26A: Type 1 diabetes

History

Points to be Noted

- Onset of symptoms and their course
- Ask any history of fever, cough, expectoration, hemoptysis, pain chest, night sweats, fatigue, etc.
- Ask for history of dysuria, pyuria, increased frequency, burning micturition
- History of chronic diarrhea, vomiting, gastric distention
- History of breathlessness, orthopnea, PND, etc.
- Ask for edema feet or legs
- History of menstrual irregularity, sterility, vaginal discharge etc.
- History of paraesthesias, loss of sensations, motor deficit (monoplegia, paraplegia, etc), facial asymmetry, deafness, mental features, disturbance in consciousness
- Ask for symptoms of hypoglycemia such as profuse sweating, palpitation, air hunger, nausea and convulsions, etc.
- History of visual disturbance or visual loss or decreased vision.

General Physical Examination

- Body habitus/fat distribution
- Dry mouth/dehydration (dry tongue)
- Air hunger
- Skin and mucosal sepsis, candidiasis
- Skin pigmentation, vitiligo, dermopathy
- Weight loss (insulin deficiency)
- Obesity-may be abdominal (insulin resistance)
- White spots on shoes (glycosuria)
- Deep sighing respiration (Kussmaul breathing)
- Eyes for xanthelasma (Fig. 1.26B), evidence of infection

Fig. 1.26B: Type 2 diabetes

- Ear for infection and deafness
- Neck examination for JVP, lymph nodes enlargement and carotid pulsations
- Record pulse, BP, temperature and respiration.

Insulin Injection Sites

Main areas used and the abnormalities thereof
- Anterior abdominal wall
- Upper thighs/buttocks
- Upper outer arms
- Lumps (lipodystrophy)
- Subcutaneous fat deposition (lipohypertrophy)
- Subcutaneous fat loss (lipoatrophy; associated with injection of unpurified animal insulins—now rare)
- Erythema, infection (rare)

Examination of the Hands

- Limited joint mobility (sometimes called *cheiroarthropathy*) may be present. This is the inability to extend (150° to 180°) the metacarpophalangeal or interphalangeal joints of at least one finger bilaterally. The effect can be demonstrated in the *prayer's sign*. causes painless stiffness in the hands, and it occasionally affects the wrists and shoulders.
- *Dupuytren's contracture* is common in diabetes and may include nodules or thickening of the skin and knuckle pads
- *Carpal tunnel syndrome* is common in diabetes and presents with wrist pain radiating to the hand
- *Trigger finger* (flexor tenosynovitis) may be present in people with diabetes
- Muscle-wasting /sensory changes may be present as features of a peripheral sensorimotor neuropathy, although this is more common in the lower limbs.

Examination of the Feet

- Look for evidence of callus formation on weight-bearing areas, clawing of the toes (a feature of neuropathy), loss of the plantar arch, discoloration of the skin (ischemia), localized infection and the presence of ulcers.
- Deformity of the feet may be present, especially in Charcot neuroarthropathy.
- Fungal infection may affect skin between toes, and nails.

Examination of Legs

- Muscle wasting, sensory abnormality
- Granuloma annulare, lipoid dystrophica diabeticorum
- Hair loss
- Tendon reflexes lost

Systemic Examination

I. Nervous System

- Test higher mental functions.
- Cranial nerve examination.

Visual acuity
- Distance vision using Snellen chart at 6 metres
- Near vision using standard reading chart
- Impaired visual acuity may indicate the presence of diabetic eye disease, and serial decline may suggest development or progression in severity.

Lens opacification
- Look for the red reflex using the ophthalmoscope held 30 cm from the eye

- The presence of lens opacities or cataract should be noted.

Fundus examination
- The pupils must be dilated with a mydriatic (e.g. tropicamide) and examined in a dark clear room.
- Features of diabetic retinopathy should be noted including evidence of previous laser treatment which leaves photocoagulation scars.

Sensations; test the followings;
- Light touch.
- Vibration sense: use of 128 Hz tuning fork over big toe/malleoli
- Pin-prick: use pin.
- Pain: pressure over Achilles tendon, calf tenderness on squeezing
- Proprioception: test position sense at big toe
- Test for distal anesthesia/hypoaesthesia in glove-stocking distribution.

Reflexes
- Test plantar and ankle reflexes.
- Test other reflexes also.

II. Cardiovascular System

- Pulses. Palpate all the peripheral pulses. Capillary refill should be tested
- Examine the heart for cardiomegaly. Auscultate the heart for any murmur or rub or an abnormal sound.

III. Respiratory System

- Examine for any evidence of tuberculosis, pneumonia, pleural effusion or empyema.

IV. Examination of Abdomen

- Palpate for liver, spleen or kidney enlargement
- Palpate for any other mass.

V. Genitourinary System

- Examine the penis for evidence of infection or discharge per urethra. Examine scrotum and epididymus for tenderness or swelling
- Examine vulva and vagina for evidence of infection and discharge. Peform per vaginal examination also.

Q. What is your clinical diagnosis?

Ans. Type 1 DM with ketoacidosis in case no. 1
Type 2 DM with nephropathy in case no. 2

Q. What are the points in favor of your diagnosis?

Ans. Case No 1
- Young adult (30 yrs)
- H/o polyuria, polydipsia and polyphagia
- Presence of ketoacidosis

Case No 2
- Middle aged female
- Obesity
- Polyuria, polydipsia and polyphagia
- Xanthalesma
- Puffiness of face, edema and hypertension indicate nephropathy.

Q. What bedside test would you like to perform to confirm the diagnosis?

Ans.
- Urine exam for sugar, proteins and ketone bodies
- Bedside blood sugar by glucometer, if possible.

Q. How do you define diabetes mellitus and impaired glucose tolerance (IGT)?

Ans. A clinical syndrome of hyperglycemia with or without glycosuria either due to lack of insulin (type 1) or insufficiency of insulin with insulin resistance (type 2) is termed diabetes mellitus.

Impaired glucose tolerance (IGT): is defined as an abnormal response to 75 g of oral glucose on glucose tolerance test. Fasting blood sugar < 126 mg and postprandial glucose between 180 and 200 mg indicate IGT.

Q. What is gestational diabetes mellitus (GDM)?

Ans. Glucose tolerance is impaired during pregnancy, results as a result of insulin resistance related to metabolic changes of late pregnancy, increases insulin requirement and may lead to impaired glucose tolerance and GDM. GDM occurs in about 4% women during pregnancy which reverts to normal glucose tolerance in postpartum, but there is risk of developing permanent DM later in life.

Q. What is classical triad of type 1 DM?

Ans. Polyuria, polydipsia and polyphagia is clinical triad and hallmark of Type 1 DM.

Q. What is the clinical presentations of type 2 diabetes?

Ans. See the Table 1.78.

Q. How do you classify diabetes?

Ans. The broad categories of DM are type 1 and type 2. Type I is divided into A and B. A means immunological destruction of pancreas leading to insulin deficiency (autoimmune type) while B is nonautoimmune idiopathic (Table 1.79). Type 2 DM is heterogenous group of disorders characterised by variable degree of insulin resistance, impaired glucose secretion and increased glucose production. Type 2

Table 1.78: Clinical presentation of type 2 DM (NIDDM)

These patients present to different specialities or superspecialities with following features which arise as a result of complications. The organs/systems involvment and their presenting features are as follows:

Organ/system affected	Clinical presentation
• Eye	• Recurrent styes, chalazion, anterior uveitis (hypopyon), frequent change of glasses due to error of refraction, visual impairment due to premature development of cataract or retinopathy
• Urinary tract	• Urinary tract infections, acute pyelitis or pyelonephritis, nephrotic syndrome
• GI tract	• Chronic diarrhoea, malabsorption, gastroparesis (dilatation of stomach)
• Genital tract	• Females present with pruritus vulvae, vaginal discharge, menstrual irregularities, recurrent abortions, infertility, etc.
• Cardiovascular	• Ischemic heart disease, hypertension, peripheral vascular disease (cold extremities, absent peripheral pulses, gangrene or diabetic foot)
• Nervous	• Peripheral neuritis (tingling sensations in the extremities with numbness) symptoms of autonomic neuropathy (Table 1.93), cerebral ischemic episodes and strokes.
• Skin	• Multiple boils, carbuncles, abscesses, non-healing wounds, mucocutaneous candidiasis
• Respiratory	• Pneumonias, lung abscess, tuberculosis, etc.

Table 1.79: Classification of DM based on etiology

I. **Type 1 diabetes mellitus** (beta-cell destruction with absolute insulin deficiency)
   A. Immune-mediated
   B. Unknown mechanism (idiopathic)
II. **Type 2 DM** (either due to insulin resistance with relative insulin deficiency or insulin secretion defect with insulin resistance)
III. **Other specific types of diabetes**
   A. Genetic defect of beta-cell function leading to gene mutation)
      • MODY I (hepatocyte nuclear transcription factor (HNF-4-alpha)
      • MODY 2 (Glucokinase). MODY3 (HNF-1-alpha) MODY4 (insulin promotor factor, MODY5 (HNF-1-beta), MODY 6(Neuro DI)
      • Proinsulin or insulin conversion
   B. Genetic defect in insulin action
      • Type I insulin resistant.
      • Lipodystrophy syndromes
   C. Pancreatic diabetes (pancreatitis, hemochromatosis, cystic fibrosis)

Contd...

Contd...

   D. Endocrinopathies (acromegaly, Cushing's syndrome, thyrotoxicosis, pheochromocytoma)
   E. Drug and chemical induced
   F. Other genetic syndromes, e.g. Down's and Klinefelter's syndrome, DIDMOAD (diabetes insipidus, DM, optic atrophy and deafness) Turner's syndrome, hereditary ataxia, Huntington's chorea, Laurence-Moon-Biedl and dystrophic myotonia
IV. Gestational diabetes mellitus (GDM)

DM is preceded by a period of abnormal glucose homeostasis classified as impaired fasting glycaemia or impaired glucose tolerance also called prediabetic states.

Q. What are prediabetic states?

Ans. • Impaired fasting glucose (IFG)
• Impaired glucose tolerance (IGT)
Both are prediabetic states.

Q. What is pathogenesis of type 1 diabetes?

Ans. It is considered as an autoimmune disorder. The various criteria of autoimmunity are given in the Box 26.1. Genetic susceptibility is a major determinant while environmental factors act as a trigger to initiate autoimmune destruction of beta cells of the pancreas. The genetic predisposition is HLA linked class II genes at D locus (DR_3 and D_4) on short arm of chromosome 6. Immunological response results in production of class II beta cell specific molecules which play a role in autoimmune destruction. Beta cell mass declines, insulin secretion becomes progressively impaired although normal glucose tolerance is maintained. The rate of decline of beta-cell mass varies with some patients progressing rapidly to clinical diabetes, while other evolving slowly. Features of diabetes will appear once > 80% of beta cells have been destroyed. At this point, residual functional existing beta cells are insufficient in number to maintain glucose tolerance. Thus, there is a transition period between impaired glucose tolerance with increase in requirement of insulin to frank diabetes. After the onset of type IA diabetes, there is *"honey-moon"* period of 1 to 2 years during which glycemic control is achieved with modest dose of insulin or rarely, insulin is not required. This is a transient or fleeting phase of endogenous

BOX 26.1: POINTS IN FAVOR OF AUTOIMMUNITY

• HLA linkage
• Its association with other autoimmune disorders
• Lymphocytic infiltration of beta cells pancreas
• Circulating anti-insulin antibodies
• Recurrence of beta cells destruction in pancreas

insulin production from beta cells, which subsequently disappears as the autoimmune process progresses and ultimately individual becomes completely insulin deficient.

Q. What is pathogenesis of clinical features of type 1 diabetes and ketoacidosis?

Ans. Lack of insulin stimulates counter-regulatory hormone release, e.g. glucagon, GH and catecholamines in addition to stimulation of catabolism of nutrients producing neoglucogenesis, glycogenolysis and liposis and subsequently ketoacidosis. Lack of insulin results in hyperglycemia due to increased hepatic output of glucose and poor peripheral utilization of glucose. Glycosuria, osmotic diuresis and salt and water loss are its consequences which produce various clinical features of type I diabetes. Diabetic ketoacidosis is an acute metabolic complication, requires urgent diagnosis and management.

Q. What are the differences between type 1 and type 2 DM?

Ans. Table 1.80 deals with general clinical characteristics of type 1 and type 2 DM.

Q. How do you diagnose DM?

Ans. Table 1.81 describes criteria for diagnosing diabetes mellitus and other related complications.

Q. What are characteristics of hyperosmolar Non-ketotic Diabetic Coma?

Ans. It is common in elderly people with type 2 diabetes with several weeks history of polyuria, weight loss and diminished oral intake followed by confusion and coma. The physical examination reveals marked dehydration, hypotension, tachycardia and altered mental status. The GI symptoms and Kussmaul acidotic breathing are notably absent.

The **biochemical characteristics** of this coma include:

- Hyperglycaemia (blood glucose >600 mg%)

Table 1.80: General clinical characteristics of type 1 and type 2 DM

Features	(Type 1) (Fig. 1.26A)	(Type 2) (Fig. 1.26B)
1. Gene locus	Chromosome 6	Chromosome 11
2. Age of onset	< 30 years	> 30 years
3. Onset of symptoms	Rapid	Slow
4. Body weight	Thin, lean	Normal weight or obese
5. Duration of symptoms	Weeks	Months or years
6. Presenting features	Polyuria, polydipsia polyphagia	Present with different compli-cations
7. Ketonuria	Present (Ketone-prone)	Absent (Ketone-resistant)
8. Complications at the time of diagnosis	Absent	Present (10-20%)
9. Family history	Negative	Positive
10. Plasma insulin	Low or absent	Normal to high
11. Choice of treatment	Insulin	Oral hypoglycemics
12. Mortality if untreated	High	Low

- Hyperosmolality (>350 mOsm/l). Normal osmolality 280-290 mOsm/l.
- Absent or minimal ketone body in the blood or urine. The marked dehydration and relative deficiency of insulin are presumed to be factors for absence of ketosis in this coma. Acidosis is also absent.
- Pre-renal azotemia

Q. What are factors which push a contolled patient of diabetes into uncontrolled state or coma?

Ans.
- Acute concurrent illness
- Infection, sepsis
- Acute catastrophic event, e.g. MI, stroke
- Hemodialysis or any other procedure

Table 1.81: American Diabetic Association (1997) criteria endorsed by WHO (1998) for diagnosis of diabetes or other related conditions

Condition	Venous plasma glucose concentration in mg% (mmol/L)	
	Fasting	Postprandial (2 hr GTT)
Normal	<110 (6.1)	<140 (7.3)
Diabetes	>126	>200
	Or	
	Symptoms of diabetes plus random blood sugar ≥ 200 mg% (11.1 mmol/l)	
Impaired fasting glycemia	110-126 (6.1-7.0)	<140 (7.8)
Impaired glucose tolerance	<126 (7.0)	≥140 but <200 (7.8-11.1)

Note: 2 hours GTT means following 75 g glucose load. Venous blood glucose concentration is lower than capillary blood. Whole blood glucose is lower than plasma because RBC contain little glucose.

Q. Name the various types of coma in DM.

Ans. These are:

1. Diabetic ketotic coma (common in type 1 diabetics)
2. Hyperosmolar hyperglycemic, nonketotic coma (common in type 2 diabetics)
3. Hypoglycemic coma (common in both type 1 and type 2 diabetics)
4. Lactic acidosis coma.

Q. What are chronic or late complications of DM?

Ans. Chronic complications can be divided into vascular and nonvascular (Table 1.82); the vascular are further divided into microvascular and macrovascular. Since type 2 DM has a long asymptomatic period of hyperglycemia, many individuals with type 2 DM have complications at the time of diagnosis.

Q. What are pathogenic mechanisms for complications of DM?

Ans. The pathogenic mechanisms are:

- Activation of polyol pathway
- Formation of advanced glycation end products (AGEs) leading to endothelial dysfunction
- Activation of protein kinase-C-second messanger system
- Oxidative stress

All these mechanisms lead to endothelial dysfunction and development of vascular complications.

Table 1.82: Chronic or long-term complications of DM

I. Vascular

  A. *Microvascular*

   i. Eye disease
    - Retinopathy (see Table 1.85)
    - Macular edema

   ii. Neuropathy, e.g. sensory, motor, mixed, autonomic (see Table 1.84)

   iii. Nephropathy

  B. *Macrovascular*
   - Coronary artery disease
   - Peripheral vascular disease
   - Cerebrovascular disease
   - Diabetic foot
   - Hypertension

II. Others/nonvascular
   - Gastrointestinal, e.g. gastroparesis, diarrhoea
   - Genitourinary (nephropathy (Fig. 1.26C)/sexual dysfunction)
   - Dermatologic
   - Infections/pressure sore (Fig. 1.26D)
   - Cataracts
   - Glaucoma

Q. What are various neurological complications in DM? How do you manage them?

Ans. These may be somatic or autonomic (Table 1.83).

Q. What are the autonomic disturbances in diabetes?

Ans. Read the Table 1.83.

Table 1.83: Classification, clinical features and steps of management of diabetic neuropathy

Classification	Symptoms and signs	Treatment
1. Somatic a. **Symmetric sensory and distal (Large fiber, small fiber, mixed type)**	• Tingling or burning sensation in the extremities (hands and feet), nocturnal pain in limbs, numbness and coldness of extremities. • Glove and stocking type of anesthesia • Loss of tendon reflexes and muscle wasting • Disorganisation of joints (Charcot's joints) • Abnormal gait (wide based, thumping gait) • Nerve conduction velocity delayed in distal parts	• To maintain near or near normal metabolic control on long-term basis with insulin • Insulin is better for control than OHA • Symptomatic relief of pain in extremities is achieved by anti-depressants (imipramine or amitriptyline) or by anti-epileptics (dilantin or carbamazepine or gabapentine or valproate)
b. **Asymmetric, motor, proximal (diabetic amyotrophy)**	• Lower motor neuron paralysis with wasting of muscles • Hyper- or hypoasthesia may be present on anterior aspect of thighs. • Lower limbs are commonly involved than upper limbs. • Tendon reflexes are lost on affected side • Lumbosacral area is site of involvement	• Aldolase reductase inhibitors may be useful, if available. • Optimal control will not only delay the progress of neuropathy but metabolic complications may even be reversed
Mononeuropathy • Mononeuritis or cranial poly neuritis	• 3rd and 6th cranial nerves involvement common	

Contd...

Classification	Symptoms and signs	Treatment
• Mononeuritis multiplex (entrapment of ulnar, median and popliteal nerves)	producing diplopia and loss of eye movements • Carpal tunnel syndrome with ulnar and median nerve involvement (wrist drop) • Foot drop; due to sciatic or popliteal nerve involvement	
2. **Autonomic (visceral)**		
a. Cardiovascular	• Vertigo, giddiness and blurring of vision due to postural hypotension, resting tachycardia and fixed heart rate	• Support the limbs by stockings • Fludrocortisone therapy to raise BP • Monitor Na^+, K^+ and BP
b. Gastrointestinal	• Nausea, vomiting, abdominal distention, nocturnal diarrhea, constipation due to colonic atony, gastroparesis, dysphagia due to esophageal atony	• For gastroparesis use metoclopamide • Itopride or mosapride (prokinetic) 5-15 mg/day • For diarrhea, tetracycline 250 mg after every 6 hours
c. Genitourinary	Loss of libido, impotence, urinary incontinence, difficulty in micturition (atony of bladder)	• Penile prosthesis (silicon rods) • Injection of papaverine into corpora cavernosa • Avoid betablockers, methyldopa, other antihypertensives
d. Pseudomotor plus Vasomotor	• Abnormal or gustatory sweating, anhydrosis, fissuring of feet, cold extremities, dependent edema	• Propantheline 15 mg t.i.d. may relieve gustatory sweating
e. Eye (Pupils)	• Constriction of pupils, absent or delayed light reflex	

Q. What is glycosylated hemoglobin? What is its significance?

Ans. The hemoglobin (Hb) gets glycosylated due to formation of a covalent bond between glucose molecule and β-chain of hemoglobin. Glycosylated Hb is related to prevailing glucose concentration, hence, hyperglycemia and its excursions lead to increased glycosylation. Glycosylated Hb is expressed as percentage of normal hemoglobin (4-6% depending on the technique of measurement).

It is parameter of long-term control (i.e. past 6 weeks) of DM because it is an index of average blood glucose concentration over the life of the hemoglobin molecule (e.g. approx 6 weeks). Its higher values reflect various grades of control of DM. The target value of glycosylated Hb ($HbA1_c$) for control of diabetes is < 7% so as to retard or delay the onset of complications.

Q. What is diabetic retinopathy? What are ocular fundi changes in DM?

Ans. The involvement of retina (basement membrane, blood vessels) in diabetes is called *diabetic retinopathy*. It is an important cause of blindness among diabetics. Early detection and early management are essential. Ocular fundi should be checked regularly to detect asymptomatic disease. The fundosocopic findings are given in Table 1.84.

Table 1.84: Fundoscopic findings in diabetic retinopathy

- Increase in capillary permeability.
- Microaneurysms (earlier to appear as dark spots/dots)
- Retinal hemorrhage (blot hemorrhage)
- Hard and soft exudates (cotton wool exudates)
- Neovascularization (new vessels formation)
- Pre-retinal hemorrhage
- Vitreous hemorrhage
- Retinitis proliferans, fibrosis and retinal detachment

The dot (microaneurysms) and blot (leakage of blood into deeper layer) hemorrhages are the characteristic findings of background retinopathy in DM.

Q. What is the earliest sign of diabetic retinopathy?

Ans. An increase in capillary permeability evidenced by leakage of dye into the vitreous humour after fluorescein injection.

Q. What are the clinical stages and time course of diabetic nephropathy?

Ans. The clinical stages and their time course is as follows:
1. *Stage of microalbuminuria* (incipient nephropathy). It takes 5 years for its appearance

2. *Overt proteinuria* (non-nephrotic range). They take 5-10 years for development

3. *Nephrotic syndrome* (Fig. 1.26C). It takes 5-10 years for development

4. *Renal failure/insufficiency*	Both these stages take
5. *End stage renal disease (ESRD)*	10-15 years for their development

Q. Why dose of insulin decreases in diabetic nephropathy?

Ans. It is due to:
- Excretion of insulin binding antibodies with albumin in urine
- Decreased degradation of insulin
- CRF tends to impair neoglucogenesis.

Q. What are GI complications of DM?

Ans. Gastrointestinal complications in DM are:
- Candidiasis or fungal infections of oral cavity (an opportunistic infection)
- Diabetic esophageal hypomotility and gastroparesis
- Chronic gastritis
- Diabetic enteropathy
- Pancreatitis (chronic) causing steatorrhea
- Hepatomegaly (fatty infiltration)
- Acalculous cholecystitis.

Q. Name the various microvascular complications of diabetes.

Ans. Read the Table 1.82.

Q. What is microalbuminuria? What is its significance?

Ans. Microalbuminuria is defined as:
 i. Loss of < 300 mg of albumin in urine over 24 hrs
 ii. Albumin excretion rate in urine is 20 μg/min

It indicates early diabetic nephropathy, a stage from which nephropathy can be reversed with tight metabolic control.

Q. What is diabetic foot? What are its types?

Ans. Examination of foot is an important part of clinical evaluation of a case with diabetes (Fig. 1.26E).

The clinical features of diabetic foot are given in Table 1.85. Diabetic foot results as a result of neuropathy, vasculopathy and infections.

Diabetic foot is either neuropathic or ischemic or both

Q. What is diabetic vasculopathy (Ischemic foot)?

Ans. It refers to occlusive vascular disease involving both microangiopathy and atherosclerosis of large and medium sized arteries.

Fig. 1.26C: Nephrotic syndrome in a patient with diabetes of > 10 years duration. Note the gross edema and puffiness of face

Fig. 1.26D: Pressure sore. The wound is infected (↓)

126

Table 1.85: Features of diabetic foot

Neuropathy	Vasculopathy
• Paraesthesia	• Claudication
• Numbness	• Rest pain
• Pain	• Loss of dorsalis pedis and or
• Loss of sensations	posterior tibial pulsations.
• Decreased tendon Jeeks	
Structural damage	• Feet are cold to touch
• Ulcer on the foot	• Skin is shining and atrophic
• Sepsis, abscess	with sparse hair
• Loss of the arch of foot	
• Osteomyelitis	
• Digital gangrene (loss of peripheral pulses)	
• Charcot joint	

Q. What is pathogenesis of neovascularization?

Ans. It is due to production of following factors by ischemic retina
- Angiogenic factors
- Vascular endothelial growth factor.

Q. How will you manage a case of type 2 DM?

Ans. The essential steps in the management of type 2 diabetes are represented in the flow chart (Fig. 1.26F).

Q. How would you manage diabetic foot?

Ans.
- Debridement of necrotic tissue and antiseptic dressing daily.
- Control of hyperglycemia with insulin.
- Antibiotics for infection.

Fig. 1.26E: Diabetic foot

- Removal of weight bearing and friction from ulcerated area, e.g. avoid crutches, use appropriate foot wear.
- Patient education. Avoid smoking and alcohol, inspect foot daily for blisters. Do not walk bare footed. Avoid tight shoes, cut toenails across.
- Chiropody.
- Surgical and orthopedic consultation.

Q. How will you classify oral hypoglycemics?

Ans. Read Unit IV—Commonly used drugs

Q. What do you understand by the term insulin sensitizers? Name them. What are their advantages?

Ans. Insulin sensitizers are the drugs which lower the blood sugar in type 2 DM by sensitizing the insulin receptors to insulin hence, overcome insulin resistance and hyperinsulinemia in type 2 DM. They are:
- Biguanides, e.g. *metformin*
- Thiazolidinedione derivatives, e.g. rosiglitazone, pioglitazone.

Advantages are:
- Hypoglycemia is rare as compared to insulin secretagogues, e.g. sulphonylureas
- They lower the blood lipid
- They lower the mortality and morbidity
- They can be used to lower blood sugar in patients with impaired glucose tolerance (IGT).

Warning: The insulin sensitizers need the presence of insulin for their action, hence, cannot be used in type 1 diabetes mellitus.

Q. What are key points (Do's and Don'ts) in the management of type 2 DM?

Ans. The Do's and Don't's are tabulated (Table 1.86) and illustrated in the Figure 1.26G.

Q. How will you investigate a case with DM?

Ans. The various investigations done are:
1. *Blood*
   - TLC, DLC, ESR for an evidence of infection
   - Sugar (fasting and PP) for diagnosis and monitoring of diabetes
   - HbAlc (glycosylated Hb) for long-term management of diabetes
   - Serum lipids for hyperlipidemia – a common finding in DM.
2. *Urine examination* for specific gravity, pus cells, RBCs, proteins, sugar, casts and culture and sensitivity.
3. *ECG* for diagnosis of silent myocardial infarction or hypertension.
4. *Chest X-ray* for pulmonary tuberculosis, fungal infections, cardiomegaly.
5. *Fundus examination* for diabeteic retinoapthy.

Fig. 1.26F: Management of type 2 diabetes mellitus

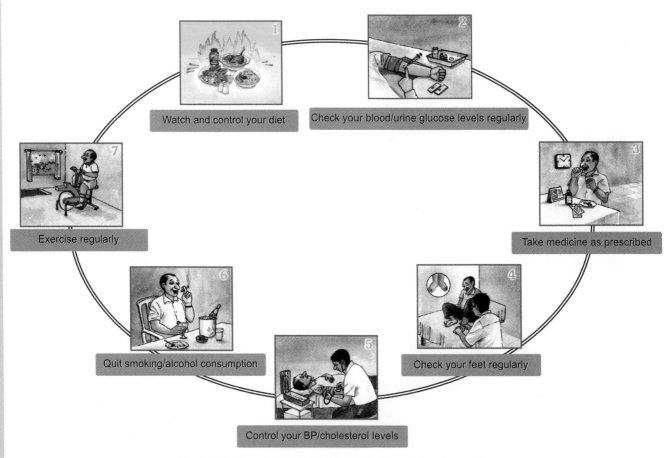

Fig. 1.26G: Key points in the management of type 2 diabetes mellitus

	Do's	Dont's
Diet	Eat a balanced diet Eat fiber rich foods Consume small, frequent meals	Avoid consumption of sweetened beverages, fried foods, alcohol, red-meat, honey, jaggery, sugar, and bakery products Do not skip your meal
Exercise	Exercise should be low to moderate in intensity Consult your doctor before starting any exercise Remember to walk and exercise daily Keep sugar or something sweet, e.g. candy, to avoid low blood sugar levels	Do not exercise if your blood sugar values are low or high and diabetes is not under control Do not exercise on an empty stomach
Foot	Keep your feet clean, warm and dry Change daily clean, soft socks and wear well fitting shoes Examine your shoes daily for cracks, pebbles, nails and other irregularities	Do not use alcohol based solutions. It makes your feet dry. Never walk barefooted Never apply heat of any kind to your feet Do not cut corns or calluses yourself
Eye	Consult your doctor if you have pain in your eyes Have an yearly eye examination done by your doctor	Do not neglect any infection in your eyes.

*Adapted from 2004 clinical practice recommendations by ADA

6. *Other investigations* are specifically performed depending on the system involved.

Q. What are parameters used for control of DM?

Ans. Parameters of control are:
  i. Urine sugar (negative or just positive)
  ii. Blood sugar, e.g.
     F. < 126 mg% PP < 200 mg%
  iii. Serum lipids
     HDL M > 40 mg/dl and F > 60 mg/dl
     LDL < 100 mg/dl
     Triglycerides < 150 mg/dl
  iv. Hb A1c (glycosylated Hb)
     • < 7% with a check once in 3 months

Q. What is hypoglycemia?

Ans. It is defined as blood glucose level<55 mg% (3.1 mmol/L). Hypoglycemia is classified traditionally into (i) postprandial (occurs in response to meals) and (ii) fasting. Fasting hypoglycemia usually occurs in the presence of disease while postprandial occurs in the absence of a recogniseable disease (Table 1.87). The factors responsible for hypoglycemia are given in Table 1.88.

Q. What is whipple triad?

Ans. • Symptoms and signs suggestive of hypoglycemia
  • Documentation of hypoglycemia
  • Reversal of hypoglycemia with administration of glucose

Q. What are the symptoms and signs of hypoglycemia?

Ans. Symptoms and signs of hypoglycemia occur due to effects of low levels of glucose *per se* as well as stimulation of sympathetic system. These are given in Table 1.89.

Table 1.87: Classification of hypoglycemia

1. **Postprandial hypoglycaemia**
   • Alimentary, e.g. dumping syndrome (following gastric surgery) due to hyperinsulinemia and idiopathic (true or pseudohypoglycemia)
   • Galactosemia and hereditary fructose intolerance (common causes of hypoglycemia in children)
2. **Fasting hypoglycemia**
   i. Hyperinsulinism
      • Insulinoma (pancreatic beta-islet cell tumor)
      • Non-pancreatic tumor secreting insulin-like growth factor I
      • Excessive exogenous insulin
      • Drugs, e.g. sulphonylurea, quinine, salicylates, propranolol, pentamidine
   ii. Endocrinal causes
      • Hypopituitarism. Addison's disease.
      • Glucagon and catecholamines deficiency
   iii. Liver diseases
      • Severe hepatitis
      • Cirrhosis of liver
   iv. Renal disease
      • Renal failure
   v. Enzymatic defects
      • G_6 phosphatase
      • Liver phosphorylase
      • Pyruvate carboxylase
      • Glycogen synthetase
   vi. Substrate deficiency
      • Malnutrition
      • Pregnancy

There is a great degree of variation among individuals in awareness of symptoms of hypoglycemia in diabetes. Some patients may feel symptoms when blood sugar is <70 mg% while others may not appreciate the symptoms even when blood glucose

Table 1.88: Factors responsbile for hypoglycemia in diabetes

The factors are:
1. Intake of too little food or no food but insulin is taken as regular
2. Unaccustomed exercise is attempted but preceding dose of insulin is not reduced
3. Alcohol intake
4. Poorly designed insulin regimen. There is mismatch between insulin administration and food habits
5. Defective counter-regulatory mechanisms such as release of glucagon and catecholamines in diabetes. They are anti-insulin in action.
6. Impaired gastric emptying. This produces mismatch between intake of food and insulin action
7. Malabsorption of food
8. Factitious (self-induced) hypoglycemia
9. An unrecognised low renal threshold for glucose. Attempts to render the urine sugar-free will inevitably produces hypoglycemia
10. Renal failure. The kidneys are important sites for the clearance of insulin which tends to accumulate if renal failure is present.

Table 1.89: Symptoms and signs of hypoglycemia

- **CVS:** Palpitation, tachycardia, anxiety, cardiac arrhythmias
- **CNS:** Tremors, confusion, headache, tiredness, difficulty in concentration, incordination, slurred speech, drowsiness, convulsions, plantars extensors, coma
- **GI tract:** Nausea, vomiting
- **Skin:** Sweating, hypothermia

level is less than 55 mg%. Occasionally, a few patients feel symptoms when blood sugar is even > 55 mg%. Actually these are the patients who are aware of these symptoms, hence may feel them early before glucose levels fall to low levels. The mechanism of this variation is not understood. Hypoglycemia is reversible with administration of glucose, symptoms and signs may disappear rapidly if it is insulin induced but may take sometime if induced by oral hypoglycemics.

Q. What are the causes of fasting hypoglycemia?
Ans. Read Table 1.87.

Q. What are causes of postprandial hyperglycemia?
Ans. Read Table 1.87.

Cardiovascular Disorders

The patient (not shown) present with history of exertional dyspnea and off and on chest pain and syncope. There was history of pain in right hypochondrium and edema legs and feet. The auscultatory findings of the patient are depicted in Figure 1.27A.

Clinical Presentations

1. Asymptomatic. It may be asymptomatic, detected on examination as an incidental finding. Congenital or mild. AS remain asymptomatic throughout life.
2. Patients of moderate or severe AS may complain of palpitation, dyspnea, anginal pain etc.
3. Patients with severe AS may also complain of syncope or giddiness and vertigo.

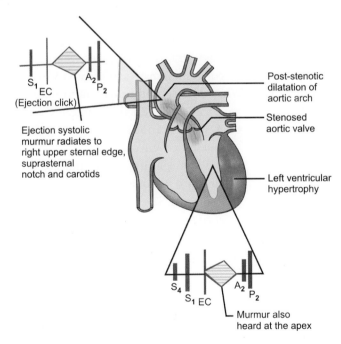

Fig. 1.27A: Aortic stenosis. Auscultatory findings and hemodynamic consequences

History

Points to be Noted

- Exertional dyspnea
- Angina pectoris
- Cough, hemoptysis, dyspnea, orthopnea, PND due to left heart failure
- Exertional syncope due to low cardiac output
- Sudden death.

General Physical Examination

- Pulse is low volume, anacrotic, slow rising in moderate severe stenosis, normal in mild stenosis.
- Pulse pressure is low
- Jugular venous pressure is raised if right heart failure develops. Prominent 'a' wave may be seen
- Ankle edema may be present if heart failure develops.

Systemic Examination

Inspection

- Apex beat may be normally placed or displaced down beyond left 5th intercostal space outside the mid-clavicular line due to left ventricular hypertrophy/enlargement. It is forceful and sustained (heaving).

Palpation

- Apex beat may be normally placed or displaced downwards and outwards due to left ventricular hypertrophy. It is forceful and sustained (heaving)
- Left ventricular thrust may be palpable
- P_2 may become palpable if pulmonary hypertension develops
- Systolic thrill over the aortic area and carotids.

Percussion

- Cardiac dullness is within normal limits.

Auscultation

- A mid-systolic ejection murmur which is diamond-shaped (crescendo-decrescendo) often with thrill best heard at right 2nd space (A1 area) or left 3rd space (A2 area), is radiated to carotid vessels and downwards to apex. Murmur is best heard in sitting position with patient bending forward
- An ejection click (EC) is heard in valvular aortic stenosis (Fig. 1.27A).
- Second heart sound is short and feeble, normal or paradoxically split.
- An atrial sound (S4) may be heard
- *Other systems examination*
  1. *Respiratory system*
     Basal rales at both the bases of the lungs
  2. *Abdomen*
     - Hepatomegaly may be present
     - No ascites, no splenomegaly

Q. What is your probable diagnosis?

Ans. The patient has pure aortic stenosis either rheumatic or congenital in origin. It is moderate in severity with CHF with sinus rhythm without SABE.

Q. What are points in favor of your diagnosis?

Ans. 1. H/O exertional dyspnea, syncope, chest discomfort
2. Signs of CHF, e.g. raised JVP, cyanosis, edema and tender hepatomegaly
3. Displaced apex beat (down and out) with heaving character.
4. Signs of pulmonary hypertension, e.g. loud P2 with narrow splitting
5. An ejection click and ejection systolic murmur over A1 and A2, best heard in sitting position and leaning forward. It radiates to carotid. A2 is soft.
6. Systolic thrill over aorta and carotids.

Q. What is aortic stenosis? What are its types?

Ans. Aortic stenosis is defined as narrowing of the aortic orifice due to valve or wall involvement leading to left ventricular outflow obstruction (pressure overload).

Types and Forms

1. *Valvular aortic stenosis (bicuspid aortic valve).* It is the commonest type of congenital aortic stenosis.
2. *Congenital subvalvular AS.* This congenital anomaly is produced by either a membraneous diaphragm or a fibrous ridge just below the aortic valve, or asymmetrical hypertrophy of the interventricular septum—called idiopathic hypertrophic subaortic stenosis (IHSS).
3. *Supravalvular AS.* This uncommon congenital anomaly is produced by narrowing of the ascending aorta or by a fibrous diaphragm with a small opening just above the aortic valve. It is commonly seen in William's syndrome (Table 1.90). It is probably due to mutation in the elastin gene

Table 1.90: William's syndrome

- *Elfin facies*, e.g. broad forehead, pointed chin, upturned nose, hypertelorism, peg-shaped incisors, low set ears.
- Supravalvular aortic stenosis
- Mental retardation
- Hypercalcemia

Q. What are causes of aortic stenosis?

Ans. The likely etiology varies with the age of the patient (Table 1.91).

Table 1.91: Causes of aortic stenosis

1. **Infants, children, adolescents**
   - Congenital aortic stenosis (valvular)
   - Congenital subvalvular aortic stenosis
   - Congenital supravalvular aortic stenosis
2. **Young adults and middle-aged persons**
   - Calcification and fibrosis of congenitally bicuspid aortic valve
   - Rheumatic aortic stenosis
3. **Old age**
   - Senile degenerative aortic stenosis
   - Calcification of bicuspid valve
   - Rheumatic aortic stenosis

Q. What are important features of aortic stenosis?

Ans. Common features of AS are:
- Dyspnea, angina and syncope on exertion
- Slow rising sustained low volume pulse called anacrotic pulse, occurs in severe stenosis, pulse is normal in mild AS.
- Low systolic pressure with low pulse pressure (< 20 mmHg)
- Apex beat down and out or may be normal with heaving in character
- Cardiomegaly
- Ejection click and ejection systolic murmur and a thrill in aortic area conducted to carotids. The same murmur is also heard at apex
- Basal crackles and rales. Signs of pulmonary congestion may be present (LVF).

Q. What does second heart sound tell us in AS?

Ans.
- A soft and muffled S2 indicates valvular stenosis
- A single S2 indicates fibrosed/fused cusps or fenestrated valve
- Reverse splitting of S2 indicate mechanical or electrical prolongation of ventricular systole.
- A normal S2 rules out the possibility of critical aortic stenosis.

Q. How will you investigate a patient with AS?

Ans. Following investigations are done:
1. *Electrocardiogram (ECG)* may show left atrial and left ventricular hypertrophy with strain, i.e. ST-T wave changes due to myocardial ischemia may be present. Heart blocks and bundle branch block in calcific aortic stenosis may occur sometimes.
2. *Chest X-ray.* It may be normal. Sometimes, heart is enlarged due to a left ventricular hypertrophy. Post-stenotic dilatation of aorta may be seen in some cases. Lateral view may show calcification of aortic valve.

Fig. 1.27B: Aortic stenosis. Color Doppler Echocardiogram showing aortic stenosis with gradient of 50 mm across the valve

3. *Echocardiography (Fig. 1.27B).* It will show left ventricular enlargement and hypertrophy, severity of AS, calcification of valve and decreased left ventricular function.

4. *Doppler echocardiography*: demonstrates the systolic gradient across the valve, detects presence and absence of aortic regurgitation.

Q. **How would you grade AS on electrocardiography?**

Ans. It is graded as mild (valve area >1.5 cm), moderate (valve area 1-1.5 cm^2) and severe (valve area < 1 cm^2).

Q. **How will you differentiate among three common types of AS?**

Ans. The differential diagnosis of aortic stenosis lies among its three types:

1. *Valvular AS* (its important features have already been listed)

2. *Subvalvular aortic stenosis* (idiopathic hypertrophic subaortic stenosis –IHSS). The features are:

   • Dyspnea, angina pectoris, fatigue and syncope
   • Double apical impulse (apex beat)
   • A rapidly rising carotid arterial pulse
   • Pulsus bisferience (double upstroke)
   • A harsh, diamond-shape ejection systolic murmur without ejection click is best heard at lower left sternal border as well as at the apex. It does not radiate to neck vessels. It becomes louder with valsalva maneuver.
   • Early diastolic murmur of aortic regurgitation may also be heard in some patients.
   • No post-stenotic dilatation
   • Second heart sound is normal, single.

3. *Supravalvular aortic stenosis*

   • Unequal BP in both arms, i.e. right arm > left arm

   • May be associated with other features of William's syndrome
   • No ejection click, only ejection systolic murmur
   • Systolic thrill is more pronounced and radiates to the neck vessels but not to the apex
   • A$_2$ is accentuated
   • No poststenotic dilatation.

Q. **What are the complications of AS?**

Ans. Common complications are as follows:

   • Left ventricular failure
   • Hemolytic anemia
   • Systemic embolization
   • Congestive cardiac failure
   • Infective endocarditis
   • Arrhythmias (ventricular) and conduction disturbances (heart blocks)
   • Precipitation of angina
   • Sudden death. It is more common in hypertrophic cardiomyopathy (HOCM).

Q. **How will you differentiate between aortic stenosis and pulmonary stenosis?**

Ans. Differences between AS and PS are dealt with in Table 1.92.

Table 1.92: Differentiation between aortic stenosis and pulmonary stenosis (PS)

Features	AS	PS
Pulse	Small amplitude, anacrotic, parvus et tardus	Normal
BP	Low systolic	Normal
Apex beat	Heaving	Normal
Second heart sound	A$_2$ soft	P$_2$ soft
Splitting of S$_2$	Reverse	Wide
Location of systolic murmur	Aortic area, conducted to carotids	Pulmonary area. No conduction
Relation to respiration	No change	Increases on inspiration
Associated ventricular hypertrophy	LVH	RVH

Q. **What are characteristics of severe aortic stenosis?**

Ans. Aortic stenosis is said to be severe when:

   • Pulse character is slowly rising plateau
   • Pulse pressure is narrow
   • Signs of LVF present
   • S$_2$ is soft, single or paradoxically split
   • Presence of S$_4$

- Systolic thrill and late peaking of ejection systolic murmur
- Cardiac catheterization reveals transvalvular gradient >60 mmHg

Q. What are causes of systolic murmur in aortic and pulmonary area?

Ans. The murmurs in this area are ejection or mid systolic. The causes of ejection systolic murmur (ESM) are given in Table 1.93.

Table 1.93: Systolic murmurs at base of the heart

Aortic area (A1 and A2) (right 2nd and left 3rd space)
- AS
- Systemic hypertension
- Coarctation of the aorta
- Aneurysm of the ascending aorta
- Atherosclerosis of the aorta (old age)
- Functional flow murmur in AR

Pulmonary area (left 2nd interspace)
- Pulmonary stenosis
- Pulmonary hypertension
- Cor pulmonale (acute or chronic)
- Hyperkinetic states, e.g. anemia, thyrotoxicosis, fever, pregnancy
- Congenital heart diseases, e.g. ASD, VSD, Fallot's tetralogy
- Innocent (benign) murmur

Q. What are benign (innocent) murmurs?

Ans. These murmurs are flow murmurs without organic cause, commonly seen in children due to;
- Hyperkinetic circulatory state in children especially during exercise, crying or fever.
- Increasd resistance of the pulmonary vascular bed

Characteristics:
- Usually systolic localized to pulmonary outflow tract
- There is no associated thrill
- Best heard in supine position, may disappear in upright position
- Heart sounds are normal.

Q. What is a hemic murmur?

Ans. It is an ejection systolic murmur heard at the pulmonary area due to rapid blood flow in a patient with severe anemia. It is due to hyperkinetic circulatory state combined with dilatation of pulmonary artery and its vasculature.

Note: Hemic murmurs are also functional ejection systolic murmur similar to hear in various hyperkinetic states.

Q. What are functional murmurs?

Ans. These murmurs occur in the absence of organic heart disease, are due to turbulence produced by rapid flow of blood across a normal valve (flow murmurs). These may be systolic and diastolic (Table 1.94). These murmurs are not loud, are localized in nature, and usually not associated with thrill. They are hemodynamically insignificant, do not produce cardiomegaly.

Table 1.94: Functional murmurs

Systolic
- Systolic murmur across pulmonary valve in left to right shunt, e.g. ASD, VSD
- Functional systolic murmur in aortic area in patients with severe AR

Diastolic
- Grahm-Steell murmur (early diastolic) due to pulmonary regurgitation in pulmonary hypertension
- Apical mid-diastolic murmur (Austin-Flint murmur) in severe AR.

Q. How would you manage this condition?

Ans. Mild asymptomatic AS with valvular gradient <50 mm Hg needs observation only. Moderate AS with symptoms needs medical management of LVF with salt restriction, diuretics and vasodilators. Digoxin should not be used. These patients need valve replacement.

Q. What are indications of valve replacement?

Ans.
- Symptomatic AS with valvular gradient > 50 mm Hg. It is an absolute indication.
- Asymptomatic patients with severe AS (gradient > 50mm Hg. LVH, Left ventricular systolic dysfunction and valve area <0.6 cm^2)
- Asymptomatic moderate AS in patients who are undergoing mitral or aortic root surgery or coronary artery bypass surgery.

Q. Which valve would you prefer for replacement?

Ans. Mechanical prothetic valve in young age and tissue valve (bioprosthetic value) in old age.

CASE 28: AORTIC REGURGITATION (AR)

A patient (not shown) presented with palpitation, dyspnea and off and on chest pain. The auscultatory findings are depicted in Figure 1.28. The patient had mild edema feet.

Clinical Presentations

I. Mild to moderate AR

- Often asymptomatic
- Palpitation—pounding of heart is a common symptom
- Symptoms of left heart failure appear but late

II. Severe AR

- Symptoms of heart failure, i.e. dyspnea, orthopnea, PND are present at onset
- Angina pectoris is frequent complaint
- Arrhythmias are uncommon.

History

Points to be Noted

- Onset of symptoms and their course
- Ask the history of cough, dyspnea, orthopnea, PND
- Ask for history of hemoptysis, anginal pain, headache
- History of fever
- History of edema feet and legs
- History of loss of function of any part, i.e. paralysis
- Past history of sore throat, skin infection or arthralgia (fleeting) or joint pain (arthritis).

General Physical Examination

- Face for appearance, i.e. dyspneic or orthopneic, ill-look. Note puffiness
- Look for Argyll-Robertson pupils of syphilis
- Mouth. Look for anemia or bleeding or evidence of infection, high-arch palate
- Neck examination for arterial pulsation, JVP and lymph nodes
- Pulse, BP, respiration and temperature
- Note the following other peripheral signs in case of AR
  i. Collapsing or good volume pulse (wide pulse pressure)
  ii. Bounding peripheral pulses
  iii. Dancing carotids (Corrigan's sign)
  iv. Capillary pulsations in nailbeds (Quincke's sign)
  v. Pistol shots sound and Duroziez's sign/murmur (to and fro systolic and diastolic murmur) produced by compression of femoral by stethoscope
  vi. Head nodding with carotid pulse—de Musset's sign
  vii. Hill's sign (BP in lower limb > upper limbs)

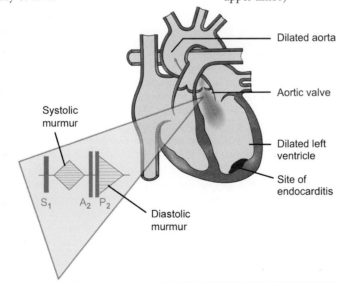

Lean the patient forward with breath held in expiration to hear the early diastolic murmur, best heard in A₂ area (left 2nd intercostal space)

Fig. 1.28: Aortic regurgitation

- Cyanosis (peripheral, central or both) may be present
- Pitting ankle edema may be present
- Tender hepatomegaly if right heart failure present.
- Look for stigmatas of Marfan's syndrome.
- Look for joint deformity for rheumatoid arthritis and ankylosing spondylitis

All these peripheral signs may not be evident in mild AR. In our case, they were present indicating severe AR.

Examination of CVS

Inspection

- Apex beat is displaced down and outside the midclavicular line and is forceful
- Left ventricular thrust
- Pulsations in suprasternal notch and epigastrium are usually seen.

Palpation

- Apex beat is forceful and sustained
- No thrill is palpable
- Tender hepatomegaly if right heart failure present.

Percussion

- Cardiac dullness is within normal limits.

Auscultation

- An *early diastolic murmur* is best heard in A₂ area (3rd left intercostal space) or A₁ area (2nd right intercostal space) in sitting position with patient leaning forward and during held expiration
- An *ejection systolic murmur* in the same area. It is due to increased stroke volume. It may also radiate to neck vessels
- Ejection click suggests bicuspid aortic valve.
- *Austin flint* (soft, middiastolic) murmur at apex in severe AR.
- Second heart sound is soft and feeble
- Loud pulmonary component in second left space indicates pulmonary hypertension
- Signs of left heart failure (fine end-inspiratory rales at bases of lungs).
- A 3rd heart sound at apex is present in severe AR.

Q. What is your provisional diagnosis?

Ans. In view of clinical features and ausculatory findings, the provisional diagnosis is aortic regurgitation with congestive cardiac failure without evidence of endocarditis or thromboembolic complication. The cause of AR is to be found out.

Q. Is it severe or moderate AR?

Ans. The presence of all the signs of wide pulse pressure indicates severe AR in this patient. However, the signs of severity are described in Table 1.95.

Q. How do you define AR?

Ans. When blood is pushed by left ventricle into the aorta during systole, a part of it regurgitates back into same ventricle during diastole due to inadequate closure of the aortic valve, called *aortic regurgitation*. It leads to volume overload of the left ventricle resulting in its hypertrophy and enlargement.

Q. What are causes of chronic AR?

Ans. The causes are:
   I. *Congenital*
   - Bicuspid valve
   II. *Acquired*
   - Rheumatic heart disease
   - Infective endocarditis (acute regurgitation)
   - Trauma leading to valve rupture
   - Atherosclerosis, hypertension
   - Marfan's syndrome (aortic dilatation)
   - Syphilitic aortitis
   - Ankylosing spondylitis, rheumatoid arthritis
   - Dissecting aneurysm of ascending aorta.

Q. What are causes of acute AR?

Ans. Causes of acute AR
   - Acute bacterial endocarditis
   - Rupture of sinus of valsalva
   - Failure of prosthetic valve.
   - Trauma to the chest.
   - Acute dissection of the aorta.

Q. What are clinical features of acute AR?

Ans. The clinical features of acute AR will be:
   - An acutely ill patient with severe breathlessness, chest discomfort
   - Acute left ventricular failure (LVF)
   - Peripheral signs of AR will be absent.

Q. Differential diagnosis of AR.

Ans. The common causes of AR are compared clinically in the Table 1.96 for differential diagnosis.

Q. What are differences between AR and PR (pulmonary regurgitation)?

Ans. These are summarized in Table 1.97.

Q. How will you decide whether MDM in mitral area is due to severe AR or due to associated MS?

Ans. The mid-diastolic murmur in AR may be confused with MDM of MS though both lesions may coexist. The differentiation are given in Table 1.98.

Q. How will you investigate a patient with AR?

Ans. Following investigations are done:
   1. *Chest X-ray (PA view) may show;*
   - Cardiomegaly (LV enlargement-boot shaped heart)
   - Dilatation of ascending aorta, valvular calcification
   - Aortic knuckle prominent

Table 1.95: Signs of aortic regurgitation (AR) and its severity.

Sign of severity AR	Signs of moderate AR
• All signs of moderate AR • Wider pulse pressure (normal 20-40 mm) wider the pulse pressure, severe is AR. • Soft second heart sound • Signs of left heart failure • Duration of the decrescendo diastolic murmur; longer the murmur, sever is AR • Hill's Sign (normal difference in BP of LL and UL is <20 mm Hg) Larger the difference, severes is the AR. A difference of 20-40 mm indicates moderate AR and >60 mm difference suggest severe AR. • Presence of third heart sound. It indicates severe AR. • Austin flint murmur – a low pitched, soft mid-diastolic murmur caused by vibration of the anterior mitral cusp by the regurgitant jet and is heart at the apex. It indicates severe AR.	*Peripheral signs** • Collapsing or good volume pulse (wide pulse pressure) • Bounding peripheral pulses • Dancing carotids *(Corrigan's sign)* • Capillary pulsation in nailbeds *(Quincke's sign)* • Pistol shot sound and *Duroziez's sign/ murmur* • Head nodding with carotid pulse de *Musset's sign* • *Hill's sign* (BP in lower limbs >upper limbs) • Cyanosis (peripheral, central or both) may be present • Fundus examination will reveal capillary pulsations • Pitting ankle edema may be present • Tender hepatomegaly if right heart failure present

*All these peripheral signs may not be evident in mild AR because these indicates wide pulse pressure due to significant aortic run-off into the heart.

Rheumatic AR	Syphilitic AR	Aortic dilatation (Marfan's syndrome)
Young age group	Older age group	Young age
History of rheumatic fever in the past	History of sexual exposure	Eunuchoidism (lower segment >upper segment, arachnodactyly)
Other valves may be involved	Usually an isolated lesion	Mitral valve may be involved (floppy mitral valve syndrome)
Diastolic thrill absent	Thrill may be present	Aortic pulsation in suprasternal notch. No thrill
A_2 diminished or absent	A_2 may be loud (tambour like)	A_2 normal
Murmur best heard in left 3rd space (A_2 area)	Murmur best heard in right second or 3rd space along right sternal border	Murmur heard in second right and third left intercostal space
Peripheral signs present	Peripheral signs are marked, Austin-Flint murmur may be present	Peripheral signs are usually absent.

Table 1.97: Differentiation between AR and PR

Feature	AR	PR
Peripheral signs of wide pulse pressure	Present	Absent
Apex beat	Hyperdynamic	Normal
Site of early diastolic murmur	Best heard in aortic area	Best heart in pulmonary area
Relation of murmur to respiration	None	Increases with inspiration
Ventricular enlargement	LVH	RVH

Table 1.98: Differential diagnosis of MDM in AR

Feature	Severe AR (Austin-Flint murmur)	AR with MS
Peripheral signs of AR	Florid	Masked
Character of murmur	Soft	Rough and rumble
First heart sound (S_1)	Normal	Loud
Opening snap (OS)	Absent	Present
LA enlargement	Absent	Present
Calcification of mitral valve	Absent	May be present
Echocardiogram	Normal	Suggestive of MS

2. *ECG may show*
   - LVH and left atrial hypertrophy in moderate to severe AR
   - ST segment depression and T wave inversion due to left ventricular strain
3. *Echocardiogram. It detects;*
   - Left ventricular enlargement, hyperdynamic left ventricle and assessment of severity of AR
   - Fluttering of anterior mitral leaflet in severe AR
   - Aortic root dilatation and valve morphology.
   - Vegetations may be detected in a case with endocarditis

- Assessment of LV (dimension, size systolic function)
4. *Color Doppler flow studies* detect the reflux through aortic valve and its magnitude
5. *Radionuclide imaging* in asymptomatic patients where echocardiographic images are of poor quality
6. *Cardiac catheterization* is necessary when coronary artery disease is suspected
7. *MRI* and *spiral CT* scan for assessment of aortic root size.

Q. What are complications of AR?

Ans. Following are common complications:
- Acute LVF
- Infective endocarditis
- CHF
- Cardiac arrhythmias
- Heart blocks (calcific aortic valve)
- Precipitation of angina.

Q. What are the causes of an ejection systolic murmur in aortic area? How would you differentiate them?

Ans. The ejection systolic murmur in aortic area occurs either in severe AR or when AR is associated with AS or isolated AS. The AS has already been discussed. The diffrences between severe AR or AR with AS are compared in Table 1.99.

Q. How will you decide the dominance of a lesion in combined AS and AR?

Ans. The features of dominant AS or AR in combined aortic lesion are given in Table 1.100.

Q. How would you treat AR?

Ans. *Mild asymptomatic* disease does not require treatment
- *Moderate to severe disease* is treated by salt restriction, diuretics, digitalis and vasodilators (ACE inhibitors). Surgery is the final answer.
- *Severe AR* needs surgery (valve reconstruction or replacement) in addition to medical management.

Table 1.99: Differential diagnosis of an ejection systolic murmur (ESM) in AR

Feature	Severe AR	AR with AS
Signs of wide pulse pressure (water-hammer pulse, Corrigan's sign, dancing carotids and pistol shot sounds etc).	Present	Absent
Systolic BP	High systolic	Normal or low systolic
Ejection click	Absent	Present
Radiation of murmur	Usually localized, may radiate to neck vessels	Widely radiated to neck vessels as well as to apex
Systolic thrill	Absent	Present

Q. What are indications of surgery in AR?

Ans.
- Severe AR with concomitant angina
- Severe AR with heart failure and reduced ejection fraction (e.g between 30-50%). A reduction in exercise ejection fraction by 50% or more even in the absence of symptoms
- When end-systolic dimension of aorta or aortic root diameter is > 55mm.

Q. Which valve would you prefer for replacement in AR?

Ans.
- If patient is young, mechanical prosthetic valve would be preferred as they are more durable.
- Bioprosthetic (tissue valve) valve is used in elderly because they are prone to degeneration and calcification may need re-operation after 7-10 years.

Table 1.100: Dominant aortic stenosis vs aortic regurgitation in combined AS and AR

Features	Dominant AS	Dominant AR
I. *Symptoms* • *Exertional angina* • *Dyspnea on effort* • *Fatigue* • *Syncope* • *Palpitation*	All are marked	Chest pain, dyspnea, palpitation common
II. *Signs*		
Pulse	Low volume Pulsus bisferiens (tidal wave prominent than percussion wave)	High volume collapsing pulse Pulsus bisferiens (percussion wave prominent than tidal wave)
BP	• Low systolic BP • Low pulse pressure	• High systolic BP • Wide pulse pressure
Peripheral signs of AR	Masked	Marked
Apex beat	Heaving	Hyperdynamic
Thrill	Systolic	No thrill
S_3	Absent	Present
S_4	May be present	Absent
Ejection click	Present	Absent
Diastolic murmur	Short early diastolic	Prominent early diastolic
Systolic murmur	Marked, radiating to neck vessels	Present, does not radiate to neck vessels

The patient (not shown) presented with off and on cough and expectoration with dyspnea and PND for the last 4-5 years. There was history of pain abdomen, edema feet and hemoptysis off and on. His auscultatory findings are depicted in Figure 1.29. Loud 1st heart sound, opening snap and a rough rumbling mid-diastolic murmur were present in this case.

Clinical Presentations

1. The patients of mild MS may be asymptomatic and a presystolic murmur may be an evidence which increases on exercise.
2. Patients of mild to moderate MS present with symptoms of low cardiac output, e.g. syncope, fatigue, weakness. They may have exertional dyspnea only.
3. Patients of moderate to severe MS present with symptoms and signs of left heart failure followed by right heart failure and congestive cardiac failure.
4. These cases of MS of any severity may present with features of embolization (e.g. hemiplegia, recurrent hemoptysis, gangrene of peripheral parts) due to thrombus either in left atrium or peripheral venous system; the formation of which is triggered by either a transient arrhythmias (e.g. AF) or LVF or CHF.

History

Points to be Noted

- History of exertional dyspnea, orthopnea, PND
- Any history of pain chest, hemoptysis, hoarseness of voice.
- History of dizziness, vertigo or syncope
- History of fever, joint pain or urinary disturbance
- History of pain abdomen, edema feet or legs, distention of abdomen.
- History of any paralysis (motor or sensory deficit)
- History of missing of heart beat.

Past history

- History of sore throat, joint pain, rash or abnormal movement or skin infection
- History of recurrent chest pain or hemoptysis.

Physical Signs

- Mitral facies – A characteristic bilateral, cyanotic or dusky pink hue (malar flush) on cheeks.
- Low volume pulse, which may be irregularly irregular if atrial fibrillation is present.
- Low pulse pressure
- Raised jugular venous pressure and 'a' wave on jugular venous pulse will be absent in atrial fibrillation

- Cold extremities: Extremities are usually warm but may be cold in severe mitral stenosis or due to embolization.
- Pitting ankle edema

Note: Always look for the signs of bacterial endocarditis (Read Case 31) or acute rheumatic activity in a case of MS, if complicated.

I. Estimation of Heart (CVS)

Inspection

- Apex beat is normally situated or apex beat is displaced outwards but not downwards
- Pulsation of pulmonary artery may be visible in 2nd left intercostal space.
- Epigastric pulsations may be visible due to right ventricular hypertrophy.
- Left parasternal lift may be visible.

Palpation

- Apex beat is palpable and tapping in character
- An apical diastolic thrill may be palpable in left lateral position
- Ist heart sound at apex (mitral area) may become palpable, best demonstrated in left lateral position.
- Parasternal heave is usually present
- Second sound (pulmonary component) may become palpable at left 2nd intercostal space
- Right ventricular pulsations may be palpable in epigastrium.

Percussion

- Left border of heart corresponds with apex beat
- 2nd and 3rd left intercostal spaces may become dull due to pulmonary hypertension.

Auscultation

1. *Mitral area (apex)*
   - Heart beats may be irregular due to atrial fibrillation
   - First heart sound is loud and banging, short and snappy
   - A mid-diastolic murmur, best heard in left lateral position with the bell of stethoscope. It is rough and rumble. It is accentuated during late diastole called 'presystolic accentuation'. A presystolic murmur without mid diastolic murmur is an early sign of mitral stenosis, and in mild mitral stenosis this may be the only finding.

Fig. 1.29: Mitral stenosis. Hemodynamic effects and auscultatory findings in MS Roll the patient to the left to hear MDM (low pitched mid-diastolic rumbling murmur, which is best heard with the bell of stethoscope

- Opening snap (OS) is present. It is snapping sound heard after 2nd heart sound. Its proximity to S2 determines the severity of mitral stenosis. Nearer the opening snap to 2nd heart sound, more severe is the mitral stenosis. It is absent if valve becomes calcified.

2. *Pulmonary area* (left 2nd intercostal space)
   - Loud 2nd heart sound due to pulmonary arterial hypertension
   - There may be an ejection systolic or an early diastolic murmur (*Graham-Steell murmur*) due to pulmonary regurgitation.
   - Splitting of 2nd heart sound becomes narrow

3. *Tricuspid area* (lower left parasternal border)
   There may be a pansystolic murmur due to functional tricuspid regurgitation which may develop in cases with severe mitral stenosis.

4. *Aortic area* (right 2nd intercostal space)
   Normal 2nd heart sound heard. No abnormality detected in this area.

II. Examination of Other Systems

i. **Examination of lungs**
   There may be fine crepitations (end-inspiratory crackles) at both the bases of lungs due to LHF. There may be hydrothorax (pleural effusion)

ii. **Examination of abdomen**
   Liver is enlarged, soft and tender. Ascites may be present. Spleen gets enlarged in presence of subacute bacterial endocarditis.

iii. **Examination of nervous system**
   - Monoplegia/hemiplegia due to embolism
   - Sydenham's chorea
   - Optic fundi for Roth's spots.

Q. What is the clinical diagnosis?

Ans. In view of symptoms and physical signs described in this case, the patient appears to have RHD with MS, sinus rhythm (say AF if present), CHF without infective endocarditis or acute rheumatic activity.

Note: In cardiac cases, one has to tell the basic cardiac disease (e.g. valvular, hypertensive, cardiomyopathy, congenital, thyroxicosis etc.) first followed by sequence of the heart disease (e.g. with or without pulmonary hypertension and with/without LHF or CHF and then its complication/sequale (e.g. normal sinus rhythm/abnormal rhythm, presence/absence of SABE and/or acute rheumatic activity).

Q. What are points that favor your diagnosis of MS? How would you explain them?

Ans. *Points in favor of mitral stenosis* are:
1. *History* of cough, dyspnea, orthopnea and PND. *Hemoptysis* was present.
2. *Palpable apex beat.* Apex beat is palpable and tapping in character (tapping character is due to palpable first heart sound)
3. *Loud first heart sound(S_1).* Due to persistent rise in left atrial pressure, the diastolic gradient across the mitral valve is increased that keeps the valve cusps wide open at the end of diastole with the result when ventricular systole starts, the widely opened mitral valve cusps close rapidly like a thud producing a loud S_1.
4. *Mid-diastolic murmur (MDM) with presystolic accentuation.* The murmur is rough, rumbling, low-pitched, low frequency, of variable duration, best heard at the apex in left lateral position with bell of the stethoscope.

   There is presystolic accentuation of the murmur. The last part of the ventricular filling in diastole depends on the atrial boost which normally is small but increased in MS due to raised left atrial pressure, hence, accentuation of the murmur.

5. *Opening snap (OS).* This is a snappy, sound produced due to sudden forceful opening of the mitral valve during diastole due elevated left atrial pressure. It is heard in expiration with diaphragm of stethoscope at or just medial to cardiac apex. This sound follows aortic component of second heart sound (A_2) by 0.05 to 0.1 sec.

Q. What are common clinical features of MS?

Ans. The common features of MS and their pathogenesis is described in the Box 29.1.

Q. What are the common causes of mitral stenosis?

Ans. The causes are:
1. *Rheumatic:* MS is invariably rheumatic in origin.
2. *Congenital,* e.g. parachute mitral valve where all chordae tendinae are inserted into a single papillary muscle.
3. Rarely-carcinoid syndrome, SLE, endomyocardial fibrosis, Hurler's syndrome, RA (Rheumatoid arthritis) and calcification of mitral annulus and leaflets.

Q. What is normal cross-sectional area of mitral valve? When do symptoms and signs of MS appears? What is tight MS?

Ans. The normal mitral valve orifice is 4-6 cm^2 (average 5 cm^2) in diastole in adults. Narrowing of the mitral

BOX 29.1: CLINICAL MANIFESTATIONS OF MS

1. **Symptoms due to low cardiac output,** e.g.
   - fatigue
   - tiredness
   - weakness
   - lethargy
2. **Symptoms of pulmonary congestion (left heart failure),** e.g.
   - dyspnea,
   - orthopnea,
   - paroxysmal nocturnal dyspnea (PND)
   - hemoptysis
3. **Symptoms of right heart failure,** e.g.
   - puffiness of face and edema of legs
   - pain in right hypochondrium due to hepatomegaly
4. **Symptoms due to embolization,** e.g.
   - right sided embolization leads to hemoptysis and pain chest
   - left sided or systemic embolization leads to hemiplegia, acute pain abdomen (infarction of viscera), loss of peripheral pulses or gangrene, etc.
5. **Symptoms related to arrhythmias,** e.g.
   - palpitation,
   - missing of beat(s).

valve is called *mitral stenosis*. The symptoms arise due to hemodynamic disturbances such as rise in left atrial pressures, pulmonary arterial pressure when valve orifice is reduced to half of its original size (2.0 cm² approx). Mitral stenosis is severe when orifice is 1 cm² or less and said to be *critical*. The hemodynamic consequences in severe stenosis include rise in left atrial, pulmonary venous pressure and pulmonary edema (LVF) followed by pulmonary arterial hypertension and right heart failure. This is called *backward failure theory of heart failure*.

Q. What is functional MS?

Ans. *Functional Mitral Stenosis* refers to functional obstruction to inflow of blood from left atrium to left ventricle, is due to rapid flow through a normal valve as seen in (i) hyperdynamic circulation (VSD, ASD, PDA, thyrotoxicosis, anemia etc) and (ii) in severe mitral regurgitation. Severe aortic regurgitation produces functional MS by partially narrowing the valve by regurgitant jet.

In organic lesion, the valve is deformed while in functional MS, the valve is normal.

Q. What is significance of OS?

Ans.
- The presence of OS indicates organic MS
- The OS indicates that mitral valve is still pliable (i.e. not calcified). It disappears if valve is calcified
- It also decides the severity of MS. Diminishing A2-OS gap (gap between second heart sound and OS) indicates increasing severity of the MS.
- It disappears following valvotomy.

Q. What conditions simulate MS?

Ans.
1. Atrial myxoma – Read features of atrial myxoma further in this case.
2. Ball valve thrombus in left atrium
3. Cortriatum – a rare congenital heart condition

N.B. These conditions constitute the differential diagnosis of MS.

Q. What are the causes of loud S1?

Ans. Following are causes:
- Mitral stenosis
- Tricuspid stenosis
- In tachycardia. S1 is loud due to short P-R.
- Hyperkinetic circulation (exercise, anemia, thyrotoxicosis, fever, pregnancy, etc). This is due to rapid flow across the valves which keeps them wide open (functional MS), hence, their closure produces loud S1.
- *Short P-R interval.* P-R interval influences the heart rate, short P-R causes loud S1 while long P-R causes muffling of S1. The short P-R interval is seen in WPW syndrome and in tachycardias.
- Children or young adults (physiological)

Q. What are the causes of muffling of S1 in MS? What are the causes of changing S1?

Ans. Certain conditions/diseases when associated with MS produce muffling of S1 (Table 1.101). The causes of changing 1st sound are given in the footnote of the table.

Q. What are causes of mid-diastolic murmur (MDM) at the apex?

Ans. In addition to MS, the other conditions/diseases that lead to mid-diastolic murmur are;
1. *Active rheumatic carditis (valvulitis).* It produces a soft mid-diastolic (Carey-Coombs') murmur without loud S1, opening snap and diastolic thrill. It is due to edema of valve cusps just producing obstruction. The murmur disappears as soon as the acute condition is over.
2. *Severe aortic regurgitation* (Austin-Flint murmur). It is due to functional MS produced by the aortic regurgitant jet striking against the anterior mitral leaflet forcing its partial closure. The murmur has following characteristics:
   - It is neither associated with loud S1 or presystolic accentuation
   - Opening snap is absent
   - No thrill
   - The patient has florid signs of severe AR (read aortic regurgitation)
3. *Functional mid-diastolic murmur* (increased flow through a normal valve). This is seen in left to right shunts (VSD, ASD, PDA) or in hyperdy-

Table 1.101: Diseases /conditions causing muffling of S₁ in MS

Diseases/condition	Mechanism
1. Mitral regurgitation or aortic regurgitation	Valve cusps do not close properly due to dilatation of the valve ring
2. Mitral valve calcification	Valve cusps are immobile
3. Acute rheumatic carditis and digitalis toxicity or overdosage	P-R interval is prolonged
4. Myocardial infarction or dilated heart (gross CHF)	The valve does not close completely as the forces that close the valve are diminished
5. Emphysema, pericardial effusion, obesity, rotation of the heart	All these conditions do not affect the mitral valve, hence production of S_1 is normal, but its transmission through the chest is diminished.

Note: Atrial fibrillation and complete heart block produce varying intensity of the first heart sound

namic circulation. The murmur is soft, not associated with thrill and opening snap. The third heart sound (S_3) due to rapid filling of the heart may be present.

4. *Severe mitral regurgitation*
   - A soft mid-diastolic murmur with a pansystolic murmur and S_3 indicates severe MR.
5. *Left atrial myxoma.* A pedunculated myxoma may strike against the valve in diastole producing signs of MS with mid-diastolic murmur. The characteristic features of atrial myxoma are:
   - Tumor plop—a sound produced by striking of myxoma against the valve.
   - Disappearance or change in the intensity and character of the murmur during lying down. The murmur is best heard in sitting position.
   - No associated thrill or opening snap.
   - Constitutional symptoms (fever, weight loss, arthralgia, rash) or embolic episodes may occur
   - Confirmation of diagnosis is done by 2-D-echocardiography
6. *Tricuspid stenosis.* The murmur has similar characteristics as in MS, but is best heard at left sternal edge.
7. *Ball valve thrombus.* It floats in the left atrium and produces functional MS similar to atrial myxoma from which it is differentiated by 2-D echocardiography.

Q. What are the causes of split S1?
Ans. Normally the two components of 1st sound (e.g. mitral and tricuspid) cannot be heard separately. However, the S1 gets split under following conditions:
   i. RBBB
   ii. Mitral or tricuspid stenosis
   iii. Ventricular pacing.

Q. What does presystolic murmur in MS indicate? What do you mean by presystolic accentuation of MDM in MS?
Ans. Presystolic murmur vs presystolic accentuation of MDM in MS is as follows:

The presystolic murmur is due to forceful atrial contractions against the stenotic mitral valve. The presystolic murmur without other auscultatory findings of MS, indicates mild MS; on the other hand in sinus rhythm presystolic accentuation of the mid-diastolic murmur indicates severe mitral stenosis. Presystolic accentuation of MDM disappears in AF and big atrial thrombus.

Q. What are the causes of opening snap?
Ans. Following are the causes:
   - Mitral stenosis
   - Tricuspid stenosis
   - Left to right shunt (VSD, ASD, PDA)
   - Sometimes in severe MR.

Q. What is Lutembacher's syndrome?
Ans. It comprises of:
   - Atrial septal defect ASD)
   - MS (rheumatic in origin)

Q. How do you decide the severity of mitral stenosis?
Ans. The auscultatory findings that determine the severity of MS are:
   - Lower volume pulse and low pulse pressure
   - Cold peripheral extremities
   - Longer duration of the mid-diastolic murmur with the pre-systolic accentuation.
   - Proximity of the OS to second heart sound. More near is the OS to the aortic component of second heart sound, more severe is the MS.

Q. What is Ortner's syndrome?
Ans. It is hoarseness of voice due to compression of recurrent largyngeal nerve by enlarged left atrium in MS

Q. What is juvenile mitral stenosis?

Ans. In the West, MS is seen usually in 4th or 5th decade, but in India, it develops early and may be seen in children commonly. The criteria for juvenile MS are:
- Occurs below 18 years of age
- It is usually severe (pin-point mitral valve)
- Atrial fibrillation is uncommon.
- Calcification of valve uncommon
- Needs immediate surgical correction.

Q. What are signs of pulmonary arterial hypertension?

Ans. The signs are limited to second left intercostal space (pulmonary area). There is prominent '*a*' wave in neck veins which are distended. The examination of the heart shows:

Inspection
- There may be visible pulmonary arterial pulsations
- Parasternal heave may be visible
- Right ventricular pulsations may be seen in epigastrium

Palpation
- P_2 may be palpable
- Left parasternal heave is palpable

Percussion
- The pulmonary area (second left intercostal space just lateral to sternal edge) may be dull on percussion

Ausculation
- P_2 is loud
- Second heart sound is narrowly split
- The *Graham-Steel murmur* of pulmonary regurgitation—a high pitched diastolic decrescendo blowing murmur along the left sternal edge
- Pulmonary ejection click
- A soft ejection systolic murmur and right-sided S_3 may be heard in severe pulmonary hypertension

Development of pulmonary hypertension is protective mechanism as it relieves pulmonary edema.

Q. How will you investigate a case with MS?

Ans. The investigations are as follows:
1. *ECG*: It may show left atrial hypertrophy (P mitrale), right ventricular hypertrophy and atrial fibrillation.
2. *Chest X-ray*: *Mitralised heart;* Left atrium is conspicuously prominent on left border of heart which is straightened. There is double atrial shadow. Signs of pulmonary congestion present. Pulmonary conus is prominent.
3. *Echocardiogram shows;*
   - Thickened immobile mitral cusps.
   - Reduced rate of diastolic filling (EF slope is flattened)
   - Reduced valve orifice area
   - Left atrial thrombus, if present
4. *Cardiac catheterization*
   Pressure gradient between LA and LV.

Q. In which trimester do the patients of MS usually become symptomatic and why?

Ans. Patient usually becomes symptomatic in second trimester of pregnancy. This is due to increase in blood volume which increases pulmonary pressure. The symptoms improve late in the 3rd trimester due to decrease in blood volume.

Q. What are the complications of mitral stenosis?

Ans. Common complications are as follows:
1. *Acute pulmonary edema* (left heart failure). In patients with MS, the left ventricle is hypoplastic (under-filled) hence, pulmonary edema is due to elevated left atrial pressure transmitted to pulmonary veins resulting in transudation.
   In mitral stenosis, there is initial left heart failure – left atrial failure with congestion of the lungs followed by right ventricular failure or congestive heart failure.
2. *Pulmonary hypertension* and *right heart failure*
3. *Arrhythmias,* e.g. atrial fibrillation, atrial flutter, VPCs
4. *Left atrial thrombus* with systemic embolization leading to stroke, Lerische's syndrome – occlusion of bifurcation of aorta
5. *Recurrent massive hemoptysis* leading to hemosiderosis
6. *Infective endocarditis* – rare. It is common in mitral regurgitation than stenosis
7. *Recurrent pulmonary infections* due to chronic passive venous lung congestion
8. *Complications produced by enlarged left atrium*
   - *Ortner's syndrome.* Hoarseness of voice due to compression of recurrent laryngeal nerve.
   - Dysphagia (compression of esophagus)
   - Clot in the left atrium gives rise to embolization in sinus rhythm
   - Collapse of the lung due to pressure on left bronchus
9. Sudden death due to *ball valve thrombus* – a big thrombus fits like a ball into mitral valve.
10. Interlobar effusion *(phantom tumor)* or hydrothorax *(pleural effusion).*

Q. What are clinical signs of acute pulmonary edema?

Ans. Read mitral regurgitation.

Q. What are the causes of pulmonary edema?

Ans. The pulmonary edema may be *cardiogenic* (left ventricular or left atrial failure, high CVP, and PCWP, and engorged neck veins) or *noncardiogenic* (normal left ventricular and atrial pressure, normal CVP and PCWP and neck veins). The noncardiogenic pulmonary edema is also called *adult respiratory distress syndrome (ARDS)*. The causes are given in Table 1.102.

Table 1.102: Causes of pulmonary edema

1. **Cardiogenic**
   - Left heart failure (e.g. mitral and aortic valve disease, HT)
   - Acute MI
   - Cardiac arrhythmias
   - Acute pulmonary thromboembolism
2. **Noncardiogenic**
   - Severe sepsis
   - Inhalation of toxic and irritant gases (phosgene, phosphine (PH_3), hyperbaric O_2)
   - High altitude pulmonary edema
   - Drowning or near drowning
   - Aspiration of gastric contents or corrosive poisoning
   - Aluminium phosphide poisoning (insecticide, pesticide)
   - Acute hemorrhagic pancreatitis
   - Narcotic overdose
   - Snake bite
   - Acute fulminant hepatitis (hepatic failure)
   - Sudden removal of air (pneumothorax) or fluid (pleural effusion) from thoracic cavity
   - Fluid overload
   - Chronic renal failure (CRF), Goodpasture's syndrome

Q. How would manage the patient?

Ans. The patient is managed as follows:
- If the patient is in acute LVF, then it is an emergency requiring parenteral diuretics, bronchodilators, vasodilators along with oral digoxin (0.5 mg stat) or I.V. digoxin (not preferred now a days) In addition, patient needs prop up position and O_2 inhalation
- Mild stenosis is treated with salt restriction and diuretics.

- Moderate to severe MS needs, propped up position, O_2 inhalation, oral digoxin and diuretics. Vasodilators are needed to reduce afterload. As patient improves, he/she is prepared for surgery.
- Treatment of atrial fibrillation if present, by digitalis or calcium channel blocker, beta blocker. Anticoagulant is also needed to prevent thromboembolism.
- Prophylaxis against bacterial endocarditis by penicillin, benzathine penicillin 12.5 lac units/ every 3-4 weeks for 5 years or up to 25 years of age depending on the age of onset of MS.
- Surgery

Q. What are indications for surgery?

Ans.
- Severe or significant symptomatic MS with pliable valve
- Patient with recurrent hemoptysis and pulmonary hypertension
- Recurrent thromboembolism despite anticoagulation.

Q. Name the surgical procedures for MS.

Ans.
1. *Closed commissurotomy*: (closed mitral valvotomy by mechanical dilators or valvuloplasty by balloon dilatation of the mitral valve)
2. *Open commissurotomy*: It requires cardio-pulmonary bypass and allows surgical repair of valve under direct vision.
3. *Valve replacement*: It is done when valve is fibrosed, disorganized, calcified or when there is associated mitral regurgitation.

Q. What are complications of surgery?

Ans.
- Mitral regurgitation may occur
- Risk of thromboembolic event
- Restenosis

Q. What factors determine the success of balloon valvuloplasty?

Ans.
- Pliable valve cusps
- No or little calcification
- Good left ventricular function

CASE 30: MITRAL REGURGITATION

The patient (not shown) presented with complaints of palpitation, dyspnea, PND and chest discomfort. There was history of cough with no hemoptysis. Patient had history of pain abdomen and edema feet.

Examination revealed normal pulse, BP and raised JVP. Apex beat was down and outside the midclavicular line in 5th intercostal space, forceful and diffuse. Left parasternal heave present. A systolic thrill present at apex. The auscultatory findings included soft and muffled S1, a pansystolic murmur, a third heart sound (Fig. 1.30A).

Clinical Presentations

- The patient may be entirely asymptomatic, murmur is often detected in medical board examination more often in young females without any apparent disability
- These patients may present with symptoms of left heart failure (cough, dyspnea, PND, hemoptysis, etc.)
- These patients in addition to above symptoms may present with complications, e.g. hemiplegia, gangrene of finger, toes

Fig. 1.30A: Mitral regurgitation. Hemodynamic effects and auscultatory findings

- Acute mitral regurgitation may present as acute LHF in a patient with acute MI due to rupture of papillary muscle or chordae tendineae.

History

Points to be Asked/Noted

Ask for the followings:

- Exertional dyspnea, nocturnal dyspnea, palpitation
- Symptoms of acute pulmonary edema, e.g. cough, frothy sputum, dyspnea at rest and hemoptysis
- Fatigue, weakness, tiredness due to reduced cardiac output
- Puffiness of face, ankle or leg swelling, ascites due to right heart failure
- History of trauma to chest or cardiac surgery, MI, connective tissue disease, infective endocarditis.

Past History

- Ask for history of sore throat, skin infection, rheumatic fever (joint pain)
- History of recurrent chest infections, fever, paralysis.

General Physical Examination

- Pulse may be good volume or normal volume or jerky. It is usually regular but becomes irregular in presence of atrial fibrillation or ventricular ectopics
- Pulse pressure may be wide or normal Note BP, temperature and respiration
- Cyanosis (peripheral or central or both) may be present
- Raised jugular venous pressure with prominent 'a' wave in severe pulmonary hypertension and 'v' wave if TR develops
- Pitting pedal edema
- Look for signs of bacterial endocarditis, e.g. fever, splinter hemorrhage, Janeway's lesion, palmar erythema, clubbing of fingers, painful fingertips or gangrenous finger(s), cold extremities, red coloration of urine
- Look for signs of acute rheumatic activity, e.g. arthritis, fever, erythema marginatum, subcutaneous nodules, etc.

- Note for the presence of features of Marfan's syndrome, e.g. tall stature arachnodactyly, high-arched palate, ectopia lentis.

Systemic Examination

I. Cardiovascular System

Inspection

- Apex beat is displaced down beyond 5th intercostal space outside the midclavicular line and is diffuse but forceful.
- Pulmonary artery pulsations in 2nd left intercostal space may be seen.
- Left parasternal heave may be visible.

Palpation

- Left parasternal heave may be palpable.
- Displaced down and out forceful apex beat.
- Systolic thrill at apex may be palpable
- P_2 may be palpable in pulmonary area in pulmonary hypertension.

Percussion

- Left border of heart corresponds to apex beat, i.e. dullness does not extend beyond apex beat.

Auscultation

- First heart sound soft or muffled and buried in the pansystolic murmur
- Pansystolic murmur at apex, high-pitched soft and radiates to left axilla, heard with diaphragm of the stethoscope in expiration
- Third heart sound (S_3) may be present, is caused by rapid flow of blood causing tensing of papillary muscle, chordae tendineae and valve leaflets
- P_2 may be loud and narrowly split. Ejection systolic and/or diastolic murmur (Graham Steell) at 2nd left space. These are signs of pulmonary arterial hypertension.

II. Examination of Other Systems

1. **Respiratory system**
   - Tachypnea may be present
   - Crackles and rales at bases of lungs
2. **Abdominal examination**
   - Mild tender hepatomegaly
   - No ascites, no splenomegaly.

Q. What is the clinical diagnosis in this case?

Ans. The symptoms and signs suggest the diagnosis of mitral regurgitation (MR) with CHF with normal sinus rhythm without SABE and acute rheumatic activity in this case.

Q. What are points in favour of your diagnosis?

Ans. 1. *H/O dyspnea*, orthopnea and PND.
2. *Signs of MR*, i.e. down and out apex beat, parasternal heave, a pansystolic murmur radiating to axilla, muffled S$_1$ and a S$_3$.
3. *Signs of pulmonary hypertension*, e.g. loud P$_2$, narrow split S$_2$.
4. *Signs of CHF*, e.g. raised JVP, tender hepatomegaly and edema feet.

Q. Could it be mitral valve prolapse (MVP)?

Ans. No, there is no click and murmur is holosystolic instead of mid and late systolic.

Q. What is prevalence of MVP in general population?

Ans. About 9–10%. More common in young females (15-35 years).

Q. What is mechanism of click in MVP?

Ans. It is due to sudden tensing of mitral valve apparatus as the leaflet prolapse into the left atrium during systole.

Q. How do you define mitral regurgitation? What are its hemodynamic consequences?

Ans. Regurgitation of blood through the mitral valve during systole is called *mitral regurgitation*.

Hemodynamic Consequences: Normally mitral valve closes during ventricular systole, but in mitral regurgitation, a small volume of blood regurgitates back into left atrium during systole in addition to left ventricular ejection into the aorta, leading to left atrial enlargement due to volume overload. During diastole, a large volume of blood from overloaded left atrium rushes to the left ventricle producing its subsequent enlargement, hence, the consequences of MR are:

- Dilatation of left atrium (*giant atrium*). It occurs first of all.
- Dilatation of left ventricle due to volume overload leading to subsequent LVF.
- The back flow of blood from overloaded left atrium produces lung congestion, pulmonary edema and subsequent pulmonary arterial hypertension.
- Ultimately pulmonary arterial hypertension leads to right ventricular hypertrophy, then its failure leading to congestion of various viscera called congestive heart failure.

Q. What are the causes of mitral regurgitation?

Ans. The mitral regurgitation occurs commonly from the dilatation of the mitral ring in rheumatic heart disease or due to diseases of myocardium and endocardium producing insufficient closure of the valve, though structurally valve may be normal. It may be acute, either due to papillary muscle dysfunction or chordae tendineae rupture in patients with MI. The causes are given in Table 1.103.

Table 1.103: Causes of mitral regurgitation

1. **Rheumatic (less common)**
   - Rheumatic heart disease, acute rheumatic fever
2. **Non-rheumatic (common)**
   - Mitral valve prolapse
   - Myocarditis
   - Acute MI (due to papillary muscle dysfunction or rupture of chorae tendineae producing acute mitral regurgitation)
   - Infective endocarditis
   - Dilated cardiomyopathy
   - Trauma during valvotomy
   - Marfan's syndrome
   - SLE (Libman-Sack's endocarditis)
   - Rarely congenital
3. **Left ventricular dilatation (volvering dilatation) Secondary to:**
   - Aortic valve disease, e.g. AS, AR or both
   - Systemic hypertension

Note: Isolated mitral regurgitation is commonly non-rheumatic in origin.

Q. What are the frequencies with which various valves get affected by rheumatic heart disease?

Ans.
- Mitral valve disease (80%). MS is the commonest lesion followed by combined MS and MR
- Aortic valve (50%)
- Combined mitral and aortic valve lesion (20%)
- Tricuspid valve involvement (10%)
- Pulmonary valve involvement rare (<1%)

Q. What are congenital causes of MR?

Ans.
- Ostium primum atrial septal defect (cleft mitral valve)
- Endocardial cushion defect (partial atrioventricular canal)
- Corrected transposition of great vessels

Q. Where are characteristic features of severe MR?

Ans. Characteristic features of severe MR are as follows:
i. *General physical signs*
   - A good volume pulse with wide pulse pressure
   - Raised JVP with prominent 'a' wave due to severe pulmonary hypertension, and a prominent 'v' wave if there is associated TR
   - Bilateral pitting pedal edema

ii. *Signs of left ventricular hypertrophy/failure*
- Apex beat is hyperdynamic and goes down and out. A systolic thrill may be palpable.
iii. *Signs of RVH*
- Left parasternal heave
- Epigastric pulsation
- Signs of severe pulmonary hypertension (Read signs of pulmonary hypertension in MS).
iv. *Auscultatory signs of mitral regurgitation*
- The S_1 is generally muffled, soft or buried within pansystolic murmur
- A pansystolic murmur radiating to left axilla
- S_3 may be audible due to rapid filling of left ventricle
- A short-soft diastolic murmur even in the absence of MS (functional MS) may be heard
- An S_4 is audible in acute severe MR
- An OS may be heard in the absence of MS. Usually OS indicates associated MS but can be heard in severe MR.

Electrocardiogram
- P mitral, P- pulmonale or bifid P wave of biatrial enlargement with severe LVH
- Atrial fibrillation common.

Color Doppler is the most accurate noninvasive technique for detection and estimation of severe MR.

Q. How would you grade systolic murmurs?
Ans. Read Clinical Methods in Medicine by Prof SN Chugh.

Q. What is pansystolic murmur and what are its causes?
Ans. Definition: A pansystolic or holosystolic murmur starts with the first heart sound (S_1) and continues throughout the systole and embraces S_2. It has uniform intensity hence called holosystolic.

Mechanism: As the left ventricle in MR is overloaded, its pressure exceeds LA pressure just after the first heart sound, hence, the regurgitant jet of blood starts flowing from LV to LA producing systolic murmur that continues throughout systole up to S_2 until LA pressure exceeds the LV pressure to stop the jet.

Causes
1. *MR* due to any cause (read the causes in the Table 1.118).
2. *TR:* The pansystolic murmur is best audible in the tricuspid area (left parasternal), increases in intensity with inspiration (*Carvallo's sign*) and does not radiate to axilla. There may be prominent 'v' waves in JVP and liver may be pulsatile.
3. *Ventricular septal defect (malade Roger):* The murmur is rough, pansystolic, best heard across the chest (on both sides of sternum). Very often, there is an associated thrill.

4. *Dilated cardiomyopathy* sometimes myocarditis
5. *Functional murmur* (Left ventricular dilatation): These murmurs are usually soft, mostly midsystolic, may be pansystolic and do not radiate to the axilla. No change with posture and respiration.
6. *Papillary muscle dysfunction.*

Q. What does mid-diastolic murmur in MR indicate?
Ans. It indicates:
1. Associated MS (i.e. MR with MS)
2. Severe MR with functional MS.

Q. What are causes of acute MR?
Ans. Causes of acute MR are:
- Acute myocardial infarction with either rupture of papillary muscle or chordae tendineae.
- Acute bacterial endocarditis with rupture/perforation of valve cusps or chordae tendineae.
- Traumatic rupture of chordae tendineae.
- Myxomatous degeneration of the valve

Q. What are the characteristics of mitral valve prolapse syndrome (Barlow's syndrome, midsystolic click-murmur syndrome, floppy mitral valve syndrome)?
Ans. The characteristic features are:
- This is myxomatous degeneration of the mitral leaflets resulting in redundant mitral leaflets that prolapse into LA during systole.
- It is commonly seen in young females.
- It is asymptomatic and mid-systolic murmur or the click or both may be the only evidence. Valsalva maneuver and standing increase the murmur while squatting decreases it.
- The prolapse of the posterior cusp (common) radiates the murmur towards right side while prolapse of anterior cusp radiates the murmur to left axilla.
- It is commonly associated with ventricular arrhythmias, hence, β-blockers are indicated for symptom relief and prophylaxis.
- Other associated conditions include Marfan's syndrome, RHD, Ehlers-Danlos syndrome, SLE, Psoriatic arthritis.

Q. When does the murmur of MR radiates to neck (or base of heart) instead of axilla?
Ans. Rarely involvement of posterior mitral leaflet in mitral valve prolapse syndrome or ruptured chordae tendineae, reflects the regurgitant jet that strikes the left atrial wall adjacent to the aortic root towards the base of heart, hence, murmur is heard at this site.

Q. What are the causes of mitral valve prolapse?
Ans. Following are causes:
- Marfan's syndrome
- Ehlers-Danlos syndrome

- Collagen vascular disorders (genetically determined)
- Straight-back syndrome (a thoracic cage abnormality)
- As a sequel of acute rheumatic fever
- Ischemic heart disease
- Cardiomyopathy.

Q. What is Cooing or 'Seagull' murmur?

Ans. When a patient of MR either develops SABE or rupture of chordae tendineae, a systolic murmur appears that has either a cooing or musical or sea-gull quality – here the chordae tendineae act like strings of a musical instrument. This type of murmur is also found in acute myocardial infarction with rupture of chordae tendineae and rarely in acute rheumatic carditis.

Q. What is effect of Valsalva maneuver on MR?

Ans. The systolic murmur of MR is increased by isometric strain (hand – grip) but is reduced during the Valsalva maneuver.

Q. What are clinical signs of congestive heart failure?

Ans. Following are signs of congestive heart failure:
- Extremities may be cold or pale.
- Tachycardia and tachypnea.
- Profuse sweating or perspiration.
- Central cyanosis.
- Low volume pulse or pulsus alternans.
- Cheyne–Stokes breathing.
- Third heart sound (S_3). Ventricular gallop rhythm means triple rhythm (S_1, S_2, S_3 sounds) with tachycardia – is so named because it resembles with the cadence produced by galloping of a horse).
- Fine basal pulmonary rales/crackles.
- Expiratory wheezing.
- Hydrothorax or pleural effusion.
- Oliguria and nocturia.
- Cardiomegaly with other signs of basic heart disease (For signs of basic heart disease, one should read the specific disorder).

Q. How will you arrive at the diagnosis of congestive heart failure (CHF)?

Ans. The diagnosis of CHF is based on presence of some combinations of the clinical manifestations described in Table 1.104, together with the findings characteristics of one of the underlying forms of heart disease.

Q. What are the causes of right heart failure?

Ans. Following are the causes:
1. *Pulmonary valve disease*
   - Pulmonary stenosis
   - Pulmonary hypertension due to any cause

Table 1.104: Framingham criteria for diagnosis of CHF

Major criteria
- Paroxysmal nocturnal dyspnea (PND)
- Distended neck veins
- Cardiomegaly
- Rales
- Acute pulmonary edema
- S_3 gallop
- Increased venous pressure (>16 cm H_2O)
- Positive hepatojugular reflux

Minor criteria
- Peripheral pitting edema
- Night cough
- Dyspnea on exertion
- Hepatomegaly
- Pleural effusion (hydrothorax)
- Reduced vital capacity by 1/3 of normal
- Tachycardia ($\geq$ 120 bpm)

NB: To establish the diagnosis of CHF, at least one major and two minor criteria are required

- Acute cor pulmonale (pulmonary thromboembolism)
- Chronic cor pulmonale
2. *Tricuspid diseases*
   - Tricuspid stenosis
   - Tricuspid regurgitation (dilated cardiomyopathy)
   - Ebstein anomaly
3. *Depressed myocardial contractility*
   - Right ventricular infarction
   - Right ventricular dysplasia (right ventricular cardiomyopathy)
   - Myocarditis
4. *Secondary to left heart failure.* The left ventricular failure ultimately may lead to right ventricular failure.

Q. What are the complications of MR?

Ans. Complications of MR are:
- *Acute LVF* (acute pulmonary edema). It is characterized by persistent coughing with bringing out of small amount of frothy pink colored sputum with increasing breathlessness, orthopnea, PND, tachypnea, tachycardia and central cyanosis. The chest shows diffuse bilateral crackles and rales throughout both lungs. The X-ray is diagnostic.
- *Infective endocarditis.*
- *CHF* and *deep vein thrombosis.*
- *Arrhythmias,* e.g. ventricular ectopics, atrial fibrillation common. Atrial fibrillation is due to giant left atrium.
- *Giant left atrium* may produce pressure symptoms, e.g. hoarseness, dysphagia.

- *Thromboembolism*
- *Atypical chest pain.*

Q. How will you investigate a patient with MR?

Ans. Investigations required are as follows:

1. *Chest X-ray.* It may show:
   - Cardiac shadow is enlarged and occupies >50% of transthoracic diameter.
   - The left atrium may be massively enlarged and forms the right border of the heart.
   - The left ventricle is also enlarged producing *boot-shaped heart.*
   - There may be pulmonary venous congestion (e.g. upper lobar veins prominent producing increased bronchovascular marking or there may be diffuse haze from hilum to periphery – pulmonary edema), interstitial edema (*Kerley's B lines)* and sometimes interlobar fissure effusion or hydrothorax.
   - Mitral valve calcification may occur, seen in penetrating films.

2. *ECG.* It may show:
   - Right atrial, left atrial or biatrial hypertrophy
   - LV or biventricular hypertrophy
   - AF
   - Inferior or posterior wall ischemia/infarction if CAD is the cause.

3. *Echocardiogram and Doppler imaging.* The 2D-echocardiogram is useful for assessing the cause of MR displacement of one or both cusps into left atrium during systole in AVP and for estimating the LV function and ejection fractions. Left atrium are left ventricle enlarged. Vegetations may be seen in infective endocarditis. The echocardiogram M-mode shows characteristic feature of MVPS (incomplete coaptation of anterior and posterior leaflets during mid and late systole).

4. *Color Doppler flow study* is most accurate diagnostic technique for detection and quantification of MR. It shows a characteristic regurgitant jet.

5. *Trans-esophageal echocardiography* is useful in those in whom transthoracic echocardiography provides non-diagnostic images.

6. *Cardiac catheterization* It is useful to determine coronary artery disease or aortic valve disease, may be needed prior to surgery.

Q. What are the causes of LVH? What are its ECG characteristics?

Ans. Read Practical Electrocardiography by Dr SN Chugh.

Q. How will you treat a patient with MR?

Ans. Treatment consists of symptomatic relief to be provided by medical treatment and permanent relief by surgical treatment (valve replacement).

1. *Medical treatment*
   - Asymptomatic disease does not require treatment except penicillin prophylaxis such as mitral valve prolapse.
   - Salt restriction
   - Digitalis and diuretics
   - Bronchodilatation if there is severe bronchospasm
   - Vasodilators (ACE-inhibitors) to reduce the regurgitant flow in severe cases.
   - *Prophylaxis.* Penicillin prophylaxis is must.

2. *Surgical treatment* is valve replacement

Q. What is indication of surgery in MR?

Ans. Moderate to severe symptomatic disease with good left ventricular function.

Q. How will you decide clinically the dominance of mitral valve lesion in a patient with combined mitral valve disease (MS and MR)?

Ans. The dominance is decided by features described in Table 1.105.

Q. What does 3rd heart sound in MR indicate?

Ans. The presence of 3rd heart sound in MR indicates rapid ventricular filling due to free flow of blood through mitral valve. It signifies moderate to severe MR and in combined mitral valve lesion (MS with MR), it indicates dominance of MR over MS.

Q. What are signs of digitalis toxicity?

Ans. The signs are as follows:

1. *GI manifestations,* e.g. anorexia, nausea, vomiting. These are earliest to appear.

2. *Cardiac arrhythmias and conduction disturbances*
   - Premature ventricular complexes (VPCs) usually ventricular bigeminy or multiforme.
   - Nonparoxysmal atrial tachycardia with block
   - Varying degrees of AV block
   - Sinoatrial block (SA block)
   - Ventricular tachycardia; bidirectional ventricular tachycardia is mainly due to digitalis
   - Ventricular fibrillation

3. *Miscellaneous effects*
   - Weight loss
   - Cardiac cachexia
   - Gynecomastia
   - Yellow vision (xanthopsia)
   - Mental features, e.g. agitation

Table 1.105: Features of dominant MS or MR in combined valvular lesion

Feature	Dominant MS	Dominant MR
1. Clinical presentations	Dyspnea on exertion, orthopnea and PND. Palpitation is uncommon occurs if AF present	Palpitations common, followed by dyspnea, orthopnea and PND
2. Symptoms • Hemoptysis and PND • Symptoms of CHF • Systemic embolization • Lung congestion	Marked	Mild
3. Signs		
Pulse	Low volume	Normal volume
BP	Low systolic	Within normal limits
Apex	Tapping, not displaced	Heaving and displaced down and out
Left parasternal heave	Grade III	Grade I
First heart sound	Short, loud and snappy	Soft or muffled
Opening snap	Present	Absent
Third heart sound (S_3)	Absent	Present
Murmur and thrill	• Rough and rumbling diastolic murmur with thrill • Pansystolic murmur present, does not radiate to axilla	• Soft pansystolic murmur radiating to axilla with a systolic thrill • Soft mid-diastolic murmur
4. Chest X-ray	Mitralized heart	Cardiomegaly with giant left atrium forming right heart border
5. ECG	RVH with left axis deviation	LVH with right axis deviation

Q. How will you treat digitalis toxicity?

Ans. The steps of treatment are:

- Stop digoxin
- Stop diuretic
- Give potassium
- Give phenytoin for digitalis-induced arrhythmias
- Give digitalis Fab antibody

Q. How would you differentiate MR from TR?

Ans.

Feature	Mitral regurgitation	Tricuspid regurgitation
Pulse	Good volume Jerky or normal volume	Normal pulse
JVP	Raised with prominent 'a' wave	Raised with 'VY' Collapse
Palpation	Left ventricular heave	Left parasternal heave
Auscultation	• Pansystolic murmur	• Pansystolic murmur at apex at left parasternal edge or eping astrium
	• Murmur radiates to axilla	• Murmur may be heard in epigastrium and right sternal border.
	• Intensity increases with expiration	• Intensity increases with inspiration
	• 3rd heart sound present	• 4th heart sound present
Other features	• Liver may be enlarged without pulsation	• Liver enlarged with pulsations (Pulsatile liver)
	• Lungs congested with crackles	• Lungs may or may not be congested, depend on its cause–Isolated or associated

Q. Mention recent Jones Criteria for acute rheumatic fever.

Ans. Table 1.106 explains the John's criteria for acute rheumatic fever.

Q. What are various types of prosthetic valves?

Ans. I. *Mechanical valves*

- Ball and cage (*Starr-Edwards*)
- Titting disc valve i.e. Single tilting disc (*Bjork-Shirley*) and double tilting disc (*bileaflet valve-St Jude*)

II. *Tissue (biological valves)*

Xenografts (porcine valves and pericardial valves derived from animal tissue)

Homograft

- Cadaveric aortic or pulmonary valve (human valve)

Q. What are indications of valve replacement?

Ans.
- Severe calcified mitral stenosis
- Calcific aortic stenosis
- Severe mitral regurgitation
- Severe aortic regurgitation

Q. What kind of valve would you use to replace mitral valve ? and why ?

Ans. Mechanical valve because of durability. Anticoagulant is to be used to protect them.

Q. Why mechanical valves are preferred over bioprosthesis?

Ans. Mechanical valves are preferred because of two reasons:

- Lower rate of reoperation
- Lower chances of anticoagulant related bleeding.

Q. Which bioprosthesis is commonly used?

Ans. Porcine heart valve.

Q. What are complications of porcine heart valve?

Ans.
- Degeneration with time
- Calcification

Q. What are the complications of mechanical valves?

Ans.
- High incidence of hemolysis leading to anemia
- Thromboembolism
- Bleeding due to anticoagulants use
- Endocarditis
- Valve dysfunction, e.g. valve leak, valve dehiscence and valve obstruction by thrombus or clogging
- Structural dysfunction, e.g. fracture, cuspal tear and calcification.
- Nonstructural dysfunction e.g. perivalvular leak, suture entrapment.

Q. How would you recognize that patient had prosthetic valve?

Ans.
i. Mid-sternal vertical thoracotomy scar
ii. Metallic heart sounds in mitral area (mitral valve replaced) or at both sites if both valves have been replaced.

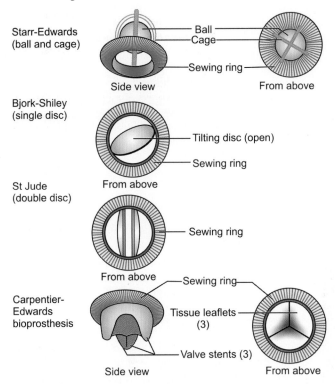

Starr-Edwards (ball and cage)
Ball
Cage
Sewing ring
Side view
From above

Bjork-Shiley (single disc)
Tilting disc (open)
Sewing ring
From above

St Jude (double disc)
Sewing ring
From above

Carpentier-Edwards bioprosthesis
Sewing ring
Tissue leaflets (3)
Valve stents (3)
Side view
From above

Fig. 1.30B: Type of valves

Q. Which patients should receive bioprosthetic valve?

Ans.
- Those unable to take anticoagulants.
- Those not expected to live longer than predicted lifespan of prosthesis (7-10 yrs).
- Patients over the age of 70 years who require an aortic valve replacement as the rate of degeneration is slow in these patients.

Q. In women of child bearing age, which valve would you prefer?

Ans. Until recently bioprosthetic valves were being preferred to avoid risk of anticoagulation on the fetus and spontaneous abortion but the major disadvantage of these valves is degeneration requiring reoperation. Nowadays mechanical valves are preferred because studies have now shown low risk of warfarin and spontaneous abortion in women.

Q. Which valve would you use in presence of AF?

Ans. Mechanical valve as these patients need warfarin treatment.

Table 1.106: Jone's diagnostic criteria for acute rheumatic fever

1. **Major**
   - Carditis
   - Polyarthritis
   - Chorea
   - Erythema marginatum
   - Subcutaneous nodules
2. **Minor**
   - Fever
   - Arthralgia
   - Previous rheumatic fever
   - Raised ESR or C-reactive protein
   - Leukocytosis
   - First degree or second degree AV block
   - Echocardiographic evidence of endocarditis

The diagnosis is *definite* if;
- Two or more major manifestations are present, or
- One major and two or more minor manifestations
  Plus
- Supporting evidence of preceding streptococcal infection, recent scarlet fever, raised ASO titers or other streptococcal antibody titer, positive throat culture, or echocardiographic evidence of carditis.

CASE 31: INFECTIVE ENDOCARDITIS

The patient presented with palpitation, cough, breathlessness and chest discomfort. There was history of PND and edema of feet off and on for the last few years. He was taking treatment and edema and breathlessness relieved. Now he complained of fever with chills, rigors and diaphoresis. He developed gangrene of the fingers (Fig. 1.31A) suddenly

Clinical Presentations

1. *Acute endocarditis* caused by more virulent organisms mostly *Staphylococcus aureas* involves normal heart valves or cardiac structures, produces acute febrile illness with fever, chills, diaphoresis and acute onset of regurgitant murmur due to damage to valves and cardiac structures, with septic embolization to various viscera and peripheral structures.
2. *Subacute infective endocarditis* caused by less virulent organisms such as bacteria i.e. (*Streptococci, pneumococci, Staphylococci, fastidious gram-negative coccobacilli, HACEK group-Hemophilus, Actinobaccilus, Corynebacterium, Eikenella and Kingella*), fungi (*candida*) or rickettsia cause insidious onset of fever with chills and rigors, changing or new cardiac murmurs, precipitation of CHF and embolization to viscera and peripheral structures in a patient who is already suffering from either a congenital heart disease or acquired rheumatic heart disease or has undergone cardiac surgery or has prosthetic valve.

History

Points to be Noted

- Dyspnea, palpitation, cough, chest discomfort due to basic heart disease, i.e. valvular or congenital lesion
- Fever with chills, diaphoresis
- Symptoms of complications such as CHF or systemic embolization, e.g. cold extremity, hemiplegia, hematuria
- Visual disturbance or visual loss
- Onset, duration of symptoms.
- History of fever, sore throat
- History of procedure or dental extraction in a patient with underlying congenital or acquired valvular heart disease
- History of recent cardiac surgery
- History of I.V. drug misuse
- History of sepsis, skin infection
- Ask about past history of rheumatic or congenital heart disease.

General Physical Examination

- General look-toxic. Patient is febrile
- Weight loss
- The skin may show purpuric spot, ecchymosis, Janeway lesion
- Neck for JVP and lymphadenopathy
- *Extremities.*
  - Clubbing of fingers
  - Janeway lesion
  - Digital gangrene
  - Petechial
  - Splinter hemorrhage
  - Osler's nodes
  - Coldness of extremities
  - Painful fingertips
- Eyes for subconjunctival hemorrhage, Roth's spots

- Look for anemia, cyanosis, jaundice, edema
- Examine vitals, e.g. pulse, BP, respiration and temperature
- Palpate all the peripheral pulses. Pulsation in right brachial artery absent in this case.

Systemic Examination

1. CVS

- Inspection. Look for signs of LHF.
- Palpation. Look for signs of LHF.
- Percussion for cardiac dullness.
- Auscultation. Auscultate for any murmur, change in previous murmur and appearance of new murmur in addition to findings of heart disease.

2. Other Systems

- Nervous system for motor or sensory deficit due to embolization (stroke). Examine ocular fundi
- Respiratory system for pulmonary embolism, infection, LVF
- Kidneys for pain and tenderness in renal area or hematuria.
- Palpate for splenomegaly and hepatomegaly

N.B. Look for signs of heart failure. Auscultate for any murmur, change in murmur and appearance of new murmur in addition to basic findings of underlying disease

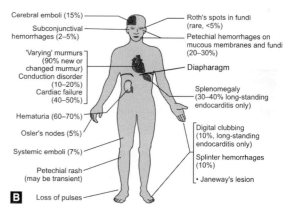

Figs 1.31A and B: Infective endocarditis A. Gangrenous fingers, hand and forearm on left side due to embolic occlusion of brachial artery on Doppler study. The patient had cold extremities with absent brachial and radial pulses on left side. B. Clinical features of endocarditis (diagram)

Q. What is your clinical diagnosis and why?

Ans. In view of history suggestive of some heart disease with CHF combined with embolic occlusion of brachial artery with gangrenous fingers, the provisional diagnosis is infective endocarditis due to underlying cardiac disorder which will be apparent on physical signs and on investigations.

Q. Name the conditions that produce clinical feature similar to endocarditis.

Ans.
- Atrial myxoma
- Sickle cell disease
- SLE
- Nonbacterial endocarditis.

Q. How you do define endocarditis? What are common causative organisms?

Ans. Infective endocarditis is due to microbial infection of a heart valve (native, prosthetic), the lining of a cardiac chamber, or blood vessels or a congenital septal defect or a congenital anomaly. The causative organism is either a bacterium (S. *viridans, Staph. aureus, Strep. fecalis*) or a fungus or a rickettsia (*Q fever endocarditis*).

Acute endocarditis is usually bacterial in origin, has rapid onset, fulminant course causing destruction of cardiac structures, perforation of valve cusps and hematogenously seeds the extracardiac sites, and if untreated, progresses to death within weeks.

Subacute endocarditis follows an indolent course, causes structural cardiac damage slowly and rarely causes metastatic infection, and is gradually progressive unless complicatd by a major embolic event or rupture of mycotic aneurysm.

Q. What are symptoms and signs of endocarditis? What is their pathogenesis?

Ans. The symptoms and signs (Table 1.107) are due to
- Infection and fluctuating toxemia
- Embolization
- Immune-complex mechanism
- Anemia.

Table 1.107: The symptoms and signs of infective endocarditis

Organ	Symptoms and signs (Fig. 1.31B)
General	Fever, nausea, anorexia, sweating, weakness Temperature is raised, weight loss is present
Heart	Dyspnea, palpitations, cough, pain chest • Tachycardia • Changing or appearance of new murmurs • Conduction defects • CHF • Muffling of heart sounds

Contd...

Contd...

Organ	Symptoms and signs (Fig. 1.31B)
Lung	Hemoptysis, chest pain Pleuritic rub due to embolic pulmonary infarct may be present
CNS	Headache, toxic encephlopathy, meningitis Monoplegia or hemiplegia due to embolization
Blood vessels	Coldness of extremities • Loss of peripheral pulses due to embolization
Hands	• Digital gangrene • Clubbing of the fingers • Splinter hemorrhages • Osler's nodes (painful tender swellings at fingertips) Janeway's lesion (large nontender maculopapular eruptions in palm and sole)
Skin	• Petechial hemorrhage • Purpuric spots Eyes, i.e. redness of eyes, visual disturbance • Subconjunctival hemorrhage blindness • Roth's spots
Kidneys	• Hematuria • Renal angle tender • Acute flank pain, pain in splenic area • Splenomegaly • Splenic infarct (rub)
Blood	Pallor, lassitude, fatigue • Anemia

Q. What are complications of endocarditis?

Ans. Common complications are:
1. *Heart failure*. Endocarditis may precipitate or aggravate the heart failure which may occur following a tear in a leaflet, ruptured chordae tendineae, dehiscence of a prosthetic valve or perforation of interventricular septum.
2. *Embolization* to any organ producing an infarct
3. *Neurological complications*. Embolic stroke is the most common neurological complication. Intracranial hemorrhage may occur due to ruptured mycotic aneurysm or rupture of an artery due to septic arteritis. Meningitis and brain abscess can occur.
4. *Septicemia*.
5. *Valve destruction*, e.g. acute regurgitation.
6. *Local extension*, e.g. myocarditis (abscess) and purulent pericarditis.
7. *Glomerulonephritis*.

153

8. *Conduction disturbance* caused by an abscess in ventricular septum.

Q. What are clinical features of acute bacterial endocarditis?

Ans. Clinical features are as follows:

- Often involves the normal heart valves and has rapid downhill course.
- *Staphylococcus* is the commonest pathogen
- Right sided involvement is common because it is common in IV drug users. Pneumonia is common.
- Clubbing is not a feature.
- Source of infection is evident, i.e. Staphylococcal abscess or pneumococcal meningitis.
- Cardiac and renal failure develop rapidly.
- Perforation of cusps (aortic, mitral) may occur leading to acute valvular regurgitation.

Q. What is right sided endocarditis?

Ans. Main features are as follows:

- Commonly caused by *S. aureus*.
- Tricuspid valve is commonly affected producing regurgitation. Pulmonary valve involvement is rare.
- Involvement of right ventricular wall is common in VSD.
- Common in drug addicts using IV line for drug delivery. It may occur in immuno-compromised patients and those with burns
- Prognosis is better
- Systemic embolization is rare. Lung infarction or pulmonary infection (lung abscess, empyema, pneumonias) are common.

Q. When do you suspect infective endocarditis in a patient with heart lesion?

Ans. Diagnosis of infective endocarditis is suspected in each and every patient of rheumatic valvular heart disease or a congenital heart disease developing fever, tachycardia, worsening dyspnea or congestive heart failure or an embolic episode, e.g. monoplegia/hemiplegia, hematuria, etc.

The clinical supportive features include:
- Fever (swinging temperature)
- Pallor, anemia, toxic look, tachypnea and tachycardia
- Clubbing of the fingers
- Splenomegaly (mild)
- Microscopic hematuria
- Embolic manifestations.

Q. Name the predisposing factors for endocarditis.

Ans. Predisposing factors are:

1. *Valvular heart disease.* Mitral and aortic valvular lesion predispose to infective endocarditis. Regurgitant lesions are more prone to produce endocarditis as the regurgitant jet damages the mural endocardium and predisposes to seeding of the organism. The mitral valve involvement is commoner than aortic. The tricuspid valve is involved in right sided endocarditis. Pulmonary valve is rarely involved.

2. *Congenital heart disease.* The VSD, PDA and bicuspid aortic valve are common predisposing lesions. It occurs on low pressure side of the ventricular septum, i.e. on right ventricular endocardium in VSD.
   The ASD does not lead to endocarditis.

3. *Prosthetic valve or a foreign body* also predispose to endocarditis.

4. *Immunocompromised state* either due to disease (diabetes, malignancy) or due to drugs (steroids and immunosuppressive drugs) predispose to it. In such patients acute bacterial endocarditis is common.

5. *Intravenous drug abusers*

6. *Prior heart surgery* (valvotomy, balloon dilatation and valve replacement).

Q. How will you investigate a patient suspected of endocarditis?

Ans. Investigations required are as follows:

1. *Blood examination.* There may be anemia (normocytic normochromic) leukocytosis and raised ESR and high C-reactive protein levels

2. *Urine examination* reveals mild albuminuria and microscopic hematuria. Gross hematuria is rare

3. *Immune-complex titer and rheumatoid factor titers* may be elevated

4. *Blood culture.* Isolation of the micro-organism from blood cultures is crucial not only for diagnosis but also for determination of antimicrobial sensitivity and planning the management. In the absence of prior antibiotic therapy; a total of 3 blood culture sets, ideally with the first separated from the last by at least 1 hour from different sites should be obtained from different venipuncture sites over 24 hour. If the cultures remain negative after 48 to 72 hours; two or three additional blood culture, including a lysis–centrifugation culture, should be obtained, and the laboratory should be asked to pursue fastidious microorganisms by prolonging the incubation time and performing special subcultures.

   It is likely that 95-100% of all cultures obtained will be positive and that one of the first two cultures will be positive in at least 98% of patients. Blood culture obtained just prior to temperature peak will give a higher yield. Blood culture is likely to be sterile if patient has already received antibiotic.

5. *Echocardiogram.* Vegetations may be identified as small, sessile or polypoidal masses on heart valves or congenital defects. Transthoracic echocardiography is noninvasive and exceptionally specific, but has sensitivity of 65%. Transesophageal echocardiography offers the greatest sensitivity for detection of vegetations.

6. *Serological tests.* Serological tests including polymerase chain reaction can be used to identify some organisms that are difficult to recover from the blood culture.

Q. **What are the diagnostic criteria for endocarditis?**

Ans. The diagnosis of infective endocarditis is established with certainty only if culture from the vegetations is positive. Nevertheless, a highly sensitive and specific diagnostic criteria – *Duke's criteria* has been developed on the basis of clinical, laboratory and echocardiographic findings (Table 1.108).

Table 1.108: The Duke criteria for the clinical diagnosis of infective endocarditis

Infective endocarditis is definite if following criteria using specific definitions listed below are met;
Two major criteria **or**
One major and three minor criteria **or**
Five minor criteria
Major criteria
1. *Positive blood culture*
i. Typical microorganism for infective endocarditis from two separate blood cultures
• Viridans streptococci, *Streptococcus bovis,* HACEK group, *Staphylococcus aureus* **or** Community-acquired enterococci in the absence of a primary focus, **or**
ii. Persistently positive blood culture, defined as recovery of a microorganism consistent with infective endocarditis from:
• Blood cultures drawn >12 hour apart; **or**
• All of three or a majority of four or more separate blood cultures, with first and last drawn at least 1 hour apart
• Single positive blood culture for Coxiella burnetii *or* phase 1 IgG antibody titer of >1:800

Contd...

Contd...

2. *Evidence of endocardial involvement*
• Positive echocardiogram, i.e. Oscillating intracardiac mass on a valve or supporting structures or in the path of regurgitant jet or in implanted material, in the absence of an alternative anatomic explanation, **or**
• Abscess, **or**
• New partial dehiscence of prosthetic valve, **or**
• New valvular regurgitation (increase or change in preexisting murmur not sufficient)
Minor criteria
1. *Predisposition:* predisposing heart condition or injection drug use
2. *Fever* = 38°C (=100.4°F)
3. *Vascular phenomena:* major arterial emboli, septic pulmonary infarcts, mycotic aneurysm, intracardial hemorrhage, conjunctival hemorrhage, Janeway lesions
4. *Immunologic phenomena:* glomerulonephritis, Osler's nodes, Roth's spots, rheumatoid factor
5. *Microbiologic evidence:* positive blood culture but not meeting major criterion as noted previously for serologic evidence of active infection with organism consistent with infective endocarditis
• Excluding single positive culture for coagulase-negative staphylocci and diphtheroids, which are common culture contaminants, and organisms that do not cause endocarditis frequently, such as gram-negative bacilli
Abbrev: HACEK, Hemophilus, Actinobacillus, Cardiobacterium, Eikenella, Kingella.

Q. **What precautions would you take to prevent bacterial endocarditis?**

Ans. Antibiotic prophylaxis before conducting a procedure in a patient with rheumatic heart disease, congenital heart diseases (except ASD secundum type), and prosthetic heart valve.

Q. **How would you treat a patient suspected to have endocarditis?**

Ans. Until culture report become available, I.V. benzylpenicillin and gentamicin will be given on empirical basis. In severely ill patients cloxacillin would be added to the regimen.

Q. **What is marantic endocarditis?**

Ans. Marantic or Libman-Sacks endocarditis is seen in SLE. It is a postmortem diagnosis. It is rarely detected clinically.

A-60-year male (Fig. 1.32A) presented with cough, breathlessness, progressive in nature for the last 7 years. He has been taking treatment and getting relief on and off. Now for the last 1 month, he complains of increase in breathlessness, cough and oedema of legs and feet. Examination revealed emphysematous chest (barrel shaped) with hyper – resonant note on percussion. Auscultation revealed vesicular breathing with prolonged expiration, crackles and rhonchi on both sides.

Clinical Presentation

- Patients suffering from chronic lung disease (obstructive or suppurative or interstitial) present with signs of right ventricular failure (distended neck veins, cyanosis, tender hepatomegaly and pitting edema).
- A patient with chronic chest deformity, e.g. kyphoscoliosis may present with symptoms of progressive dyspnea, worsening cough over the last few years. They may complain of pain abdomen and edema feet due to right heart failure.

History

Points to be Noted

Ask about:

- Cough, its frequency, seasonal relation, nocturnal, etc.
- Sputum production, quantity, color, smell, consistency and history of hemoptysis
- Any recent change in the symptoms. History of recent fever, sore throat or loose motions
- History of swelling feet, abdomen (hepatomegaly)
- Ask for any aggravating or relieving factors
- Take full drug history, drug being taken and their effect

Past history

- Cough or expectoration in the past
- History of allergy or rhinitis or asthma in the past

Personal history

- History of smoking, alcoholism, exposure to dust or fumes

Occupational history.

General Physical Examination

- Patient is orthopnoic, sitting with hands on cardiac table or legs dangling/hanging from the bed to relieve breathlessness

- Cyanosis present
- Neck veins distended. JVP raised. There may be v and y collapse due to TR. (present in this case)
- Pulse and respiratory rate increased
- Warm extremities, clubbing of fingers and edema feet may be present (present in this case)
- Purse-lip breathing may be present (present in this case)
- Action of extra-respiratory muscles, i.e. there may be hyperactivity.

Systemic Examination

1. Examination of Respiratory System

- Inspection ⎫ There will be evidence
- Palpation of ⎬ of COPD or other
- Percussion ⎭ chronic lung disease
- Auscultation – reveals vesicular breathing with prolonged expiration. Crackles and rhonchi were scattered all over the chest.

2. Examination of CVS

Inspection

- Apex beat may be normally placed or centrally placed or displaced outwards but not downwards or may not be visible
- No other visible pulsation

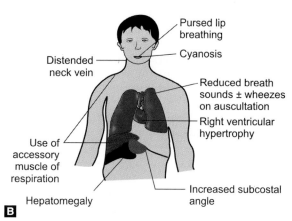

Figs 1.32A and B: A. Chronic cor pulmonale. The patient has signs of COPD. Note the purse lip breathing, cyanotic spells. The patient has edema and raised JVP. Note the common position adopted by patient with COPD and acute exacerbation with cor pulmonale to get relief from breathlessness. B. Clinical signs of chronic cor pulmonale (diagram).

Palpation
- Apex beat may be palpable outside the midclavicular line (not palpable in this case)
- Parasternal heave present
- Right ventricular pulsations palpable in epigastrium

Percussion
- Cardiac dullness may be masked or just limited to center (cardiac dullness was masked)

Auscultation
- Heart sounds normal
- Second heart sound narrowly split
- There may be an ejection systolic murmur in P$_2$ area and a pansystolic murmur in tricuspid area

3. Abdominal Examination
- Liver is enlarged, soft, tender and may be pulsatile if TR present (liver was enlarged & tender in this case)

- There may be signs of ascites (fluid thrill and shifting dullness present).

Q. **What is your clinical diagnosis?**

Ans. The symptoms and signs suggest COPD with pulmonary hypertension with chronic cor pulmonale and congestive heart failure without respiratory failure.

Q. **What is differential diagnosis in your case?**

Ans. When all the signs of CHF such as raised JVP, cyanosis, dyspnea/ tachypnea, ascites and edema are present then following conditions will constitute the differential diagnosis.

1. *Valvular heart disease*: The presence of cardiomegaly, presence of precordial pulsations, murmurs and thrill and added heart sounds make the diagnosis clear.

2. *Cardiomyopathies*: The cardiomegaly with or without murmurs when there is no cause to explain cardiomegaly constitute myocardial disease.

3. *Primary pulmonary hypertension*: In this condition, symptoms and signs of lung disease will be absent. These patients usually present with progressive dyspnea commonly in females, occurs due to repeated pulmonary vascular resistance. All signs of pulmonary hypertension (loud P2, narrow split S2 and Graham-Steell murmur, signs of TR) are present with RV failure.

4. *Constrictive pericarditis*: The precordial chest pain, distended neck veins with raised JVP and prominent x descent with muffled heart sounds, enlarged cardiac shadow on X-ray chest suggest the diagnosis of pericardial disease.

5. *Eisenmenger's syndrome*: Long history of symptoms of cough, dyspnea, fever since childhood/adolescence suggestive of left to right shunt will be present. The presence of signs of heart failure combined with signs of reversal of shunt i.e. clubbing of fingers, cyanosis and decreased intensity and duration or absence of previous murmurs with signs of pulmonary hypertension (loud P2, narrow spliting of S2 and Graham-Steell murmur) make the diagnosis most likely.

6. *Cor pulmonale secondary to pulmonary disease*: Features of cor pulmonale has been described as separate question.

Q. **How do you define cor pulmonale?**

Ans. *Chronic cor pulmonale* is defined as right ventricular hypertrophy or dilatation secondary to the disease of the lung parenchyma, pulmonary vasculature, thoracic cage and ventilatory control.

Q. **What are positive features in favor of your diagnosis?**

Ans. Sir, first of all history is suggestive of COPD, i.e. history of cough for most of the days in a week for 3 months in a year for 2 consecutive years.

Secondly symptoms such as breathlessness, cough, sputum production, hemoptysis and signs such as purse lip breathing, cyanosis, action of extra respiratory muscles, excavation of suprasternal and supraclavicular fossae, barrel shaped chest or change in AP and transverse thoracic diameter ratio, decreased respirating movement, diminished expansion and recession of intercostal spaces, reduced vocal fremitus, hyper-resonant note on percussion with pushing down of liver dullness to 7 th intercostal space suggest COPD. On auscultation, harsh vesicular breathing with prolonged expiration, crackles and rhonchi favor obstruction to the respiratory passage.

Findings of distended neck veins with pulsations and raised JVP, enlarged liver, edema of legs and feet indicate right ventricular failure, therefore, after combining the two conditions the diagnosis become COPD with cor pulmonale with congestive heart failure:

Q. What are the other conditions that produce right heart failure (RHF)?

Ans. 1. Severe pulmonary stenosis (congenital)
2. Pulmonary hypertension due to any cause (valvular heart disease, cor pulmonale, pulmonary vascular disease, etc.)
3. Eisenmenger's syndrome, i.e. reversal of left to right shunt (VSD, ASD, PDA) due to development of pulmonary hypertension.
4. Secondary to left heart failure due to any cause.
5. Cardiomyopathy especially right ventricular type or dilated cardiomyopathy.
6. Constrictive pericarditis or chronic or acute myocarditis.

Q. What are the causes of chronic cor pulmonale?

Ans. Chronic cor pulmonale is secondary to development of pulmonary arterial hypertension which may be primary (idiopathic) or secondary due to disease of pulmonary vasculature or pulmonary parenchyma or thoracic cage. The causes are described in Table 1.109.

Q. What are clinical features of chronic cor pulmonale due to COPD?

Ans. The clinical features (Fig. 1.32B) are divided into two parts;

The presenting symptoms of chronic cor pulmonale include dyspnea which occurs during exertion or at rest (orthopnea) and is not relieved by sitting posture. There is tachypnea. Unproductive cough with or without hemoptysis is another common symptom followed by chest discomfort/pain abdomen,

Table 1.109: Causes of cor pulmonale

I. **Parenchymal lung disease**
- COPD, cystic fibrosis
- Hypertrophic emphysema
- Diffuse bilateral bronchiectasis
- Diffuse interstitial lung disease
- Occupational lung diseases, e.g. Pneumoconiosis

II. **Occlusion of pulmonary vascular bed**
- Pulmonary thromboembolism (recurrent, medium sized vessel embolization)
- Primary pulmonary hypertension
- Pulmonary angitis or chronic widespread vasculitis such as occurs in collagen vascular disease, CRES syndrome and polyarteritis nodosa
- Sickle cell disease

III. **Diseases of thoracic cage affecting lung function, i.e. produce chronic hypoventilation**
- Obesity (Pickwickian syndrome)
- Sleep apnea
- Neuromuscular disease, e.g. Poliomyelitis
- Chest wall dysfunction, e.g. Kyphoscoliosis, ankylosing spondylitis
- Idiopathic

distension of abdomen and swelling of legs occurs due to right heart failure.

Clinical signs of COPD (read case discussion on COPD). However, few important clincal signs are:
- Pursed-lip breathing
- Use of accessory muscles of respiration
- Barrel-shape chest
- Retraction of supraclavicular fossae with inspiration
- Cyanosis
- Restricted chest movements and expansion
- Reduced palpable length of trachea
- Intercostal indrawing
- Vocal fremitus reduced
- Percussion note hyper-resonant, cardiac dullness and liver dullness masked
- Harsh vesicular breathing with prolonged expiration
- Crackles and rhonchi/rales.

Clinical signs of pulmonary arterial hypertension (PH) Here due to presence of COPD, some signs of PH will be masked such as pulsations of pulmonary artery in second left interspace and cardiac apex beat and dullness. The physical signs which will be present include:

A. *General physical*
- Pulse-low volume
- Neck veins – distended. JVP raised and 'a' wave prominent

B. *Signs on chest examination*

Inspection
- Epigastric pulsations due to RV hypertrophy
- Pulmonary artery pulsations in 2nd left interspace may not be visible due to hyperinflated lungs covering the artery

Palpation
- Apex beat may not be visible
- P_2 is palpable
- Left parasternal heave may be present due to RVH.

Percussion
- Cardiac dullness will be masked due to hyperinflated lungs or limited to center (heart is pushed centrally by the overdistended lungs).

Auscultation
- Loud P_2 – an ejection click in left second intercostal may be present
- Ejection systolic murmur
- Close or narrow splitting of S_2
- Graham-Steel murmur
- Right sided S_3.

Q. Does definition of cor pulmonale include right heart failure? What are its signs?

Ans. Right heart failure is not included in the definition of chronic cor pulmonale. It is a complication of cor pulmonale.

The signs of right ventricular failure are:
- Raised JVP/distended neck veins with v and y collapse
- Hepatojugular reflux will be positive
- Liver will be enlarged and tender, may be pulsatile if functional TR present
- A pansystolic murmur of TR, heard best in left parasternal edge or in epigastrium
- Pitting pedal edema and/or ascites.

Q. How do you classify pulmonary arterial hypertension?

Ans. See Table 1.110.

Table 1.110: Classification of pulmonary hypertension

I. **Primary pulmonary hypertension**
• Idiopathic
II. **Secondary pulmonary hypertension**
• Passive or reactive (from left sided heart lesions) such as MS, MR, AS and AR
• Hyperkinetic (left to right shunt), e.g. ASD, VSD, PDA
• Vasoconstrictive (hypoxic) chronic cor pulmonale
• Obstructive (reduction in vascular bed), e.g. pulmonary thromboembolism (acute cor pulmonale)
• Obliterative, e.g.
• Pulmonary angiitis/vasculitis
• Sickle cell disease
• SLE, PAN, CREST syndrome

Q. What is normal pulmonary arterial pressure? What is pressure in pulmonary hypertension?

Ans. Normal pulmonary arterial pressure 18-25/6-10 mmHg.

In pulmonary hypertension;
- Pulmonary artery systolic pressure is >30 mmHg
- Mean pulmonary artery wedge pressure is >20 mmHg

Q. What are causes of TR? Name its two characteristics?

Ans. The causes of TR are given in the box:

Causes of TR

1. Right ventricular dilatation secondary to pulmonary hypertension
2. Rheumatic heart disease
3. Right sided endocarditis in drug abusers
4. Right ventricular infarction
5. Carcinoid syndrome

The characteristic signs of TR are:
1. A pansystolic murmur in tricuspid area (right parasternal area/epigastrium) is heard which increases with inspiration.

2. Signs of RVH: There will be parasternal heave. Right ventricular pulsation may be felt in epigastrium.
3. Distented neck veins with typical 'V' and 'Y' collapse.
4. Pulsatile liver.
5. Hepatojugular reflux is positive.

Q. How will you investigate a patient with cor pulmonale?

Ans. Investigations required are as follows:
1. *Chest X-ray.* It will show:
   - Cardiomegaly
   - Pulmonary conus is prominent
   - Hilar bronchovascular markings prominent with pruning of the peripheral pulmonary vessels
   - Signs of COPD (emphysema) on X-ray will be evident (read radiology section)
2. *ECG.* It will show
   - Low voltage graph
   - Right axis deviation, clockwise rotation
   - Right atrial hypertrophy (P- pulmonale)
   - Right ventricular hypertrophy (R>S orR:S >1 in lead V1 but both complexes being small)
   - SI, SII, and SIII syndrome
   - ST-T wave changes
   - Arrhythmias (MAT—multifocal atrial tachycardia is common)
3. *Echocardiography.* It will show increased right atrial and right ventricular wall thickness and enlargement of cavity. Interventricular septum is displaced leftward. Color Doppler may reveal functional TR.
4. *MRI* is useful to measure RV mass, wall thickness, and ejection fraction.
5. *Ventilation and perfusion scan are helpful in confirming the diagnosis of chronic pulmonary vascular disease.*
6. *Systemic venography* and Doppler study may reveal deep vein thrombosis.
7. *Cardiac catheterization* for measurement of pulmonary vascular pressures, calculation of pulmonary vascular resistance and response to vasodilator therapy.

Q. What are the complications of cor pulmonale?

Ans. Following are complications:
- Right heart failure
- Secondary polycythemia
- Deep vein thrombosis
- Cardiac arrhythmias (multifocal atrial tachycardia, ventricular arrhythmias)

159

Q. Is cor pulmonale high output failure. What are other causes of high output failure ?

Ans. Initially, cor pulmonale is high output failure when hypoxia dominates leading to wide pulse pressure, later on due to involvement of myocardium, it becomes low output failure. Other causes of high output failure are:

i. Aortic regurgitation
ii. Severe anaemia (Hb<4g%)
iii. Severe thyrotoxicosis
iv. Arteriovenous fistula
v. Paget's disease
vi. Cirrhosis of liver
vii. Beriberi heart disease

Q. What is treatment of cor pulmonale?

Ans. • *General measures,* i.e. Back rest or prop up position, salt restriction and O2 inhalation. Long term domiciliary O2 therapy is helpful in patients with severe COPD as it reduces pulmonary artery pressure and lowers pulmonary vascular resistance.

• *Antibiotics* Acute respiratory infection is common precipitant of RV failure. Broad spectrum antibiotic may be used initially followed by antibiotic on the basis of sputum culture and sensitivity.

• *Bronchodilators* are used to relieve obstruction and to improve oxygenation.

• *Diuretics* are used to relieve edema.

• *Vasodilators* may be used to reduce preload.

• *Digitalis* should be used cautiously as it may induce arrhythmias in hypoxic myocardium.

• *Phlebotomies* to be done to reduce hematocrit, if there is polycythemia.

• *Inhalation of NO* and *infusion of prostacycline* are undergoing evaluation as agents to lower pulmonary hypertension.

Q. What are the signs of acute cor pulmonale?

Ans. Sudden onset of dyspnea, cough, hemoptysis and cardiovascular collapse (tachypnea, tachycardia, sweating, hypotension) in a patient with or predisposed to venous thrombosis suggest acute pulmonary embolism leading to acute cor pulmonale.

Signs of RV failure, i.e. small volume pulse, low pulse pressure, distended neck veins with prominent 'V' waves, a pansystolic murmur on left sternal border a soft S4 and pulsatile liver appear due to development of severe pulmonary hypertension due to medium or massive pulmonary vascular embolization.

On cardiac auscultation, signs of pulmonary hypertension, i.e. loud P2, narrow splitting of S2, a Graham-Steell or a soft systolic murmur suggest the diagnosis. ECG (right ventricular hypertrophy) and Echocardiogram showing dilatation of RV cavity and low RV output further support the diagnosis of pulmonary embolism.

Pulmonary angiography or ventilation and perfusion scan confirm the diagnosis.

Q. Which diuretic is preferred in Cor pulmonale?

Ans. You can use any diuretic but loop diuretics should be used with caution as it may cause metabolic alkalosis and thereby blunt the respiratory drive. Thiazides are better than loop diuretics.

Q. What is indication of beta blocker in heart failure?

Ans. Usually beta blockers are contraindicated in heart failure but to slow the heart rate in AF or otherwise, beta blockers are used in diastolic heart failure as they provide more time for ventricular filling.

The betablockers used in heart failure include carvedilol, bisoprolol, nevibilol and metoprolol.

Q. What are precipitants for Cor pulmonale?

Ans. The precipitant of cor pulmonale are:

• Acute respiratory infection
• Thyrotoxicosis
• Salt intake
• Mental stress
• Arrhythmias
• Noncompliance to treatment
• Pulmonary embolism
• Anemia.

Q. What is primary pulmonary hypertension (PPH)?

Ans. When the cause of elevated pulmonary vascular resistance responsible for cor pulmonale cannot be defined, the condition is referred to as primary pulmonary hypertension.

CASE 33: CHEST PAIN

The patient (Fig 1.33) 55-year-old male presented with chest pain on exertion, relieved on rest. No radiation of pain. No associated symptoms. Examination was normal.

Presenting Symptoms

- Patients with chest pain present with typical anginal symptoms, or atypical anginal symptoms, e.g. angina equivalents, gastroesophageal reflux disease (GERD)
- They may present with musculoskeletal disease where pain is related to movements
- Patient with neurosis have cardiac symptoms (cardiac neurosis).

History

Points to be Asked

- Have you ever had such type of pain or discomfort in the chest before?

- How would you describe the pain (burning, heaviness or tightness, stabbing, pressure)?
- Do you get this pain chest during walking at normal pace or does it come when you walk fast or in a hurry?
- Does the pain get relieved by rest or by nitroglycrine?
- Is this pain localized or radiate to some other sites?
- Can you pinpoint the pain with your finger?
- Does the food has any relation with pain?
- Are there any associated symptoms of retching, nausea, vomiting, sweating, syncope, palpitation, dyspnea.
- Ask about risk factors such as smoking, diabetes, HT, alcohol, oral contraceptive.
- Is there any family history of ischemic heart disease? Did the patient has MI in the past?
- Is there any aggravating or relieving factor known?

General Physical Examination

- Facial appearance, e.g. depressed or normal
- Pulse (rate and rhythm) and BP (all the four limbs). Feel all other pulses (Carotids, femoral)
- Eyes for xanthelasma, fundus examination for evidence of Hypertension.
- Neck for thyroid enlargement and JVP
- Skin for xanthomas.
- Hands for nicotine staining (smoking)
- Look for signs of any cardiac or extracardiac disease
- Look for anemia.

Systemic Examination

CVS Examination

Inspection
- No abnormality detected

Palpation
- Apex beat normal
- Chest expansion/movement normal
- Tenderness over chest

Percussion
- Percussion note/cardiac dulness (normal/abnormal)

Auscultation
- Auscultate for the presence of a pansystolic murmur of papillary muscle dysfunction or a pericardial rub or a fourth heart sound.

Respiratory System

Examine respiratory system for any consolidation or evidence of pulmonary infarction or COPD.

Abdomen Examination

- For any evidence of mass
- For aortic pulsations.

Fig. 1.33: Chest pain: A. Patient with ischemic chest pain (diag), B. Evidence of coronary thrombosis

Q. What is your clinical diagnosis and why?

Ans. In view of middle aged male having central chest pain, constricting/squeezing in quality with no rodiation, occurs on exertion, relieved by rest, my provisional diagnosis is acute coronary syndrome, or angina pectoris.

Q. What is differential diagnosis?

Ans. As the pain chest is central in location, it could be due to cardiovascular, gastrointestinal and musculoskeletal cause (Table 1.111)

Q. What are differences between cardiac and noncardiac chest pain?

Ans. Read Clinical Methods by Dr SN Chugh

Q. What is mechanism of angina pectoris?

Ans.
- It is caused by increased myocardial oxygen demand triggered by physical activity.
- Coronary vasospasm is the other mechanism which causes transient decrease in O_2 supply.
- Nonocclusive intracoronary thrombi cause unstable angina pectoris.

Q. How would you grade angina?

Ans. The Canadian Cardiovascular Society has graded angina into 4 functional classes

Class I: Angina occurs on strenous or prolonged exertion.

Class II: Angina with slight limitation of ordinary normal activity.

Table 1.111: Differential diagnosis of central chest pain

Cause	Site	Quality/Severity/Timing	Aggravating/relieving factors
Angina pectoris	Retrosternal or across the chest, radiating to left arm, neck, shoulder, lower jaw, upper abdomen	Squeezing/pressing/tightness in chest, moderate in intensity lasting for few minutes (1-3 min)	• Exertion, cold, heavy meal and psychological upset exacerbate it • Rest, nitroglycerine selieve it.
Myocardial infarction	Same as above	Same as above. Pain is more severe and prolonged, associated with diaphoresis.	• No aggravating or relieving factor • Underlying risk factor may be evident
Pericarditis	Central limited to precordium may radiate to shoulder or back	Sharp, cutting (knife like) pain, often severe and persistent	• Breathing, change in posture, coughing lying may exacerbate it. • Sitting and forward blenolling relieve it
Aortic dissecting aneurysm	Anterior chest wall radiating to back between scapula	Tearing pain severe and persistent	• Hypertension aggravate it • No relieving factor • Associated feature, e.g. syncope, aortic diastolic murmur help in the diagnosis
GASTROINTESTINAL CAUSES			
Reflex esophagitis /gastrointestinal reflux disease/ diffuse esophageal spasms	Retrosternal, may radiate to back	Burning/squeezing, mild to moderate in intensity	• Large meals, bending, emotional upset, spicy food aggravate it • Lying down and antacid relieve it • Heart burn and acid taste in mouth are common accompaniments
MUSCULOSKELETAL CAUSES			
Myalgia	Often below the left breast	Stabbing or dull ache of fleeting nature, severity variable	• Movement of the chest, aggravate it
Teitz' syndrome	Pain along the left costal margins	Sticking/stabbing, variable severity	• There is local tenderness – do – • There may be tenderness of costochondral junctions (2nd to 4th ribs)
PSYCHOGENIC			
Cardiac neurosis	Precordial, below the left breast or whole of anterior crest	Stabbing, variable intensity, fleeting in nature	• Stress and effort precipitate it • Mental rest and anxiolytic relieve it • Anxious look, palpitations hyperventilation, frequent sighs are common associated symptoms.

Class III: Angina with marked limitation of ordinary activity.

Class IV: Angina at rest with inability to perform any physical activity.

Q. What is Prinzemetal's angina?

Ans. It is a variant angina that occurs at rest, frequently at night and coronary vasospasm over and above athero-sclerosis is the underlying cause. It is characterized by transient elevation of ST segment (>4 mm) during pain which resolves with relief of pain.

Q. What are the risk factors for acute coronary syndrome?

Ans. Risk factors are:
- Genetic (deletion polymorphism in the ACE gene (DD)
- Advancing age and male sex
- Smoking
- Alcohol
- Diabetes
- Hypertension
- Hyperlipidemia
- Lack of exercise (sedentary lifestyle)
- Deficiency of antioxidant vitamins
- Homocysteinemia (Homocysteinuria)
- Oral contraceptive
- High levels of fibrinogen and factor VIII.

Q. What do you understand by the term acute coronary syndrome?

Ans. Acute coronary syndrome refers to coronary events that occur due to atherosclerosis. It includes unstable angina/Non-ST elevation myocardial infarction and ST elevation myocardial infarction (STEMI).

Q. What is metabolic syndrome (syndrome X, Reaven's syndrome)?

Ans. It is a syndrome of clusters of factors which otherwise act as independent risk factors consisting of obesity (visceral), insulin resistance, hypertension, increased very low density lipoprotein (VLDL) and reduced high density lipoprotein (HDL) in blood.

Q. What is microvascular angina (cardiac syndrome X)?

Ans. It refers to classic anginal symptoms with ST depression on stress ECG testing and a normal coronary angiogram in the absence of any demostable cardiac abnormality.

Q. What is prevalence of angina?

Ans. The prevalence of angina is approx 2% with an incidence of new cases each year approximately 1 per 1000.

Q. What are common clinical patterns of angina?

Ans. • *Classical or exertional angina pectoris.*

- *Decubitus angina* (angina on lying down) indicates angina with impaired LV function.
- *Nocturnal angina* (critical coronary artery disease or vasospasm are the causes)
- *Variant (Prinzmetal's) angina* (Rest angina without any provocation).
- *Unstable angina* (angina of recent onset <1 month, worsening angina or angina at rest).

Q. What are anginal equivalents?

Ans. These are symptoms of myocardial ischemia other than angina, carry same significance as angina. These include dyspnea, fatigue and faintness. They are more common in elderly and in diabetic patients.

Q. What do you understand by the term unstable angina?

Ans. It refers to more severe and frequent angina superimposed on chronic stable angina, angina at rest or minimal exertion or new onset angina < 1 month which is brought about by minimal exertion.

Q. What is postprandial angina? What is its mechanism and significance? What is its treatment?

Ans. Angina following meals is called postprandial angina. It results from the carbohydrate content of the meal. It indicates severe coronary artery disease and could occur as a result of intramyocardial stealing of blood from stenotic territories to normal territories.

Q. How would you investigate a case of angina?

Ans. • **Hemoglobin** for anemia (anemia aggravates angina)
- **Resting ECG** (LV hypertrophy, ST-T changes, prior Q- wave MI).
- **Exercise ECG** for ST change (Horizontal or downsloping ST segment depression > 1 mm staying for 60-80 ms or ST elevation) or an arrhythmia or production of symptoms.
- **Rest Echocardiogram** for any evidence of asymptomatic aortic stenosis or hypertrophic cardiomyopathy.
- **Exercise myocardial perfusion imaging/ exercise echocardiography** in patients having abnormal ECG at rest.
- **Coronary angiography** for coronary anatomy for any abnormality (atherosclerotic occlusion) or non-atherosclerotic causes (e.g. vasospasm, coronary anomaly/ dissection/vasculopathy).

Q. How would you treat a patient with chronic stable angina?

Ans. Treatment is denoted by Mnemonic ABCDE
- **A**spirin
- **B**etablocker and **B**lood pressure control

- Cigarette smoking abstinence and Cholesterol reduction.
- Diet and Diabetes control
- Education and Exercise.

Q. What is the prognostic significance of stress testing in evaluation of chest pain?

Ans. Stress testing determines high risk and low risk population of patients with chest pain suggestive of ischemic heart disease.

I. **Low risk group:** These are patients who can complete 1 minute of exercise using Bruce protocol without any change in ST segment and can achieve a maximum heart rate >160/min without discomfort. These were found to have good prognosis (1 year survival in 99% and 4 years in 93%) and cardiac catheterization and CABG can be deferred.

II. **High risk group:** These are patients who were forced to stop exercise in Stage I and II (under 6 minutes). Survival rate was reduced to 85% at one year and 63% at 4 years.

Q. What are glycoprotein II/IIIb inhibitors?

Ans. Glycoprotein II/IIIb inhibitors are antithrombotic agents useful for preventing thrombotic complications in patients with STEMI undergoing PCI.

Q. Name the cardiac markers. What is their significance?

Ans. Cardiac markers are:
- CPK-MB
- Troponins I and T
- Myoglobin

Troponins are useful for early diagnosis before enzymes rise.

Q. What is Tietze syndrome?

Ans. Read Table 1.114

Q. What is gastroesophageal reflux disease? What are its causes?

Ans. Gastroesophageal reflux disease is defined as reflux of gastric contents into the oesophagus resulting in inflammation of esophagus (reflux esophagitis caused by H^+ ion, pepsin and bile salts). The causes are:
- Old age and smoking
- Fat, chocolate, coffee, spicy food and alcohol
- Hiatus hernia
- Gastric stasis (e.g. gastroparesis in diabetes, due to anticholinergics and systemic sclerosis).
- Raised intra-abdominal pressure (e.g. pregnancy, ascites, straining at stool/urination)
- Obesity and sedentary habits.

Q. What are angina precipitants?

Ans. Angina precipitants are:
- Physical exertion
- Heavy meals
- Recumbency (angina decubitus)
- Emotional disturbance
- Cold exposure
- Vivid dreams (nocturnal angina)
- Thyrotoxicosis
- Asymptomatic aortic valve disease
- Drugs, e.g. beta adrenergic stimulants
- Tachycardia and tachyarrhythmias.

CASE 34: DILATED CARDIOMYOPATHY

The patient presented with history of breathlessness on exertion for the last 3 years (Fig. 1.34). It was progressive in nature and interfered with normal activities. Now for the last 2 months, patient develops dyspnea on minimal exertion and there is history of orthopnea and PND off and on. For the last 15 days patient is having swollen legs and distended abdomen. On symptomatic enquiry, there is history of palpitations, headache, weakness and fatigue. Examination revealed raised JVP, hepatomegaly, ascites and edema. There was cardiomegaly with pansystolic murmur heard over whole of the precordium with 'vy' collapse. A soft 3rd heart sound was also heard. There were end-inspiratory crackles at both bases of the lungs.

Clinical Presentation

- Patient suffering from dilated cardiomyopathy present with palpitation, dyspnea and CHF.

Fig. 1.34: A patient of rheumatic heart disease with mitral stenosis and mitral regurgitation showing signs of congestive heart failure

- Patients of alcoholism may present with cirrhosis, neuropathy and cardiomyopathy.
- Patients of postpartum cardiomyopathy present with symptoms and signs of CHF within 6 months following delivery.

History

Points to be Noted

Ask about:

- Cough, its frequency, nocturnal, etc.
- Sputum production, quantity, color, smell, consistency and history of hemoptysis
- Any recent change in the symptoms. History of recent fever, sore throat or loose motions
- History of swelling feet, abdomen (hepatomegaly)
- Ask for any aggravating or relieving factors
- Take full drug history, drug being taken and their effect.

Past history

- History of delivery or abortion
- H/O diabetes

Personal history

- History of smoking, alcoholism
- Family history.

General Physical Examination

- Patient is orthopneic, lying in prop up position.
- Cyanosis present
- Neck veins distended. JVP raised. There may be v and y collapse due to TR (present in this case)
- Pulse and respiratory rate increased
- Cold extremities and edema feet may be present (present in this case)
- Record BP, pulse and temperature

Systemic Examination

1. Examination of CVS

Inspection

- Apex beat may be normally placed or centrally placed or displaced outwards but not downwards.
- No other visible pulsation all over the precordium

Palpation

- Apex beat may be palpable outside the midclavicular line (palpable in this case)
- Parasternal heave present
- Right ventricular pulsations palpable in epigastrium (present in this case)

Percussion

- Cardiac dullness area increased due to dilated heart. Dullness corresponds with apex beat.

Auscultation

- Heart sounds normal/feeble.
- Second heart sound normally split
- There may be an ejection systolic murmur in P₂ area and a pansystolic murmur in tricuspid and mitral areas.

2. Abdominal Examination

- Liver is enlarged, soft, tender and may be pulsatile if TR present (liver was enlarged & pulsatile in this case)
- There may be signs of ascites (fluid thrill and shifting dullness present).

Q. What is your clinical diagnosis?

Ans. In view of clinical findings, patient has features of congestive heart failure probably due to dilated cardiomyopathy (primary).

Q. What are the points in favor of your diagnosis?

Ans. • H/O dyspnea, progressive in nature, orthopnea and PND
- A middle aged female patient.
- Signs of congestive heart failure without signs of pulmonary hypertension, e.g. raised JVP, tender hepatomegaly, ascites and pitting edema. There were end inspiratory crackles in the lungs.
- Signs of cardiomegaly, e.g. dilated heart with heaving apex beat which is down and out.
- Exclusion of other causes of heart failure such as valvular, hypertensive, thyrotoxic and ischemic heart disease.
- The features suggestive of mitral and tricuspid regurgitation (pansystolic murmur in both the areas) indicates dilated cardiomyopathy as simultaneous occurrence of both regurgitant lesions commonly occur in dilated cardiomyopathy.

Q. Could it be rheumatic mitral regurgitation leading to tricuspid regurgitation?

Ans. No. There are no signs of pulmonary hypertension (loud P_2, narrow splitting of 2nd heart sound, Graham-Steell murmur or an ejection systolic murmur).

Q. What are the signs of tricuspid regurgitation in this patient?

Ans. • Raised JVP with 'vy' collapse
- Signs of RVH, e.g. left parasternal heave and pulsations in the epigastrium
- Liver is enlarged and pulsatile
- There is pansystolic murmur heard at left parasternal border and also heard ar right sternal edge and epigastrium which increases on inspiration.

Q. What is your differential diagnosis?

Ans. Following myocardial diseases come into the differential diagnosis of idiopathic dilated cardiomyopathy:
- *Peripartum cardiomyopathy* in female (there will be history of delivery followed by signs and symptoms of CHF within 6 months)
- *Alcoholic cardiomyopathy* (H/O alcoholism, stigmatas of alcoholism and other associated diseases, e.g. cirrhosis or neuropathy).
- *Neuromuscular disease associated cardiomyopathy,* e.g. Friedrich's ataxia, Duchenne's muscular dystrophy, myotonic dystrophy, etc. (features of these neurological diseases will be present)
- Myocarditis-viral.

- *Diabetic cardiomyopathy* (H/O long duration of diabetes with other complications).

Q. What are clinical types of cardiomyopathy?

Ans. WHO classified cardiomyopathy clinically into 3 main groups:
i. **Dilated cardiomyopathy** characterized by ventricular enlargement, CHF, inpaired systolic function, arrhythmias and embolization.
ii. **Restrictive cardiomyopathy** characterized by restriction to left and/or right ventricular filling. It resembles constrictive pericarditis.
iii. **Hypertrophic cardiomyopathy** characterized by left ventricular free wall hypertrophy along with septal hypertrophy without any dilatation of the ventricular cavity.

Q. Name few common causes of dilated cardiomyopathy.

Ans. The common causes are:
- *Primary* (unknown cause)
- *Secondary* due to:
  - Alcohol induced cardiomyopathy
  - Peripartum cardiomyopathy
  - Ischemic cardiomyopathy
  - Metabolic cardiomyopathy, e.g. thyrotoxic, diabetic.
  - Viral: chronic myocarditis, Chagas disease
  - Drug induced, e.g. doxorubicin, cocaine, cyclophosphamide.

Q. What is peripartum cardiomyopathy?

Ans. It develops during the last trimester or within 6 months after delivery, hence, the patient usually a multiparous woman over the age of 30 yrs develops symptoms and signs of CHF either 1 month before or immediately after delivery. The investigations revealed a dilated heart with depressed ejection fraction. Treatment is that of heart failure, i.e. salt restriction, diuretics, digitalis and ACE inhibitors. These patients if have dilated heart should avoid subsequent pregnancies which are likely to produce additional myocardial damage.

Q. How would you investigate such a case?

Ans. i. *ECG.* It will often show sinus tachycardia or atrial fibrillation, ventricular arrhythmias, left atrial enlargement, nonspecific ST-T changes and sometimes conduction defects and low voltage graph.
ii. *Chest X-ray* will show cardiomegaly. There will be pulmonary venous congestion and interstitial/alveolar edema (Kerley's lines).
iii. *Echocardiogram.* It will show ventricular dilatation with normal or thinned walls. The ejection fraction is markedly reduced.

iv. *Radionuclide ventriculography*, usually, not required, may confirm ventricular dilatation and thinning/thickening of the walls.

v. *Brain natriuretic peptide* levels are elevated.

vi. *Cardiac catheterization and coronary angiography:* They are often performed to exclude ischemic heart disease (ischemic cardiomyopathy).

vii. *Transvenous endomyocardial biopsy.* It is usually not necessary in idiopathic or familial cardiomyopathy. However, it is helpful in recognition of secondary cardiomyopathy due to amyloidosis and chronic myocarditis.

Q. How would you treat?

Ans. Treatment is symptomatic with:

- Salt restriction, diuretics, digitalis and ACE inhibitors
- Anticoagulation for systemic embolization
- Antiarrhythmics in case of arrhythmias
- Sophisticated therapy such as biventricular pacing (resynchronization therapy for intraventricular conduction delay, bundle branch blocks) and insertion of implantable cardioverter-defibrillator (ICD) for symptomatic ventricular arrhythmias
- Avoid alcohol and NSAIDs.

Q. What are the characteristic features of alcoholic cardiomyopathy?

Ans.
- It occurs in chronic alcoholic who are heavy drinkers.
- It presents with all symptoms and signs of congestive heart failure with dilated cardiomyopathy.
- The arrhythmias, e.g. atrial and ventricular commonly occur after a drinking binge.
- The progression of disease may stop following cessation of alcohol use.

Neurological Disorders

CASE 35: HEMIPLEGIA

A young female (18 yrs—Fig. 1.35) presented with cough and breathlessness on exertion for the last 4 yrs. She was well on treatment. There was no history of orthopnea, PND, hemoptysis or pain chest. Now for the last 2 days, she is complaining of weakness of right half of the body with deviation of face. After recovery, she was able to walk and the picture was taken to show the gait. Examination revealed signs of UMN paralysis on right side.

Fig. 1.35: A young female with hemiplegia walking with circumducting gait. She has recovered recently from stroke

Clinical Presentation

- Patient usually complain of weakness of one half of the body with asymmetry of face. There may be complaints of sensory and speech disturbance.
- In addition to weakness, patient may complain of symptoms of the underlying disorder if it is the cause, i.e. hypertension, diabetes, TIA, rheumatic heart disease (valvular lesion Fig. 1.33), cardiomyopathy, etc.

History

Points to be Noted

- Note the date and time of onset of stroke
- Mode of onset, e.g. sudden or gradual
- Evaluation of paralysis, i.e. whether it was TIA, stroke-in-evolution or complete stroke
- Any known precipitating factor(s)
- Progress or course of paralysis, e.g. improving, stationary or deteriorating or waxing and waning
- Any associated motor and sensory symptoms
- Any disturbance of consciousness/ convulsion, visual disturbance, speech disturbance
- Symptoms of raised intracranial tension

Past History

- History of similar episodes in the past which recovered completely (TIA)
- History of head injury or epilepsy
- History of HT, diabetes, RHD, meningitis, tuberculosis, migraine, exposure to sexually transmitted diseases
- Intake of oral contraceptive.

Family history, e.g. HT, DM, Epilepsy, migraine and similar illness in other family members.

Personal history. History of overweight or obesity, smoking, alcoholism.

Examination

1. **General physical**
   - Is patient conscious or cooperative?
   - Posture of the patient
   - Neck examination for pulsations, lymph node, thyroid
   - Vitals, e.g. pulse, BP and temperature
   - Edema
   - Any obvious deformity.

2. **Nervous system** *(read proper nervous system examination)*
   - Higher functions
   - Cranial nerves (UMN or LMN paralysis of 7th nerve), fundus for papilloedema
   - Neck rigidity absent
   - *Motor system examination*
     - There will be UMNs signs on the side of the body involved (i.e. opposite to the CNS lesion) if lesion is above the cervical cord
     - Gait will be spastic
     - Cerebellar and autonomic functions normal
     - Speech involved if dominant hemisphere is the site of lesion
     - Sensory system may show hemi-anesthesia or may be normal.

3. **Other systems examination**
   - CVS
   - Respiratory
   - GI tract and genitourinary
   - Lymphoreticular system.

Q. What is your clinical diagnosis?

Ans. In view of the presentation of weakness of right half of the body, the patient appears to be a case of young CVA (left) with right sided hemiplegia. The cause of stroke is cerebral embolism.

Q. What are the points in favor of diagnosis?

Ans. 1. Patient is a case of RHD with MS and AF.
2. Sudden onset of hemiplegia without convulsion and speech disturbance.
3. 7th supranuclear palsy on right side and hemiplegia on right side (uncrossed hemiplegia)
4. UMN signs present in right upper and lower limbs.

Q. What do you think the cause of hemiplegia in this case and why?

Ans. Embolic stroke. Points in favor are:
- Catastrophic onset
- Underlying RHD with MS

- Atrial fibrillation present
- Complete uncrossed hemiplegia
- More or less complete recovery.

Q. What is your complete diagnosis in this case?

Ans.
- The clinical diagnosis is CVA left side with hemiplegia right side.
- Site of the lesion is internal capsule
- Neurological deficit is pyramidal tract only
- Etiology is embolic stroke due to underlying RHD with MS and atrial fibrillation.

Q. What is hemiplegia? What are its various types?

Ans. *Hemiplegia* is defined as complete loss of motor functions (paralysis) on one half of the body; whereas partial loss of motor function is designated as *hemiparesis*. It is usually due to UMN lesion at any level from the cerebrum to spinal cord. The tracts involved are ascending and descending motor tracts especially the pyramidal tracts.

Hemiplegia is said to be complete if UMN 7th nerve palsy accompanies the hemiplegia and is considered incomplete in the absence of its involvement.

Terminology used for Hemiplegia

1. *Crossed hemiplegia*. It refers to ipsilateral LMN paralysis of one of the cranial nerves with contralateral (opposite side) hemiplegia. It signifies the brainstem as the site of the lesion.
2. *Uncrossed hemiplegia*. It refers to UMN 7th nerve palsy on the side of hemiplegia (i.e. both being opposite to cerebral lesion). For example, if UMN 7th nerve palsy and hemiplegia are on the left side, the cerebral lesion is on the right side.
3. *Dense hemiplegia*. The complete loss of voluntary functions (weakness) of equal magnitude in both upper and lower limbs on the side of the body involved constitutes dense hemiplegia. This signifies an internal capsular lesion as corticospinal fibers are condensed there.
4. *Pure motor hemiplegia*. Isolated unilateral involvement of corticospinal tract gives rise to pure motor hemiplegia. Usually, internal capsular lesion produces hemiplegia associated with hemianesthesia. A lacunar (small vessel) infarct of posterior limb of the internal capsule produces pure motor hemiplegia.

   Pure motor hemiplegia, pure sensory hemiplegia, ataxic hemiballismus syndrome and syndrome of pseudobulbar palsy are few examples of small vessel (lacunar) infarct.
5. *Stuttering hemiplegia*. Transient speech disturbance (aphasia, dysarthria) with hemiplegia indicates stuttering hemiplegia, is due to progressive occlusion of internal carotid artery (stroke-in-evolution). It ultimately results in complete stroke.
6. *Transient ischemic attack or transient hemiplegia*. It is sudden transient loss of motor function (paralysis) on one side of the body which recovers completely within 24 hours.
7. *Homolateral hemiplegia*. It means hemiplegia occurring on the same side of the lesion, is seen in unilateral cervical spinal cord lesion (Brown-Sequard's syndrome) because descending corticospinal tracts have already crossed at the level of the medulla, hence, they now represent the same side of cerebral hemisphere.

Q. What are the causes of hemiplegia?

Ans. The vascular diseases of the cerebrum (thrombosis, embolism, hemorrhage) exceed all other causes of hemiplegia. Trauma to the brain is second common cause followed by uncommon causes such as tumors, infections, demyelination and degenerative disorders (Table 1.112).

Q. What do you mean by stroke?

Ans. A stroke is defined as a neurological deficit occurring as a result of CVA (atherosclerosis, thrombosis, embolism and hemorrhage) and lasting for more than 24 hrs. Stroke in clinical practice is used for hemiplegia but actually it implies more than that.

Q. What is TIA and What is RIND? What is completed stroke?

Ans.
1. *TIA*. It means transient hemiplegia or neurological deficit occurring as a result of ischaemia which recovers within 24 hours.

Table 1.112: Causes of hemiplegia

1. **Organic causes**
A. *Cerebrovascular disease*
• Transient ischemic attack (TIA)
• Progressive atherosclerosis (stroke-in-evolution, completed stroke)
• Internal carotid artery aneurysm or AV malformations
• Cerebral thrombosis, embolism, hemorrhage
• Cerebral arteritis
• Dural sinus thrombosis
B. *Traumatic disorders*
• Brain contusion (concussion)
• Subdural hematoma
C. *Brain tumors*
D. *Infective disorders,* e.g. brain abscess, meningitis, encephalitis, tuberculosis, syphilis
E. *Demyelinating disorders*
• Multiple sclerosis
2. **Functional, e.g. hysteria**

2. *Stroke-in-evolution.* The neurological deficit worsens gradually or in a step-wise pattern over hours or days.

3. *Completed stroke.* Neurological deficit is complete at the onset and persists for days to weeks and often permanently.

4. *Reversible ischemic neurological deficit (RIND).* It means neurological deficit persisting for more than 24 hours but recovers totally within a week.

5. *Partial nonprogressive stroke.* As the name suggests, the neurological deficit is partial that persists for more than 3 weeks without any further progression.

Q. How would you classify stroke?

Ans. Based on Bomford clinical classification; stroke is divided into

1. **Total anterior circulation syndrome**
   i. Hemiplegia (motor deficit of face, arm and leg)
   ii. Homonymous hemianopia
   iii. Higher cortical dysfunction (aphasia, memory, neglect)

2. **Partial anterior circulation syndrome**
   Any two of the following may be present:
   i. Hemiplegia (motor and/or sensory deficit)
   ii. Ipsilateral hemianopia or higher cerebral dysfunction
   iii. Higher cerebral dysfunction alone
       or
       Isolated motor and/or sensory deficit restricted to one limb (monoplegia) or the face

3. **Posterior circulation syndrome**
   One or more of the following features present:
   i. Bilateral motor or sensory signs not secondary to brainstem compression by a large supratentorial lesion
   ii. Cerebellar signs (ataxic hemiparesis)
   iii. Unequivocal diplopia with or without external ocular muscle palsy
   iv. Crossed sign, for example, left facial and right limb weakness
   v. Hemianopia alone or with any of the 4 features described above.

Q. How will you localise the lesion in a case with hemiplegia?

Ans. The site or the level of lesion can be deduced from associated neurological signs.

1. ***Cortical or subcortical (corona radiata) lesion***
   The cortical lesions usually produce monoplegia, hence, hemiplegia is of rare occurrence, but can occur if the cortical lesion extends downward into subcortical area (corona radiata). The characteristic features of cortical/subcortical lesion are:
   i. Contralateral hemiplegia of uncrossed type
   ii. Convulsions (Jacksonian) may occur
   iii. Speech disturbance (aphasia) if dominant hemisphere is involved. The dominant hemisphere is decided from handedness of a person. If a person is right-handed, the left hemisphere is dominant and contains the speech area.
   iv. Cortical type of sensory loss (astereognosis, loss of sense of position, tactile localisation, and two-point discrimination)
   v. Anosognosia, visual field defect
   vi. Supranuclear 7th nerve palsy.

2. ***Internal capsular lesions***
   • Contralateral hemiplegia of uncrossed type
   • Contralateral hemianesthesia
   • Dense hemiplegia – complete paralysis of face, upper and lower limbs
   • UMN paralysis of 7th nerve
   • No convulsion, no speech, taste or visual disturbance.
   A pure motor isolated dense hemiplegia affecting simultaneously the face, arm and leg indicates a lesion in the posterior limb of internal capsule – a lacunar infarct.

3. ***Midbrain lesion***
   • Contralateral hemiplegia of crossed type
   • The 3rd nerve nuclear paralysis with contralateral hemiplegia constitutes *Weber's syndrome*
   • Contralateral hemianesthesia and analgesia

4. ***Pontine lesion***
   • Contralateral hemiplegia of crossed type
   • Contralateral hemianesthesia and analgesia
   • Ipsilateral 6th or 7th cranial nerve paralysis (LMN type) with contralateral hemiplegia is called *Millard-Gubler syndrome*
   • Constriction of pupil (*Horner's syndrome*) on the same side of the lesion due to involvement of sympathetic fibers
   • Ataxic hemiplegia with or without dysarthria indicates a lacunar infarct

5. ***Medulla oblongata lesion***
   A. *Features of medial medullary syndrome*
      Ipsilateral
      • Paralysis of half of tongue (XII nerve palsy)
      Contralateral
      • Upper and lower limbs UMN paralysis sparing face

- Impaired tactile and proprioceptive sensations.
  B. *Features of lateral medullary syndrome (Wallenberg's syndrome)*
  Ipsilateral (same side of lesion)
  - Facial numbness (Vth nerve involvement)
  - Ataxia, nystagmus (cerebellar involvement)
  - Horner's syndrome (sympathetic involvement)
  - IX and X nerve palsy
  - Loss of posterior column sensations
  Contralateral (Opposite side)
  - Spinothalamic (pain, touch, temperature) sensory loss
  - Hemiparesis (mild, unusual)
6. *Spinal cord (C1-C4) lesion*
   - Brown-Sequard syndrome (Read spinal cord lesion).

Q. How will you evaluate an unconscious patient for evidence of hemiplegia?

Ans. The evaluation includes:

Head and Neck

Patient should be examined for evidence of trauma and neck stiffness.

Pupils

1. *Fixed dilatation of one pupil* indicates herniation of uncus of temporal lobe (coning) and compression of third nerve. This could be due to raised intracranial tension or may be observed during lumbar puncture in a patient with raised intracranial tension if precautions are not exercised for slow decompression.
2. *'Pin-point' pupils.* 'Fixed pin-point pupils' occur in pontine lesion (pontine hemorrhage) due to sympathetic involvement.
3. *Mid-dilated pupils.* Fixed mid-dilated pupil may be seen in midbrain lesion.
4. *Horner's syndrome* (Ipsilateral pupillary constriction, ptosis, enophthalmos, anhidrosis, loss of ciliospinal reflex) occurs with lesions of the hypothalamus and also in "coning".

Ocular Fundi

These should be examined for papilloedema.

Vestibulo-ocular Reflex (Doll's Head Reflex)

Passive head rotation causes conjugate deviation of eyes in the direction opposite to the induced head movement (doll's head reflex). This reflex is lost in deep coma. It is absent in brainstem lesions.

Abnormalities of Conjugate Deviation

i. Sustained conjugate lateral gaze occurs towards the side of a destructive hemispheric lesion (i.e. the eyes look towards normal limbs)
ii. In pontine lesion, sustained conjugate lateral gaze occurs away from the side of lesion, i.e. 'towards the paralysed limbs'
iii. Skew deviation (one eye rolled upwards and the other downwards) is a rare sign, indicates brainstem lesions
iv. Ocular bobbing. These are sudden, brisk, down–ward—diving eye movements seen in pontine or cerebellar hemorrhage.

Motor System Examination

- In hemiparesis, there is abnormal flaccidity of the limbs on the affected side. Raise both the upper limbs and then release them suddenly, the paralysed limb falls to the ground with a thud rapidly than non-paralysed limb
- Facial asymmetry (drooping of one side of face), unilateral dribbling, or blowing in and out of the paralysed cheek indicate 7th nerve palsy
- Asymmetry of tendon reflexes. In deep coma, the reflexes may be absent and even plantars are extensor. Occasionally, asymmetry of reflexes helps to point out the side of lesion
- Decerebrate or decorticate posture indicates cerebral lesion.

Q. What is hysterical hemiplegia?

Ans. In hysterical hemiplegia, the patient drags the affected leg along the ground behind the body and does not circumduct the leg or use it to support the body weight. At times, hemiplegic leg is pushed ahead of the patient and used mainly for support. The arm on the affected side remains limp and is kept by the side of the body and does not develop flexed posture commonly seen in hemiplegia from organic causes (Fig. 1.33). The characteristic signs of hysterical hemiplegia are:

1. *Hysterical gait*
2. *Normal tone.* The affected limbs show normal resistance to passive manipulation or there may be increasing resistance being offered by the patient as limb is being moved. The patient is asked to move the limb, the movement is seen to be slow and jerky, often with contraction of both agonist and antagonist muscles simultaneously or intermittently.
3. The *tendon reflexes* are normal on both the sides

4. *Plantars* are flexor or down-going
5. Often there is *loss of all forms of sensations* (touch, pain, smell, vision and hearing) on the paralysed side— a group of sensory changes that is never seen in organic brain disease.
6. *Hoover's sign and Babinski's combined leg flexion tests* are helpful in distinguishing hysterical from organic hemiplegia.

"To elicit *Hoover's sign*, the supine patient is asked to raise one leg from the bed against resistance. In a normal individual the back of heel of contralateral leg presses firmly down, and the same is true for organic hemiplegia when attempts are made to lift the paralysed leg. The hysterical patient will press down the supposedly paralysed limb more strongly under these circumstances which can be appreciated by placing a hand below the normal heel.

In *Babinski's combined leg flexion test*, the patient with organic hemiplegia is asked to sit up on the bed from lying down position without using his/her arms; in doing this, the paralysed leg flexes (if power is good) at the hip and heel is lifted from the bed, while the heel of the normal leg is pressed into the bed which is appreciated by putting the hand below the heel. This sign is absent in hysterical hemiplegia".

Q. How will you proceed to diagnose a case of hemiplegia? What clinical conditions will you keep in mind in a case with hemiplegia?

Ans. Clinical evaluation of hemiplegia rests on history, clinical examination and investigations. A protocol of questionnaire is given in Table 1.113. The differential diagnosis includes to find out its cause and to localise the site of the lesion. Functional disorders such as hysterical hemiplegia should be differentiated from organic one.

Q. How will you describe the complete diagnosis in a case with hemiplegia?

Ans. The complete diagnosis includes:
- Clinical diagnosis such as CVA left side with hemiplegia right side
- Site of lesion—internal capsule
- Net neurological deficit, e.g. Pyramidal tract, Posterior column, Spinothalamic tract
- Type of lesion, e.g. vascular (middle cerebral artery thrombosis, embolism, etc.)
- Etiology—atherosclerotic or embolic from heart lesion.

Q. How would you decide vascular lesion in hemiplegia?

Ans. The common clinical conditions that come to the mind are cerebral thrombosis, cerebral hemorrhage,

Table 1.113: Clinical evaluation of a case with hemiplegia

Note the followings:
- Age
- Onset-acute (sudden, catastrophic), subacute or chronic Acute onset suggests cerebral hemorrhage
- *Disturbance in consciousness.* Majority of the patients with cerebral thrombosis and embolism retain consciousness
- Disturbance of speech (aphasia, dysarthria, dysphonia)
- History of nasal regurgitation, drooling of saliva from the angle of the mouth, facial asymmetry
- Trauma
- Convulsions-Generalized convulsions preceding the paralysis; Todd's paralysis (postictal) indicate ICSOL (intracranial space occupying lesion), hypertensive encephalopathy. Convulsions, fever and paralysis indicate meningitis, cerebral abscess, encephalitis
- Disturbance of smell, taste, vision (visual field defect, diplopia)
- Headache – severe, persistent or mild. Severe headache associated with hemiplegia points out either subarachnoid hemorrhage or cerebral hemorrhage or hypertensive encephalopathy. Headache preceding paralysis suggests ICSOL or subdural hematoma
- History of diabetes, hypertension, familial hyperlipidemia, obesity, pregnancy, delivery (puerperium), bleeding or coagulation disorders, hypercoaguable states, etc.
- Symptoms and signs of cardiovascular and pulmonary disease
- Symptoms and signs of infections
- Symptoms and signs of raised intracranial tension.

cerebral embolism. The three common cerebrovascular lesions that can produce hemiplegia are compared in Table 1.114.

Q. What are the characteristic features of hemiplegia due to a brain tumor? What are false localising signs?

Ans. They are given in Table 1.115.

Q. What are features of hemiplegia due to chronic subdural hematoma?

Ans. The features of hemiplegia in chronic subdural hematoma are:
i. There may be history of injury or fall. Patient may have underlying liver disease, bleeding diathesis or may be on anticoagulants
ii. Slow or chronic onset with fluctuating headache, slow thinking, confusion, drowsiness, personality changes, seizures, etc
iii. There may be lucid interval (weeks, months or more than a year) between the onset of injury and symptoms
iv. Hemiplegia is uncrossed, due to compression effect on pyramidal tracts

Table 1.114: Differential diagnosis of cerebrovascular accidents with hemiplegia

Features	Cerebral thrombosis	Cerebral embolism	Cerebral hemorrhage
Onset	Sudden, may be slow (stroke-in-evolution)	Abrupt like bolt from the blue	Sudden, catastrophic
Premonitory symptoms	May be present in the form of TIA	Absent	May be present in the form of speech disturbance or attacks of weakness in a limb
Consciousness	Preserved or there may be slight confusion	Preserved, sometimes patient may be dazed or drowsy	Usually semiconscious or unconscious
Headache	Absent but occurs if cerebral edema develops	Absent	Severe, persistent
Neck stiffness	Absent	Absent	Present if bleed leaks into subarachnoid space
Neurological deficit	Slowly developing	Maximum at the onset, followed by initiation of recovery	Rapidly developing and progressive
Precipitating or predisposing conditions	Hypertension, diabetes, dyslipidemia, hypothyroidism, hypercoagulable states (pregnancy, puerperium, oral contraceptives), dehydration or shock	Evidence of source of embolization, i.e. heart disease (ischemic, rheumatic), aneurysm (arterial, ventricular), thrombosis (atherosclerosis, atrial)	Precipitated by stress, exertion, physical act, sudden rise in BP. Atheromatous arteries, aneurysm of arteries or AV malformations predispose to hemorrhage
Symptoms and signs of raised intracranial tension	Absent	Absent	May be present if bleed leaks into subarachnoid space
Recovery	Slow, may be partial or complete	Rapid, recovery is the rule	Slow, if patient recovers. Residual damage persists

---

Table 1.115: Hemiplegia due to brain tumor

1. Slow onset and slow progression
2. *Focal symptoms* – Jacksonian fits (focal epilepsy), aphasia, hemiplegia or monoplegia
3. *Symptoms and signs of raised intracranial tension, e.g.*
   - Headache, vomiting, papilloedema
   - Bradycardia, slight rise in BP, rise in respiratory rate
   - Mental features – confusion, disorientation, emotional apathy, depression, somnolence, urinary and fecal incontinence
   - Epileptic seizures
   - *False localizing signs*
     - Unilateral 6th nerve palsy (diplopia with lateral deviation of the eye), sometimes it may be bilateral
     - Bilateral plantar extensor response
     - Bilateral grasp reflexes
     - Cerebellar signs
     - Fixed dilated pupils

v. Symptoms and signs of raised intracranial tension
vi. Hemianopia, hemianesthesia, aphasia, epilepsy are seldom observed as structures subserving these functions are deeply situated and are not compressed easily.

Q. List the predisposing factors for CVA (hemiplegia).

Ans. The following are the risk factors for accelerated atherogenesis prodisposing to cerebral thrombosis (CVA). These must be taken into account in the past/present history (Table 1.116).

Q. What are features of atherosclerosis?

Ans. Following are the features:
- Age >60 years
- There may be past history of IHD/TIA/intermittent claudication

Table 1.116: Risk factors in CVA

- Systemic hypertension
- Heart disease, e.g. ischemic, rheumatic with atrial fibrillation, cardiomyopathy.
- Diabetes
- TIA
- Hyperlipidemia (familial or nonfamilial), atherosclerosis
- Homocysteinemia and homocysteinuria
- Deficiency of proteins C and S
- Strong family history
- Smoking
- Obesity
- Oral contraceptives
- Hyperviscosity syndrome, e.g. polycythemia, antiphospholipid syndrome
- Increasing age (old age)

- Risk factor may be present (Table 1.116)
- The radial pulse or other vessel walls may be thickened and palpable
- There may be suprasternal pulsations
- Weak carotids and even a bruit may be present
- Signs of hyperlipidemia (e.g. xanthomas or xanthelasma) may be evident occasionally
- Signs of senility, e.g. wrinkled face, corneal arcus, frontal baldness may be present
- Fundus examination may reveal arteriosclerotic changes (A:V nipping)
- BP may show systolic hypertension
- Chest X-ray may reveal unfolding or calcification of arch of aorta (ring shaped calcification).

Q. What are causes of recurrent CVA/hemiplegia?

Ans. Causes are:
- TIA (transient ischemia attack) is common cause
- Post-epilepsy – Todd's paralysis
- Hypertensive encephalopathy
- Migrainous hemiplegia (vasospastic hemiplegia)
- Hysterical hemiplegia.

Q. What are the causes of stroke in young?

Ans. Causes are:
- Cerebral embolism from a cardiac source, commonly rheumatic valvular disease
- Subarachnoid hemorrhage (rupture of Berry aneurysm or AV malformations or anticoagulant therapy)
- Hyperviscosity syndrome, e.g. polycythemia, post-partum state, oral contraceptive
- Arteritis, e.g. tubercular, syphilitic, Takayasu's disease, collagen vascular disease
- Premature or accelerated atherogenesis, e.g. familial hyperlipidemia, hypertriglyceridemia, diabetes, nephrotic syndrome, hypothyroidism
- Demyelinating disease, e.g. multiple sclerosis
- Head injury
- Inflammatory disease, e.g. meningitis, encephalitis, cerebral abscess, tuberculoma, cerebral malaria
- Migrainous
- Intracranial neoplasm, e.g. primary or secondary
- Procoagulant states, e.g. protein C and S deficiency, homocysteinemia, antithrombin –1 deficiency, antiphospholipid syndrome, puerpurium.

Q. What are bladder and bowel disturbances in the hemiplegia?

Ans. Unilateral involvement of bladder usually does not produce much symptoms, hence, in hemiplegia, there can be either hesitancy or precipitancy. In unconscious patient with hemiplegia, condom drainage or indwelling catheterization is necessary to prevent bed-wetting.

Q. What is the usual clinical course of hemiplegia?

Ans. A patient of hemiplegia may pass through the following stages:

1. *Stage of neuronal shock.* It is state when the reflex activity is suppressed, i.e. there is hypotonia. Jerks are absent and plantars are silent. This stage may not be seen in all cases of hemiplegia, but commonly seen in acute onset hemiplegia. This lasts for 2-3 weeks

2. *Stage of recovoery:* After 2-3 weeks the recovery starts. The face recovers first. Power returns in the extensors of lower limb and flexors of the upper limb. Finer movements of the fingers and hand recover last to a variable extent.

3. *Stage of residual paralysis.* The only deficit is little spasticity and a hemiplegic gait.

Q. What is blood supply of internal capsule?

Ans. Blood supply of internal capsule is described in Table 1.117.

Table 1.117: Blood supply of internal capsule

Limb	Upper half	Lower half
Anterior	Middle cerebral artery	Anterior cerebral artery
Posterior	Middle cerebral artery	Anterior choroidal and Posterior communicating artery

Q. What is lacunar syndrome? What is small vessel infarct?

Ans. The term lacunar syndrome or infarction implies atherothrombotic or lipohyalinotic occlusion of a small vessel (<300 μm) in the brain; most of such infarcts being small are not picked up on CT Scan. Now, it has been replaced by another term called *small-vessel infarct or stroke* which denotes occlusion of a small penetrating artery and >50% of these infarcts are picked up on CT scan. Small vessal stroke accounts for > 20% of stroke.

Q. Name the various lacunar syndromes.

Ans. 1. *Pure motor hemiparesis*
- It results from infarct in posterior limb of internal capsule.
- The face, arm and leg are almost always involved on one side

2. *Pure sensory hemiparesis*
- It results from lesion in ventrolateral thalamus
- Unilateral pure sensory symptoms involving face, arm, legs on one side.

3. *Ataxic hemiparesis*
   - It results from infarction in the pons
   - Ipsilateral cerebellar (ataxia) and corticospinal (hemiparesis) signs
   - There may or may not be dysarthria
   - There is no higher cerebral dysfunction or visual field defect.
4. *Dysarthria and clumsy hand or arm syndrome*
   - It results from infarction in the base of pons or in the genu of internal capsule
   - There is involvement of one arm
   - Dysathria is present.
6. *Aphasic hemiparesis syndrome*
   - It results due to infarction of internal capsule and adjoining corona radiata.
   - There is Broca's (motor) aphasia
   - There is pure motor hemiparesis.

Q. How would you manage a case of TIA?

Ans.
- Differentiate TIA from stroke by history, examination and CT scan.
- Perform duplex ultrasonography of the carotid vessel and/or carotid artery DSA
- Evaluate clinical risk profile and institute life style modifications i.e.
  - Stop smoking and alcohol.
  - Dietary management.
  - Exercise as advised by the doctor
  - Weight control.
  - Maintain the BP and sugar control in diabetes
  - Antiplatelets e.g. aspirin or aspirin plus clopidogrel or dipyridamole.
- Statins: Several trials have confirmed that statin drugs reduce the risk of TIA and stroke even in patients without elevated LDL or low HDL. Therefore, all patients of TIA must receive one of statins.
- Angiotensin-converting enzyme inhibitors or angiotensin- receptor blockers. Lowering of blood pressure to levels below those traditionally defining hypertension with these drugs reduce the risk of stroke further, hence they also can be included in medical regimen of TIA

Q. What is anterior cerebral artery syndrome?

Ans. Occlusion of anterior cerebral artery (anterior cerebral artery syndrome) produces certain clinical features depending on the site of block such as:

Symptoms and signs	Area involved
Monoplegia involving lower limb and paresis of opposite arm to lesser degree (incomplete hemiplegia)	Motor leg area. Arm area of cortex or its descending fibers in corona radiata
Loss of cortical sensations over lower limb involved	Sensory leg area
Urinary incontinence	Paracentral lobule (bladder area)
Contralateral primitive reflexes, e.g. grasp, sucking present	Supplemental motor area
Akinetic mutism	Cingulate gyrus
Gait apraxia	Frontal cortex near leg area

Q. How will you investigate a patient with hemiplegia?

Ans. Investigations are done for diagnosis, to find out the underlying cause and risk factors. They are given in Table 1.118.

Table 1.118: Investigations for a patient with hemiplegia

	Purpose	Test(s)
1.	For vascular episode	CT scan/MRI
2.	For underlying vascular cause	ECG, cardiac ultrasound, MRA, (MR angiography), Doppler ultrasound, carotid angiography
3.	For risk factors	Blood count, serum cholesterol, blood glucose, clotting or thrombophilia screen

CASE 36: PARAPLEGIA

A patient (not shown) presented with weakness of both lower limbs which was slowly progressive with difficulty in passing urine. There was history of numbness of both the lower limbs below the umbilicus. There was no history of fever or trauma preceding to this illness. The physical signs of the patients are represented in Figure 1.36.

Clinical Presentations

- Weakness of both lower limbs
- Numbness of both lower limbs
- Difficulty in passing urine and stool

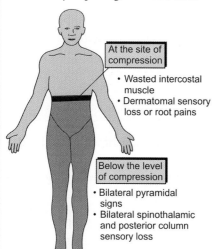

At the site of compression
- Wasted intercostal muscle
- Dermatomal sensory loss or root pains

Below the level of compression
- Bilateral pyramidal signs
- Bilateral spinothalamic and posterior column sensory loss

Fig. 1.36: Compression paraplegia with transverse thoracic spinal cord lesion with definite level. There are UMN signs below the site of compression. There is bilateral loss of all sensory modalities below the level of compression

History

Points to be Noted

- Note date and time of onset of paralysis
- Mode of onset (sudden or gradual)
- Precipitating factors, e.g. spinal trauma, vaccination
- Progress of paralysis, e.g. increasing, stationary, progressive, waxing or waning type
- Motor symptoms including inability or difficulty in walking
- Sensory symptoms, e.g. root pain, sensation of pins and needles, numbness, history of a constriction band around the waist.

Past History

Ask for:

- History of fever, tuberculosis, exposure to STD
- History of similar episodes in the past
- History of spinal trauma
- History of diabetes, HT
- History of alcoholism
- Pain in back

Family History

- Diabetes, HT
- History of paraplegia in other members of the family
- Tuberculosis

Unilateral Compression

(Brown-Sequard syndrome) The signs are:

i. Ipsilateral in the side compression) pyramidal signs

ii. Contralateral (opposite to the side involved) spinothalamic sensory loss of pain, touch and temperature.

Examination

I. **General physical: Note the following:**
- Consciousness or cooperative, posture
- Neck for lymphadenopathy
- Vitals, e.g. pulse, BP and temperature
- Skin, e.g. pigmentation, neurofibroma

II. **Nervous system. Examine:**
- Higher functions
- Neck rigidity
- Cranial nerves
- Cerebellar functions
- Motor system including gait
- Sensory system

III. **Examination of spine**
- Kyphosis, scoliosis, gibbus, tenderness and spina bifida (a tuff of hair)

IV. **Other systems**
- *Respiratory system examination* for tuberculosis, bronchogenic carcinoma and lymphoma
- *CVS-*as discussed in hemiplegia
- *GI tract* for hepatosplenomegaly, ascites
- *Lymphoreticular system* for sternal tenderness, hemorrhagic spots and lymphadenopathy.

Q. What is your clinical diagnosis?
Ans. Presence of UMN signs in both lower limbs with localised LMN signs over the lower part of chest, suggest the provisional diagnosis of compression (spastic) paraplegia.

Q. Where is the site of lesion?
Ans. Site of lesion is upper thoracic region between T2-T5. The points in favor are:
1. Presence of upper limb reflexes which indicate intactness of all cervical segments and first thoracic.

2. Loss of abdominal reflexes indicate lesion above T6.
3. Weakness of intercostal muscles of T4, T5 and a dermatomal sensory loss points the lesion at this site. However there was no bony deformity of spine at this level.

Q. What is net neurological deficit in your case?
Ans.
- Bilateral pyramidal tract involvement
- Bilateral sensory involvement of all modalities (spinothalamic and posterior column involvement)
- Sphincter involvement (autonomic involvement)

Q. **What does paraplegia mean?**

Ans. It refers to complete loss of motor functions (paralysis) of both lower limbs. Partial weakness is designated as *paraparesis.*

Q. **What is the type of lesion in your case?**

Ans. Extramedullary compression due to spinal tumor. The points in favor are:

1. Slowly progressive paraplegia, symmetric involvement.
2. History of root pain and dermatological sensory loss.
3. Brisk reflexes and sensory loss of all modalities below the level of compression.
4. Bowel and bladder involvement.
5. There is no sacral sparing.

Q. **Why do you say compression paraplegia in your case?**

Ans. It is a case of compression paraplegia because:

1. There is evidence of LMN paralysis and dermatomal sensory loss (weakness of intercostal muscles and loss of sensation at $T_4 - T_6$).
2. UMN signs are present below the level of compression (spasticity, exaggerated reflexes and plantar extensors).

N.B. To decide the site of lesion, Read Table 1.125.

Q. **What is cerebral paraplegia? What are its causes?**

Ans. The lower limbs and bladder (micturition centre) are represented in paracentral lobule (about upper one inch of cerebral cortex), hence, lesion of this area produces paraplegia with bladder disturbance (retention of urine) and cortical type of sensory loss. There may be associated headache, vomiting and convulsions or Jacksonian fits.

The **causes** are:

• Cerebral diplegia
• Superior sagittal sinus thrombosis
• Parasagittal meningioma
• Thrombosis of unpaired anterior cerebral artery
• Gun shot injury of paracentral lobule
• Internal hydrocephalus.

Q. **What are the causes of UMN paralysis of one leg?**

Ans. 1. Cerebral lesion e.g. unilateral parasagittal hematoma.
2. Brown- Sequard syndrome at thoracic level.

Q. **What is spastic paraplegia?**

Ans. The involvement of spinal cord and cerebrum produces spastic (UMN) paraplegia. Spastic paraplegia is of two types;

• *Paraplegia-in-extension*
• *Paraplegia-in-flexion*

The difference between paraplegia-in-extension and paraplegia-in-flexion are summarised in Table 1.119.

Q. **What is clinical course of compression paraplegia?**

Ans. Initially, due to involvement (compression) of pyramidal tracts, there is *paraplegia-in-extension* due to increased tone of antegravity muscles as a result of intact extrapyramidal system. When extrapyramidal system is involved (tectospinal, rubrospinal, vestibulospinal), the paraplegia-in-flexion develops resulting in flexors spasms, contractures and deformity (Table 1.119).

Q. **What is flaccid paraplegia?**

Ans. Flaccid paralysis means lower motor neuron type of paralysis resulting from the diseases involving anterior horns cells, radicals, peripheral nerves and muscles (Table 1.120). Acute onset of UMN type of paralysis may be flaccid instead of spastic if patient is in shock state. A hysterical patient may also present with LMN type of paraplegia. The cause are summarised in Table 1.120.

Q. **What are the causes of spastic paraplegia?**

Ans. It may be due to compression of the spinal cord or without it. Spinal cord tumors are the most common cause of compression (Table 1.121).

The central causes of spastic paraplegia have already been listed.

Q. **What is neuronal (spinal) shock?**

Ans. It refers to depression or loss of reflex activity (absent tendon reflexes) in acute lesion of spinal cord. It is transient, may last for few days followed by recovery. This explains the loss of deep tendon reflexes in acute onset UMN lesion of the cord.

Q. **What are common causes of hypertonia?**

Ans. • UMN lesion
• Tetanus
• Strychnine poisoning
• Hysterical
• Voluntary in noncooperative patients
• Extrapyrimidal lesion except chorea
• Myotonia
• Catatonia
  Decerebrate rigidity

Q. **How will differentiate between extramedullary and intramedullary spinal cord compression?**

Ans. Table 1.122 differentiates between these two spinal cord compressions.

Q. **How will you calculate the level of spinal segments in relation to vertebra in a case with compression paraplegia?**

Ans. In case of compression, if vertebra involved is known, then calculation of spinal segment is done as follows:

Vertebra	*Spinal segment*
• For cervical vertebrae	: Add 1
• For 1-6 thoracic vertebrae	: Add 2

Table 1.119: Distinction between paraplegia-in-extension and paraplegia-in-flexion

Feature	Paraplegia-in-extension	Paraplegia-in-flexion
Posture	Lower limbs adopt an extension posture and extensor muscles are spastic. Extensor spasms occur	Lower limbs adopt flexed posture. Intermittent flexor spasms occur in which there is flexion of both lower limbs
Neurological deficit	Only pyramidal tracts involved	Both pyramidal and extrapyramidal tracts are involved
Clinical features		
Positions of limbs	Hip extended and adducted, knee extended and feet plantar-flexed	Thigh and knee flexed, feet dorsiflexed
Tone	Clasp-knife spasticity in extensor groups of muscles	Rigidity in flexor groups of muscles
Tendon jerks	Exaggerated	Diminished
Plantar response	Extensor	Extensor but evokes flexor spasms
Incontinence of bowel and bladder	Absent	Present
Mass reflex*	Absent	Present

N.B. *Mass reflex* is an enlarged area of hyperexcitability of reflex activity. Just stroking the skin of either lower limbs or lower abdominal wall, produces the reflex evacuation of the bladder and bowel with reflex flexor spasms of the lower limbs and lower trunk muscles.

Table 1.120: Causes of flaccid paralysis

Sites	Causes
• Anterior horn cells	Poliomyelitis
• Nerve root	Radiculitis, polyradiculoneuro-pathy, tabes dorsalis, Cauda equina
• Peripheral nerves	GB syndrome, peripheral neuropathies
• Myoneural junction	Myasthenic gravis, Myasthenia-myopathic syndrome (Lambert-Eaton syndrome) periodic paralysis (hypo or hyperkalemic)
• Muscles	Myopathy

- For 7-9 thoracic vertebrae : Add 3
- The T10 vertebra overlies : L1 and L2
- The T11 vertebra overlies : L3 and L4
- The T12 vertebra overlies : L5 segment
- The L1 overlies the sacral and coccygeal segments.

N.B: If spinal segment involved is known then vertebral level can be calculated as detailed above.

Q. What is hemisection of spinal cord?

Ans. *Brown-Sequard syndrome.* It is hemi-section of spinal cord, commonly due to gun shot injury.

It consists of:
- Contralateral loss of pain and temperature with ipsilateral loss of posterior column sensations
- Monoplegia or hemiplegia on the same side of the lesion below the site of involvement
- UMNs signs below the level of lesion, i.e. exaggerated tendon jerks and plantar extensors. Superficial reflexes are lost
- A band of hyperesthesia or a zone of anesthesia at the level of compression.

Table 1.121: Common cause of spastic paraplegia

I. **Compressive**
  A. Extramedullary
    i. **Intradural**
      • Meningioma, neurofibroma, arachnoiditis
    ii. **Extradural**
      • Pott's disease (caries spine)
      • Vertebral neoplasms, e.g. metastases, myeloma
      • Pachymeningitis
      • Prolapsed intervertebral disc
      • Epidural abscess or hemorrhage
      • Fracture dislocation of vertebra, Paget's disease, osteoporosis
  B. Intramedullary
      • Syringomyelia, haematomyelia
      • Intramedullary tumor, e.g. ependymoma, glioma
      • Spinal cord abscess (e.g. pyogenic, tuberculosis)

II. **Non-compressive**
  • Motor neurone disease especially amyotrophic lateral sclerosis
  • Multiple sclerosis, postvaccinal myelitis
  • Acute transverse myelitis
  • Subacute combined degeneration (Vit. B_{12} deficiency)
  • Lathyrism
  • Syringomyelia
  • Hereditary spastic paraplegia
  • Tropical spastic paraplegia
  • Radiation myelopathy

- Segmental signs, i.e. muscle atrophy, redicular pain and loss of a reflex on the side involved.

Q. What are the causes of Brown-Sequard syndrome?

Ans.
  • Syringomyelia
  • Cord tumor
  • Bullet or stab injury
  • Hematomyelia
  • Degenerative disease of spine
  • Multiple myeloma

Table 1.122: Differentiation between extramedullary and intramedullary spinal cord compression

Feature	Extramedullary	Intramedullary
Root pain	Common	Rare
UMN signs	Early and prominent	Late feature and are less prominent
LMN signs	Segmental at the site of compression	Extends to involve few segments with atrophy and fasciculations
Reflexes	Brisk, early feature	Less brisk, late feature
Sensory deficit	Contralateral loss of pain and temperature with ipsilateral loss of proprioception	Dissociated sensory loss
Sacral sparing	Absent	Present
Bowel and bladder involvement	Late	Early
Trophic changes	Unusual	Common
Vertebral tenderness	May be present	Absent
CSF changes	Froin's syndrome common	Rare

Q. How will you distinguish compressive from noncompressive myelopathy?

Ans. The absolute characteristic of compression of the cord is either motor loss (loss of tendon jerk, muscle wasting, fasciculations) or a sensory sign (hyperesthesia, analgesia) at the site of compression while no such phenomenon is seen in noncompressive myelopathy. The distinction between the two is described in Table 1.123.

Read Neurological Examination in Clinical Method in Medicine by Dr SN Chugh

- Grading of power
- UMN signs
- LMN signs

Table 1.123: Distinction between compressive and noncompressive myelopathy

Compressive	Non-compressive
Bone changes, i.e. deformity, tenderness present	No bony change
Girdle-like pain present (root pain)	No root pain
Upper level of sensory loss present	No definite level
Zone of hyperesthesia may be present	Absent
Usually of gradual onset	Usually of acute onset
Asymmetrical involvement of limbs	Symmetrical involvement of limbs
Flexor spasms common	Absent
Bowel and bladder involvement is early	Late involvement
Commonest cause is caries spine	Commonest cause motor neuron disease

Q. What are the causes of cord compression at multiple sites?

Ans. Following are the causes:
- Arachnoiditis (tubercular—there is patchy involvement)
- Neurofibromatosis
- Multiple discs prolapse
- Secondary deposits
- Cervical spondylosis.

Q. What are the causes of paraplegia without sensory loss?

Ans. Causes are:
- Hereditary spastic paraplegia
- Lathyrism
- GB syndrome
- Amyotrophic lateral sclerosis
- Fluorosis.

Q. What are the causes of paraplegia with loss of deep tendon jerks?

Ans. In paraplegia, the tendon jerks are brisk. They can only become absent when either patient is in spinal shock or there is involvement of afferent or efferent side of the reflex arc. The causes are:
- Neuronal shock (spinal shock). All jerks are absent
- Radiculitis—the jerk whose root is involved will be absent
- Peripheral neuropathy—bilateral ankle jerk will be absent
- Presence of bedsores or complicating UTI. The reflex activity in this complication may be suppressed leading to loss of most reflexes
- Hematomyelia (sudden hemorrhage from AV malformation) or myelomalacia cause loss of reflexes
- Hypokalemic periodic paralysis.

Q. What are the causes of Quadriplegia?

Ans. Quadriplegia means weakness of all the four limbs. Therefore, cause may lie in the brain or spinal cord anywhere from the cortex to spinal level T1. The cranial lesion must be bilateral. The *causes* are:

1. Cerebral palsy
2. Bilateral brainstem lesion
3. High cervical cord compression, e.g. craniovertebral anomaly, high spinal cord injury, etc.
4. Multiple sclerosis
5. Motor neuron disease
6. Acute anterior poliomyelitis
7. Guillain-Barré syndrome
8. Peripheral neuropathy
9. Myopathy or polymyositis
10. Periodic paralysis (transient quadriplegia).

Q. What are the causes and clinical features of high cervical cord compression?

Ans. The features of high cervical cord compression are tabulated in Table 1.124.

Q. How will you localise of the lesion in compressive myelopathy?

Ans. Diagnostic clues to lesions at different sites are depicted in Table 1.125.

Q. What are symptoms and signs of spinal cord compression?

Ans. In spinal cord compression, certain symptoms and signs (motor and sensory) appear at the site of compression as well as below the compression (Tables 1.126A and B).

Q. What are classical features of acute transverse myelitis?

Ans. Following are classical features:

- Acute onset of fever with flaccid paralysis. There may be neck or back pain
- Cause is mostly viral
- Bladder involvement is early
- Girdle constriction (constriction band) around the waist is common indicating mid-thoracic region as the common site of involvement
- Variable degree of sensory loss (complete or incomplete) below the level of the lesion. A zone of hyperesthesia may be present between the area of sensory loss and area of normal sensation
- There is loss of all tendon reflexes (areflexia) due to spinal shock. Abdominal reflexes are absent. Plantar are silent. As the spinal shock passes off, hyper-reflexia returns with plantar extensor response.

Q. What are causes of episodic weakness?

Ans. Causes are:
- Myasthenia gravis

Table 1.124: Features and causes of high cervical cord compression

Causes

1. *Craniovertebral anomalies,* e.g. platybasia, basilar impression, atlantoaxial dislocation, Klippel-Feil anomaly, Arnold-Chiari malformation
2. *High cervical cord (C1-C4) lesion,* e.g. due to craniovertebral anomaly, fracture dislocation, hematomyelia, cervical spondylosis, cord tumors, caries spine.

Features

- A triad of short neck, low hair line and restricted cervical movements
- Spastic quadriparesis of gradual onset, involving one limb followed by the other or
- Spastic paraplegia with:
  Horner's syndrome
  XI nerve palsy
  V nerve palsy (spinal tract of Vth nerve) leading to loss of sensation over face, e.g. 1st and 2nd division of V)
  Vertical nystagmas
- Cerebellar signs may be present
- Mirror image movement, impaired sense of position and vibration

- Hyperthyroidism
- Periodic paralysis (hypokalaemic, hyperkalaemic)
- Conn's syndrome (primary hyperaldosteronism)
- Botulinum poisoning
- Guillain-Barré syndrome

Q. What is Lathyrism?

Ans. It is a slowly evolving epidemic spastic paraplegia due to consumption of *'khesari dal'* (lathyrus sativus) for prolonged period. It occurs in areas where drought are commonly seen, e.g. UP, Bihar, Rajasthan and MP where poor people consume often a mixture of wheat, Bengal gram and Khesari dal – called *"birri"*. It may involve many families in a locality. The causative factor is BOAA – a neurotoxin. Initially, patients complain of nocturnal muscle cramps, stiffness of limbs and inability to walk. Ultimately due to increasing spasticity they pass through one-stick stage (scissor type gait), two-stick stage (patient uses two sticks to walk) and crawler stage (patient crawls on hands).

Q. What are causes of optic atrophy and paraplegia?

Ans. Optic atrophy may be part and parcel of the disease causing paraplegia.

- Hereditary (Friedreich's) ataxia
- Neuromyelitis optica (Devic's disease—a demyelinating disorder)
- Eale's disease
- Subacute myelo-optic neuropathy, alcohol-induced
- Infections like tuberculosis and syphilis
- Deficiency states, e.g. subacute combined degeneration, pellagra.

Table 1.125: Lesions at different sites and their signs

Site of lesion (spinal segment)	Symptoms and signs
High cervical cord lesion e.g. at C_1-C_4	• UMN quadriplegia • There may be weakness of respiratory muscles or diaphragmatic palsy • There may be suboccipital pain radiating to neck and shoulder • Sensory loss over upper part of chest

	Sensory	*Motor*
C_5	• Radicular pain/paresthesia over neck, shoulder, outer brachioradialis arm, forearm • Sensory deficit over outer aspect of upper arm	• Muscle weakness of deltoid, supraspinatus brachioradialis • Jerks affected, e.g. biceps, supinator lost
C_6	• Radicular pain/paresthesia over neck, shoulder, outer arm, forearm, thumb and index finger • Sensory loss over thumb and index finger	• muscle weakness, e.g. biceps brachio radial is extensor carpiradialis longus • Dept tendon jerks affected, e.g. biceps, supinator lost
C_7	• Radiator pain/paresthesia neck, shoulder, arm, forearm to index and middle finger • Superficial sensory loss of middle and index finger	• Muscle weakness of triceps and muscle of forearm • Jerk affected is loss of tricep jerk
C_8	• Radicular pain/paraesthesia over neck shoulder, arm, ring and index fingers • Sensory loss ring and little fingers	• Muscle weakness of flexors of forearm • Finger flexion jerk is lost
T_1	• Radicular pain/paresthesia over neck, axilla, medial aspects of arm, forearm, little and ring finger • Sensory loss over medial arm and little finger	• Muscle weakness of small muscle of hand • Finger flexion jerk is lost.

Note: Horner's syndrome may occur at any level of cervical cord compression

Lesion above T_6	• Paraplegia with loss of all abdominal reflexes • There is a level of sensory loss over the chest • Deep tendon reflexes below compression are exaggerated and plantars are extensor
Lesion T_7-T_9	• Paraplegia (UMN) with loss of upper abdominal reflexes
Lesions at T_9-T_{10}	• Umbilicus is turned downwards during rising test (Beever's sign)
Lesion T_{10}-T_{12}	• Paralysis of both lower limbs (UMN type of paraplegia) • Upper abdominal reflexes are spared but lower abdominal reflexes are lost • Umbilicus is turned upwards during rising test due to paralysis of lower part

(continued) of rectus abdominis. Beever's sign actually indicates lesions at T_9 and T_{10}

Lesion of L_1 and L_2	• Paraplegia (UMN) with loss of cremasteric reflex • Superficial sensory loss over sacrum • Deep tendon jerks below the level of compression exaggerated • Radicular pain/paresthesia limited to anterior aspect of thigh, grain and testicle
Lesion of L_3-L_4	• Paraplegia with loss of knee jerks and preservation of ankle jerks • Radicular pain/paresthesia over anteromedial aspect of the leg • Superficial sensory deficit over anteromedial aspect of leg
Lesion of L_5 and S_1	• Paralysis of movements of foot and ankle, flexion at knee and extension of thigh. There is loss of ankle jerks • Radicular pain/ paresthesia over dorsum of foot and anterolateral aspect of leg (L5) or radicular pain/ paresthesia over buttock, back of thigh, calf and lateral border of foot.

Table 1.126A: Symptoms of spinal cord compression

Symptoms
1. *Pain:* Localised pain over the spine or in a root distribution which may be aggravated by coughing, sneezing or straining Girdle-like sensation or sense of constriction band at the level of lesion suggests posterior column involvement.
2. *Sensory:* Paresthesia or numbness in the lower limbs which spreads upwards.
3. *Motor:* Weakness, heaviness or stiffness of the limbs most commonly the legs.
4. *Sphinctors:* Urgency or hesitancy of micturition leading eventually to urinary retention.

Table 1.126B: Signs of spinal cord compression

Signs
1. **Sensory deficit**
   A. *At the level of compression:* A zone of hyperesthesia or hyperalgesia points towards the level of compression
   B. *Below the level of compression:* There is loss of sensations carried by spinothalamic tracts and posterior columns.
2. **Motor**
   A. *At the level of compression*
   • Atrophy of a muscle
   • Loss of a deep tendon reflex, if the segmental supply of the reflex is interrupted
   • The loss of lower abdominal reflex with preservation of upper abdominal reflex indicates the lesion at T_9-T_{10}
   B. *Below the level of lesion*
   • All deep tendon reflexes exaggerated
   • All superficial reflexes lost
   • Tone increased, power decreased
   • Plantars are extensor
   • Retention of urine

Q. How does tuberculosis cause paraplegia?

Ans. This is as follows:

1. Compression of the cord by cold abscess (extradural compression)
2. Tubercular arachnoiditis or pachymeningitis
3. Tubercular endarteritis (vascular phenomenon) producing myelomalacia of the cord
4. Tubercular myelitis, i.e. extension of the lesion from outside to within.

Q. How will you investigate the case with paraplegia?

Ans. Investigations are:

1. *Routine blood tests* (TLC, DLC, ESR)
2. *Urine examination,* urine for culture and sensitivity
3. *Blood biochemistry,* e.g. urea, creatinine, electrolytes
4. *Chest X-ray* for tuberculosis or malignancy lung or lymphoma
5. *Lymph node biopsy –* if lymph node enlarged
6. *CSF examination.* Features of *Froin's* syndrome below the level of compression will be evident if spinal tumor is the cause of spinal block.
   – Low CSF pressure
   – Xanthochromia
   – Increased protein
   – Normal cellular count
   – Positive Queckensted test (i.e. no rise in CSF pressure following compression of internal jugular vein)
7. *CT myelography* to determine the site and type of compression. Nowadays it has been replaced by MRI.

The CT myelography may show;
   i. *Meniscus sign* in intradural compression
   ii. *Brush border sign* in extradural tumors
   iii. *Candle-wax or Candle-guttering appearance* in arachnoiditis
   iv. *Expansion sign* in syringomyelia
8. *MRI to* find out the cause of compression
9. *Other tests* depending on the cause or disease.

Q. What is albumino-cytological dissociation?

Ans. It refers to increased protein content in CSF with no parallel rise in cell count, hence, the word dissociation is used. The causes are:
   • GB syndrome
   • Froin's syndrome (spinal block due to a spinal tumor)
   • Acoustic neurofibroma
   • Cauda equina syndrome.

Q. What are causes of xanthochromia (yellow coloration of CSF)?

Ans. Following are the causes:
   • Old subarachnoid hemorrhage
   • GB syndrome
   • Froin's syndrome
   • Acoustic neuroma
   • Deep jaundice.

Q. What is tropical spastic paraplegia (HTLV-1 associated myelopathy)?

Ans. It is common in females (3rd, 4th decades) associated with HTLV-1 infection where the patient develops gradual onset of weakness of legs (paraplegia) which progresses and patient becomes confined to wheel chair within 10 years. This is UMN spastic paraplegia without sensory disturbance. Bladder disturbance and constipation are common. This is an example of noncompressive progressive myelopathy. The diagnosis is suggested by seropositivity for HTLV-1.

CASE 37: CAUDA EQUINA SYNDROME

The patient (Fig. 1.37) an electrician while at work fell down and developed sudden onset of weakness, of both the lower legs without bladder and bowel dysfunction.

Fig. 1.37: Testing for sensations

History

Points to be Noted

- History of root pain projected to perineum and thighs
- History of trauma
- History of neurogenic classification
- Pain in anterior thigh
- Any trophic change
- History of leukemia or prostatic carcinoma
- History of disc prolapse
- Patient present with paraplegia without sphincter involvement
- With sensory loss over the buttocks
- Paralysis is lower motor neuron type e.g. muscle weakness wasting and loss of tendon jerks

Examination of Lower Limbs

Motor System

- There is wasting of quadriceps muscles and weakness of inverter of foot
- Nutrition of muscle is normal
- Tone is decreased in the muscles of foot and thigh muscles
- Bilateral foot drop
- Bilateral ankle jerks and knee jerks are absent.

Sensory System

- Saddle distribution of sensory loss
- Sensory loss over the dorsum and sole of the foot, lateral aspect of the leg and a part of back of the leg
- Plantars are flexors (downgoing)
- Sphincters are involved.

Q. What is your probable diagnosis and why?

Ans. Sir, my provisional diagnosis is LMN type of paraplegia due to cauda equina syndrome.
The points in favor of the diagnosis are:
1. Sudden and symmetrical involvement of both lower limbs.
2. History of root pain, radiating to the distribution of L3, L4, L5, S2-3 segments.
3. Saddle shaped distribution of sensory loss
4. Flaccid paraparesis with loss of knee and ankle jerks
5. Plantars are flexors (downgoing)
6. Bowel and bladder function are spared.

Q. What is differential diagnosis?

Ans. All causes of acute onset LMN paraplegia will come into differential diagnosis such as:
1. Guillain-Barre syndrome
2. Diabetes mellitus producing symmetrical neuropathy and amyotrophy
3. Porphyria
4. Paraneoplastic conditions.

Q. What is the cause of cauda equina syndrome in your case?

Ans. As there is history of trauma to the spine, therefore, the cause in my case is traumatic compressive lesion, involving cauda equina.

Q. What are the causes of cauda equina syndrome?

Ans. Centrally placed lumbosacral disc or spine involvement or spondylolisthesis at the lumbosacral junction produce cauda equina syndrome. Causes include:
  i. Prolapse disc due to degeneration, tuberculosis, trauma, etc.
  ii. Leukemic infiltration of the roots of cauda equina.
  iii. Tumors of the cauda equina (e.g. ependymoma, neurofibroma).
  iv. Secondaries in the spine causing compression of roots of cauda equina.

Q. Which vertebral level is the lesion in the cauda equina syndrome?

Ans. Spinal cord ends at the level of L1, after that roots of cauda equina emerge. All the lumbar segments (L2 to L5) lie opposite to T10 to T12. First lumbar vertebra overlies the sacral and coccygeal segments. Therefore, a lesion in the spinal cord at any level below the 10th thoracic vertebra can cause cauda equina syndrome.

Q. What is relationship of the spinal cord to the vertebra?

Ans. Read the Examination of nervous system in Clinical Methods in Medicine by Prof SN Chugh.

Q. What are the various types of cauda equina syndromes in adults?

Ans. 1. *Lateral cauda equina syndrome*: It is characterized by:
  - Pain in the anterior thigh
  - Wasting of quadriceps muscle (L2 – L4)
  - Weakness of foot invertors (L4)
  - Absent knee jerk (L2 – L4)
  Cause e.g. disc prolapse or neurofibroma
  2. *Midline cauda equina syndrome*
  - Bilateral lumbar (L2 – L4) and sacral roots (S1 – S2) lesions leading to (i) wasting of the quadriceps and absent knee jerks,(ii) wasting of the foot invertors and evertors (L4–L5 and S1) with loss of ankle jerk (L5 – S1) and (iii) saddle shaped anesthesia over the buttocks
  Causes: e.g. disc prolapse, sacral bone tumors (chordomas), secondaries in the bone and leukemic infiltration of the roots.

Q. What are differences between cauda equina and conus medullaris lesion?

Ans. The conus medullaris is the terminal portion/point at which spinal cord ends and cauda equina (a bunch of roots) starts. Therefore, the main distinctions

Table 1.127: Differentiating features between conus medullaris and cauda equina syndrome

Conus medullaris lesion	Cauda equina syndrome
Bilateral symmetrical involvement of both lower limbs	Asymmetric involvement of both lower limbs
No root pain	Severe low back or root pain
No limb weakness	Asymmetric limb weakness
Bilateral saddle anaesthesia	Asymmetric sensory loss
The bulbocavernous (S_2-S_4) and anal reflexes (S_4-S_5) are absent	Variable areflexia depending on the roots involved
Bladder and bowel disturbance common	They are relatively spared
Plantars are extensor but not always	Plantars are normal or not elicitable

between the two is the plantars extensor and symmetrical LMN signs in conus medullaris; while plantar are flexor or not elicitable with asymmetric LMN paralysis in cauda equina syndrome (Table 1.127).

Q. Name the conditions where ankle jerk is absent but knee jerk is preserved.

Ans. • Peripheral neuropathy
• Tabes dorsails
• Subacute combined degeneration.

Q. Name the conditions where knee jerk is absent but ankle jerk is present. Where is the site of lesion?

Ans. Absent knee jerk indicates LMN involvement of L_2 to L_4. Causes are:
 i. Diabetic amyotrophy
 ii. Proximal myopathy
 iii. Disc prolapse compressing L_2 - L_4 due to trauma or bone disease.
 iv. Radiculitis involving L_2 - L_4

Q. What are root values of deep tendon jerks of lower limbs?

Ans. Read Clinical Methods in Medicine by Prof SN Chugh.

Q. How would you elicit the different tendon jerks of lower limb?

Ans. Read Clinical Methods in Medicine and practise the various jerks in the class over the patients and in the hostel over your colleagues.

Q. What do you know about the term neurogenic claudication?

Ans. It implies that patient develops root pain and leg weakness usually a foot-drop while walking which rapidly recovers on resting.

Q. What is sciatica syndrome?

Ans. It is characterized by low back pain that radiates along the sciatic nerve, occurs due to irritation of roots or nerve anywhere in the spinal canal, intervertebral foramina, in the pelvis or buttocks. Straight leg raising test is positive. There may be sensory or motor deficit with absent or depressed ankle jerk on the side involved. Causes include lateral protrusion of the disc, spinal tumors, or spondylolisthesis. Spinal canal stenosis can lead to bilateral sciatica with neurogenic claudication.

Q. How would you elicit straight leg raising test?

Ans. Read Clinical Methods in Medicine by Prof SN Chugh.

Q. What is spondylolisthesis?

Ans. It is anterior slippage of vertebral body, pedicles and superior articular facet leaving behind the posterior element: A 'Step' may be present on deep palpation of posterior elements of the segment above the spondylolisthetic joint.

Spondylolithesis is associated with degenerative spine disease and spondylosis and occurs more frequently in women. It can be asymptomatic. Symptomatic disease produces back pain, root pain and sometimes cauda equina syndrome.

Q. What is spina bifida occulta?

Ans. It is a failure of closure of one or several vertebral arches posteriorly. The meninges and spinal cord are normal. A dimple or a tuff of hair or lipoma may overlie the defect. Most cases are asymptomaitc and discovered incidently on X-rays spines during evaluation of back pain.

Q. What is tethered cord syndrome?

Ans. It presents either as progressive cauda equina syndrome or as myelopathy (cord lesion) or both. The patient is usually young adult who complains of perineal or perianal pain, sometimes following minor trauma. Neuroimaging studies reveal a low lying conus (below L1-L2) and a short and thickened filum terminale.

Q. How would you investigate a patient with cauda equina syndrome?

Ans. 1. *Routine laboratory investigations,* e.g. complete blood count, ESR, biochemistry profile and urinalysis.
 2. *Plain X-ray films* of lumbosacral regions.
 3. *CT myelography* and *MRI* are the radiological tests of choice for evaluation of cauda equina syndrome.
 4. *EMG* and *nerve conduction velocities.* They are usually of uncertain values.

Q. What is the treatment of cauda equina syndrome?

Ans. 1. To relieve pain, NSAIDs and paracetamol are effective. Opiates analgesic are not better than NSAIDs, but can be used for short-term if patient is unresponsive to NSAIDs.
 2. Exercise program: The early resumption of normal physical activity is beneficial, Person should avoid maneuvers which produce stress e.g. bending, weight lifting, etc.
 3. Traction can be employed during acute back pain but is not much effective.
 4. Facet joint, trigger point and ligamentous injections are not recommended.
 5. Proof is lacking regarding the benefit of accupuncture, transcutaneous electrical nerve stimulation, massage, ultrasound, diathermy, or electrical stimulation. Similarly use of ice or heat is not beneficial to relieve pain.
 6. Therapeutic nerve root blocks with corticosteroids and local anesthesia is an optimal therapy when conservative measures to relieve acute pain fail.
 7. Similarly a short course of spinal manipulation or physiotherapy for symptomatic relief in uncomplicated cases is an option.
 8. Find out the cause and treat it accordingly.

Figs 1.38A and B: Peripheral neuropathy. **A.** A patient with bilateral foot drop due to peripheral neuropathy.
B. Glove-stocking type of anesthesia (diagram).

The patient (Fig. 1.38A) presented with following complaints:
1. Sensations of pins and needles (tingling and numbness) in the distal parts of all the four limbs
2. Weakness of all the limbs especially distal parts
3. Thinning of legs.

Clinical Presentations

- These patients may present with acute onset of areflexic paralysis of all the four limbs called post-infective polyneuritis (Guillain-Barré syndrome)
- Chronic cases of peripheral neuropathy present with paresthesias (tingling and numbness) of hands and feet with weakness and thinning of legs with or without wrist or foot drop.

History

Points to be Noted

- Note the duration and onset of symptoms
- Initiation and distribution of sensory disturbance (i.e. glove-stocking anesthesia)
- Evolution of weakness (proximal or distal). Was there any difficulty in holding the things?
- Progression of symptoms, e.g. stationary, progressive, recovering or waxing and waning
- Is there any history of weakness of respiratory muscles or facial muscles. Difficulty in coughing or breathing?
- History of taking drugs (e.g. INH)
- Any precipitating factor or illness
- Bowel and bladder disturbance.

Past History

Ask for:

- Alcoholism
- Headache, vomiting, convulsions
- Diplopia, dysphagia, nasal regurgitation
- Past history of spinal trauma
- History of fever, contact with a patient of tuberculosis, exposure to STD, vaccination
- History of systemic illness, i.e. diabetes, renal failure, chronic liver disease, diarrhea or malabsorption, etc.
- History of exposure to solvents, pesticides or heavy metals.

Family History

- History of similar illness in other family members.

General Physical Examination

- Consciousness and behavior
- Look for anemia, jaundice, edema
- Look for signs of vitamin deficiencies i.e. tongue, eyes, mucous membranes
- Look for alcoholic stigmata, e.g. gynaecomastia, testicular atrophy, muscle wasting, parotid enlargement, palmar erythema or flushing of face. Look at the skin for hypopigmented or hyperpigmented patches, scar or burn mark
- Record pulse, BP and temperature.

Systemic Examination
(Read CNS Examination)

- Higher functions
- Cranial nerves
- Neck rigidity.

Motor Function

- Look the posture (usually decubitus) and foot drop
- Note the nutrition, tone, power and coordination of the muscles
- Elicit the tendon jerks. Bilateral ankle jerks are usually absent.

Sensory System

- Test superficial and deep sensations including cortical sensations. They are lost in the peripheral parts
- Palpate the various long nerves (ulnar, radial, common peroneal). They may be palpable in diabetes, leprosy, hereditary polyneuropathy

Other System Examination

1. CVS for sounds, bruits and murmurs
2. Respiratory system for evidence of tuberculosis, sarcoidosis, malignancy
3. GI tract for hepatosplenomegaly
4. Lymphoreticular system for lymph node enlargement.

185

Q. What is your probable diagnosis and why?

Ans. Sir, my provisional diagnosis is peripheral neuropathy, distal and symmetric. The points in favor of my diagnosis are:

- History of pins and needles in distal parts of all limbs
- Loss of all types of sensations, i.e. superficial and deep (spinothalamic and posterior column) in peripheral parts of all the four limbs.
- Weakness of distal parts of all four limbs with hypotonia, loss of deep tendon jerks and superficial reflexes (plantar response) in the peripheral parts of all limbs.
- Presence of bilateral foot drop.
- Presence of trophic changes.

Q. What is differential diagnosis of polyneuropathy?

Ans. The differential diagnosis lies between its various causes. The characteristics of some common causes of neuropathies are discussed here.

1. **Guillain-Barré Syndrome.** The characteristic features are:
   - It is an acute, frequently severe and fulminant polyradiculopathy of autoimmune origin
   - Peak incidence between 20-50 years
   - It manifests as rapidly evolving areflexic (LMN type) motor paralysis with or without sensory disturbance
   - It usually starts from the lower extremities followed by upper extremities or all the four limbs may be involved simultaneously (uncommon). The legs are more affected than arms
   - The lower cranial nerves are also frequently involved, causing bulbar weakness. The VII cranial nerve is frequently involved producing LMN type of paralysis. Bilateral involvement is common though it can occur unilaterally
   - Deep tendon reflexes are diminished in the limbs
   - Bowel and bladder are rarely involved
   - Plantars are either flexor or not elicitable
   - Sensorium is clear throughout the illness
   - The usual variant is *Miller-Fischer syndrome* which comprises of a triad of ophthalmoplegia, ataxia and areflexia.

   The diagnostic criteria are listed in Table 1.128.

Table 1.128: Diagnostic criteria for Guillain-Barré syndrome

Essential	Supportive
• Progressive weakness of 2 or more limbs due to neuropathy • Areflexia (loss of reflexes) • Disease course <4 weeks • Exclusion of other causes of LMN type of paraplegia or quadriplegia	• Relative symmetric weakness • Mild sensory involvement • Facial and other cranial nerve involvement • Absence of fever • Typical CSF changes (acellularity, rise in protein) • Electrophysiologic evidence of demyelination

2. **Diabetic peripheral neuropathy**
   - History of diabetes, i.e. type 1 (polyuria, polydipsia or polyphagia) or type 2 (impaired wound healing, infections, etc.)
   - History of intake of either insulin or OHA
   - Duration of diabetes is longer
   - A triad of retinopathy, neuropathy and nephropathy may occur but these complications can occur individually also
   - History of susceptibility to infection, weakness, impaired wound healing
   - The various types of neuropathy in diabetes have already been described.

3. **Leprosy**
   - Typical 'Leonine' facies
   - Typical hypopigmented and anesthetic skin lesions
   - Palpable peripheral nerves with peripheral neuropathy
   - Trophic changes

4. **Diphtheric neuropathy**
   - Common in children, but now rarely observed due to effective immunization against diphtheria
   - Palatal weakness followed by pupillary paralysis and sensorimotor neuropathy
   - Cranial nerves 3rd, 6th, 7th, 9th and 10th may be involved
   - The condition develops 2-6 weeks after the onset of disease
   - Myocarditis may occur in two-thirds of patients with diphtheria. It manifests on ECG as arrhythmias, conduction blocks, ST-T changes and CHF.

5. **Prophyric neuropathy**
   - Acute intermittent porphyria produces attacks of paroxysmal neuropathy simulating G.B. syndrome
   - This is associated with abdominal colic, confusion, autonomic disturbances and later coma
   - Alcohol and barbiturates precipitate the attacks.

6. **Arsenical neuropathy**
   - Rain-drop skin lesions with hyperkeratosis of palms and soles
   - People of known geographical area using deep tube-well water are mainly affected
   - Mee's line (white transverse ridges on nails) are diagnostic
   - Presence of anemia with or without jaundice (hepatic involvement)
   - Diagnosis is confirmed by estimation of arsenic in skin, nails, hair and urine.

7. **Neuropathies with HIV infection**
   - Distal, symmetric, mainly sensory polyneuropathy which evolves slowly in symptomatic HIV disease, is associated with encephalopathy and myelopathy
   - GB syndrome or chronic inflammatory demyelinating polyneuropathy (CIDP) may occur following conversion to seropositivity and during the asymptomatic phase of the disease.

8. **Neoplastic neuropathy.** Polyneuropathy is sometimes seen as a non-metastatic manifestation of a malignancy (paraneoplastic syndrome) which may be motor or sensorimotor.

   In multiple myeloma and other dysproteinemias, the polyneuropathy occurs due to demyelination associated with allergic reaction within peripheral nerves. The POEMS syndrome is an example of polyneuropathy in multiple myeloma in which,

   P stands for chronic inflammatory demyelinating polyneuropathy
   O stands for organomegaly (hepatomegaly)
   E stands for endocrinopathy (gynaecomastia and atrophic testes)
   M stands for M band on electrophoresis
   S stands for skin pigmentation.

9. **Hereditary neuropathy (Charcot-Marie-Tooth disease)**
   - An autosomal dominant/recessive/X-linked transmission. It occurs in first and second decades of life.
   - Sensorimotor neuropathy characterised by distal muscle weakness and atrophy, impaired sensations, absent or hypoactive deep tendon reflexes
   - Pattern of involvement is feet and legs followed by hands and forearm
   - High-steppage gait with frequent falling due to bilateral foot drop
   - Foot deformity (pes cavus, high arch feet) and hand deformity due to atrophy of intrinsic muscles of the hands.

10. **Chronic inflammatory demyelinating polyneuropathy (CIDP)**
    - It is a chronic GB syndrome, affects young adults
    - Onset is gradual, sometimes subacute, and the initial episode is indistinguishable from that of GB syndrome
    - It is a sensorimotor neuropathy with predominant motor findings, but a small number of patients may present with pure syndrome of sensory ataxia
    - Some patients experience a chronic progressive course, whereas, others have a relapsing and remitting course
    - Some patients may have cranial nerve involvement including external ophthalmoplegia.

    The diagnosis is confirmed on typical CSF findings and electrophysiological studies which show findings similar to GB syndrome.

11. **Triorthocresylphosphate (TOCP) neuropathy**
    It is called *'ginger paralysis'* owing to consumption of fluid extract of ginger which was used in the manufacture of bootleg alcohol and was adulterated with TOCP. It is pure motor neuropathy characterized by bilateral foot and hand drop. It occurs 10-20 days after consumption of adulterated food (cooking - oil) or drink.

Q. **What is clinical presentations of peripheral neuropathy?**

Ans. Clinical presentations are:
   - Distal paresthesias (pins and needles sensation) is the presenting symptom usually first affecting the feet and then the hands and subsequently progressing upwards but stopping short below the knees and elbows.
   - Loss of all types of sensations in a glove-stocking distribution (Fig. 1.38B). Patient may be unaware of injury or burn marks on the hands in smokers and on the feet in labourers.

- Distal weakness of all the four limbs leading to bilateral foot drop and/or bilateral wrist drop.
- There may be autonomic disturbances in peripheral parts, i.e. postural edema, cold extremities, etc.

Q. Could your case be of Guillain-Barre syndrome?

Ans. Yes. The points in favor are:
- Short duration and acute onset of symptoms.
- Progressive weakness
- Areflexia with bilateral footdrop
- Peripheral neuropathy
- Bowel and bladder not involved

Q. How would you confirm the diagnosis of Guillain-Barre syndrome?

Ans.
- CSF examination for rise of proteins and albuminocytological dissociation
- Immunoelectrophoresis of CSF proteins for rise in immunoglobulin
- Nerve conduction velocities of peripheral nerve
- Sural nerve biopsy and histopathology.

Q. What is the tone of muscles in your case?

Ans. There is hypotonia of all peripheral muscles (feet and hands) otherwise tone is preserved in other muscles. Bilateral footdrop in my case is an example of hypotonia.

Q. Name the terms used in relation to neuropathy?

Ans. Terminology Used in Relation to Neuropathy

Neuropathy means a pathological process affecting a peripheral nerve or nerves.

Mononeuropathy refers to a process affecting a single nerve (radial, ulnar, median, etc).

Multiple mononeuropathy (mononeuritis multiplex) refers to a process involving several or multiple long nerves.

Polyneuropathy or peripheral neuropathy refers to a diffuse symmetrical disease process involving the peripheral parts and progressing proximally.

Radiculopathy means a disease process affecting the nerve roots (motor or sensory).

Q. What are the causes of peripheral neuropathy?

Ans. There are numerous causes of peripheral neuropathy, out of which some are common such as diabetes, toxins (alcohol or drug induced), Guillain-Barre syndrome, leprosy and chronic renal failure (Table 1.129).

Q. What are the causes of acute onset peripheral neuropathy?

Ans. Causes are:
- GB syndrome
- Diabetes mellitus
- Drugs (TOCP, Arsenic)
- Diphtheria
- Porphyria
- Paraneoplastic syndrome

Table 1.129: Etiology of peripheral neuropathy

Cause	Common conditions	Uncommon conditions
Metabolic/ endocrinal	• Diabetes • Chronic renal failure • Amyloidosis • Hypothyroidism • Liver cell failure *Toxic Neuropathy* Alcohol induced	• Multiple myeloma • Cryoglobulinemia • Porphyria Drug induced (e.g. INH, vincristine, phenytoin, NFT) Heavy metals (Pb, As, Hg) and organic solvents (TOCP)
Inflammatory or infective	Guillain-Barre syndrome	Chronic inflammatory demyelinating polyneuropathy, connective tissue diseases, e.g. SLE, PAN, Sjögren's syndrome and infective (leprosy diphtheria, typhoid fever, HIV)
Hereditary/ Genetic	Genetic Deficiency states	Hereditary motor and sensory neuropathies (Charcot Marie-Tooth) • Vit. B_1 deficiency • Vit. B_{12} deficiency • Others
Others	Pyridoxine deficiency —	Malignant disease (paraneoplastic neuropathy) Critical illness neuropathy

Q. What are the causes of predominant motor neuropathy?

Ans. Causes are:
- GB syndrome (70%) and CIDP (Chronic inflammatory demyelinating polyradiculoneuropathy)
- Porphyria
- Connective tissue diseases, e.g. SLE, PAN
- Hereditary polyneuropathy
- Acute motor axonal neuropathy
- Delayed neurotoxicity due to organophosphates (TOCP, TCP)
- Diphtheria
- Lead intoxication
- Hypoglycemia
- High doses of dapsone.

Q. What are the causes of predominant sensory neuropathy?

Ans. Causes are:
- Hereditary sensory neuropathy
- Paraneoplastic syndrome
- Leprosy
- HIV
- Sjögren's syndrome
- Dysproteinemia
- Vitamin B_1 and B_{12} deficiency

- Thalidomide toxicity
- Pentamidine sensory neuropathy
- Cisplatin (antineoplastic)
- Chronic renal failure
- Alcoholic Poly-neuropathy

Q. What are the causes of recurrent neuropathy?

Ans. These patients may have several attacks of neuropathy. The common causes are:
- Porphyria
- Chronic inflammatory demyelinating polyneuro-pathy (CIDP)
- Alcoholic neuropathy
- Occupational toxic neuropathy.

Q. What are the causes of peripheral neuropathies with predominant autonomic neuropathy?

Ans. Most varieties of polyneuropathy affect autonomic functions to a mild extent, but certain neuropathies may have predominant autonomic dysfunction. The causes are:
- Diabetes mellitus
- Porphyria
- Alcoholism
- Leprosy
- Amyloidosis
- GB syndrome

Q. What are the causes of palpable thickened peripheral nerves?

Ans.
- Amyloidois
- Guillain - Barre syndrome
- Leprosy
- Charcot - Marie Tooth disease
- Refsum syndrome (retinitis pigmentosa, deafness and cerebellar degeneration)
- Dejerine-Sottas disease (hypertrophic peripheral neuropathy)
- Diabetes.

Q. How do you classify neuropathy in diabetes mellitus?

Ans. Neuropathy is a microvascular complication of diabetes, occur commonly in type 2 than in type I diabetes. It may be symmetric or asymmetric, motor, sensory or mixed. Read case discussion on diabetes.

Q. What do you know about diabetic amyotrophy?

Ans. It is asymmetrical motor polyneuropathy characterized by asymmetric weakness and wasting of the proximal muscles of the lower limbs and sometime upper limbs, diminished or absent knee jerk and sensory loss in the thigh. It is usually accompanied by severe pain in the thigh, often awakening the patient at night. Patient usually recovers, hence, prognosis is good.

Q. How do you diagnose peripheral neuropathy?

Ans. The diagnosis of peripheral neuropathy is based on the peripheral signs which are:
1. *Sensory loss of all modalities* in glove-stocking fashion in both upper and lower limbs, i.e.
   - Loss of sensations carried by spinothalamic tract, e.g. pain, temperature, crude touch
   - Loss of sensations carried by posterior column, e.g. vibration sense, joint position sense, deep pressure and fine touch.
2. *Loss of motor functions, i.e.*
   - Wasting of small muscles of hands and feet
   - Loss of deep peripheral jerks in lower limbs, e.g. ankle
   - Loss of deep peripheral jerks in upper limb, e.g. supinator and finger flexion
   - Bilateral wrist or footdrop.
3. *Autonomic dysfunction* (read features of autonomic neuropathy p. 125)
4. **Confirmation of diagnosis** is made by nerve conduction studies. Nerve conduction studies can distinguish demyelinating neuropathy from axonal neuropathy.
   - In *demyelinating neuropathy*, there is slowing of conduction velocity, dispersion of evoked compound action potentials, conduction block and marked prolongation of distal latencies.
   - In contrast *in axonal type*, there is reduction in amplitude of evoked compound action potentials with preservation of nerve conduction velocity.

Q. What are various symptoms of axonal and demyelinating neuropathies? What are their causes?

Ans. The distinction between axonal and demyelinating polyneuropathy is mainly based on the electro-physiological studies. Both axonal and demyelinating neuropathies present in a similar manner, can be acute, subacute and chronic. The causes are given in Table 1.130.

Table 1.130: Major types of neuropathy (axonal vs demyelinating)

Type	Axonal	Demyelinating
Acute	Porphyria, toxic (As) GB syndrome	All forms of GB syndrome
Subacute	Toxic/metabolic	Relapsing form of CIDP
Chronic	Toxic or metabolic Hereditary Diabetic Dysproteinemia	Hereditary Inflammatory Autoimmune Dysproteinemia Toxic/metabolic

Q. What are the characteristic features of alcoholic neuropathy?

Ans.
- It is nutritional neuropathy due to deficiency of B_1, B_6 and B_{12} induced by alcohol

- It is predominantly sensory neuropathy
- Other stigmatas of alcoholism may be present
- Features of other alcohol-induced conditions e.g. hepatomegaly, cardiomyopathy.

Q. What are other effects of alcohol on CNS?

Ans. 1. Wernicke's encephalopathy (ophthalmoplegia, nystagmus, confusion and neuropathy)
2. Korsakoff psychosis (recent memory loss and confabulation)
3. Cerebellar degeneration.
4. Marchiafava- Bignami disease
5. Central pontine myelinosis
6. Amblyopia
7. Epilepsy
8. Myopathy and rhabdomyolysis.

Q. What are the causes of footdrop?

Ans. Paralysis of extensors of foot and peronei muscles produces footdrop. The common causes are:
- Peripheral neuropathy (bilateral footdrop)
- Common peroneal nerve palsy (unilateral foot-drop)
- PIVD (lesion involving L5) produces unilateral or bilateral footdrop
- Motor neuron disease (bilateral footdrop)
- Sciatic nerve lesion (unilateral footdrop)
- Peroneal muscle atrophy (bilateral footdrop)

Q. What are the causes of wristdrop?

Ans. Paralysis of the extensors of wrist produces wrist-drop. The patient is not able to extend the wrist and fingers when asked to do so. In an attempted extension of fingers, there will be flexion of metacarpophalangeal joints and extension of the interphalangeal joints due to unopposed action of lumbricals and interossei.

Causes
- Radial nerve palsy
- Lead neuropathy
- Other peripheral neuropathies.

Q. What are the characteristics of root (radicular) lesion?

Ans. Following are the characteristics:
- Lesion of the anterior (motor) root(s) produces weakness and atrophy of the muscles innervated by these roots.
- Irritative lesion of posterior (sensory) root produces root pain (increases with coughing), hyperalgesia (calf tender on squeezing) or hyperesthesia related to the segment irritated.

In compressive lesion (radiculopathy), there is segmental sensory loss such as in PIVD or cauda equina syndrome (saddle-shape anesthesia).

Q. What is entrapment neuropathy? What are common entrapment neuropathies?

Ans. Entrapment means traping of the nerve in a tight anatomical compartment leading to compression of the nerve. The common entrapment neuropathies are:
1. Meralgia paresthetica (lateral cutaneous nerve trapped)
2. Carpal tunnel syndrome (median nerve trapped)
3. Tarsal tunnel syndrome (posterior tibial nerve trapped)
4. Common peroneal nerve entrapment at head of fibula
5. Elbow tunnel syndrome (ulnar nerve trapped).

Q. What is mononeuritis? What are characteristics of various mononeuropathies?

Ans. Involvement of a single nerve (mononeuritis) is either acute (compression) or chronic (entrapment). In both, the demyelination predominates, but some axonal degeneration also occurs.

Acute compression usually affects nerves which are superficially placed at some points/regions (e.g. the common peroneal nerve at the head of fibula). Entrapment occurs when a nerve passes through a relatively narrow or tight anatomical compartment (e.g. carpal tunnel). These conditions are diagnosed by clinical features and confirmation is done by conduction studies and EMG.

The symptoms and signs of various mono-neuropathies are given in Table 1.131.

Q. What are the causes of carpal tunnel syndrome (median nerve compression)?

Ans. These are:
- Hypothyroidism or myxedema
- Diabetes mellitus
- Pregnancy, oral contraceptives
- Obesity
- Acromegaly
- Rheumatoid arthritis
- Idiopathic
- Chronic renal failure
- Amyloidosis.

Q. What are features of carpal tunnel syndrome?

Ans. Read Table 1.131

Table 1.131: Symptoms and signs of mononeuropathies

Nerve	Symptoms	Muscle weakness	Sensory loss
1. Upper extremities			
Median (carpal tunnel syndrome)	Nocturnal pain and tingling sensations on the palm and fingers waking the patient from sleep. Pain may extend to arm and shoulder	Abductor pollicis brevis	Lateral palm and thumb, index, middle and half ring finger (radial three and half fingers)
Ulnar	Tingling on medial (ulnar) border of hand; wasting and weakness of hand muscles	All hand muscles except abductor pollicis brevis	Medial palm and little and half ring finger (one and half medial fingers)
Radial	Wrist drop, weakness of fingers extension and hand supination	Wrist and finger's extensors, and supinator	Dorsum of the thumb
2. Lower extremities			
Common peroneal	Footdrop	Dorsiflexers and everter of foot	Nil or dorsum of foot
Lateral cutaneous (Meralgia paresthetica)	Tingling and paresthesia on lateral aspect of thigh	Nil	Lateral border of thigh
Femoral (L2-L4) (diabetic amyotrophy)	Hip flexion and knee extension difficult	Anterior thigh muscles and loss of knee jerk	Front of thigh and lateral aspect on the back of thigh
Sciatic (L4-S3)	Severe leg weakness below knee, flail foot and severe disability	Hamstring muscles, hip abductor and all muscles below knee	—
Posterior tibial (tarsal tunnel syndrome)	Pain and numbness of sole, weak toe flexors	Calf muscles, toe flexors and intrinsic foot muscles	—

Q. **What is meralgia paresthetica?**

Ans. It is involvement of lateral cutaneous nerve of thigh (Read Table 1.131).

Q. **What do you understand by the term mono-neuritis multiplex (multiple mononeuropathy)?**

Ans. Mononeuritis multiplex refers to simultaneous or sequential involvement of individual non-contiguous nerve trunks either partially or completely evolving over days to years. Usually there is ischemia of long nerves due to vasculitis involving vasa nervosa which renders the nerves prone to mechanical compression. The causes are:
- Diabetes mellitus
- Leprosy
- Collagen vascular disorders, rheumatoid arthritis
- Sarcoidosis
- Amyloidosis
- Malignancy
- Neurofibromatosis
- AIDS
- Hypereosinophilic syndrome
- Cryoglobulinemia
- Wegener's granulomatosis.

Q. **Which drugs are effective for painful neuropathy in diabetes?**

Ans. • Tricyclic antidepressants

- Antiepileptics, e.g. phenytoin, carbamazepine, valproate, gabapentine/pregabalin
- Topical capsaicin.

Q. **What are the causes of brachial plexus lesions? What are the characteristic features of these lesions?**

Ans. Trauma or injury (stab or gun shot) is the commonest cause of damage to the brachial plexus. The injury commonly occurs during forced separation of head and shoulder, during a fall, or following excessive abduction of the arm. Other causes include invasion of the plexus by neoplasia involving cervical lymph nodes or pulmonary apex (Pancoast's tumor), compression of the thoracic outlet (cervical rib or a fibrous band) and damage due to radiation to the axillary area. One or more spinal nerves may be involved by lesion of the cervical spine such as Klippel-Feil syndrome, fusion of vertebrae, fracture dislocation, prolapsed intervertebral disc, caries spine or malignant deposits. The plexus may be damaged by stabs or gun-shot wounds, by fracture of clavicle and by dislocation of upper end of the humerus. The clinical signs of brachial plexus lesions are given in Table 1.132.

Q. **What is neuronopathy? What are its causes.**

Ans. Involvement of anterior horn cell producing motor paralysis is called *neuronopathy*. It is characterized by

Table 1.132: Physical signs in brachial plexus lesions

Location	Root(s) affected	Weakness of muscles	Sensory loss
1. *Upper plexus (Erb's paralysis)*	C_5 (C_6)	Biceps, deltoid, spinati, rhomboids, brachioradialis, triceps, serratus anterior. Biceps and supinator jerks are lost	Small area over deltoid

Causes. Indirect violence resulting in the nerve being torn by undue separation of head and shoulder, such as birth injury. In adults, it may occur during fall from a motor cycle on one side. Occasionally, it occurs following general anesthesia in patients in whom, during the operation the arm has been held abducted and externally rotated.

2. *Lower plexus (Dejerine-Klumpke paralysis)*	T_1 (C_8)	All small muscles of hand, claw hand (ulnar/wrist flexors)	Ulnar border of hand/forearm

Causes: Birth injury or may be produced by a fall during which patient tries to save himself by clutching something with the hand

3. *Thoracic outlet syndrome (cervical rib or a fibrous band)*	C_8/T_1	Small muscles of hands, ulnar/ forearm muscles	Ulnar border of hand/forearm (upper arm)

weakness, muscle denervation atrophy, areflexia and fasciculations. It is difficult to distinguish between neuropathy and neuronopathy because both share same clinical features. Electrophysiological study may help in their differentiation.

Causes

1. Motor neuron disease
2. Poliomyelitis
3. Hereditary spinal muscle atrophies
4. Adult variant of hexosaminidase A deficiency.

Respiratory Diseases

CASE 39: DEEP VEIN THROMBOSIS—SWOLLEN LEGS

Examine the Lower Limbs

The patient developed swelling of the right leg following delivery (Fig 1.39).

History

Points to be Asked

- Onset: acute or chronic
- History of pain, fever
- History of drugs, e.g. oral contraceptives
- Recent history of delivery, surgery, CVA, MI
- History of trauma, insect bite
- Past history of diabetes, hypertension, DVT
- Past and family history of DVT and pulmonary embolism

Examination

Inspection

- Right leg is swollen along with right foot.
- Skin is shining

Fig.1.39: Deep vein thrombosis of right leg in a postvertebral female

- Superficial veins are engorged but they are not varicose.
- No ulcer, No tropic changes, no sign of injury or infection, gangrene

Palpation

- Temperature over the skin is normal
- Calf is tender
- Edema is pitting
- Homan's sign is positive (there is pain in the calf on dorsiflexion of the foot)
- Femoral and popliteal pulses are normal on right side. Dorsalis pedis and posterior tibial pulses could not be palpated due to edema
- Knee and ankle jerks could not be elicited due to pain.

Note: Always tell the examination of involved limb in comparison to non-involved limb. Expose both the limbs.

Systemic Examination

- Examine the cardiovascular system for MI or signs of CHF
- Examine respiratory system for consolidation/collapse, wheezes, rales for pulmonary embolism (acute cor pulmonale), chronic cor pulmonale
- Examine nervous system for CVA

Advice

When you are to examine the legs/lower limb, please do not jump to see the limb. Sit calmly and quietly and recollect what you have to examine. Ask appropriate questions on the history and examine the limb systematically.

Q. What is your probable diagnosis?
Ans. Sir, my provisional diagnosis on history and examination of lower limbs is swollen right leg and foot due to deep vein thrombosis

Q. Why do you say deep vein thrombosis?
Ans. • A female patient
- Recent history of delivery (predishosing factor)
- Red, swollen leg with prominent superficial veins
- Pitting edema over the feet and above the ankle
- Positive Homan's sign

Q. How do you perform Hofman's sign? What is its significance?

193

Ans. Read the clinical methods in medicine by Prof S N Chugh. This sign is nowadays not elicited because there is risk of dislodging the thrombus in the vein.

Q. What are the causes of unilateral swelling of leg?

Ans. • Superficial thrombophlebitis following trauma, injection or infection/inflammation, malignancy
- Deep cellulitis
- Deep vein thrombosis
- Elephantiasis/lymphangitis/lymphedema
- Coagulation disorder (Hemophilia)
- Venous compression due to enlarged inguinal lymph node.

Q. What are the causes of non-pitting edema?

Ans. • Lymphedema due to any cause
- Elephantiasis due to microfilaria
- Myxoedema

Q. What are the predisposing factor for DVT?

Ans • *Prolonged immobilization* following surgery, fracture, stroke, paraplegia
- *Following CVA* (about 50% develop DVT) and myocardial infarction (30% patients develop DVT)
- *Obesity*
- *Internal malignancy* (pancreas, stomach, lung, etc)
- *Drugs*, e.g oral contraceptive
- *Older age.*
- *Pregnancy, puerperium, postmenopausal hormone replacement therapy*
- *Previous DVT*
- *Tissue trauma*
- *Hypercoagualable states*
    - Antithrombin C deficiency
    - Protein C and S deficiency, thrombophilia
    - Antiphospholipid syndrome, SLE, Hypertension
    - Excessive plasminogen activator inhibitor
    - Polycythemia vera.
    - Secondary polycythemia due to hypoxia
    - Erythrocytosis
- *Disease of the vein*, e.g. varicose vein
- *Use of chronic indwelling central venous catheters, insertion of permanent pacemakers and internal cardiac defibrillator* are the common cause of DVT of upper extremity.

Q. What are the complications of DVT?

Ans. • Pulmonary embolism
- Venous ulceration
- Venous gangrene
- Extension of the thrombosis to ileofemoral vein

Q. How would you confirm your diagnosis?

Ans. For confirmation of the diagnosis and to assess the extent of thrombosis, following investigations are done;

1. Duplex ultrasonography scanning.
2. Color Doppler studies
3. Venography
4. Coagulation studies

Q. When would you suspect pulmonary embolism in DVT?

Ans. Dyspnea, syncope, hypotension or cyanosis of acute onset in a patient with DVT suggests PE. Cough, hemoptysis and pleuritic rub suggest small distal thrombi near the pleura. However, Well's diagnostic scoring system is used for suspected PE (Table 1.133)

Table 1.133: Well's diagnostic scoring system for suspected PE

Features	Points
• Clinical symptoms and signs of DVT (Pain on deep palpation and leg swelling)	3
• An alternative diagnosis is less likely than PE	3
• HR> 100/min	1.5
• Immobilization or surgery in previous 4 weeks	1.5
• Hemoptysis	1
• Malignancy (on treatment, treated in past 6 months or palliative)	1

The Well's scoring system has a maximum of 12.5 points. If the score is ≤ 4 points, the likelihood of PE is only 8%.

Q. What is the incidence of pulmonary embolism in DVT?

Ans. About half of the patients with pelvic vein thrombosis or proximal leg vein thrombosis (DVT) have pulmonary thromboembolism. However, nowadays, DVT of upper extremity due to increased use of indwelling central venous catheter, pacemaker insertion and **internal cardiac defibrilator** insertion (ICD) also become an important cause of PE.

Q. What are the causes of recurrent venous thrombosis?

Ans • Pregnancy, oral contraceptives
- Surgery, trauma
- Anti-thrombin III, protein C, protein S or factor V
- Anti-phospholipid syndrome
- Occult malignancy, myeloproliferative disorders
- Vasculitides
- Potential abnormalities such as thrombomodulin, tissue factor pathway inhibitors, vitronectin associated with heparin and antithrobin III and fibrinolytic receptors.

Q. What do you know about antiphospholipid syndrome?

Ans. This question has been answered in case discussion SLE. All questions regarding antiphospholipid syndrome have been answered there.

Bedside Medicine

194

Q. How would you prevent DVT?

Ans. 1. Subcutaneous low dose heparin or low molecular weight heparin (LMWH) should be given to patients:
   - who are undergoing surgery on the leg, pelvis, or prostatectomy
   - with myocardial infarction
   - with cardiac failure.
2. Warfarin in a dose that yields INR of 2.0 to 3.0 is effective in preventing DVT associated with bone fracture and orthopedic surgery
3. External pneumatic compression devices applied to legs to prevent DVT in patients where heparin or warfarin might cause serious bleeding.
4. Early mobilization within 72 hr after surgery
5. Encourage exercise in patients following surgery or in patients who are bed ridden due to illness or patients with CHF or MI
6. Elastic supports/stockings to patients with history of thrombosis or obesity.

Q. How would you treat such a case?

Ans. • *Pain relief with analgesics*
- *Control of edema by:*
  - Intermittent elevation of foot above the level of heart during night with pillows.
  - Avoid long periods of standing
  - Elastic stockings from mid-foot to just below the knee, worn during the day
- *To prevent thromboembolism and to restore venous patency*
  - Aspirin 150 mg daily
  - Anticoagulation with unfractionated heparin or low molecular heparin
  - Recent data suggest that synthetic penta-saccharide with antithrombotic effects may be superior to LMWH in prevention of DVT
  - Warfarin therapy with the aim of maintaining the international normalized ratio (INR) at 2-3 is recommended for treatment of venous thromboembolic disease, Remember, anti-coagulation does not affect thrombosis that is already formed but prevents extension of thrombosis
- *Duration of therapy should be;*
  a. For 3-6 months with first episode
  b. About 6 weeks to 3 months in postoperative cases with any risk factor
  c. 6-12 months in patients with persistent risk factors and recurrent venous thromboembolic events.
  d. Life-long only rarely if recurrent thrombo-embolic episodes.
- *Inferior vena caval filters* may be required when there is a higher risk of pulmonary embolism.

Q. What are clinical clues to development of acute cor pulmonale?

Ans. The sudden development of pulmonary hypertension in a patient with DVT who develops progressive dyspnea, fatigue, syncope, cough and hemoptysis with chest pain indicates the development to acute cor pulmonale. The classical signs to be observed for acute cor pulmonale are:
1. Raised JVP with prominent 'a' wave.
2. A reduced carotid pulse
3. Parasternal lift
4. A loud S2 with narrow split. There may be a S4
5. Tricuspid regurgitation, i.e. a pansystolic murmur that increases with inspiration, is heard over the right parasternal area. There is V and Y collapse in JVP. Liver may or may not be pulsatile.
6. Signs of RV failure, e.g. raised JVP, hepatomegaly, cyanosis and peripheral pitting edema

Q. How would you investigate for acute thrombo-embolism?

Ans. 1. *Chest X-ray:* There may be enlarged central pulmonary arteries. The lungs are oligemic.
2. *ECG:* Shows right axis deviation, RVH. Sometime there may be S1, QIII, TIII syndrome.
3. *Echocardiogram:* Demonstrates RV and RA enlargements, reduction in left ventricular cavity size and a tricuspid regurgitation on colour doppler study.
4. *Pulmonary function tests:* Show hypoxemia and abnormal diffusing capacity for CO due to pulmonary hypertension.
5. A *perfusion scan:* Is always abnormal, shows perfusion defect. A lung perfusion and ventilation scan is helpful in diagnosis.
6. *D-dimers:* D-dimers in blood are highly suggestive of PE.
7. *CT, MRI angiography:* It is confirmatory.

Endocrinal Diseases

CASE 40: CUSHING'S SYNDROME

The male patient (Fig. 1.40) presented with puffiness of face, headache and weight gain. Examination revealed moon face (plethoric face), hypertension, and edema. There were truncal obesity and abdominal striae. His left lower limb was in plaster (visible) due to fracture.

EXAMINE THE PATIENT

How would you proceed?

History

Points to be Noted

- Onset of symptoms
- H/o steroid therapy
- Weight gain
- Excessive hair growth (hirsutism)
- Acne over face
- H/o easy bruisability
- Weakness of proximal muscles, difficulty in climbing stairs.
- Loss of libido, menstrual irregularity
- Depression, sleep disturbances

Fig. 1.40: Cushing's syndrome

- Back pain, H/o trauma
- There is history of fracture and left limb is in plaster in this patient.

Examination

- Patient face is moon shaped
- Buffalo hump at the back present
- Central obesity present
- Pink striae over abdomen present
- Redistribution of fat, more in the centre than periphery
- Weakness of shoulder and hip girdle muscles (proximal myopathy) present
- There is fracture of left lower limb which is in plaster. Look for kyphoscoliosis, vertebral collapse.
- BP is normal.
- There is no evidence of asthma, rheumatoid arthritis, SLE, nephrotic syndrome

Q. What is your diagnosis? What are the causes of moon face?

Ans. The symptoms and signs suggest the diagnosis of Cushing's syndrome in the patient in picture which could be iatrogenic (steroid-induced) or due to disease (excess secretion of corticosteroids).

Points in favor of diagnosis

- Moon face
- Acne
- Pink/purple striae over the abdomen
- Truncal obesity
- Fracture of left leg due to osteoporosis
- Weakness of proximal groups of muscles.

Q. What is differential diagnosis Cushing's syndrome?

Ans. All the conditions that produce pseudocushing syndrome come in the differential diagnosis.

1. *Obesity*

   Extreme obesity is uncommon in Cushing's syndrome. Obesity due to exogenous cause is generalized not truncal. It is not associated with hirsutism, hypertension and pink striae. Adrenocortical abnormalities in obesity are modest. Basal urine steroid excretion is either normal or slightly elevated and diurnal pattern in blood and urine level is normal.

2. *Chronic alcoholism and depression*

   Both these conditions share some features of cushing's syndrome, i.e. moon facies, obesity, etc.

They have some abnormalities in adrenocortical functions which are similar to cushing's syndrome, i.e. increased steroid output, elevated urinary excretion of steroids, absent diurnal variation of cortisol level and positive overnight dexamethasone suppression. All these tests return to normal after discontinuation of alcohol and following treatment of depression with improvement in mental status.

3. *Iatrogenic Cushing's Syndrome*

Clinically it resembles Cushing's syndrome. The distinction can be made however by measuring blood and urine cortisol levels in basal state; in iatrogenic syndrome, these levels are low secondary to suppression of pituitary adrenal axis by exogenous steroids.

Q. What is differential diagnosis of moon face?

Ans. 1. *Cushing's syndrome*

The characteristic features include:

- Moon face, obesity (truncal or centripetal), camel hump
- Weight gain, hypertension, edema
- Cutaneous striae, easy bruising, back pain, muscle weakness, osteoporosis
- Acne, hirsutism, menstrual irregulairty
- Emotional changes
- Pigmentation and hypokalemic alkalosis
- Raised blood cortisol levels (loss of diurnal pattern), raised urinary excretion of 17-OH corticosteroid and dexamethasone suppression test will confirm the diagnosis

2. *Nephrotic syndrome*

Read the features in clinical case discussion No. 18

3. *Nephritic syndrome* (read case discussion no. 17)

4. *Myxoedema* (Read case discussion no. 25)

5. *Superior mediastinal syndrome* (read case discussion no. 64). The characteristic features are:

- Cough, dyspnea, chest pain
- Engorged but nonpulsatile neck veins
- Puffiness of face or moon face, cyanosis
- Hoarseness of voice, Horner's syndrome, vocal cord paralysis
- Paralysis of hemidiaphragm

6. *Angioneurotic edema*

- Type I hypersensitivity reaction, commonly due to drugs, e.g. ACE inhibitor
- Diffuse swelling of the eyelids, face (moon face), lips, tongue, hands, genital or other parts of the body

- Associated with itching
- Congenital variety is due to C1 esterase deficiency
- Wheezing, shortness of breath, headache, nausea, vomiting, arthalgia may occur as systemic manifestations
- Glottis may be involved producing suffocation
- The condition reverses with use of adrenaline, antihistamine and a steroid.

Q. Mention 5 important causes of Cushing's syndrome.

Ans. 1. Iatrogenic (steroid or ACTH use)
2. Pituitary adenoma (Cushing's disease)
3. Adrenal adenoma
4. Adrenal carcinoma
5. Ectopic ACTH production (small-cell carcinoma lung)

Q. What are common indications of steroid therapy?

Ans. The indications of steroids therapy depending on mechanisms of action are enlisted in Table 1.134.

Table 1.134: Actions and indications of steroid therapy

Action	Uses
• Anti-inflammatory agents	• Rheumatoid arthritis, acute rheumatic carditis
• Antiallergic agent	• Allergic skin conditions (urticaria), anaphylactic shock, acute severe asthma
• Antilymphocytic	• Acute lymphatic leukemia
• Immunosuppressive	• Nephrotic syndrome, SLE and other collagen vascular disorders, interstitial lung disease, in organ transplantation to prevent rejection
• Antifibroblastic agent to prevent adhesions	• Used locally or systemically in joint disease, pericardial and pleural effusion
• As replacement therapy in its deficiency	• Addison's disease, Sheehan's syndrome
• To lower intracranial tension	• Cerebral edema, CVA, benign raised intracranial tension
• As a diagnostic test to suppress raised levels	• Dexamethasone or steroid suppression test of endogenous steroids

Q. What are its contraindications?

Ans. The 'check list' prior to use of steroids include:

- Presence of tuberculosis or other chronic infection
- Glucose intolerance or history of gestational diabetes or presence of diabetes

197

- History of peptic ulcer, gastritis or hematemesis or malena (positive occult blood in stool)
- Hypertension
- Osteoporosis or postmenopausal women
- Previous history of psychological disorders.

Q. What are side effects of steroids?

Ans. Read Unit 3–Commonly used drugs.

Q. What is Cushing's disease and what is Cushing's syndrome?

Ans. *Cushing's disease* is increased production of steroids by adrenals secondary to excess of pituitary ACTH. *Cushing's syndrome* is excess of steroids from any cause including steroid therapy.

Q. What are characteristics of Cushing's syndrome due to ectopic ACTH production?

Ans. The features are:
- Acute onset of symptoms
- Hyperpigmentation
- Hypertension and edema are more common
- Hypokalemic alkalosis a characteristic feature
- The diagnosis is confirmed by markedly elevated ACTH level (> 300 ng/L)

Q. What is pseudo Cushing syndrome?

Ans. Pseudo Cushing means some abnormalities in steroid output without involvement of pituitary adrenal axis. It includes certain conditions such as obesity, chronic alcoholism, depression and acute illness of any type which share abnormalities in steroid output, modestly elevated urine cortisol, blunted circadian rhythm of cortisol level (absent diurnal variation of plasma cortisol) and positive overnight dexamethasone suppression test similar to cushing's syndrome but these tests returns to normal with withdrawl of alcohol or improvement in emotional status.

Q. What is Nelson's syndrome?

Ans. This is characterized by increased ACTH production, hyperpigmentation and erosion of sella turcica due to development of chromophobe adenoma in patients with Cushing's disease who have undergone bilateral adrenalectomy. This syndrome will not occur if pituitary has also been irradiated after bilateral adrenalectomy.

Q. How do you classify steroids?

Ans. Read Unit 3, Commonly used drugs.

Q. How will you investigate a case with Cushing's syndrome?

Ans. Investigations are:
1. *Blood examination* for eosinopenia and neutrophilia
2. *Serum sodium* (hypernatraemia), K⁺ (hypokalemia) and pH (alkalosis)

3. *24-hour urinary free cortisol*: This is most direct and release index of cortisol secretion. It may be increased in Cushing's syndrome.
4. *Glucose tolerance test* may show impaired tolerance or frank diabetes (seen <20% cases)
5. *X-ray skull and spine*: X-ray skull may show enlargement of pituitary fossa if a pituitary tumor is suspected to be the cause. X-ray spines may show cord-fish vertebrae or fish-mouth appearance of intervertebral disk spaces
6. *CT scan abdomen* for adrenals may show a adrenal mass (adenoma or carcinoma) if adrenal is the cause
7. *Plasma cortisol level elevated*: There is loss of circadian rhythm
8. *Plasma ACTH levels*: They are high in ectopic ACTH production by a nonpituitary tumor, may be normal to high in pituitary tumor Pituitary radiography and MRI gadolinium enhancement confirms the diagnosis of pituitary tumor
9. *Dexamethasone suppression test*: There is no suppression of cortisol secretion in Cushing's syndrome where as high dose dexamethasone (2 mg burly for 48 hr) suppresses at least 50% of urinary steroid secretion.
10. *Metyrapone test*: It differentiates between ACTH dependent Cushing's disease (exaggerated response) and non-ACTH dependent Cushing syndrome (no response)
11. *Corticotrophin releasing hormone (CRH) test* is helpful in distinguishing pituitary led cushing's disease from ectopic ACTH production.

Q. Name the abdominal striae.

Ans. The striae are named as follows:
- *Silvery white striae/striae gravidarum* due to pregnancy or following delivery.
- *Pink striae* due to Cushing's syndrome or steroid excess.

Q. What is Conn's syndrome? What are differences between primary and secondary hyperaldosteronism?

Ans. Conn's syndrome is primary hyperaldosteronism due to adenoma or hyperplasia of adrenal cortex or idiopathic in origin.

Secondary hyperaldosteronism means raised aldosterone levels due to edematous states or low sodium such as seen in nephrotic syndrome, cirrhosis of the liver and congestive heart failure.

The differences between the two are given in the Table 1.135.

Table 1.135: Distinction between primary and secondary hyperaldosteronism

Primary hyperaldosteronism	Secondary hyperaldosteronism
• It is due to involvement of adrenal cortex	It is secondary to edematous states or low sodium
• Hypertension is a characteristic feature	No hypertension
• Hypokalemia is a characteristic feature with all its symptoms and signs	Hypokalemia occurs, commonly due to use of diuretics
• Plasma aldosterone levels elevated but renin activity is suppressed	Plasma aldosterone and plasma renin activity elevated

Q. What is normal serum K^+ level? What are the causes of hypokalemia?

Ans. Normal serum K^+ level is 3.5 to 5.5 mEq/L. Hypokalemia is said to be present when serum K^+ is <3.0 mEq/L. The common causes are:
1. Diuretics
2. GI tract diseases, e.g. diarrhea or malabsorption
3. Metabolic alkalosis
4. Renal tubular acidosis
5. Deficient dietary intake
6. Cushing's syndrome
7. Conn's syndrome
8. Bartter's syndrome
9. Insulin effect as well as diabetic ketoacidosis.

Q. What are characteristic features of hypokalemia?

Ans. These are:
I. *Neuromuscular*
   • Muscle weakness, fatigue
   • Abdominal distention, adynamic ileus
   • Distention of bladder, constipation
   • Hyporeflexia
II. *Renal*
   Metabolic alkalosis
III. *Cardiac*
   • ECG changes, e.g. appearance of U waves, prolonged QTc, ST depression and T wave inversion
   • Arrhythmias, e.g. ectopics, torsade de pointes.

Q. What is the pathogenesis of truncal obesity in Cushing's syndrome?

Ans. It is due to redistribution of fat to central part under the effect of glucocorticoids.

Q. Name the hormones secreted by adrenal cortex and their effects.

Ans. The hormones secreted and their effects are tabulated (Table 1.136).

Q. What are endocrinal causes of obesity?

Ans.
   • Cushing syndrome
   • Hypothyroidism
   • Hypogonadism (e.g. Frohlich's syndrome, Laurence-Moon-Biedl syndrome, Prader-Willi syndrome)
   • Type 2 diabetes
   • Following pregnancy and postpartum.

Table 1.136: Adrenocortical hormones

Hormone	Effect	Symptoms & signs
1. Aldosterone (mineralo-corticoid)	Retention of Na^+ and H_2O	Edema, hypertension, weight gain
2. Glucocorticoids	Redistribution of fat	Truncal obesity, moon faces, camel hump
	• Mobilization of proteins from supportive tissues, e.g. subcutaneous, bone and muscles	• Striae • Easy bruising • Back pain, fracture, osteoporosis
	• CNS effects	• Emotional changes and personality changes
	• ↑ACTH in Cushing's disease	• Pigmentation • Hypokalemic alkalosis
3. Adrenal androgens	Virilization	• Hirsutism and menstrual irregularity

Q. What is android and gynoid obesity? What is their significance?

Ans. Android obesity (e.g. abdominal or central obesity) is due to collection of fat in the abdomen above the waist producing apple-shaped body. It is associated with increased risk of CHD, HT, DM and dyslipidemia. **Gynoid obesity** is due to collection of fat below the waist, i.e. on the hips and buttocks producing pear-shaped body. It predisposed the individual to mechanical complications, e.g. OA, varicose veins, etc.

Q. How would you manage Cushing's syndrome?

Ans. *For Cushing's disease*
   • Trans-sphenoidal microadenalectomy, pituitary irradiation, total bilateral adrenalectomy.

For Adrenal tumor
   • Surgical resection,
   • Mitotane therapy
   • Resection of recurrent tumor

For Ectopic ACTH tumor
   • Surgical resection of tumor

For exogenous corticoids (iatrogenic syndrome)
   • Taper off corticosteroid

CASE 41: ADDISON'S DISEASE

Examine the patient whose case summary and figure is given below.

The female patient presented with weakness, weight loss and pigmentation of face, buccal mucosa and palms. There is history of diarrhea off and on. BP was 80/60 mm Hg. The clinical findings of the patient are depicted in Figure 1.41.

How would you examine such a case?

History

Points to be Asked on History

- H/o dizziness, syncope
- H/o skin pigmentation
- Ask history of fatigue, weakness, apathy, anorexia, nausea, vomiting, weight loss, abdominal pain
- H/o Depression
- H/o delivery and postpartum hemorrhage.
- H/o Stoppage of lactation after delivery
- History of adrenalectomy or adrenal irradiation.

Examination

- Look for pigmentation at different sites i.e.
  - Creases of palm
  - Compare the pigmentation with your own hand
  - Mouth (mucous membranes) and lips (inner surface)
  - Covered areas such as nipples, areas under belts, straps, collar, rings.
- Look for vitiligo
- Take blood pressure in sitting and standing position for postural hypotension
- Look for sparse, axillary and pubic hairs.
- Look for scar of adrenectomy on the abdomen

Fig. 1.41: Addison's disease. A young female presented with shunken cheeks, breast atrophy following postpartum bleeding (Sheehan's syndrome—postpartum pituitary necrosis)

Q. What is your clinical diagnosis?

Ans. The symptom triad of weakness, weight loss (glucocorticoids insufficiency), hypotension (mineralocorticoids insufficiency) and pigmentation of face and other sun-exposed areas (ACTH excess) suggests the diagnosis of Addison's disease.

Q. What are the causes of Addison's disease?

Ans. The causes are:

I. *Common*
- Autoimmune or idiopathic (90%)
- Congenital adrenal hyperplasia
- Pituitary necrosis (Sheehan's syndrome)
- MEN Type I, II syndromes
- Tuberculosis, fungal infections (histoplasmosis, coccidioidomycosis, etc.) and HIV involving adrenals
- Bilateral adrenalectomy

II. *Rare*
- Metastatic tumors (bilateral)
- Amyloidosis, sarcoidosis
- Waterhouse-Friderichsen's syndrome (adrenal hemorrhage in meningococcemia), HIV disease
- Hemochromatosis
- Adrenal infarction

Q. What are the causes of pigmentation?

Ans. Read case discussion of hyperpigmentation.

Q. What is primary or secondary Addison's disease? How do they differ?

Ans. *Primary Addison's disease* indicates adrenal involvement with high ACTH level due to feedback mechanism.

Secondary Addison's disease means involvement of either pituitary (hypopituitarism) or hypothalamus with decreased ACTH levels.

The differences are given in the Box 41.1.

BOX 41.1: DIFFERENCES BETWEEN PRIMARY AND SECONDARY ADDISON'S DISEASE	
Primary	*Secondary*
• Autoimmune disorder	Secondary to pituitary tumor (chromophobe adenoma), post partum hemorrhages or removal of pituitary or irradiation.
• *Adrenocortical* secretion (gluco and mineralocorticoids and androgens) suffer	there may be insufficiency of other pituitary hormones, i.e. protection, TRH.
• Hyperpigmentation is common	Hypopigmentation is common. Loss of axillary and pubic hair is marked.
• Symptoms such as apathy, weight loss, depression are marked	Less marked
• Breast atrophy absent	Breast atrophy present
• ACTH levels high, other hormones level normal	ACTH levels are low other without involvement of other hormone

Q. **What are MEN type I and MEN type II syndromes?**

Ans. MEN means multiple endocrinal neoplasia causing syndromes of hormone excess.

MEN Type I (Werner's syndrome). It is characterised by neoplasia of parathyroid, pituitary and pancreatic islet cells.

MEN Type II (Medullary thyroid carcinoma, pheochromocytoma *plus* other neoplasia)

A (Sipple syndrome): It consists of medullary thyroid carcinoma, pheochromocytoma, parathyroid adenoma.

B (Mucosal neuroma syndrome): It includes medullary thyroid carcinoma, pheochromocytoma, mucosal and gastrointestinal neuromas, marfanoid features.

Q. **What is Schmidt's syndrome?**

Ans. It is combination of Addison's disease and hypothyroidism.

Q. **What is the size of heart in Addison's disease?**

Ans. Small

Q. **What other autoimmune diseases are associated with Addison's disease?**

Ans. • Graves' disease
• Hashimoto's thyroiditis
• Primary ovarian failure
• Pernicious anemia.

Q. **What is adrenal crisis? What are its causes?**

Ans. The rapid and overwhelming intensification of chronic adrenal insufficiency usually precipitated by stress or sepsis is called *adrenal crisis*. Alternatively, acute adrenal insufficiency means acute involvement of bilateral adrenal glands in previously healthy subjects.

The *causes* are:

1. Septicemia with *Pseudomonas* or *meningococcaemia* (*Waterhouse-Friderichsen syndrome*)
2. Coagulation defect or anticoagulant therapy
3. Birth trauma in newborn
4. Idiopathic adrenal vein thrombosis or following venography
5. Sudden withdrawl of steroids in a patient with adrenal atrophy owing to chronic steroid administration.
6. Congenital adrenal hyperplasia or those with poor adrenal reserve precipitated by steroid synthesis inhibiting drugs (ketoconazole).

Q. **How will you treat adrenal crisis? (Read Emergency Medicine by Dr SN Chugh)**

Ans. Treatment is as follows:

• Find out the cause or precipitating factor and remove or treat it appropriately.

• *Replacement of glucocorticoids.* Intravenous hydrocortisone (100 mg bolus) followed by continuous infusion of 10 mg/hr. Alternatively 100 mg bolus IV followed by same dose after every 6 hours.

• *Replacement of sodium and water deficit* by 5% glucose in normal saline solution. If patient has dehydration, several litres of saline solution may be infused over few hours.

• *Treatment of hypotension:* Replacement of fluid, sodium and glucocorticoids is sufficient to treat hypotension. Dopamine/dobutamine infusion may be indicated as an adjunct to volume depletion in severe cases.

• Once patient is stablised, steroids dosage is tapered over next few days to maintenance doses orally.

Q. **How will you diagnose Addison's disease?**

Ans. The diagnosis depends on clinical features and investigations. The clinical suspicion arises when patient presents with hypotension with:

• Weight loss, malaise, nausea, vomiting, weakness
• Diarrhea—painless and progressive
• Pigmentation of sun-exposed areas, elbow, knees, creases of palm, knuckles, mucous membrane of the mouth, scars, etc.

The diagnosis is confirmed on investigations (Box 41.2).

• Total leukocytes count for lymphoytosis and eosinophilia.
• Adrenal autoantibody
• Chest X-ray for tuberculosis
• Plain X-ray abdomen for adrenal calcification
• CT scan of adrenals

BOX 41.2: INVESTIGATIONS FOR ADDISON'S DISEASE

Test	Primary Addison's	Secondary Addison's
1. Basal plasma cortisol levels, e.g. morning and evening	Low	Low
2. ACTH	High	Low
3. ACTH stimulation test	Cortisol level does not rise	Subnormal rise
4. Serum Na$^+$	Low	Low
5. Serum K$^+$	High	Normal to high
6. Plasma glucose	Normal to low in severe disease	Normal
7. Aldosterone level	Low	Low to normal

Q. What are the common conditions associated with hypotension?

Ans. The common conditions are:

I. *Hypovolemia*
- Excessive blood loss, e.g. external or internal hemorrhage, ruptured ectopic pregnancy, etc
- *Excessive fluid loss,* e.g. vomiting, diarrhea, burns, diabetes mellitus or inspidous or diuresis and internal sequestration of fluid (e.g. peritonitis, pancreatitis, intestinal obstruction)

II. *Hypotension due to cardiac origin*
Acute MI, arrhythmias, myocarditis, rupture of interventricular septum, acute aortic regurgitation or dissection and myocardial depression due to drugs

III. *Hypotension due to vasodilation*
Septic shock, neurogenic shock, anaphylaxis, drug-induced (e.g. nitrates, Ca^{++} channel blockers, ganglion blockers, postural hypotension)

IV. *Extracardiac obstructive shock/hypotension*
- Pericardial effusion, constructive pericarditis, pulmonary embolism, coarctation of aorta

V. *Miscellaneous*
- Thyroid crisis, myxedema coma, Addison's disease, cyanide and CO poisoning and endotoxemia.

Q. How would you treat hypopituitarism?

Ans. Hypopituitarism is characterized by deficiency of one or more pituitary hormones, usually, there is deficiency of TSH, ACTH and GnRH, hence, end-organ hormone deficiencies (thyroid, adrenal and gonads) are replaced life long with thyroxin, steroids and sex hormones.

Perform General Physical Examination

CASE 42: TETANY

The patient is 30 years female who presented with weakness, weight loss, intermittent muscle spasms especially involving the hands, feet and face. While taking the BP, the patient developed carpel spasms as shown in Figures 1.42A and B.

Fig. 1.42A: Tetany. A patient with hypoparathyroidism showing provoked carpopedal spasms (Trousseau's sign)

Fig. 1.42B: Spontaneous carpopedal spasm in tetany. Note the main D' accoucher's or obstetrician's hand

Q. What is your diagnosis?

Ans. In view of induced carpopedal spasms (Trousseau's sign) as well as history of muscle spasms, the patient appears to have tetany.

Q. What important points would you like to ask in this patient?

Ans. 1. History of thyroid surgery because hypoparathyroidism is common following thyroid surgery.

2. Paresthesias of hands, toes and circumoral regions (These are common presenting features of hypoparathyroidism)

3. History of muscle cramping, laryngeal stridor, convulsions, carpopedal spasms involving hands and feet will also be asked.

Q. How would you proceed to examine this case?

Ans. • Examine the hands and feet for carpopedal spasms.

• If spontaneous spasm is not evident but there is history of carpopedal spasms then, perform **Chvostek's sign** (Tap over the facial nerve in front of tragus of the ear and look for facial spasms) or **Trousseau's sign** (Inflate the BP cuff just above the systolic BP of the patient for 3 minutes, and look for carpopedal spasms).

• Look into the mouth for any evidence of oral candidasis (*Candida* endocrinopathy)

• Check for any scar of thyroid surgery.

• Look at the finger nails.

Q. What do you understand by carpopedal spasms?

Ans. Low ionized calcium results in carpal spasm (there is extension of interphalangeal joints and adduction and flexion of metacarpophanlangeal joints with adduction of the thumb) and pedal spasms.

Q. Name the position of the hand in Figure 1.42B.

Ans. It is called *obstetrician's hand or D' accoucher's hand.*

Q. Does the patient has spasms or cramps? What is the difference between the two?

Ans. Patient has carpopedal spasms. Spasm and cramps both refer to episodes of involuntary contractions of one or more muscles. The only difference is that cramps are painful while spasms are painless, and do not cause any discomfort.

533. What are the causes of hypocalcemia?

Ans. The functional classification of hypocalcemia based on the mechanisms of production is tabulated (Table 1.137). The parathormone (PTH) is responsible for minute-to-minute regulation of plasma calcium. Therefore, hypocalcemia can only occur when there is failure of homeostatic action of PTH. Failure of PTH response can occur due to:

i. Hereditary or acquired parathyroid gland failure

ii. PTH is either ineffective in target organs or its action is overwhelmed by the loss of calcium from the extracellular fluid at a rate faster than it can be replaced leading to hypocalcemia.

Table 1.137: Causes of hypocalcaemia

A. *PTH absent*
  i. Hereditary hypoparathyroidism- DiGeorge syndrome (a rare disorder), candidiasis endocrinopathy associated with familial autoimmune polyglandular deficiency syndrome
  ii. Acquired hypoparathyroidism, e.g. following surgical removal or irradiation damage
  iii. Hypomagnesemia due to any cause
B. *PTH ineffective*
  i. Chronic renal failure
  ii. Vit. D deficiency, e.g. rickets, osteomalacia, drug-induced (phenytoin)
  iii. Vit. D resistance
    – Vit. D resistant rickets (type II)
    – Intestinal malabsorption
  iv. Pseudohypoparathyroidism, e.g. Albright's syndrome (short stature, round face, brachydactyly and heterotopic calcification
C. *PTH overwhelmed*
  i. Severe, acute hyperphosphatemia
    • Tumorlysis
    • Acute renal failure
    • Rhabdomyolysis
  ii. Osteitis fibrosa cystica following parathyroidectomy

Q. Name few common clinical conditions associated with chronic hypocalcemia.

Ans. 1. Hypoparathyroidism or pseudohypoparathyroidism
2. Rickets, osteomalacia (vit. D deficiency)
3. Chronic renal failure
4. Chronic diarrhea, malabsorption syndrome
5. Hyperphosphatemia due to any cause, e.g. tumour lysis, ARF
6. Acute pancreatitis

Q. What are causes of transient hypocalcemia?

Ans. Transient hypocalcemia does not produce tetany, occurs due to;
• Severe sepsis
• Burns
• ARF
• Repeated transfusions with citrated blood
• Medications such as protamine, heparin, dilantin and glucagon.

Q. Does the low calcium levels are always associated with tetany?

Ans. No. Total low calcium is not associated with tetany because ionised calcium may be normal in such a case. Low ionised calcium irrespective of calcium levels is associated with tetany. Transient hypocalcaemia is also asymptomatic, i.e. does not produce tetany.

Q. What is differential diagnosis of hypocalcemia?

Ans. I. Low calcium and high phosphate occurs in
  • Chronic renal failure

• Massive tissue destruction
• True hypoparathyroidism and psudohyper-parathyriodism
  II. Low calcium and low phosphate occur in:
    • vit D deficiency
    • vit D resistant racket

Q. What are the causes of tetany?

Ans. Tetany could be hypocalcemic, hypomagnesemic or alkalotic. Every hypocalcemia is not associated with tetany. The low levels of ionised calcium with or without low total calcium lead to tetany (neuromuscular excitability). Idiopathic normocalcemic tetany, spasmophilia occurs in both hereditary and acquired forms. The causes of tetany are given in Table 1.138.

Table 1.138: Causes of tetany
(Low ionised Ca^{++} <1.1 mmol/L or 4.5 mg%)

I. *Hypocalcemia*
  • Malabsorption
  • Rickets and osteomalacia
  • Hypoparathyroidism
  • Chronic renal failure (usually tetany is prevented by acidosis)
  • Acute pancreatitis
  • Drugs, e.g. dilantin (Phenytoin)
II. *Hypomagnesemia*
III. *Alkalosis and hypokalemia*
  • Repeated prolonged vomiting
  • Excessive intake of alkali
  • Hysterical hyperventilation
  • Primary hyperaldosteronism
  • Acute anion load

Q. What is normal serum calcium level? How will you define hypo- and hypercalcemia?

Ans. Normal level is:
• Total plasma calcium is 2.2 to 2.6 mmol/L (9-10.5 mg/dl)
• Ionised calcium is 1.1-1.4 mmol/L (4.5 to 5.6 mg/dl)

Usually **hypocalcemia** is said to be present when serum calcium is <8.5 mg/dl. On the other hand, **hypercalcemia** is said to present when calcium is >11.0 mg/dl.

Q. What are the actions of paratharmone (PTH)?

Ans. 1. Increased osteoclastic activity resulting in mobilization of calcium and phosphorous from the bone to the extracellular compartment
2. Enhances renal tubular absorption of calcium
3. Inhibits the absorption of phosphates and bicarbonate by the renal tubule
4. Stimulates the synthesis of 25-dihydroxy-cholecalciferol (Vit D) by the kidneys

Q. How would you collect blood sample for calcium?

Ans. Blood sample for calcium should be taken without the help of compression of the arm or tourniquet, otherwise false reading will be obtained.

Q. What are the factors that affect serum calcium levels? How would you correct calcium levels in these condition?

Ans. • *Albumin concentration*: Low albumin concentration lowers the serum total calcium levels, hence it has to be corrected by a formula.
  – For 1 gm/dl fall in serum albumin you add 0.8 mg in calcium level
• *Serum immunoglobulin*: Fall in serum immunoglobulins also lowers the serum total calcium. Algorithm for correction is
  – For 1 gm/dl fall in serum immunoglobulin you add 0.5 mg/dl to calcium
• Acidosis also alters ionized calcium by reducing its association with proteins.

Q. What are clinical features of hypoparathyroidism?

Ans. Hypoparathyroidism is characterised by low calcium and high phosphate level either due to deficient production of parathormone (PTH) or its unresponsiveness. The clinical features are:
• Tetany   • Cataract
• Psychosis   • Basal ganglia calcification
• Epilepsy   • Papilledema
• Candidiasis of nails, skin and mucous membrane may be associated with endocrinopathy–*Candida endocrinopathy.*

Q. What are clinical features of tetany?

Ans. Tetany may be latent or manifest. In manifest tetany, symptoms and signs depend on the age of the patient.

In children a characteristic triad of *carpopedal spasm, stridor* (loud sound due to closure of glottis) and *convulsions* may occur in various combinations. The hands in carpopedal spasms adopt a peculiar posture in which there is flexion at metacarpohalangeal joints and extension at the interphalangeal joints and there is apposition of thumb (main D'accoucher hand – see the Figure 1.42). Pedal spasms are less frequent.
• In adults. Tingling sensations (paresthesias) around the mouth and in the hands and feet are common. Carpopedal spasms are less frequent. Stridor and convulsions are rare.

Q. What is latent tetany?

Ans. The absence of symptoms and signs of tetany in a patient with hypocalcemia is called *latent tetany*. The tetany becomes manifest on provocative tests.
  i. **Troussaeu's sign** (see Fig. 1.42A). Raising the BP above systolic level by inflation of sphygno-manometer cuff produces characteristic carpal spasms within 3-5 minutes
  ii. **Chvostek's sign**. A tap at facial nerve at the angle of jaw produces twitching of facial muscles.

Q. How do you classify hypoparathyroidism?

Ans. It is classified as either true (idiopathic) or pseudo-hypoparathyroidism.
  1. *True or idiopathic hypoparathyroidism:* It is due to deficient production of PTH. The symptoms and signs of hypoparathyroidism are present.
  2. *Pseudohypoparathyroidism:* It is a heritable or congenital disorder characterised by tissue resistance to the effects of PTH.
     In pseudohypoparathyroidism, in addition to symptoms and signs of hypoparathyroidism, there are distinct skeletal and developmental defects- a characteristic phenotype termed as '*Albright hereditary osteodystrophy.*'
  3. *Pseudopseudohypoparathyroidism:* A familial disorders in which skeletal and developmental defect are present without signs of hypoparathyroidism. PTH level is normal but there is resistance to its effects.

Q. What are differences between true and pseudo-hypoparathyroidism?

Ans. Table 1.139 presents differentiating features between both.

Q. How would you investigate a patient of tetany?

Ans. • Blood biochemistry, i.e. potassium, calcium, magnesium, phosphate, alkaline phosphate, urea and creatinine
• Blood pH
• Blood PTH and 1-25 dihydroxy cholecalciferol levels
• Urinary excretion of calcium
• X-ray skull for basal ganglia calcification
• ECG for QT prolongation

Q. How will you treat tetany?

Ans. The steps of treatment are:
  1. *Treatment of hypocalcemia* by calcium gluconate (10% 20 ml IM or IV) followed by oral supplementation of calcium and vitamin D analog. If not relieved by calcium, potassium and magnesium may be tried.
  2. *Treatment of alkalosis*
     • Withdraw the alkalies if it has been the cause
     • Isotonic saline IV if vomiting is the cause
     • Inhalation of 5% CO_2 in oxygen if hyperventilation is the cause
     • Psychotherapy for hysterical hyperventilation

Q. What is the effect of hypocalcemia on ECG?

Ans. There is prolongation of QT (QTc) interval which may predispose to arrhythmias similar to hypokalemia.

Table 1.139: Distinguishing features between idiopathic hypoparathyroidism and pseudohypoparathyroidism

Idiopathic hypoparathyroidism	Pseudohypoparathyroidism
• Usuaully acquired	• Congenital
• PTH levels are low	• PTH levels are high
• Autoimmunity plays a role in some cases	• Non- responsiveness to PTH either due to receptor or post-receptor defect
• Besides tetany, other features include epilepsy, psychosis, cataract, calcification of basal ganglia and papilledema	• Besides tetany, other features include skeletal and developmental abnormalities such as short stature, short 4th and 5th metacarpal or metatarsals (brachydactyly) etc. called *Albright's syndrome* or *Albright's hereditary osteodystrophy*

Q. What are changes in EMG in tatany?

Ans. EMG studies reveal single or more often grouped motor unit discharges at low discharge frequency

Q. How does hyperventilation lead to tetany?

Ans. Hyperventilation occurring frequently or if prolonged leads to tetany by producing alkalosis due to washing out of CO_2.

Q. Why does hypocalcemia in CRF does not lead to tetany?

Ans. Hypocalcemia in CRF is common but tetany is rare. It is due to the fact that ionised calcium does not fall to such a level to produce tetany because of associated metabolic acidosis in patients with CRF.

CASE 43: ACROMEGALY

The patient presented with coarse facial features and short stubby fingers and large hands (Figs 1.43A and B). There was associated hypertension.

Fig. 1.43A: A patient with acromegaly. Note the stout built, broad, short stubby fingers and spade like hands

Fig. 1.43B: Gigantism. Note the height of patient (8 feet 2 inches). The hands and feet are large. The built is stout

Q.   What is the clinical diagnosis and why?
Ans. My clinical diagnosis is acromegalic male.

The points in favor of my diagnosis are:
i. Coarse facial features, e.g. mature looks, elongated face, prognathism, larger prominent frontal ridges
ii. Thick lips, large tongue
iii. Large spade-like hands with short, stout, stubby fingers
iv. Deep husky voice
v. Thick skin

Q.   How would you proceed to examine this patient?
Ans.

History

Points to be Asked

- Ask about the history of change in size of the shoes or tightness of rings or size of the hat/cap.
- Ask about excessive sweating
- Ask for headache, visual field defects, paresthesia in hands and feet.
- Ask about any menstrual irregularity or impotence in male.
- Any history of dyspnea
- Any history of arthritis
- Any change in acral parts or face.

Examination

1. First of all, shake the hands with the patient and note the moist hands.
2. Now look at the hands, i.e. note the large size of hands or square shape hand with short and wide fingers. There is thick skin of hands. Volume of the hand is increased.
3. Look at the face and note the followings:
   - Prognathism (protruding jaw), thick lips, large tongue, large incisors, elongated face, prominent sinuses (frontal and maxillary) prominent supraorbital ridges and large nose.
4. Examine the eye and neck (for goiter)
5. Check the teeth and note the malocclusion and splaying of the teeth (interdental separation).

Systemic Examination

Examine

- Chest for heart enlargement. Take BP
- Abdomen for hepatosplenomegaly
- Joints for osteoarthritis and chondrocalcinosis
- Spine for kyphosis

Testing

- Look for bitemporal hemianopia and optic atrophy
- Test for deafness.

Q. What are your physical findings?

Ans. • Bitemporal hemianopia
   • Hypertension
   • Arthropathy (pain in joints)

Q. What bedside test would you like to perform?

Ans. • Urine for glycosuria
   • Blood sugar for IGT and diabetes.

Q. What is the most common cause of this condition?

Ans. A pituitary tumor mostly a GH secreting adenoma is the most common cause (≥60% of cases). Prolactinoma is the second common cause.

Q. What are common causes of macroglossia?

Ans. *Common causes*
   • Acromegaly/gigantism
   • Amyloidosis
   • Hypothyroidism (Cretinism)
   • Down's syndrome
   • Lymphangioma and hemangioma
   Uncommon causes
   • Angioedema
   • Lymphoma
   • Chronic infection, e.g. TB and syphilis

Q. What is pseudomacroglossia? What are its causes?

Ans. Pseudomacroglossia refers to relative enlargement of tongue secondary to small mandible with no histological abnormality. It is seen in Downs' syndrome and cerebral palsy.

Q. What are the clinical features of acromegaly?

Ans. Clinical features of acromegaly are depicted in Table 1.140.

Table 1.140: Clinical features of acromegaly

Systems/organs	Symptoms and signs
General	Normal height, stout and stocky built
Skin	Thickening, excessive perspiration, acanthosis nigricans
Soft tissues	Thick lips, macroglossia, thick nose, increase in heel pad (>22 mm)
Viscera	Visceromegaly (e.g. liver, spleen, heart, tongue)
Joints	Arthropathy
Muscles	Myopathy
Acral parts (hands and feet)	Spade like hands, thick short and stubby fingers, large feet with increase in the size of shoes, carpal tunnel syndrome (compression of median nerve)
Skull	Prominent ridges and furrows
Jaws	Prognathism (protuding lower jaw)
Sinuses	Large frontal and maxillary sinuses
Eyes	Visual field defects, e.g. bitemporal hemianopia or scotomas
Others	Hypertension, galactorrhea in females

Q. Name the diseases caused by GH excess?

Ans. 1. Gigantism due to excess of GH in prepubertal age group.
   2. Acromegaly due to excess of GH in post pubertal age groups.
   3. Gigantic acromegaly—A combination of both.

Q. What are actions of GH?

Ans. 1. GH induces protein synthesis, nitrogen retention, and impairs glucose tolerance by antagonizing insulin action.
   2. It stimulates lipolysis leading to increased fatty acid levels, enhanced lean body mass and reduced omental fat mass.
   3. It promotes Na, K and water retention.
   4. It stimulates linear bone growth.

Q. What are the disorders of GH deficiency?

Ans. The disorder of GH deficiency is dwarfism (pituitary dwarfism)

Q. How do the patients of acromegaly present?

Ans. 1. One-third patients present with a change in their features, e.g large hands and feet, facial appearance
   2. One-third of patients are brought by their parents with complaint of change in features.
   3. One-third patients complain of excessive sweating; visual difficulties, hypertension, etc.

Q. What are the neurological manifestations in Acromegaly?

Ans. Neurological manifestations are as follows:
   A. *Cranial nerve palsy*
      1. Optic nerve. Pressure on the optic chiasma leads to bitemporal hemianopia (most common), compression of optic nerve will lead to blindness due to optic atrophy.
      2. Paralysis of 3rd, 4th and 6th nerves leads to external ophthalmoplegia.
      3. VIIIth nerve involvement leads to deafness.
   B. *Peripheral nerve compression*
      • Carpal tunnel syndrome (median nerve compression).

Q. What are causes of carpal tunnel syndrome?

Ans. Following are the causes:
   • Myxedema
   • Pregnancy
   • Acromegaly
   • Amyloidosis (primary)
   • Rheumatoid arthritis
   • Diabetes mellitus
   • Compression of median nerve due to edema, tenosynovitis, fascitis, fracture, etc.
   • Osteoarthritis (rare)

- Exposure to excessive vibration, seen in tractor drivers, mobile crane drivers and in workers involved in grinding using drills.
- Idiopathic

(Read this question in peripheral neuropathy also)

Q. How can you assess activity in acromegaly?

Ans. Acromegaly is assessed for its activity as follows:
- Increasing sizes of the gloves, rings and shoes
- Ill –fitting of previous dentures
- Excessive perspiration and increasing headache
- Increasing visual loss
- Excessive sebum production
- Serial photographs of the patient may reveal progressive macrosomia
- Biochemical evidence of raised GH and somatomedian C levels.

Q. What are the complications of acromegaly?

Ans.
- Cardiomegaly and heart failure
- Hypertension
- Impaired glucose tolerance
- Arthritis of hip, knee and spine
- Hypopituitarism
- Visual field defects
- Carpal tunnel syndrome
- Spinal canal stenosis.

Q. What are the uses of octreotide therapy?

Ans. Octreotide or lanreotide, a somatostatin analog is used in:
- Treatment of variceal bleed due to portal hypertension
- For treatment of acromegaly if disease is active
- Used in treatment and prevention of development of carcinoid syndrome, during surgery, anesthesia, stress

Q. Mention some other condition in which there is excess of GH?

Ans. 1. MEN-type-I (Parathyroid hyperplasia, pituitary tumor, and gut tumor)
2. McCune-Albright's syndrome (polystotic fibrous dysplasia, sexual precocity and café-au-lait spots).

Table 1.141: GH producing tumor

Tests	Results
Basal GH or serum IgG (insulin like growth factor I levels)	High
Prolactin level	High (in 30%)
Glucose tolerance suppression test by 75 g glucose	There is either no suppression or or failure of suppression to <1µL paradoxical rise of GH
X-ray skull for pituitary fossa	There may be enlargement of pituitary fossa with destruction of clinoid processes
X-ray heel pad thickness	Increased (>22 mm)
X-ray sinuses	Large and widened sinuses
Visual fields	Bitemporal hemianopia or scotoma
CT scan	A small or large hypodense microadenoma may be seen

Q. How will you investigate such a patient?

Ans. The investigations and the test results of a GH secreting tumor are listed in Table 1.141.

Q. What is treatment of acromegaly?

Ans. Following are treatment methods:
1. *Medical:* Bromocriptine, a long-acting dopamine agonist may be used to lower the GH levels in active disease. The dose is 15-30 mg/day in divided doses; starting at a low dose of 2.5 mg/day and then gradually increasing it. Side effects include nausea, vomiting, postural hypotension, constipation and dyskinesia.

   Now-a-days a somatostatin analog, i.e. octreotide is used subcutaneously three times a day.

2. *Surgical:* Surgical treatment is indicated for pituitary tumors with compressive symptoms. Removal of adenoma by trans-sphenoidal route is preferred mode of surgery.

3. *Radiotherapy:* Pituitary is irradiated externally by gamma rays or by accelerated proton beam (linear accelerator) or internally by implanting rods of yttrium (radioactive isotope) into the pituitary gland.

An 18-year-old female presented with short stature, decreased weight and failure of development of secondary sexual characters and menstrual irregularity (Figs 1.44A and B).

Figs 1.44A and B: Pituitary dwarfism. An 18-year-old female pituitary dwarf (A) compared with age and sex matched control (B)

Q. What is your clinical diagnosis?

Ans. The patient appears to be dwarf, the cause of which appears to be endocrinal, i.e. hypopituitarism.

Q. What are points in favor of your diagnosis?

Ans. • Female patient
- Thick skin, coarse features
- Overweight
- Failure of secondary sexual character
- Menstrual irregularity.

Q. How do you define dwarfism and short stature?

Ans. *Dwarfism* means short stature where the height of person is much below the prescribed normal height in relation to his/her chronological age and sex. Short stature is defined as height of the child >2.5 SD below the mean for chronological age, or the growth velocity that falls below 5th percentile on the growth velocity curve. Dwarfism means height below 3rd percentile of normal population of same age and sex.

Q. What is significance of history taking in a case with short stature?

Ans. The natal (prenatal, intranatal and postnatal) history, the family and personal history are important.

1. *Prenatal history:* Ascertain the followings:
   - Age of mother at conception
   - Exposure to smoking and alcohol
   - TORCH infection (Toxoplasma, Rubella, CMV, Herpes)
   - Exposure to irradiation
   - Any chronic illness during pregnancy
   - Any thyroid disorder during pregnancy
   - Exposure to drug-phenytoin
2. *Intranatal*
   - Duration of gestation, e.g. premature delivery
   - Nature of delivery, e.g. vaginal, forceps used or cesarean section
   - Birth weight
   - Birth asphyxia, cry after birth
   - Persistence of neonatal jaundice
3. *Postnatal*
   - Development of milestones
   - Height gain in a year
   - History of chronic or recurrent illness
4. *Family history*
   - Parent's height, e.g. mother and father
   - Height of the siblings
   - Any family history of growth delay
   - Constitutional growth delay
5. *Personal history*
   - Dietary history—caloric intake, food faddism
   - Protein and calcium intake
   - Scholastic performance
   - Relationship with peers

Q. What are the causes of short stature?

Ans. Causes of short stature are:
1. *Heredofamilial*
2. *Constitutional delayed growth*
3. *Idiopathic*
4. *Skeletal dysplasias and rickets*
5. *Dysmorphic syndromes*
   - Noonan's syndrome
   - Down's syndrome
   - Turner's syndrome
   - Russel-Silver syndrome

Some important causes to be remembered

- *Constitutional or heredofamilial*
- *Celiac disease*
- *Isolated GH deficiency*
- *Hypothyroidism*
- *Hypopituitarism*
- *Rickets*
- *Chronic renal failure*

6. *Nutritional*
   - Celiac disease
   - Inflammatory bowel disease
   - Poor diet intake and food faddism
7. *Chronic illnesses*
   - Chronic infections
   - Chronic renal failure
   - Thalassemia major
8. *Endocrinopathies*
   - Isolated GH deficiency
   - Hypothyroidism (cretinism)
   - Hypopituitarism
   - Cushing's syndrome
   - Pseudohypoparathyroidism
   - Uncontrolled type I diabetes
9. *Intrauterine growth retardation*

Q. **What is differential diagnosis of short stature?**

Ans. The conditions and their clinical features associated with short stature are enlisted in Table 1.142.

Q. **What is Down's syndrome? What are its characteristic features?**

Ans. *Down's syndrome* is a chromosomal disorder characterised by trisomy 21 (chromosome 21 is present in triplicate) as a result of nondysjunction during meiosis.

The characteristic features are:
1. *Mongol facies (mongolism)*
   - Microcephaly
   - Upward slanting eyes with epicanthal folds
   - Small, low-set ears
   - Depressed bridge of the small nose
   - Widely-set eyes (hypertelorism)
   - Open mouth, fissured protuding tongue (macroglossia)
   - High arched palate and small teeth
   - Idiotic face, mental retardation (low IQ)
2. *Short and broad hands (Simian hand)*
   The hands have
   - Single palmar crease (simian crease)
   - Clinodactyly (hypoplasia of middle phalanx of little finger resulting in incurving of it)
   - Missing of one crease in little finger
3. *The feet* show
   - *Sandle gap*, e.g. increased gap between first and second toe
   - Single longitudinal crease in the sole
4. *The eyes* show
   - Brushfield's spot
   - Cataract
   - Squint
5. *CVS*
   - Endocardial cushion defects (e.g. VSD, ASD, PDA)
6. *GI tract*
   - Duodenal/jejunal/biliary atresia
7. *Neuromuscular*
   - Hypotonia
8. *Hematopoietic*
   - More chances of acute leukemia
9. *Skeletal*
   - Short stature

Q. **What are features of achondoplasia?**

Ans. Read the differential diagnosis of dwarfism (Table 1.142)

Q. **What is gene defect in achondroplasia?**

Ans. It is inherited as an autosomal dominant trait with complete penetrance, Mutation of the fibroblast growth factor receptor 3 (FGFR-3) gene on

Table 1.142: Differential conditions for short stature

Causes	Clinical features
GH deficiency	Chubby child, frontal bossing, central obesity, high pitched voice, midline defects
Hypothyroidism (cretinism)	Read the clinical features as a separate question
Cushing's syndrome	Moon face, central obesity, striae, hypertension, camel hump, hirsutism
Pseudohypoparathyroidism	Moon facies and obesity, short metacarpals and metatarsals, mental retardation, tetany, epileptic convulsions, basal ganglia calcification
Rickets	Craniotabes, widened wrist joint, rickety rosary, Harrison's sulcus, genu valgum, scoliosis, lordosis, kyphosis, protuberant abdomen
Down's syndrome (Trisomy 21)	Read the clinical features of Down's syndrome – separate question
Noonan's syndrome	Phenotype characteristics of Turner's syndrome, microphallus and delayed puberty are common
Achondroplasia (premature fusion of epiphyses)	Normal mental and sexual development, short limbs (shortened proximal extremites), large head with saddle nose, normal sized trunk lumbar lordosis or kyphoscoliosis. They are seen as jokers in circus.
Prader-Willi syndrome	Hypotonia, obesity, hypogonadism, mental deficiency, small hands and feet with growth retardation
Laurence-Moon-Biedl syndrome	Obesity, hypogonadism, mental retardation, polydactyly and retinitis pigmentosa

chromosome 4 with the transition from guanine to adenine or guanine to cytosine transversion at nucleoside 1138 is the defect in these patients.

Q. **Which maternal serum markers are used for prenatal screening of Down's syndrome?**

Ans. • Serum α-fetoprotein,
• Chorionic gonadotropin
• Estriol

Q. **What are features of Turner's syndrome?**

Ans. It is X-linked disorder characterized by monosomy X (45XO) and affects the females. The features of this syndrome are:
• Short stature, short neck, low-hairline on the back, receding chin, low-set ears (Fig. 1.44C).
• Primary amenorrhea
• Poorly developed secondary sexual characters
• Webbing of neck in a female patient
• Shield breast (flat breast)
• Cubitus valgus (increased carrying angle)
• Short 4th metacarpal or metatarsal
• Coarctation of aorta/aortic stenosis
• Peripheral lymphedema (hands and feet)
• Nail hypoplasia, epicanthal folds, double eyelashes, multiple pigmented nevi.

Q. **How would you examine a case of Turner's syndrome?**

Ans. Look for all the feature of Turner's syndrome described above especially, dwarfism, webbed neck, primary hypogonodism (poorly developed sexual characters), etc.

Q. **What do you understand by a web?**

Ans. It means either a fan-like fold of skin extending from shoulder to the neck or an abnormal splaying out of the trapezius.

Q. **Name cardiovascular diseases associated with webbed neck?**

Ans. • Noonan's syndrome (ASD)
• Ullrich's syndrome with pulmonary stenosis

Q. **What is karyotype in Turner's syndrome?**

Ans. Karyotype is 45 XO. Other variants include 46X (with abnormal X), 45XO/46XX mosaics and 45XO/46XY mosaics.

Q. **What are the facial features in Down's syndrome?**

Ans. Ptosis, micrognathia, low-set ear, epicanthal folds, double eyelashes.

Q. **Is pregnancy possible in Down's syndrome?**

Ans. It is possible only in mosaic individuals with a normal 46 XX cell line (45XO/46XX).

Q. **What are renal abnormalities associated with Turner's syndrome?**

Ans. Horse shoe kidney, hydronephrosis.

Q. **What are different body proportions in dwarfism?**

Fig. 1.44C: Turner's syndrome. A: Short webbed neck, receding chin and low hairline

Ans. 1. *The upper segment and lower segment are equal:* The causes are; hereditary, constitutional and hypopituitarism
2. *The upper segment is more than lower segment:* The causes are; achondroplasia and hypothyroidism (cretinism, juvenile hypothyroidism)
3. *Upper segment is less than lower segment:* It occurs in spinal deformities.

Q. **What is cretinism? What are its features? How does it differ from pituitary dwarf?**

Ans. Hypothyroidism dating from birth and resulting in developmental abnormality is termed as cretinism. The characteristic features are:
• Short stature
• Dull idiotic face
• The child is lazy and lethargic
• Coarse features with protruding tongue, broad flat nose and widely-set eyes (hypertelorism), thick lips
• Sparse hair and dry skin
• Pot belly (protuberant abdomen) with an umbilical hernia
• Impaired mental development, delayed milestones development
• Retarded bone age
• Epiphyseal dysgenesis and delayed dentition.

Q. **What are differences between cretinism and pituitary dwarfism?**

Ans. The difference between cretinism and pituitary dwrarf are given in Table 1.143.

Table 1.143: Cretinism vs pituitary dwarfism

Cretinism	Pituitary dwarfism
Coarse facies, large tongue, depressed nose	Chubby juvenile facies
Low or lack of intelligence	Normal intelligence
Normal sexual development	Sexual infantalism

Tests	For
Complete hemogram	Anemia (chronic infection, worm infestation)
ESR	Inflammatory bowel disease, tuberculosis
Urine pH	Renal tubular acidosis (RTA)
Ca^{++}, PO_4^{+++} and alkaline phosphatase	Hypoparathyroidism, metabolic bone disease
Stool for ova and cysts	Intestinal infestation (hook worm, giardiasis)
Blood urea, nitrogen, SGOT and SGPT	Renal and liver disease
Radiology (X-ray skull and hands)	Bone age and pituitary fossa assessment
Thyroid function tests	Primary and secondary hypothyroidism
Chromosomal karyotyping	Gonadal dysgenesis
GH level and provocative test	GH deficiency

Q. How does hypothyroidism manifests in neonates?

Ans. It manifests as
- Persistence of jaundice in neonates
- Constipation
- A hoarse cry
- Somnolence
- Feeding problem

Q. How will you proceed to investigate a patient with short stature?

Ans. Various tests and conditions for which they are done are tabulated in Table 1.144.

Q. How will you treat dwarfism?

Ans. Correction of primary medical disorder is the treatment of choice for growth failure. The GH or IGF-1 therapy can improve the growth of the child but complete gain of the height may not be possible without correction of underlying cause.

- *Treatment of constitutional delay of growth and adolescence (CDGA).* This condition is a normal variant in which children have short stature with normal growth rate during childhood. They have delayed puberty and attenuated pubertal growth rate. The GH is normal or low for the skeletal age but lower than normal for chronological age. The final height remains lower than predicted height in this group. These cases can be managed after careful assessment with sex steroids for few months. In girls, low dose estrogen may be used. The bone age acceleration does not occur with this therapy.

- *Treatment of GH failure:* GH can be used in growth hormone deficiency and even non-growth hormone deficient short statured children.

  The dose of human GH (recombinant) is 0.175 to 0.35 mg/kg/week subcutaneously preferably at bed time for 6-7 weeks. The growth accelerates from 3-4 cm/yr to 10-12 cm/yr in first year. It slows down in 2nd year of therapy. Treatment is continued till target height is achieved and then dose adjusted so that growth of child is maintained to >4 cm/yr. The side effects of the therapy is development of leukaemia and intracranial tumor.

- *Treatment of short stature due to other causes:* GH has been used with growth failure not due to GH deficiency with some success. It is indicated in children with dwarfism (>2.5 SD below the mean of age) who do not have GH deficiency. Many of these children show short-term increase in growth rate in response to GH therapy but whether their final target height will be achieved or not has not been established.

A 17-year male presented with increase in height with non development of facial hair and small genitalia. His height is 6″-3″ (Fig. 1.45A).

Fig. 1.45A: Tall stature. A patient with hypogonadotrophic hypogonadism—Kallmann's syndrome

Q. What is your diagnosis?

Ans. Tall stature due to hypogonadism, the cause of which has to be found out.

Q. What is stature?

Ans. Stature means total height from crown to heel. Tall stature means height above 97th percentile of normal population of same age and sex.

Q. What important points on history would you ask from such a patient?

Ans. • Age of the patient
• Height of the patient
• Family history of tall stature (constitutionally tall)
• Built of the patient (thin built in Marfan's syndrome, Kallmann's syndrome, thick and stout built in gigantism and acromegaly).
• Infertility, if person is married
• Any mental subnormality
• H/o decreased or loss of smell (anosmia)

Q. How would you proceed to examine such a patient?

Ans. • Note the age (prepubertal or post-pubertal) and total height of the patient.

• Measure both the upper and lower segments.
• Measure the arm span and deduce the ratio of arm span with total height.
• *If lower segment (pubis to heel) is equal to greater than upper segment (crown to pubis), then look for the*
  1. Marfanoid features (Marfan's syndrome) i.e. arachanodactly (spidery fingers), confirmed by thumb protrusion sign or wrist sign, hypermobility of the joints, eyes for iridodonesis (ectopia lentis), high arched palate, kyphoscoliosis or chest deformity and heart for valvular regurgitation.
  2. Features for Klinefelter's syndrome i.e. lack of beard and scanty pubic hair, female voice, gynecomastia, small atrophic testes and infertility.
  3. Features of acromegaly/gigantism, i.e. large head, prognathism, large tongue, thick stout built, short stubby fingers, large feet, etc.
  4. Features of Kallmann's syndrome, i.e. tall stature, thin built, small testes and anosmia.

If upper segment is > lower segment, then
• Look for the features of precocious puberty of adrenal virilization.

N.B. Never forget to examine primary and secondary sexual characters in a patient with tall stature. There is corollary that the longer the person, the more are chances of infertility.

Q. What is eunuchoidism?

Ans. Leydig cell failure (loss of androgens or testosterone) prior to puberty results in hypogonadism, arrest of sexual maturation and tall stature due to failure of closure of the epiphyses—a condition called *eunuchoidism*, which in addition includes an infantilism, i.e. scanty distribution of body hair and poor muscle mass.

In common sense, androgens loss implied eunuchoidism.

Q. What do you understand by the term body proportion? What are different body proportions in tall stature?

Ans. Body proportion means ratio of upper segment (vertex to pubis) to lower segment (pubis to sole or heel) which is 0.93 in adults because legs grow faster than trunk. The different body proportions in tall stature are:

1. The upper segment is equal to lower segment (1:1) in:
   • Gigantism
   • Kallmann's syndrome
   • Frohlich's syndrome
   • Constitutional cause

2. The lower segment > upper segment is seen in:
   - Marfan's syndrome
   - Klinefelter's syndrome
   - Hypogonadism
   - Homocystinuria
3. Upper segment > lower segment
   - Precocious puberty
   - Adrenal cortical tumors

Q. What are causes of tall stature?

Ans. These are:
- Constitutional
- Racial
- Marfan's syndrome
- Klinefelter's and Reifenstein's syndromes
- Gigantism, acromegaly
- Hypogonadotrophic hypogonadism (*Kallmann's syndrome, Frohlich's syndrome*)
- Homocysteinuria
- Congenital contractural arachnodactyly
- Super-males (XYY) and super-females (triple X)

Q. What is Kallmann's syndrome?

Ans. It is a congenital disorder inherited as an X-linked recessive trait, characterised by prepubertal hypogonadotrophic hypogonadism (low testosterone, low LH and FSH levels) due to GnRH deficiency associated with eunuchoidism, small testes, scanty pubic hair (Fig. 1.45A) and anosmia (loss of smell) as a result of defect in the developing olfactory tract. In some cases, cerebellar dysfunction, cleft palate and congenital deafness are present. Cryptorchidism may occur.

Q. What is Marfan's syndrome? What are its characteristic features?

Ans. Marfan's syndrome (Fig. 1.45B) is an autosomal dominant disorder characterized by two of the three (a triad) abnormalities:

Fig. 1.45B: Marfan's syndrome. Note tall stature on measurement. Height is 6'-1½"; Arm span 6'-6" upper segment 31½"; Lower segment 42"; Ratio 0.75

1. Musculoskeletal
2. Ocular
3. Cardiovascular

The clinical features are given in Table 1.145. Marfan's habitus refers to presence of some of skeletal abnormalities without other features of Marfan's syndrome.

Table 1.145: Features of Marfan's syndrome

1. Musculoskeletal
   - Tall with long slender limbs
   - Lower segment > upper segment
   - Arachnodactyly (long slender fingers)
   - Arm span > total height
   - Hypotonic muscles
   - Narrow face, high-arched palate and dolichocephalic skull
   - Hyperextensible joints and laxity of ligaments leading to recurrent dislocation of hip and femoral and inguinal hernias
   - Kyphoscoliosis, pectus carinatum or excavatum
   - *Steinberg's sign or thumb protrusion sign*- in which the thumb when apposed across the palm protrudes beyond the ulnar border of the hand
   - *Wrist sign* – the thumb and little finger overlap when elapsed around the opposite wrist.
   Metacarpal index > 8 (the average ratio of lengths/breadth of last 4 metacarpals from 2nd to 5th as seen on X-ray).
2. Ocular
   - Ectopia lentis – upward bilateral dislocation of lens, may be seen on slit lamp examination
   - Myopia with blue sclera
   - Squint, nystagmus
   - Iridodonesis may be seen
3. Cardiovascular
   - Dissecting aneurysm of aorta
   - Aortic regurgitation
   - Conduction abnormalities.

Q. What are diagnostic criteria for Marfan's syndrome?

Ans. The diagnostic criteria are:
I. Positive family history with two systems involvement out of three systems.
II. If no positive family history, then skeletal features *plus* involvement of two other systems and one of the major criteria, ectopia lentis, aortic root dilation or aortic dissection and lumbosacral duct ectasia on CT/MRI.

Q. How would you proceed to examine a patient with Marfan's syndrome?

Proceed as follows:
1. *Height and arm span:* Patient is tall, has disproportionately long and thin extremities. Arm Span is more than height on measurement.
2. *Head:* Head is long (dolichocephalic)

3. *Eyes:* Examine eyes by slip lamp examination for iridodonesis or etopia lentis (subluxation upwards)

4. *Palate:* It is dome-shaped-high arched palate. Skin for striae over shoulder, buttocks

5. *Hands:* Look for the followings:
   - Long, slender finger (arachnodactyly) which can be confirmed by thumb sign and wrist sign.

6. *Chest:* Look for deformity such as pectus excavatum, and cystic lung disease

7. *Spine:* for scoliosis and kyphosis

8. *Heart:* Examine the heart for mitral regurgitation (mitral value prolapse), aortic aneurysm and aortic regurgitation

Q. What are causes of arachnodactyly?

Ans. 1. Marfan's syndrome

2. Congenital contractural arachnodactyly.

3. Homocystinuria

Q. What are ocular manifestations of Marfan's syndrome?

Ans. Read the Table 1.145.

Q. What is differential diagnosis of Marfan's syndrome?

Ans. Read the differential diagnosis of tall stature. The only condition in which skeletal manifestations of Marfan's syndrome are present is homocysteinuria which has to be differentiated.

Q. What is the basic defect in Marfan's syndrome?

Ans. Being a heritable (autosomal dominant) disorder of connective tissues the basic defect lies in gene mutation of single allele of the fibrillin gene (FBNI).

Q. Is eunuchoidism a feature of Marfan's?

Ans. No, eunuchoidism refers to androgen deficiency leading to tall stature. The patients with Marfan's have normal sex characters and sexual development.

Q. What are cardiovascular manifestations of Marfan's syndrome?

Ans. Read the Table 1.145.

Q. What are the pulmonary manifestations of Marfan's syndrome?

Ans.
- Associated cystic lung disease
- Spontaneous pneumothorax.

Q. What are complications of pregnancy in women with Marfan's syndrome?

Ans.
- Early premature abortion
- Maternal death from aortic dissection. Pregnancy is not dangerous when aortic root diameter is < 40 mm

Q. What is the cause of death in Marfan's syndrome?

Ans. Cardiovascular complication (aortic dissection or congestive heart failure due to aortic regurgitation)

Q. What would you advise the patient of Marfan's syndrome with cardiovascular manifestations?

Ans.
- Annual echocardiography to monitor aortic diameter and mitral value function.
- Long-term beta-blockers to retard the rate of progression of aortic dilatation
- Prophylaxis against infective endocarditis.
- Prophylactic replacement of the aortic root with a composite graft when the diameter reaches 50-55 mm (normal < 40 mm).

Q. What are features of Klinefelter's syndrome (47 XXY Fig. 1.45C)?

Ans.
- Eunuchoidism (lower segment > upper segment)
- Gynecomastia
- Hypogonadism (small firm testes), lack of male distribution of pubic hair
- Phenotypically male
- Buccal smear shows Barr bodies (chromosomal pattern is 47, XXY)
- Azoospermia may occur
- Gonadotropin levels are high (hypergonadotrophic hypogonodism)
- Mental subnormality (sometimes)

The triad for Klinefelter's syndrome is eunuchoidism, gynecomastia and hypogonadism

Q. What important questions would you ask from a patient of Klinefelter's syndrome?

Ans.
- Age and height of patient.
- Condition of hair distribution in axillae and pubic region.
- Character of voice (feminine voice)
- Is he mentally subnormal? How does he perform in the school/college?

Fig. 1.45C: Klinefelter's syndrome—46 XXY (hypergonadotrophic hypogonadism). Note bilateral gynecomastia, small testes (< 1 cm), scanty pubic hair, smaller size of penis and eunuchoidism

- If married, ask about the fertility. Does he has any issue?
- Ask about sense of smell (anosmia is common in Kallmann's syndrome while sense of smell is normal in Klinefelter's syndrome)
- Ask about the size of the testes, whether small or normal

Q. **How would you proceed to examine such a case?**

Ans.
- Note the body habitus and measure all body proportions, i.e. upper and lower segments
- Note gynecomastia
- Examine the distribution of hair (face, mostachuttes, pubic region)
- Test mental IQ of the patent
- Test for sense of small
- Examine the testes for size, consistency.

Q. **What are the features of male hypogonadism in Klinefelter's syndrome?**

Ans.
- Male patient with enuchoid habitus (lack of androgenization)
- Gynecomastia, infertility
- Lack of male distribution of pubic hair, lack of beard in adult male.
- Voice is not masculine (feminine voice).

Q. **What is most common Karyotype in Klinefelter's syndrome?**

Ans. The most common karyotype is 47,XXY (80%) which results from non-dysfunction of sex chromosomes at meiosis during gametogenesis in one of the parents.

Q. **Are patients of Klinefelter's syndrome fertile?**

Ans. Classical cases of Klinefelter's syndrome are infertile. However some men having chromosomal mosacisim (46,XXY/47,XXY) are fertile called mosaic Klinefelter's. Mosaic forms result from chromosomal mitotic nondysjunction within the zygote and occurs in 10% cases.

Q. **How would you investigate Klinefelter's syndrome?**

Ans.
- *Plasma gonadotrophins levels:* FSH levels are persistently highly in hypergonodotrophic hypogonadism.
- *Plasma testosterone levels:* They are low.
- *Plasma estradiol levels:* They are raised.
- *Chromosome analysis:* It shows two or more X-chromosomes and one or more Y-chromosome.

Q. **How would you differentiate Marfan's syndrome from homocysteinuria?**

Ans. Presence of downward dislocation of lens, mental retardation and homocystein in the urine differentiates homocysteinuria from Marfan's syndrome.

Q. **What are features of homocysteinuria?**

Ans. Following are the features:
- It is genetic disorder inherited as autosomal recessive
- There is reduced activity of the enzyme – cystathionine beta synthetase
- Mental retardation
- Osteoporosis is common
- Ectopia lentis with displacement of lens downward (in Marfan's, lens is displaced upwards), glaucoma and impaired visual acquity may result
- Thrombotic episodes may occur
- Plasma methionine and homocysteine are raised and cysteine is low. The cyanide-nitroprusside test is positive.

An 18-year male presented with enlargement of breasts with scanty facial, axillary and pubic hairs (Fig. 1.46).

Fig. 1.46: Gynecomastia. A young adolescent male with bilateral gynecomastia

Q. What is the clinical diagnosis?

Ans. Bilateral gynecomastia.

Q. What is gynecomastia?

Ans. The enlargement of breast in the male like that of female is called *gynecomastia.*

Q. Why do you say it gynecomastia not pseudo-gynecomastia?

Ans. On palpation of the breast, glandular tissue is being felt which confirms the diagnosis of gynecomastia.

Q. What is differential diagnosis?

Ans. The differential diagnosis of gynecomastia is based on its cause, hence, following conditions are to be kept in mind in an adult patient:

1. Klinefelter's syndrome (testicular failure)
2. Cirrhosis of the liver
3. Thyrotoxicosis
4. Renal failure
5. Neoplasms (bronchogenic carcinoma, testicular carcinoma, hepatoma)
6. Drug-induced (spironolactone is the most common)
7. Idiopathic.

Q. What are the key points to be asked or seen in a patient with gynecomastia?

Ans. Following are the key points to be noted:
- Age of the patient
- History of taking drugs, mumps or castration or prostatic cancer in old persons

- Unilateral or bilateral
- Stature of the patient and look for eunuchoidism
- Palpate the breast tissue with fingers and then with flat of the hands to confirm glandular tissue
- Examine both the testes for size, consistency
- Look for secondary sexual characters, e.g. moustache, axillary and pubic hair
- Look for signs of chronic liver disease and hepatocellular failure
- Look for signs of superior mediastinal compression or tuberculosis or collapse of the lung
- Look for presence of leprosy

Q. What are the causes of gynecomastia?

Ans. Gynecomastia may be physiological or pathological resulting from imbalance between the circulating estrogens and androgens, i.e. either estrogen excess or androgen deficiency or insensitivity (Table 1.146).

Q. What are physiological causes of gynecomastia

Ans.
- Newborn
- Adolescence
- Old age

Q. Name the drugs causing gynecomastia.

Ans. Read the Table 1.146.

Table 1.146: Causes of gynecomastia

I. Estrogen excess
• Testicular or adrenal tumors (estrogen-secreting)
• Exogenous estrogens (estrogen use)
• Obesity
• Hereditary
II. Androgen deficiency
• *hCG producing tumor*, e.g. testes, liver,
• Endocrinopathies, e.g. hyperthyroidism, acromegaly, Cushing's syndrome, true hermaphroditism
• Miscellaneous, e.g. chronic illness, starvation/refeeding, cirrhosis of liver, renal failure, local trauma
• *Drugs*, e.g. spironolactone, oestrogen, digitalis, cimetidine, methyldopa, isoniazid, phenothiazines, diazepam, amphetamines, cytotoxic agents

Q. How will you evaluate a case with breast enlargement in a male?

Ans. Breast enlargement in a male may be due to enlargement of breast tissue (gynecomastia) or nonbreast fatty tissue (pseudogynecomastia). The clinical evaluation is depicted in Table 1.147.

Q. What are the causes of pseudogynecomastia?

Ans. Causes are:
- Fat deposition
- Neoplasm
- Neurofibromatosis
- Factitious

Table 1.147: Clinical evaluation of breast enlargement at different age groups

Newborn	Prepubertal onset	Pubertal onset		Postpubertal
		Genitalia		
		Normal	*Ambiguous*	
• Physiological bilateral gynecomastia	• Drugs • Idiopathic • Neoplasm (estrogen producing)	• Pubertal gynecomastia • Klinefelter's syndrome	• Mixed gonadal dysgenesis Androgen resistance • True hermaphroditism	• Testicular failure • Drug-induced • Cirrhosis liver • Thyrotoxicosis • CRF • Starvation/refeeding • Neoplasm • Idiopathic
• Exposure to estrogens				

Q. How would you investigate such a patient?

Ans. Investigations are done mainly to find out the cause i.e.

1. *Chest X-ray* for bronchogenic carcinoma or metastasis
2. *Plasma human chorionic gonadotrophin (hCG)-* detectable levels indicate testicular tumor or lung or liver neoplasm.
3. *Plasma testosterone and luteinising hormone (LH)* for the diagnosis of hypogonadism (Klinefelter's syndrome, etc.)
4. *Serum oestradiol* usually normal
5. *Other hormones* e.g.
   • Serum prolactin
   • Serum T3, T4, TSH for thyrotoxicosis
6. *Chromosomal analysis* for Klinefelter's syndrome

Q. How will treat a case with gynecomastia?

Ans. Treatment of gynecomastia is:

• Find out the underlying cause and treat it, i.e. treatment of leprosy, hepatocellular failure. If drug is the cause, withdraw it.

• Pubertal gynecomastia is painless, self-limiting, and disappears within 2 years.
• Therapy is indicated if gynecomastia causes pain, embarrassment and emotional discomfort
• Medical therapy with testosterone is indicated in androgen deficiency. Antiestrogen therapy with tamoxifen is indicated if estrogen excess is the cause
• Surgery (simple mastectomy or liposuction) is indicated if medical therapy fails or gynecomastia shows continued growth or for cosmetic and psychological reasons.

Q. What are the causes of feminization?

Ans. • Estrogen producing tumors
• Increased levels of estrogen as a result of cirrhosis of liver
• Increased extraglandular estrogen production (ectopic estrogen production).
• Relative increase in ratio of estrogen to androgens, e.g. testicular failure
• Drugs.

A young 20-year female presented with excessive hair growth on face and the body like a male (beard, moustache, chest) (Fig. 1.47).

Fig. 1.47: Hirsutism. A young female patient with beard (growth of hairs on chin)

Q. What is the clinical diagnosis?

Ans. Hirsutism

Q. What do you mean by hirsutism?

Ans. Hirsutism is defined as male pattern of hair growth in women.

Q. What important points have you asked on history?

Ans.
- Age of the patient
- Rate of progression of hirsutism
- History of thinning of scalp hair and deepening of voice
- History of obesity
- Drug history (corticosteroids, androgens, phenytoin, minoxidil, diazoxide, cyclosporine)
- Menstrual history, i.e. oligomenorrhea, infertility, acne, seborrhea, voice change, etc. suggest polycystic ovarian diseases an important case of hirsutism.
- Family history (familial).

Q. Where would you see for excessive growth of hair?

Ans.
- The sites include chin, sternum, upper abdomen and upper back.
- Terminal hair (excessive normal hair growth) can be seen normally on the arms, legs, periareolar area and tinea alba.

Q. Would you like to find out for the cause of hirsutism?

Ans. Yes, I would like to
- Record the BP.
- Look for the features for Cushing's syndrome.
- Look for the signs of virilization (receding hair line, muscular built, breast atrophy, clitoromegly)
- Examine the urine for sugar (diabetes)

Q. What is significance of menstrual history in this case?

Ans. If menstruation is normal, it indicates that there is no increase in testosterone production. However, if menstruation is abnormal, then cause of hirsutism is polycystic ovarian disease (POCD).

Q. What are the causes of hirsutism? What is virilization and defeminization?

Ans. Androgens are responsible for differential hair distribution in women. *Virilization* means androgen excess in women. It causes deepening of voice, temporal balding, acne, greasy skin, clitoromegaly, hirsutism and increased muscle mass. Therefore, hirsutism can be *without virilization, or with virilization* leading to diminishing female characters, e.g. decrease in breast size, loss of female body contours, amenorrhea causes are given in Table 1.148.

Table 1.148: Causes of hirsutism

• Cushing's syndrome	• Acromegaly
• Adrenal tumors	• Ovarian tumors
• Polycystic ovarian syndrome (mild)	• Congenital adrenal hyperplasia
• Drug induced	
• Familial	• Idiopathic
• Polycystic ovarian syndrome	

Note: Androgens in women are derived both from ovaries and adrenals as well as from peripheral conversion, hence, cause lies either in the ovary or adrenal

Q. How will you investigate such a case?

Ans. Following investigations are done:
1. *Serum androgens*
   Dihydroepianderosterone (DHEAS) >8000 ng/ml and serum testostterone >2 ng/ml suggest adrenal neoplasm or congenital adrenal hyperplasia
2. *Other hormones assay*, e.g. TSH, ACTH, cortisol, prolactin. A short ACTH stimulation test may be performed if needed for congenital adrenal hyperplasia.
3. *LH and FSH and their ratio.* The LH: FSH ratio >3:1 suggest polycystic ovarian disease.
4. *Glucose tolerance test (GTT) and insulin* levels for polycystic ovarian disease. This would help to establish insulin resistance that occurs in polycystic ovarian disease.

5. *USG* of ovaries for polycystic disease (10 or more ovarian cysts >2 mm in diameter, increased ovarian stroma and a thickened capsule suggest polycystic ovarian disease).

6. *Laparoscopy* and *biopsy* of the ovary for ovarian neoplasm

7. *CT scan* of adrenals for adrenal tumor.

Q. What is polycystic ovarian disease?

Ans. Polycystic ovarian disease, a severe form of which is called *Stein-Leventhal syndrome* is characterized by multiple ovarian cysts and excessive androgen production from the ovaries and adrenals.

The clinical features are:
- Symptoms onset immediate after menarche
- Ammenorrhea/oligomenorrhea
- Hirsutism or acne
- Obesity
- Mild virilization in severe cases
- Insulin resistance associated with menstrual irregularity, hypertension, hyperlipidemia
- The diagnosis is confirmed by typical ultrasonic findings and raised LH with normal or low FSH with LH: FSH ratio >3:1.

Q. What is pathophysiology of POCD?

Ans. It is due to an abnormality of pulsatile secretion of GnRH (gonodotrophin-releasing hormone) causing increased leutinizing hormone (LH) and follicle stimulating hormone (FSH) secretion. This results in hyperplasia of the ovarian theca cells leading to multiple follicular cysts formation and excessive androgen production and ovulation.

Q. What is relationship of body weight and hirsutism?

Ans. Hirsute women are more likely to be obese (POCD). Thus weight reduction must be priority in treating overweight women with hirsutism.

Q. What are other conditions associated with insulin resistance?

Ans. Besides polycystic ovarian disease, the other conditions are:
- Obesity
- Lipodystrophies
- Ataxia-telangiectasia
- Werner's syndrome
- Alstrome syndrome
- Pineal hyperplasia syndrome.

Q. How metabolism of glucose is affected POCD?

Ans. POCD is associated with insulin resistance and hyperinsulinemia which results in impaired glucose tolerance. The site of insulin resistance is skeletal muscles and adipose tissue and there is no hepatic resistance.

Q. What is treatment of impaired glucose tolerance (IGT) in POCD?

Ans.
- Life style modifications and weight reduction.
- Insulin sensitizers. e.g. metformin, pioglitazone (thiazolidinedione derivative)

Q. What is role of testosterone in hirsutism?

Ans. Testosterone is the most potent androgen and is directly derived from ovarian secretion and peripheral conversion of androstenedione. 98% of testosterone is bound and only 2% is free which can enter the target cells to produce androgen effect. In the skin, it is converted to dihydrotestosterone (DHT) which stimulates the hair follicles and cause hirsutism

Q. How will you proceed to treat such a case?

Ans. The treatment is as follows;
1. In case it is drug-induced, stop the offending drug. If it is due to a tumor, surgical removal is indicated.
2. Adrenal steroidogenic defects are treated with glucocorticoids to suppress excess ACTH and inhibit adrenal androgen secretion.
3. In idiopathic cases and in polycystic ovarian disease both cosmetic treatment (concealment or removal of hair from exposed skin areas) and suppression of androgen production or antagonism of its action by antiandrogens, e.g. cyproterone, flutamide, spironolactone, cimetidine and 5-alpha-reductase inhibitor (finasteride). GNRH analogs (leuprolide, nafarelin) have been found useful.
4. Local treatment. e.g. shaving, epilation, laser-assisted epilation, waxing, electrolysis, or bleaching

Q. Name the few drugs that produce hirsutism?

Ans. The drugs are:
- Phenytoin
- Androgens
- Psoralens
- Oral contraceptives
- Diazoxide
- Minoxidil

Q. What is adrenal virilization in female? What is its commonest cause?

Ans. Adrenal androgens excess resulting from excessive production of dihydroepiandrosterone and androstenedione get converted into testosterone and lead to virilization, hirsutism, acne and oligomenorrhea.

Congenital adrenal hyperplasia is the most common cause of virilization in female. It is characterized by excess of androgens with low or normal levels of glucocorticoids and mineralocorticoids.

CASE 48: GOITER

Perform General Physical Examination

Case Summaries

Case 1. (Fig 1.48A) An adult female is presented with swelling of the neck, irritation of throat, fever, myalgia and difficulty in swallowing. There was no history of weight gain, lethargy, slowness of activity.

Case 2. (Fig 1.48B) A young girl was brought by the mother with history of swelling in the neck. There was no other complaint on symptomatic enquiry.

Hashimoto's thyroiditis

Fig. 1.48A: Adult female with goiter

Puberty goiter

Fig. 1.48B: Adolescent girl with goiter

CASE 1

Q. **What is the diagnosis of Case 1?**

Ans. A 35 years female presenting with diffuse smooth enlargement of thyroid with fever and myalgia and no signs of thyroid underactivity or overactivity, my provisional diagnosis is goiter due to thyroiditis, may be Hashimoto's thyroiditis.

Q. **What important points would you ask on history from this patent?**

Ans.
- History of fever, myalgia, generalized body aches and pains
- H/o viral infection or congenital rubella syndrome
- H/o other autoimmune diseases, which have stronger association such as type 2 DM, Addison's disease, pernicious anemia and vitiligo.
- H/o chromosomal disorders, e.g Down's syndrome, Turner's syndrome
- H/o a high iodine intake (high iodine intake may increase the risk of autoimmune hypothyroidism by immunologic effects or direct thyroid toxicity).
- Ask for the features of hypothyroidism (Hashimoto's thyroiditis may be asymptomatic or may have features of subclinical or overt hypothyroidism)
- H/o deafness (dyshormogenetic goiter is associated with deafness called *Pendred's syndrome*)
- H/o depression
- H/o drug intake, e.g. lithium or iodine containing compounds

Q. **Describe the findings in your case?**

Ans. The patient is moderately built and well nourished with no anemia, pallor, jaundice, cyanosis and edema. Pulse is 68/min., regular and BP is 130/80 mm Hg right arm in sitting position.

Examination of Thyroid

Inspection

Thyroid is diffusely enlarged, encroaching on to the sternomastoids and suprasternal notch is full. The swelling moves with deglutition.

Palpation

- Thyroid is enlarged, surface is smooth, soft and rubbery in consistency and tender. Temperature over the thyroid is raised. There is no cervical lymphadenopathy.

Systemic Examination

CVS
CNS — Normal
Skin

Q. What is your differential diagnosis?

Ans. The differential diagnosis of this patient depends on the various types of nontoxic goiter.

1. *Diffuse nontoxic simple goiter:* This occurs in young girls at the age of puberty. It is defined as smooth enlargement of thyroid without any nodularity. It may be endemic (due to iodine deficiency) or nonendemic (sporadic) goiter. It is more common in women than men. It is not unusual particularly in iodine deficiency goiter, to find a low T4, normal T3 and TSH reflecting enhanced conversion of T4 to T3. TPO antibodies are not present. Ultrasound is generally not done but shows diffuse goiter without nodules.

2. *Nontoxic multinodular goiter:* It is also more common in women, incidence increases with age. It is also more common in iodine-deficient regions but also occurs in iodine sufficient regions. Examination reveals enlargement with nodularity of the thyroid gland which is firm in consistency and nontender. Most of these patients are asymptomatic and euthyroid. The MNG develops slowly over the years and is detected on routine physical examination or when an individual notices an enlargement in the neck. If goiter is large, patient may complain of compressive symptoms, i.e. stridor, dysphagia, hoarseness, suffusion of face, etc. USG can confirm the diagnosis and differentiates it from simple nontoxic goiter and Hashimoto's thyroiditis. Thyroid functions are normal. FNAC of nodule is indicated to exclude malignancy.

3. *Toxic multinodular goiter* (read a case discussion 49)

4. *Thyroid carcinoma:* Primary thyroid carcinoma is rare, occurs in old age, common in females. Follicular carcinoma is common in iodine deficiency area. Both differentiated carcinoma (papillary and follicular) present with solitary nodule, may spread to the regional lymph nodes (papillary) or may metastasize to other organs through blood stream (follicular). The thyroid is enlarged with single or multiple nodules which are firm to hard in consistency, may be fixed to the underlying structures.

   The diagnosis is confirmed by ultrasound, thyroid scanning and FNAC of the nodule. The thyroid function tests are usually normal.

5. *Acute suppurative thyroiditis or subacute viral thyroiditis:* Acute suppurative thyroiditis caused by bacteria (*S. aureus, Streptococcus,* and *Enterococcus*) and subacute caused by viruses (*mumps, Coxsackie, influenza, adenoviruses* and *echoviruses*) presents in adults with fever, myalgia, throat pain or thyroid pain which may radiate to ears and jaw. The thyroid gland is enlarged, palpable and tender on palpation. The temperature over thyroid is raised. Thyroid functions are usually normal. Patients of subacute thyroiditis may pass through three stages, i.e transient thyrotoxic phase, transient hypothyroid phase and recovery phase.

   The diagnosis of thyroiditis is suggested by raised ESR, C-reactive protein, leukocytosis, and low radioiodine uptake. Thyroid antibodies are negative. FNAC confirms the diagnosis.

Q. What is etiopathogenesis of Hashimoto's thyroiditis?

Ans. It is an autoimmune disorder caused by combination of genetic and environmental factors. What triggers autoimmunity is still not known. There is no convincing evidence for a role of infection (viral) in causation of this disease. Its strong association with HLA-DR3, DR4 and DR5 documents genetic influence over it. Its association with other autoimmune diseases (type 1 DM, pernicious anemia, vitiligo, Addison's disease), lymphocytic infiltration on histology and TPO antibodies confirms it to be an autoimmune disorder. Thyroid cell destruction is believed to be primarily mediated by CD8 + cytotoxic cells. In addition, local production of cytokines (i.e. TNF-α), IL-I and α-interferon may render the thyroid cells more susceptible to destruction. Antibodies to thyroglobulin (Tg) and TPO are useful marker of autoimmunity. In Hashimoto's thyroiditis, 20% patients have antibodies against. TSH-R (TSH receptors). These TSH-R blocking antibodies causes autoimmune hypothyroidism

Q. What other clinical conditions are associated with Hashimoto's thyroiditis?

Ans. I. *Endocrinal autoimmune diseases* i.e Addison's disease, Graves' disease, type 1 DM, hyperparathyroidism, ovarian failure.

 II. *Connective tissue diseases,* i.e. RA, SLE, Sjorgen's syndrome

 III. *Autoimmune GI disorder,* e.g. ulcerative colitis.

 IV. *Autoimmune hemolytic anemia* and pernicious anemia.

Q. How would investigate the patient?

1. *Complete blood count (leukocytosis),* ESR (raised) and C-reactive protein (present)

2. *Antimicrosomal (thyroid peroxidase-TPO antibodies)* Presence of TPO antibodies are diagnostic in 90 to 95% patients.

3. *RAIU studies:* They show low uptake. Usually these studies are not performed.
4. *FNAC:* In case of doubt, FNAC biopsy can be used to confirm the presence of autoimmune thyroiditis.
5. *Thyroid function tests:* They may be normal indicating euthyroid status or may be low indicating hypothyroid status of the patient.

Q. **What are histological characteristics of Hashimoto's thyroiditis?**

Ans. Histologically, it is characterized by:
- Marked lymphocytic infiltration of thyroid
- Atrophy of thyroid follicle.
- Oxyphil metaplasia, follicular cell hyperplasia.
- Absence of colloid
- Mild to moderate fibrosis. Severe fibrosis and absence of thyroid follicles indicate atrophic thyroiditis which leads to overt hypothyroidism with thyroid atrophy.

Q. **How would you treat such a case?**

Ans. *Thyroxine therapy:* It is indicated not only for hypothyroidism but also for goiter shrinkage. The dose of the thyroxine advised should be sufficient to suppress TSH to undetectable levels without inducing hyperthyroidism. The usual dose is 100-200 µg/day.

CASE 2

Q. **What is your clinical diagnosis and why?**

Ans. The clinical diagnosis is nontoxic (simple) goiter. Points in favor of the diagnosis are:
- Teenage girl (pubertal girl)
- Small goiter which is smooth
- Asymptomatic patient
- No evidence of toxic symptoms on examination.

Q. **What is your differential diagnosis?**

Ans. Read the differential diagnosis of Hashimoto's thyroiditis.

Q. **What are the differences between simple goiter and Hashimoto's thyroiditis?**

Ans. Read Table 1.76.

Q. **What is goiter and what are its causes?**

Ans. Any enlargement of thyroid is called *goiter*. The causes of goiter depending on the thyroid status are given below:

I. *Euthyroid goiter*
- Simple nontoxic goiter, puberty goiter, goiter during pregnancy
- Acute thyroiditis
- Multinodular nontoxic goiter.
- Malignancy of thyroid

II. *Goiter with hyperthyroidism*
- Graves' disease

- Solitary nodular toxic goiter
- Multinodular toxic goiter
- Thyroiditis with transient thyrotoxicosis

III. *Hypothyroidism with goiter*
- Hashimoto's thyroiditis
- Drug-induced goitrous hypothyroidism (lithium, amiodarone)
- Dyshormonogenetic goiter with nerve deafness (Pendred's syndrome).
- Postpartum thyroiditis.

Q. **How would you investigate such a case?**

Ans. Investigations to be done in simple goiter:
- Serum T3 and T4 – normal or low
- TSH levels – moderately elevated (10-30 mIU)

Patients are generally euthyroid except iodine deficiency goiter.

Q. **What is Jod-Basedow effect?**

Ans. The use of Lugol's iodine in iodine- deficient goiter and use of contrast agents and other iodine-containing preparations should be avoided for imaging nodular goiter, because of risk of Jod-Basedow effect which is characterized by enhanced hormone production by the hungry (Iodine deficient) thyroid or by autonomous nodules of nodular goiter.

Q. **What is postpartum thyroiditis (Fig 1.48C)?**

Ans. This is painless thyroid enlargement noted within 6 months of pregnancy which is attributed to modified maternal immune response during pregnancy that may unmask previously unrecognized subclinical autoimmune thyroid disease.

Fig. 1.48C: Postpartum thyroiditis without toxicity or hypothyroidism

Transient hyperthyroidism, hypothyroidism and hyperthyroidism followed by hypothyroidism have been observed in 5-10% of these women. These have antithyroid antibodies (TPO antibodies) in serum in early pregnancy. Most of these patients have asymptomatic goiter, have low to normal T4 and T3 with mildly elevated TSH. The diagnosis is confirmed by low radio-iodine uptake and FNAC of thyroid shows lymphocytic thyroiditis. Transient hyperthyroidism may be treated with beta blockers without any antithyroid antibodies and hypothyroidism may be treated with thyroxine. It tends to return in subsequent pregnancies and it ultimately leads to permanent hypothyroidism.

Q. What is sick euthyroid syndrome?

Ans. It is biochemical syndrome of normal thyroid (euthyroid) in which abnormalities of circulating TSH or thyroids hormone levels are seen in the absence of underlying thyroid disease. This syndrome is seen in any acute, severe illness and is attributed to hormonal changes induced by cytokines released in acute illness.

Warning: Routine testing of thyroids function should be avoided in acutely ill patients

The biochemical abnormities noted in sick euthryoid syndrome are:

1. *Low T3 syndrome:* This is most common hormone pattern in which T3 is low but T4 and TSH are normal. This is due to impaired peripheral conversion of T4 to T3, correlates with the severity of the illness.

2. *Low T4 syndrome:* Very sick patients may exhibit fall in total T4 and T3 levels. Free T4 and T3 (FT4 and FT3) levels are normal in such patients indicating altered binding of T4 and T3 to TBG.

3. *Fluctuations in TSH levels:* The TSH levels fluctuates from decreased to increased levels (<0.1 to 20 mIU/L) due to variations in T3 and T4 levels.

The diagnosis of sick euthyroid syndrome is arbitrary, is considered when abnormal and normal levels occur in the absence of thyroid disease. Measurement of reversed T3 (rT3) together with unbound hormones (FT3 and FT4) and TSH can help in the diagnosis, if there is documentation of provious acute illness and medications taken for it.

Treatment is controversial. Most authorities believe monitoring of these cases only as thyroid functions return to normal following recovery from acute illness.

The patient presented with a swelling in the neck (Fig. 1.49) which was slowing increasing. There was history of palpitation and sweating with no H/o diarrhea. There was hoarseness of voice and dysphasia.

Fig. 1.49: A patient with multinodular goiter

Examine the Patient

Q. What is your clinical diagnosis?
Ans. In view of multinodular goiter with toxic symptoms, my provisional diagnosis is multinodular toxic goiter.

Q. What are points in favor of your diagnosis?
Ans. • An elderly male.
• Slow onset and progressive thyroid enlargement
• Nodular enlargement of thyroid.
• Presence of toxic symptoms, e.g. palpitations, sweating, nervousness, tremors, etc.
• Presence of atrial fibrillation, e.g. irregularly irregular pulse.
• Compressive symptoms:
   – Horseness of voice
   – Dysphagia

Q. Describe your clinical findings?
Ans.

Inspection of Neck

• Lower part of the neck is full, thyroid is enlarged and suprasternal notch is full
• Swelling moves with deglutition

Palpation

• Thyroid is enlarged, nodular, firm in consistency, nontender.

• Temperature of thyroid is raised. Thyroid is not fixed to underlying or overlying structure
• There is no cervical lymphadenopathy

Auscultation

• A bruit may be heard but is absent in this case.

Examination for Toxic Symptoms

• Pulse rate is increased, it is irregularly irregular
• BP is 170/70 mm Hg, right arm in lying down position
• Extremities are warm and moist
• Fine tremors are present on outstretched hands
• Eye signs are not present

Systemic Examination

• CVS shows tachycardia, heart rate may be irregular
• Nervous system: Tendon reflexes are normal. No muscle weakness.

Q. What important points would you ask on history in such a case?
Ans. Following points will be asked on history:
   1. Onset and progression
   2. H/o stridor (for tracheal compression)
   3. Hoarseness of voice due to compression of recurrent laryngeal nerve
   4. Dysphagia due to esophageal compression.
   5. Suffusion of face due to superior mediastinal compression by substernal goiter.
   6. Acute painful enlargement due to bleeding in a nodule
   7. Deafness (8th nerve involvement suggest Pendred's syndrome)
   8. Symptoms of hyper- or hypothyroidism
   9. History of missing of beats

Q. What is your differential diagnosis?
Ans. All other conditions in which thyroid swellings are present, come into its differential diagnosis such as:
   1. **Follicular epithelial cyst adenomas (colloid, simple, embryonal, onchocystic):** These lesions are common in 5-10% adults and are detected on ultrasound. About one-third of these patients have palpable nodules which are thyroid cysts (soft to cystic and smooth contour). They are recognized easily as cysts on USG and yield large amount of pink or straw coloured fluid on aspiration. Many swellings are mixed cystic/solid lesions. FNAC of these lesions must be done to rule out malignancy.
   2. **Multinodular thyroid carcinoma:** Malignant tumors (papillary or follicular) produce firm to

hard palpable nodules, which are fixed to the underlying or overlying structures due to local tumor invasion. There may also be cervical lymphadenopathy. Tumor may metastasise into other organs. These patients do not have symptoms and signs of thyrotoxicosis. Some cases may have hypothyroidism. Diagnosis is established by USG, FNAC, thyroid scan and RAIU.

3. **Nontoxic multinodular goiter:** It is more common in women, occurs commonly in iodine deficient area (hilly areas). Thyroid is enlarged with multiple painless nodules of various sizes. Thyroid is nontender and there is no audible bruit. Sudden pain in the thyroid region indicates hemorrhage into one of the nodule. Toxic symptoms are absent. It grows slowly and slowly, produces compressive symptoms (stridor, dysphagia, hoarseness, suffusion of the face etc). The diagnosis is confirmed by nodular goiter on USG with normal thyroid functions. CT scan/MRI may be done to exclude sternal extension which is often greater than apparent on clinical examination.

Q. What are the differences between Graves' disease and multinodular toxic goiter?

Ans. Read Table 1.72 (Case discussion on thyrotoxicosis).

Q. Why is it not a case of Graves' disease?

Ans. In Graves' disease, goiter is diffuse, smooth, not nodular but sometimes nodularity may occur. Eye signs, dermatopathy and thyroid bruit are common. Compressive symptoms are rare. In my case, compressive symptoms are prominent with no evidence of eye signs, bruit over thyroid not present.

Q. What is the status of thyrotoxicosis in MNG?

Ans. Thyrotoxicosis once developed in MNG is permanent and there are no spontaneous remissions. This is the reason that antithyroid drug therapy is not effective in toxic MNG on long-term basis.

Q. How would you investigate such a case?

Ans. 1. *Ultrasonography* of thyroid to confirm the nodularity.
2. *Thyroid hormone assay* (FT3, FT4, TSH) to identify those case with subclinical or overt hyperthyroidism.
3. *Radioisotope scanning* to know the status of nodules, i.e. hot or cold. Hot nodules go in favor of toxic goiter while cold nodules indicate non-toxic multinodular goiter.
4. *CT/MRI* is done to explore the substernal extension of multinodular goiter which may not be apparent clinically or when features of compression are present.

5. *Fine needle aspiration cytology* (FNAC) for cold nodules to explore possibility of malignancy.

Q. What is common arrhythmia in toxic MGN?

Ans. Atrial fibrillation.

Q. How would you treat such a case?

Ans. • Beta-blockers to control thyrotoxicosis
• Anticoagulant (warfarin) in atrial fibrillation.
• Radio-iodine for hyperthyroidism.
• Subtotal thyroidectomy, if patient is either not fit for radio-iodine treatment or refuses to take radio-iodine.

Q. What are treatment modalities available for toxic MNG?

Ans. The treatment options are:

1. **Antithyroid drugs:** Antithyroid drugs in combination with beta-blockers can normalize thyroid function and address clinical features of thyrotoxicosis. The drug therapy is indicated in all patients with small goiter, before surgery, valuable before and after radioiodine treatment in elderly patients and long-term treatment with drugs is indicated when other therapies cannot be used. This treatment, often enlarges the growth of the goiter and spontaneous remissions do not occur, therefore, adverse effect of the drug therapy, i.e. osteoporosis, agranulocytosis are more likely to occur with long-term treatment.

2. **Surgery:** Surgery provides definite treatment of multinodular toxic goiter, hence, is gold standard treatment. It is indicated for large goiters with or without compressive symptoms and for substernal goiter. Disadvantages include mortality and morbidity, hypothyroidism, persistence or recurrence of hyperthyroidism.

3. **Radio-iodine:** It is an appealing option for majority of the patients who have completed their family, in elderly patients and patients with cardiopulmonary disease. It is highly effective to treat areas of autonomy as well as to decrease the mass of goiter and reverses hyperthyroidism. The disadvantages include more than one dose may be required and there are increased risks of hypothyroidism and radiation-induced cancer.

Q. When would you treat nontoxic multinodular goiter?

Ans. Nontoxic multinodular goiter requires treatment only when:
i. There are compressive symptoms.
ii. Goiter is retrosternal or has intrathoracic extension.
iii. Neck discomfort or cosmetic issues.

Q. What factors would you keep in mind before referring the patient to radio-iodine therapy?

Ans. 1. Age and sex
2. Diagnosis
3. Severity of hyperthyroidism.
4. Presence of other medical conditions
5. Pregnancy or desire to conceive
6. Response of thyrotoxicosis to drug therapy
7. Access to radio-iodine (I^{131}), i.e. facility of radio-active ablation
8. Patient and doctors preference.

Q. What is a hot nodule and what is a cold nodule? What is their significance?

Ans. The hot and cold nodules are the terms relatively used during RAIU studies and thyroid scanning, implies the tracer uptake by the area of nodule. The *hot nodule* is a focal area of increased uptake, indicates hyperactive nodule; the *cold nodule* is an area of decreased tracer uptake and suggests inactive or nonfunctioning area. Therefore, hot or cold state of nodule indicates its functional status.

The functional features of thyroid nodules have some prognostic significance. So called 'Cold nodules" which have diminished uptake are usually benign but become malignant (5-10%) after sometime while 'hot nodules' are almost never malignant.

Q. What is the usefulness of USG in thyroid disorders?

Ans. USG of thyroid is useful:
- To assess the size, shape and nodularity of thyroid
- In case of nodularity, it is useful to monitor the nodular size.
- To guide FNAC biopsies
- For the aspiration of cystic lesions.

Neurological Diseases

A young female (Fig. 1.50) presented with asymmetry of face, difficulty in closing the eye with dribbling of saliva from angle of the mouth on left side of face. The episode occurred following sudden exposure to cold wind in the morning. Examination revealed flattening of nasolabial fold on left side of face with inability to close the left eye. Patient could not make furrows over her forehead on the left side.

Fig. 1.50: Bell's palsy (idiopathic 7th cranial nerve infranuclear paralysis on left side)

Q. What is your clinical diagnosis?

Ans. All the above features suggest infranuclear 7th nerve palsy probably Bell's palsy on left side.

Q. What important points have you asked on history in this case?

Ans.
1. Onset whether acute followed by worsening over the next day (Bell's palsy).
2. Pain preceding or accompanying the weakness (Bell's palsy).
3. Time of paralysis. Paralysis occurs in the morning in most of the cases.
4. Difficult in closing the eye and watering of the eye.
5. Ask asymmetry of the face as face is pulled to one side.
6. Drooling of the saliva and repeated clearing of the mouth with handkerchief.
7. Disturbance of taste (involvement of fibers of chorda tympani).

8. Hyperacusis (involvement of the nerve to stapedius).

Q. How would you proceed to examine such a case?

Ans. *Inspection of face*
- Look facial expression, e.g. it is lost in Bell's palsy.
- Widened palpebral fissure on the involved side.
- Flattened nasolabial fold on the affected side.
- Drooling of saliva on the side involved and mouth on the affected side drops
- Look of the external auditory meatus for herpes zoster (*Ramsay Hunt syndrome*).

Examination
- Read the various tests for 7th nerve examination from the clinical methods in medicine by Prof SN Chugh
- In addition:
  - Examine for taste
  - Check for hearing
  - Examine the tymphanic membrane for otitis media.
- Test the urine for sugar (diabetes).

Q. What reflexes would you test for facial nerve?

Ans.
- Corneal reflex
- Palmomental reflex
- Sucking reflex

Read these reflexes from clinical methods in medicine by Prof SN Chugh.

Q. What is Bell's palsy?

Ans. It is an acute infranuclear (LMN type) palsy of 7th cranial (facial) nerve involving all the muscles of face. The cause is unknown (idiopathic) though a viral etiology is suspected. The lesion is nonsuppurative inflammation or oedema of the nerve at the level of stylomastoid foramen, hence, lacrimation and taste sensation are not reduced. Hyperacusis does not occur.

Q. What is Bell's phenomenon?

Ans. An attempt to close the involved eye by the patient with Bell's palsy producing rolling of the eyeball upwards, is called *Bell's phenomenon.*

Q. What are the differences between supranuc-lear (UMN) and infranuclear (LMN) 7th cranial nerve palsy?

Ans. Read "clinical methods in medicine" by Dr SN Chugh. In LMN paralysis, the whole half of the face on the affected side is involved. In UMN palsy, upper half of the face is spared and only lower half is involved.

229

Q. How will you localize the lesion in infranuclear 7th cranial nerve paralysis?

Ans. In a lower motor neuron facial paralysis, it is important to obtain a history of diplopia, lacrimation, hyperacusis and taste sensation to localise the level of the lesion (Table 1.149).

Table 1.149: Localization of lesion in facial nerve paralysis.

Site of lesion	Features
A. Stylomastoid foramen (Bell's palsy)	A. Paralysis of all muscles of facial expression only.
B. Facial canal (chorda tympani branch is involved)	B. Features described above (A) *plus* loss of taste sensation from anterior two-thirds of tongue
C. A higher lesion in facial canal (nerve to stapedius is damaged)	C. Features described above in A plus hyperacusis
D. Geniculate ganglion	D. In addition to features of A, there is loss of lacrimation and salivation. 8th nerve may also be involved
E. In pons	E. 6th and 7th cranial nerve palsy (Millard–Gubler syndrome)
F. Cerebellopontine angle	F. The facial nerve, 8th cranial nerve and nervus inter-medius involved

Q. What are the causes of facial nerve palsy?

Ans. The facial paralysis may be supranuclear (UMN type), nuclear and infranuclear (LMN type). The causes are enlisted in Table 1.150. The most common causes are put in the box within the table.

Q. What is Ramsay Hunt syndrome?

Ans. It is herpetic infection of geniculate ganglion. It is characterised by:
- Fever with headache, bodyache
- Herpetic vesicles/rash on the tympanic membrane, external auditory meatus and pinna.
- Loss of taste in anterior two-thirds of the tongue
- Hyperacusis on the affected side
- LMN type of ipsilateral facial nerve palsy.

Q. Is facial nerve a motor or a sensory or a mixed nerve?

Ans. It is a mixed nerve. Motor part supplies all muscles concerned with facial expression and the stapedius muscle; sensory part which is small, carries sensation of taste from the anterior two-third of the tongue and cutaneous impulses from the anterior wall of the external auditory meatus/canal.

Q. What are branches of facial nerve?

Ans.
- Motor branches supply to muscles of face after exit from the stylomastoid foramen
- Secretory nerve, i.e. greater superficial petrosal nerve supplies lacrimal, nasal and parotid glands
- Chorda tympani supplies taste to anterior two-thirds of tongue, submaxillary and submandibular glands
- Nerve to stapedius muscle

Table 1.150: Causes of facial nerve paralysis

A. Unilateral palsy
I. Supranuclear paralysis
- CVA (Stroke, hemiplegia)
- Neoplasm
- Demyelinating diseases, e.g. multiple sclerosis

II. Nuclear paralysis
- Brainstem infarction and neoplasm
- Poliomyelitis

III. Infranuclear paralysis
a. *Intracranial involvement*
- Cerebellopontine angle tumor (e.g. acoustic neuroma, meningioma)
- Meningitis
- Meningovascular syphilis
- Fracture of temporal bone
- Otitis media
- Herpes zoster infection of geniculate ganglion (Ramsay Hunt syndrome)
- Glomus jugulare tumor

b. *Extracranial involvement*
- Hansen's disease (leprosy)
- Mixed parotid tumors
- Sarcoidosis
- Bell's palsy (it is the most common)

B. Bilateral palsy
I. Supranuclear
- Cerebral atherosclerosis (common)
- Double hemiplegia
- Pseudobulbar palsy

II. Infranuclear and nuclear
- Acute Guillain-Barre syndrome (most common)
- Leprosy
- Sarcoidosis (common)
- Leukemia or lymphoma
- Forceps delivery
- Bilateral Bell's palsy
- Bilateral otitis media
- Myasthenia gravis

Common causes of unilateral 7th have palsy

UMN palsy	LMN paralysis
• CVA (stroke hemiplegia)	• Bell's (idiopathic) palsy
• Neoplasm	• Herpes zoster
• Multiple sclerosis	• Cerebella pentane angle tumor
• Parotid tumor	
• Otitis media	

Q. **How will you diagnose bilateral UMN type of 7th nerve paralysis?**

Ans. In bilateral supranuclear palsy, the upper part of face is not spared (i.e. total face is paralysed), hence, there will be:
- Mask like face
- Emotion preserved
- Exaggerated jaw jerk
- Absence of Bell's phenomenon
- Glabellar tap is positive
- Double hemiplegia (long tracts signs on both the sides).

Q. **What are the complications of Bell's palsy?**

Ans. Following are the complications:
- Exposure keratitis and corneal ulceration
- Hemifacial spasms
- Crocodile tears
- Social stigma

Q. **What is relationship between diabetes and Bell's palsy?**

Ans. Diabetes and impaired glucose tolerance are commonly associated with Bell's palsy

Q. **What is Mobius' syndrome?**

Ans. It consists of congenital bilateral facial palsy associated with 3rd and 6th nerve palsies.

Q. **What are crocodile tears?**

Ans. Watering of the eye (lacrimation) on the paralysed side during chewing is called *"Crocodile tears"*. These are due to aberrant re-innervation of the lacrimal gland by fibers originally meant for the salivary gland.

Q. **What is hemifacial spasm?**

Ans. Hemifacial spasm is characterized by the narrowing of the palpebral fissure on the affected side and pulling of the angle of the mouth due to contraction of facial muscles. The spasms may be *post-paralytic* or "essential". The pathogenesis is compression of the facial nerve by loops of cerebellar arteries or by AVM (arteriovenous malformation), or aneurysm or a cerebellopontine angle tumor.

Q. **How will you manage a case with Bell's palsy?**

Ans. Management of Bell's palsy includes:
1. NSAIDs for inflammation and relief of pain.
2. A short course of steroids (40-60 mg of prednisolone for few days then tapered over next 2-3 weeks) is given to reduce edema around the nerve.
3. Physiotherapy: massage, electrical stimulation, splint to prevent drooping of the lower part of the face
4. Protection of the eye with lubricating eyedrops and a patch during sleep.
5. If no improvement occurs within 6 weeks, the surgical decompression at the stylomastoid foramen is advised.
6. Facial exercises in front of a mirror are advised.
7. Acyclovir plus prednisolone is more effective in improving volitional muscle activity and in preventing partial nerve degeneration as compared to prednisolone treatment.

Q. **What is mimic facial nerve palsy?**

Ans. Mimic palsy refers to preservation of voluntary movements but the emotional movements of the facial muscles are lost. This is seen in frontal lobe lesion. It is due to the fact that UMN fibers for emotion have a different course than the pyramidal tract.

CASE 51: THIRD NERVE PALSY VS HORNER'S SYNDROME

Perform General Physical Examination

The patient in picture presented with dropping of left upper lid (narrow palpebral fissure) and diplopia in all directions except lateral gaze. These was no history of headache, hypertension, weakness of any past of the body. There was history of type 2 DM. Examination revealed isolated 3rd never palsy/paralysis (Fig. 1.51A)

Fig. 1.51A: Left third nerve palsy in a 40 yr female

Q. What is your clinical diagnosis?
Ans. Left third cranial nerve palsy due to diabetes.

Q. What would you ask on history in this patient?
Ans. *Ask for the following:*
- Is there absence of sweating on one side of the face.
- H/o migraine
- H/o cervical sympathectomy
- H/o lung cancer
- H/o diabetes, hypertension

Examine
- Look for ptosis (complete, incomplete)
- Is ptosis unilateral or bilateral?
- Look at the size of pupil (dilated or constricted).
- Test the extraocular muscles
- Is eyeball sunken, normal or prominent?
- Elicit the light reflex

- Look for scar of cervical sympathectomy
- Examine neck for cervical lymph nodes
- Tracheal shift (pan coast tumor)
- Aneurysm of aorta or carotids
- Nervous system for motor or sensory involvement

Q. Why do you say third nerve palsy?
Ans. All the signs of 3rd nerve palsy are present, i.e.
- Unilateral ptosis
- Dilated pupil slowly or incompletely reacting to light (e.g. paralysis of constrictor of pupil) on left side
- Paralysis of accommodation (paralysis of ciliary muscle)
- Paralysis of the movement due to weakness of muscles supplied by 3rd nerve.
- Position of the eye is down and out called paralytic squint (4th and 6th clinical nerves are intact).
- Diplopia on lateral gaze.

Q. What are the ocular muscles supplied by 3rd nerve?
Ans.
- Superior and inferior recti
- Medial rectus.
- Inferior oblique

Q. How would you test superior oblique muscle?
Ans. Superior oblique is supplied by trochlear (4th cranial) nerve which intorts the eye (SIN). Tilt the head of the patient to same side—the affected eye will intort if 4th nerve (superior oblique) is intact.

Q. Name few common causes of third cranial nerve paralysis?
Ans.
- Hypertension
- Multiple sclerosis
- Trauma
- Ophthalmoplegic migraine
- Tumor (parasellar neoplasm), meningioma, carcinoma at base of skull)
- Diabetes
- Aneurysm of posterior communicating artery (painful ophthalmoplegia)
- Encephatitis, basal meningitis
- Collagen vascular disorders.

Q. When would you suspect a lesion of third nerve nucleus?
Ans. It is suspected under two conditions:
i. Unilateral third nerve palsy, with contralateral superior rectus palsy and bilateral partial ptosis.
ii. Bilateral third nerve palsy (with or without internal ophthalmoplegia associated with spared elevator function)

Q. Name the movements of eyes and muscles involved.

Ans.

Movement of eye	Muscle	Cranial nerve
Adduction	Medial rectus	3rd cranial
Abduction	Lateral rectus	6th cranial
Elevation of abducted eye	Inferior rectus	3rd cranial
Depression of abducted eye	Inferior rectus	–do–
Elevation of abducted eye	Inferior oblique	–do–
Depression the adducted eye	superior oblique	4th cranial

Q. Name the syndromes associated with 3rd cranial nerve paralysis?

Ans. It can easily be remembered by the word WBC (Weber's, Benedict's and Claude's) syndrome

Syndrome	Features	Site of lesion
1. *Weber's syndrome*	• Ipsilaleral 3rd nerve palsy • Contralateral hemiplegia	Midbrain
2. *Benedict's syndrome*	• Ipsilateral 3rd nerve palsy • Contralateral involuntary movements	Red nucleus in midbrain
3. *Claude's syndrome*	• Ipsilateral 3rd nerve palsy • Contralateral ataxia, tremors.	Both red nucleus and 3rd nerve in midbrain

Q. Name the condition when eyeball is fixed (no movement).

Ans. Paralysis of all the three ocular cranial nerves (3rd, 4th and 6th)

Q. How would you test 3rd nerve?

Ans. Read clinical methods in medicine by Prof SN Chugh

Q. Examine the eye of the patent in picture (Fig. 1.51B). What is your diagnosis?

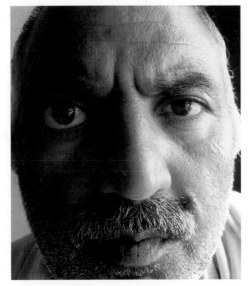

Fig. 1.51B: Horner's syndrome. There is pseudoptosis

Ans. Horner's syndrome or congenital ptosis. There is pseudoptosis without any deviation of the eyeball and there is no dilatation of pupil.

Q. What is Horner's syndrome? How does it differ form 3rd nerve palsy?

Ans. It is due to involvement of cervical sympathetic trunk. Its characteristic and differentiating features are given below.

Horner's syndrome	Third cranial nerve palsy
• Incomplete ptosis (pseudoptosis)	Complete ptosis
• No squint, no diplopic	Squint and diplopic present
• Eyeball is in center	It is deviated down and out
• Meosis	Mydriasis
• Loss of sweating	No loss of sweating
• Light reflex intact	Light reflex lost
• Eyeball sunken (enophthalmos)	Normal eyeball
• Ciliospinal reflex lost	In tact
• No extraocular muscle paralysis	Extraocular muscle paralysis present

Q. Name few common causes of Horner's syndrome?

Ans. It could be due to central or peripheral lesion.

Central causes	Peripheral causes
• *Mid brain lesion*, e.g.	Involvement of cervical sympathetic
• Vascular, Demy-elination	Enlarged lymph nodes Aortic aneurysm/carotid aneurysm
• *Medullary* lesion, e.g. lateral medullary syndrome	Pancoast's tumor Cervical sympathectomy

Q. How would decide whether lesion is above or below the superior cervical ganglion in the neck?

Ans. It is decided as per table below:

Test	Above superior ganglion	Below the superior ganglion
Sweating	No effect on sweating	Sweating is lost over the entire neck, arm and upper trunk. Lesions in the lower neck affect sweating over the entire face
Cocaine 4% in both eyes	• Dilates the normal pupil	Dilates both pupils
Adrenaline (1:1000) both eyes	• No effect on normal eye	• No effect on both eyes

Q. What is congenital Horner's syndrome?

Ans. Congenital Horner's syndrome has heterochromia of iris in addition to other features of Horner's syndrome.

Q. Which feature differentiates the central from peripheral lesion in Horner's syndrome?

Ans. Sweating is lost over entire half of head, arm and upper trunk in central lesion.

Q. **What is the cause of intermittent ptosis?**

Ans. Migraine

Q. **What is cavernous sinus thrombosis? What are its features?**

Ans. Cavernous sinus lies on each side on sphenoid bone. It contains cranial nerves (3rd, 4th and 6th), spinal nucleus of 5th nerve, ophthalmic vessels and cervical sympathetic. It is involved due to infection, thrombosis and carotid artery aneurysm. The features on the side involved are:
- Chemosis, proptosis
- 3rd, 4th and 6th cranial nerve palsies
- Horner's syndrome
- Loss of sensation over face

Q. **What is difference between supernuclear and infranuclear 3rd, 4th and 6 nerve palsies.**

Ans. Supranuclear palsies of 3rd, 4th, 6th nerves produces gaze paralysis while infranuclear palsy produces paralysis of extraocular muscles and reflex activity of the eye.

Q. **What are the causes of ptosis?**

Ans. The causes are:

Unilateral ptosis	Bilateral ptosis
• Third nerve palsy	• Myasthenia gravis
• Horner's syndrome	• Dystrophic myotonia
• Myasthenia gravis	• Ocular or oculopharyngeal
• Congenital	• Mitochondrial dystrophy
• Idiopathic	• Tabs dorsalis
	• Congenital
	• Bilateral Horner's syndrome (Syringomyelia)
	• Snake bite (Scorpion bite)

Q. **What is the difference between ptosis and pseudoptosis?**

Ans. Read Clinical Methods in Medicine by Dr SN Chugh.

The patient (Fig. 1.52) complained of diplopia on seeing to the left. She complained that she has to close the left eye to prevent diplopia. BP was 180/100 mm Hg. No H/o deafness.

Fig. 1.52: Sixth cranial nerve palsy

Examine Cranial Nerves

Q. What is your clinical diagnosis?

Ans. The patient has left 6th cranial nerve palsy probably due to hypertension.

Q. What important points would you ask on history?

Ans. *Ask for the followings:*
- H/o diplopia (double vision)
- Patient may complain that she/he has to rotate the head towards the involved side to produce single image.
- Patient may give history of closing the involved eye (left) to prevent diplopia
- Any history of deafness
- History of diabetes, hypertension

Q. How would you proced to examine such a case?

Ans. Examination of the left eye
- The eye is deviated medially
- There is failure of lateral movement on attempted abduction.
- The diplopia occurs on lateral gaze. The two images are parallel and separated in the horizontal direction. The outer image is from the affected eye which disappears when the eye is covered.
- Check BP. Examine optic fundus.
- Test for corneal sensation
- Test for deafness.

Q. What are common causes of the 6th nerve palsy?

Ans. Causes are:
- Hypertension
- Diabetes
- Multiple sclerosis
- Encephalitis
- Raised intracranial pressure (false localizing sign)
- Basal meningitis
- Acoustic neuroma, nasopharyngeal carcinoma

Q. What is the course of 6th cranial nerve in the brain?

Ans. The course is lengthy, that is the reason that it is involved in raised intracranial pressure. After its origin in the pons, it comes out at lower border of pons, then passes upwards over the apex of the petrous temporal bone and joins 3rd and 4th cranial nerves in cavernous sinus. It enters along with 3rd and 4th nerves into the orbit through superior orbital fissure. It can be involved:
- In the pons (nuclear lesion)
- Outside the pons (infranuclear lesion) at lower pons, at petrous temporal bone, in cavernous sinus and in the orbit.

Q. Where is the nucleus of 6th cranial nerve? What is its relation with 7th nerve?

Ans. Nucleus is in the pons. The fibres of 7th cranial nerve loop around the 6th cranial nerve nucleus in the lower pons.

Q. Name the structures that lies in close proximity to 6th cranial nerve nucleus and its fascicles?

Ans.
- Facial and trigeminal nerves (5th, 6th and 7th nerve nuclei lie in pons)
- Pyramidal tract (corticospinal tracts)
- Median longitudinal fasciculus (MLF)
- Parapontine reticular formation.

Q. What is Gradinego's syndrome?

Ans. It involves 5th, 6th cranial nerves and greater superficial petrosal nerve due to inflammation of the tip of temporal bone. It is characterized by:
- Unilateral 6th nerve palsy
- Pain in distribution of first division of 5th cranial nerve
- Excessive lacrimation.

Q. What are the causes of nuclear involvement of 6th cranial nerve?

Ans. As the 6th cranial nerve nucleus lies in the pons in relation to other structures, hence, nuclear involvement is associated with involvement of other structures also.
1. *Raymond's syndrome*
   - Ipsilateral 6th nerve paralysis
   - Contralateral paresis of extremities
2. *Millard-Gubler syndrome*
   - Ipsilateral 6th and 7th nerve palsies
   - Contralateral hemiplegia (crossed hemiplegia)
3. *Foville's syndrome*
   - All features of Millard-Gubler syndrome
   - Paralysis/palsy of lateral conjugate gaze

Q. Name other syndrome associated with 6th cranial nerve involvement?

Ans. *Mobius syndrome* (Read third nerve palsy)
Gehardt's syndrome
- Bilateral 6th nerve palsy

Q. What is Tolosa-Hunt syndrome?

Ans. It has seen attributed to inflammation of cavernous sinus and is characterized by:
- Unilateral recurrent pain in retroorbital region
- Extraocular muscles paralysis (3rd, 4th and 6th cranial nerve involvement)
- Vth cranial nerve involvement

Q. How would you investigate such a case?

Ans.
1. Urine and blood sugar for diabetes
2. X-ray of skull including orbit
3. CT scan/MRI brain for encephalic or meningitis or any other vascular lesion and for raised ICP.
4. Audiometry for hearing loss.

A 35 years male (Fig. 1.53A) presented with headache, generalized in nature occurring commonly during morning hours on getting up. There was history of projectile vomiting and blurring of vision. There was history of convulsions but no focal neurological deficit. Examination revealed bilateral 6th nerve palsy and papilledema. There was no disturbance in consciousness. All the reflexes were exaggerated. Sensory system was normal. No neck stiffness was detected. The CT scan of the patient is displayed (Fig. 1.53B).

Fig. 1.53A: Patient with raised intracranial pressure

Fig.1.53B: CT scan showing dilated ventricular system. The (↑) arrow indicates the causative lesion

Q. What is your probable diagnosis and why?

Ans. The persistent morning headache with projectile vomiting and papilledema in a young male with no localizing sign and no net neurological deficit suggest the diagnosis of raised intracranial tension the cause of which has to be found out.

Q. What is normal ICP?

Ans. Normal intracranial pressure within cranial cavity measured indirectly is 5-10 mm Hg. Any ICP above 15 mm Hg is taken as raised intracranial pressure.

Nowadays ICP can be measured directly by devices implanted in the lateral ventricle or intraparenchymal placement.

Q. What is benign raised intracranial tension?

Ans. The term benign or idiopathic raised intracranial pressure is used to signify increased intracranial pressure (ICP) produced by diffuse swelling of brain and characterized by a triad of symptoms (headache, vomiting, papilledema) and dilated ventricular system. The CSF pressure is raised but CSF analysis is normal. Neuroimaging is normal except dilated ventricles. The other terms used for this condition are:

- Otitic hydrocephalus
- Pseudotumor cerebri
- Serous meningitis

N.B. Benign intracranial hypertension is diagnosed by exclusion of all other causes that produce raised ICP.

Q. What is hydrocephalus?

Ans. The term *hydrocephalus* (*hydro* means excess of water, *cephalus* means head) implies dilatation of the ventricles of brain due to excessive accumulation of CSF. It may be associated with raised, normal or low ICP. Raised ICP with hydrocephalus is called *hypertensive hydrocephalus.*

Q. What are the causes of raised intracranial tension or hydrocephalus?

Ans. All the cases of hydrocephalus have increased intracranial pressure except normal pressure hydrocephalus. Raised ICP results either due to excessive production of CSF or obstruction to circulation or impaired absorption of cerebrospinal fluid in the brain. The causes of hydrocephalus and increased intracranial pressure are more or less same (Table 1.151).

Table 1.151: Causes of raised intracranial pressure (ICP) or hydrocephalus

I. *Congenital obstruction*
- Arnold-Chiari malformation
- Aqueductal stenosis
- Dandy-Walker syndrome
- Agenesis of arachnoid villi

Contd... 237

II. *Trauma to head (head injuries)*
III. *Infections*
  - Bacterial meningitis (tubercular, pyogenic)
  - Encephalitis
  - Cerebellar abscess
IV. *Intracranial bleed*
  - Cerebral hemorrhage
  - Subarachnoid hemorrhage
  - Hypertensive encephalopathy
V. *Space occupying lesions*
  - Brain tumors, e.g. craniopharyngioma, medulloblastoma, astrocytoma, ependymoma, metastases
VI. *Venous obstruction*
  - Cortical thrombophlebitis
  - Dural sinus thrombosis
VII. *Benign (idiopathic)*
  Read the causes of BIH as already discussed

Q. What are the causes of benign intracranial hypertension (BIH)?

Ans. A variety of conditions are known to produce BIH such as:
  - Hypervitaminosis A
  - Hypoparathyroidism
  - Prolonged steroid therapy
  - Addison's disease
  - Severe anemia
  - Pregnancy
  - Middle-aged female with obesity
  - Drug-induced, e.g. tetracyclines, ampicillin, amphotericin B and ciprofloxacin.

Q. What are the conditions that come into differential diagnosis of BIH?

Ans. Two important conditions that result in identical clinical picture are:
  - Neurocysticercosis
  - Cortical venous sinus thrombosis

Q. What are false localizing signs?

Ans. There are certain signs which do not have localizing value, often bilateral but can be unilateral, occur in raised ICP called *false localizing signs*. These are:
  - Bilateral or unilateral 6th nerve palsy
  - Bilateral or unilateral 3rd nerve palsy (pupillary changes)
  - Bilateral plantar extensor responses
  - Bilateral mild cerebellar dysfunction
  - Mild endocrinal dysfunction.

Q. The CT scan of the patient is displayed (Fig. 1.53B) can you point out the cause of raised ICP?

Ans. Yes. There is space occupying lesion (↑) on CT scan which explains the dilated ventricular system and raised ICP in this case.

Q. What do you understand by herniation of brain? What are various types of herniation syndromes seen in raised ICP?

Ans. The rise in ICP is equally distributed throughout the cranial cavity between supratentorial and infratentorial compartments through the tentorial opening containing the brainstem. When the tentorial opening is blocked, then there is differential distribution of ICP between the two compartments resulting in herniation (protrusion of a part of brain) syndromes.

The types of herniation are:

I. *Supratentorial (uncus herniation):* There is herniation of uncus of medial temporal lobe resulting in:
  - Contralateral hemiparesis due to compression and displacement of ipsilateral crus cerebri-*Kernohan Woltman sign*
  - Ipsilateral hemiparesis due to compression of contralateral crus against the tentorium—a *Kernohan's notch.* It is due to contracoup effect seen in a mass lesion
  - Pupillary dilatation and paresis of extraocular muscles due to stretching of ipsilateral 3rd nerve.

II. *Infratentorial (cerebellar tonsillar herniation).* Increased ICP in infratentorial compartment results in tonsillar coning compressing the medulla oblongata resulting in respiratory irregularities or distress and cardiovascular arrest.

III. *Transtentorial central herniation* in which brainstem protrudes through the tentorium resulting in:
  - Occipital headache, neck rigidity
  - Decorticate posturing
  - Bradycardia and hypertension
  - Bilateral plantar extensor responses
  - Dilated and fixed pupils
  - Brain death.

Q. How will you investigate such a case?

Ans. Following investigations are done:

1. *X-ray skull:* It may reveal sutural diastasis (separation of sutures) in infants, thinning and increased convolutional markings *(Silver-beaten appearance)* in adolescents and adults.
   In addition, the brunt of changes are seen in sellar region, e.g. destruction of anterior clinoid processes, enlargement of sella turcica.

2. *CT scan:* It reveals dilatation of ventricular system, cortical thinning, effacement of cisterns, an underlying lesion and periventricular lucency and compression of ventricle (s)

3. *MRI:* It can differentiate between vasogenic and cytopathic cerebral edema seen in patients with ICP and predicts response to shunts.

4. *Measurement of ICP:* It confirms the diagnosis. Ventriculography and pneumoencephalography are not performed nowadays.

Q. What is normal pressure hydrocephalus/occult hydrocephalus?

Ans. A syndrome of dilated ventricles with normal intracranial pressure associated with a triad of symptoms, i.e. dementia, ataxia and urinary incontinence in older persons is called normal *pressure hydrocephalus.* This is actually a misnomer. It is a communicating hydrocephalus in which CSF hemodynamics compromise and result in normal pressure. Though, it may be seen in patients with head injury, hypertensive hemorrhage or meningitis but in majority of cases no cause is identified.

Q. How will you diagnose hydrocephalus in a child?

Ans. The diagnosis is based on:

1. Abnormal enlargement of head. An increase in head circumference by >1 cm in every 2 weeks on serial measurements for the first three months of life makes the pediatrician suspicious.

2. Separation of sutures of skull

3. Buldging of anterior fontanelle

4. *"Setting-sun sign"*- the eyeballs appear to be pushed down and upper bulbar conjunctivae become visible

5. Scalp veins are dilated

6. High-pitched cry

7. The skull is resonant, gives *"cracked pot sound"* on percussion (*Macewen's sign*).

Q. What is treatment of raised ICP or hydrocephalus?

Ans. Following treatments are advocated:

1. The drug therapy to reduce the ICP include:
   • Mannitol (20%), e.g. 100 ml I.V. 4-6 hourly
   • Glycerol (10%), e.g. 1.2 g/kg over 4 hours
   • Dexamethasone (10-20 mg/day IV in divided doses)
   • Frusemide, e.g. 20-40 mg IV
   • Acetazolamide (50-75 mg/kg/day) orally

2. *Shunt surgery*
   The various shunts performed are:
   • Ventriculoperitoneal shunt (commonly used)
   • Endoscopic third ventriculostomy
   • Endoscopic placement of a stent in cerebral aqueduct in aqueductal stenosis.

3. *Repeated lumbar puncture* in a patient with benign raised intracranial pressure may be helpful to reduce ICP.

A 60-year-male presented with history of slowness of movements, difficulty in writing, disturbance in speech and slowness during activity and walking. Examination revealed mask-like face, slowness of various motor acts, tremors at rest, soft monotonous stuttering speech and abnormal (short-shuffling) gait. There was increased tone (rigidity), stooped posture and reflexes were normal (Fig. 1.54).

Fig. 1.54: Parkinsonism. There is stooped posture with short-shuffling gait

Q. What is the probable clinical diagnosis and why?

Ans. Sir, my diagnosis is parkinsonism. The points in favor of diagnosis are:
- A stooped posture
- Mask-like face
- Slowness of activity (bradykinesia)
- Resting tremors
- Rigidity
- Monotonus speech
- Fascinating gait

Q. What are your other possibilities?

Ans. The other conditions that come in differential diagnosis are
1. **Essential tremors:** Absence of other features of parkinsonism, bilateral presence of tremors, which have higher frequency and show postural dependency and abolition of tremors with alcohol favor this diagnosis
2. **Wilson's disease:** A combination of hepatic features (hepatitis, cirrhosis) and neurological features (tremors, dystopia, incoordination, parkinsonism) in young person (< 40 yr) suggest Wilson's disease. The Keyser Fleisher ring, low serum ceruloplasmin levels, higher urinary copper levels are highly suggestive of diagnosis. The confirmation is done by liver biopsy.
3. **Huntington's disease**: Although chorea is common but sometimes features of parkinsonism with positive family history and mental retardation may be presenting feature of Huntington's disease. Cognitive and behavior disturbances are common.
4. **Neurotoxin-induced parkinsonism,** e.g. carbon-monoxide and manganese poisoning.

Q. What is mask-like face? What are its causes?

Ans. It is an expressionless face with:
- Fixed stare
- Infrequent blinking
- No wrinkles

Causes are:
- Parkinsonism
- Hypothyroidism
- Dementia
- Myasthenia and myopathy involving facial muscles of expression
- Scleroderma
- Depression
- Pseudobulbar palsy

Q. What is tremor? What are its type and what are its causes?

Ans. Read all these questions in Clinical Methods in Medicine by Prof SN Chugh.

Q. What is parkinsonism? What is parkinsonian plus syndrome?

Ans. Parkinsonism is a movement disorder due to involvement of extrapyramidal system (basal ganglia) and is characterized by tremors, rigidity, akinesia or bradykinesia and postural disturbances. This is also called *akinetic* (loss or paucity of movements) *rigid* (rigidity) syndrome.

Parkinsonism plus syndrome refers to parkinsonism plus bulbar palsy (progressive supranuclear palsy), multiple system atrophies, e.g. olivopontocerebellar degeneration and primary autonomic failure (*Shy-Dragger syndrome*).

Q. What is rigidity, plasticity and Gagenhalten phenomenon?

Ans. **Rigidity** means hypertonia affecting agonistic and antagonistic muscles equally. It is present throughout the range of passive movement; when continuous and smooth, it is called *leadpipe rigidity* and when intermittent it is termed as 'cog-wheel' rigidity. It is commonly seen in extrapyramidal disease, Wilson's disease and Crutzfeld- Jacob disease.

Spasticity refers to hypertonia of clasp-knife type which is maximum at the beginning of movement and then suddenly decreases as passive movement is continued. It is seen in flexors of the upper limbs and extensors of lower limbs (antigravity muscles). It indicates pyramidal lesion.

Gagenhalten or paratonia refers to variable tone which becomes worse as the patient relaxes, seen in catatonia, dementia, CO-poisoning

Q. What are clinical features of parkinsonism?

Ans. They are described in Table 1.152.

Table 1.152: Common clinical features of parkinsonism

I. General
• Mask-like (expressionless) face
• Stooped posture/flexed posture
• Soft speech (hypophonia)
• Widened palpebral fissure and infrequent blinking
• Blepharospasm
• Drooling of saliva from the mouth
II. Bradykinesia or akinesia
• Slowness or difficulty in initiating voluntary acts such as walking, rising from an easy chair or bed
• Impaired fine movements
• Poor precision of repetitive movements
III. Disturbance of gait
• Short-shuffling (festinating) gait with difficulty in stopping
• Reduced swinging of arms during walking
• Propulsion and retropulsion
• Loss of balance on turning
IV. Tremors
• Resting tremors, suppressed by voluntary action, disappear during sleep and aggravated by fatigue and excitement
• Limited to distal parts, e.g. pill-rolling tremors of hands, or may begin with rhythmic flexion/extension of hands with pronation and supination of the forearms.
• Sometimes, there may be fast-action tremors
V. Rigidity
• Cog-wheel (more in upper limbs) Lead pipe (more in lower limbs)
VI. Miscellaneous
• Positive glabellar tap (Myerson's sign). Repetitive tapping (twice per second) over the glabella produces a sustained blink response with each tap in contrast to the normal response where blinking becomes infrequent after few taps.
• Micrographia (small hand-writing)
• Emotional lability
• Normal tendon reflexes
• Plantars are flexors

Q. What are the causes of parkinsonism?

Ans. The causes are:

1. *Idiopathic Parkinson's disease*
2. *Secondary parkinsonism* is due to:
   • *Viral infection,* e.g. encephalitis lethargica, Japanese B encephalitis, Creutzeldt-Jacob disease, subacute sclerosing panencephalitis

• Drug induced (Chlorpromazine, metoclopramide perchlorperazine, etc)
• *Toxins,* e.g. manganese, MPTP (I-methyl 4-phenyl tetrahydropyridine), carbon disulphide
• Hypoxia, e.g. cyanide, carbon monoxide
• *Vascular,* e.g. atherosclerotic
• *Metabolic,* e.g. Wilson's disease, hypoparathyroidism
• *Head injury,* e.g. Punch-drunk syndrome
• Brain tumors (They cause hemi-parkinsonism)

Q. What is the pathogenesis of clinical features in parkinsonism?

Ans. The most typical pathological hallmarks of clinical features of Parkinson's disease are:

Pathological change	Clinical feature
Degeneration of dopaminergic, nigrostrial pathway	Motor symptoms
Degeneration of dopaminergic, neocortical and mesolimbic pathways	Cognitive defects
Dopamine depletion in the dysfunction hypothalamus	Autonomic
Degeneration of the non-adrenergic locus ceruleans	Freezing phenomenon
Degeneration of the cholinergic nucleus.	Dementia

Q. What is festinating gait of parkinsonism?

Ans. It comprises of:
• Slow movements
• Narrow-based gait
• Short shuffling steps taken rapidly as if patient is chasing his/her centre of gravity
• Stooped posture with head-tilting forwards
• Sometimes, the feet may appear to be glued to the floor, so called *freezing phenomenon*
• The fall is characteristic like a telegraph pole. There is tendency to frequent forward falls due to postural instability.
• There is propulsion (*push test*) and retropulsion (*pull test*). The patient starts walking forward and backward when pushed or pulled.
• Due to postural instability, patient cannot stop himself/herself when pushed or pulled
• There is infrequent swinging of the arms during walking.

Q. What is glabellar sign (Refer to Table 1.154)?

Ans. Read Clinical Methods in Medicine by Prof SN Chugh.

Q. What autonomic disturbances occur in parkinsonism?

Ans. The common features of autonomic disturbance in parkinsonism are:
• Constipation
• Feeling of cold

- Frequency of micturition
- Postural edema
- Nocturia
- Impotence
- Excessive salivation and drooling of saliva from the mouth
- Orthostatic hypotension

Autonomic disturbances are common and early in Shy-Dragger syndrome (Parkinsonism plus syndrome).

Q. What do you understand by 'drug holidays' in L-dopa therapy?

Ans. Drug holidays means discontinuation of therapy for few days.It was practiced previously in L-dopa therapy because it was claimed to enhance the efficacy of treatment when it was resumed. This is now considered as dangerous and is of doubtful value.

Q. What are eye signs in parkinsonism?

Ans.
- Fixed stare, widened palpebral fissure
- Infrequent blinking
- Reflex blepharospasm
- Oculogyric crisis was seen in post-encephalitic variety. It is now rare.

Q. Name the components of extrapyramidal system and disease caused by them

Ans.

Name	Disease
Caudate nucleus	Chorea
Subthalamic nucleus	Hemiballismus
Putamen	Athetosis
Globus pallidus	Parkinsonism

Q. Name the various movement disorders?

Ans. Movement disorders are classified into
1. *Increased movements (Hyperkinetic disorders).* These are:
   - Tremor
   - Chorea
   - Athetosis
   - Hemiballismus
   - Myoclonus
   - Dyskinesia
   - Dystonia
2. *Decreased movement (hypokinetic disorder)* example is parkinsonism

Q. What is freezing phenomenon?

Ans. Freezing of gait momentarily occurs commonly at the onset of locomotion (Start hesitation), when attempting to change direction or turn around and upon entering a narrow space such as doorway. It is a feature of more advanced disease.

Q. How severity of parkinsonism disease graded?

Ans. The gross Parkinson's disease is graded into five stages as follows:
Stage I: New diagnosed disease or mild disease.
Stages II and III: Moderate to moderately severe disease
Stages IV and V: Advanced disease

Q. What is role of genetic in familial Parkinson's disease?

Ans. Parkinson's disease (PD) is the most common example of a family of neurodegenerative disorders characterized by a neuronal accumulation of the presynaptic protein α-synuclein. It is transmitted in autosomal manner (both autosomal dominant and autosomal recessive) .

Q. What is "wheel chair sign" in parkinsonism?

Ans. Patients with advanced disease and on-off motor fluctuations require a wheel-chair when 'off' and no chair when 'on' (are seen to walk about and sometimes pushing the chair). These patients are rarely permanently disabled (wheel chair-bound).

Q. What are changes in higher mental functions in parkinsonism?

Ans. Following changes can be observed:
- Emotional lability (e.g. spontaneous laughter is common in manganese poisoning)
- Depression-mask like face, mood disturbance
- Anxiety
- Frontal lobe dysfunction
- Dementia is uncommon

Q. What are the drugs available for treatment of parkinsonism?

Ans. The antiparkinsonian drugs are:
1. *Levodopa (1500-6000 mg/day)*
   The various combinations of L-dopa are:
   - Carbidopa/levodopa (25/100, 10/100, 25/250). Dose is 300-1000 mg of L-dopa /day
   - Benserazide/levodopa (25/100 12.5/50) dose is 600-800 mg of L-dopa/day
   - Controlled release carbidopa/levodopa (50/200). Dose is 200-800 mg/day
2. *Amantidine (100-200 mg/day)*
3. *Anticholinergics*
   - Trihexyphenidyl (4-8 mg/day)
   - Benztropine (1-1.5 mg/day)
4. *Antihistaminics*
   - Diphenyhydramine (50-100 mg/day)
   - Orphenadrine (150-200 mg/day)
5. *Dopamine agonists*
   - Bromocryptine (5-10 mg/day)
   - Pergolide (0.1-0.2 mg/day)
6. *MAO-B inhibitor*
   - Selegiline (5-10 mg/day)

Q. What is golden rule for the use of anti-parkinsonian drugs?

Ans. "Start low and go slow".

Q. What is type of speech in parkinsonism?

Ans. The voice becomes soft (hypophonic), monotonous and stuttering. The speech is rapid than normal.

In advanced cases, speech is reduced to muttering. Dribbling of saliva is common.

Q. What is Shy-Drager syndrome?

Ans. It is called *Parkinsonism plus syndrome* and includes:

- Parkinsonism. Rest tremors are early followed by gait and postural abnormality
- Autonomic disturbance (dysautonomia), e.g. orthostatic hypotension, sphincter disturbance and impotence
- In addition, patients may have laryngeal stridor and pyramidal features.

Q. What are the causes of slowness of movements?

Ans. Causes are:

- Parkinsonism
- Hypothyroidism
- Depression

Note: Read the clinical methods for answers to the following questions.

1. What is tremor?
2. What is difference between fine and coarse tremors?
3. What are the causes of tremors at rest?
4. What is benign essential tremor?

Q. Name the agents tried to delay the progression of disease?

Ans.
1. Selective in DATATOP study showed beneficial results, its metabolite desmethyl selegiline is under trial.
2. Coenzyme Q10-an antioxidant
3. Dopamine agonists
4. Nitric oxide synthetage inhibiters
5. Antiapoptotic agents
6. Minocycline—a tetracycline

Q. What is stiff man syndrome?

Ans. This rare syndrome is characterized by slowly progressive muscle stiffness involving the lower back with superadded spasms. Spasms are produced by startle, both spasms and stiffness become worse with emotional stress, disappear during sleep. The syndrome occurs in diabetes mellitus, can be paraneoplastic (lymphoma, lung cancer, breast cancer)

Most patients have a serum antibody against glutamic acid decarboxylase, an enzyme responsible for synthesis of inhibitory neurotransmitter—GABA. Stiffness results from loss of inhibition on the LMN. EMG changes are characteristic. Symptomatic relief can be obtained with baclofen or benzodiazepines.

Q. Mention some newer drugs in treatment of parkinsonism?

Ans.
1. Dopamine antagonists, e.g. cabergoline, ropinirole, pramipexole
2. Inhibitor of catechol O-methyl-transferase (COMT) e.g. entacapone, tolcapone. They are known as levodopa augmentations because they increase "on' time and reduce the duration of the "off" time and thus allow reduction of daily dose of L-dopa.
3. Inhibitors of glutamate receptors, e.g. CPP (3-6-carboxy piprazin-4-yl propyl-l-phosphonate), lamotrigine
4. GM-I ganglioside e.g. There is experimental evidence that when monkeys were treated with this drug from cow's brain, their motor function returned to normal.

Q. What is the role of fetal tissue in Parkinson's disease?

Ans. Parkinson's disease is considered to be slowly progressive disease characterized by loss of dopamine neurons of midbrain that also innervate the globus pallidus. Patients tend to have reduced response to L-dopa therapy over time (5-20 yr). On and off phenomena are common in this disease. Animal experiments have suggested that transplantation of fetal dopaminergic neurons can survive and restore neurological function. Trials are on to determine whether fetal graft to improve motor functions in patients with Parkinson's disease. Fetal ventral mesencephalic tissue is implanted in patient's postcommissural putamen.

Q. What are indications of stereotactic surgery in Parkinson's disease?

Ans. Indications are:

- Severe tremors.
- Levodopa-induced dyskinesia or levodopa failure
- Advanced parkinson's disease (Stages IV and V)
- Akinetic-rigid syndrome

Q. Name some heredodegenerative parkinsonian disorders?

Ans.
1. Hallervorden-Spatz disease (dementia, choreoathetosis, dystonia, retinitis pigmentosa)
2. Fahr's disease (Chorea, dementia palilalia)
3. Olivopontocerebellar and spinocerebellar degeneration.

A 36-years-male (Fig. 1.55) presented with wide flinging abnormal movements of upper limbs at rest. They were brief, and initiated by sudden voluntary act. They subsided during sleep. Patient had mental retardation (IQ 50-50%), and positive family history. Examination revealed no evidence of heart disease or arthritis or subcutaneous nodule or erythema marginatum. Neurological examination revealed wide-flinging, quasi-purposive involuntary movements and hypotonia. Jerks were normal. Plantars were flexor.

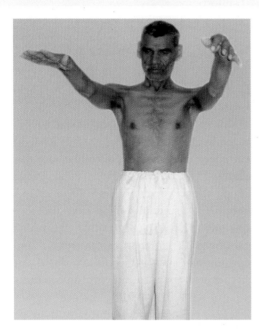

Fig. 1.55: Chorea

Q. What is your probable diagnosis and why?

Ans. Wide-flinging dancing movements of upper limbs at rest with no other finding in CVS and neurological examination suggest the diagnosis of chorea but presence of mental retardation and positive family history for the disease go in favor of Huntington's chorea

Q. What are important points to be asked in history?

Ans. • Ask the history of sore throat in adults especially if females for Sydenham's chorea (St Vitus dance) in rheumatic fever
• Ask for such a disease in the family, i.e. Huntington's chorea.
• Take a history of oral contraceptive use in young woman or recent pregnancy (*chorea gravidarum*)
• Ask for drug history, e.g. lithium, phenothiazine.
• History of fever, convulsions, stroke or systemic illness.

• Ask for history of liver disease, e.g.cirrhosis for Wilson's disease.

Q. What is chorea?

Ans. Choreiform movements are rapid, brief, jerky or wide-flinging, nonrepetitive and quasipurposive movements limited to face, limbs and tongue.

These movements are completely irregular and variable in time, rhythm, character and place of origin. The patient of chorea is clumsy and keeps dropping objects. Patient with mild disease may show increase fidgeting or restlessness.

Chorea literally means a dance, hence movements called *dancing movements*.

Q. What are the causes of chorea?

Ans. The causes are:
1. *Hereditary*
   • Huntington's chorea
   • Benign hereditary chorea
   • Ataxia telangiectasia
   • Wilson's disease
2. *Infectious*
   • Sydenham's (rheumatic) chorea
   • Postencephalitic chorea
3. *Metabolic*
   • Thyrotoxicosis
   • Hypoparathyroidism
   • Pregnancy (chorea gravidarum)
4. *Immunological*
   • SLE
   • Henoch-Schönlein purpura
5. *Drug and toxins*
   • Oral contraceptive, lithium, L-dopa, phenothiazines
   • Alcohol
   • Carbon monoxide, hypoxia, manganese
6. *Miscellaneous*
   • CVA or stroke (hemiplegic chorea)
   • Senile
   • Tumor (e.g. paraneoplastic)
   • Trauma
   • Hypernatremia
   • Remember five common causes of chorea

> • Syndenham's chorea or choreagravdarun
> • Huntington's chorea
> • Following a stroke
> • Postencephalitic chorea
> • Hyperparathyroidism
> • SLE

Bedside Medicine

Q. What are cardinal features of chorea?

Ans. Cardinal features are:

1. *Pronator sign:* Ask the patient to raise both upper limbs above the head, the hands will get pronated if chorea is present.

2. *Waxing and waning of the grip-called "milkmaid's" grip or milking sign".* It is noticed when patient is asked to squeeze the examiner's hands or fingers tightly.

3. *Dinner-fork deformity:* This refers to position of the fingers when patient is asked to stretch out the hands and spread the fingers. There is hyperextension of elbows, hyperpronation of forearms, flexion of wrists with hyperextended fingers (metacarpophalangeal joints are extended with separation of fingers). It is due to hypotonia.

4. Hypotonia and instability. It is elicited by:
   - *Pendular knee jerk* or hung-up reflex (a choreic movement is superimposed on a tendon jerk)
   - *Lizard or reptile tongue.* When patient is asked to protrude the tongue; he/she does it and takes it back with reptile speed. The tongue when projected looks like a bag of worms.

Q. How will you diagnose chorea?

Ans. The diagnosis of chorea is clinical. Perform all the signs described above.

The simplest way to diagnose chorea is to ask the patient to raise the arms above the head with hands facing each other (Fig. 1.55). If chorea is present, the patient will tend to pronate the arms and rapid jerky movements of upper limbs will appear.

Q. What is the site of lesion in chorea?

Ans. Caudate nucleus.

Q. What is hemichorea?

Ans. Choreic movements limited to one half of the body is called *hemichorea*. Usually chorea is generalized and bilateral.

Q. What is "pure chorea"?

Ans. Pure chorea means isolated rheumatic chorea when other rheumatic manifestations (Jones major criteria) are not seen. This is a due to the fact that chorea is a delayed manifestation of rheumatic fever when carditis and arthritis and other rheumatic features either have not appeared or have disappeared.

Q. What are the differences between Syndemham's chorea and Huntington's chorea?

Ans. Read Clinical Methods in Medicine by Dr SN Chugh.

Q. What are various involuntary movements?

Ans. Read clinical methods in medicine by Dr SN Chugh.

Q. What is genetics of Huntington's chorea?

Ans. It is an autosomal dominant disorder associated with random repetition of CAG. In Huntington's disease the greater is the number of CAG repeats, the earlier the onset of the disease. The protein product for gene is called *huntingtin*.

Q. What is role of assessing CAG expansion in Huntington's chorea?

Ans. Assessment of CAG expansion allows assessment of genetic risk without DNA analysis.

Q. What is treatment of Huntington's chorea?

Ans. Clozapine, risperidone and olanzapine are better tolerated drugs for this disease.

Q. What is hemibillismus? What are its causes?

Ans. It is defined as unilateral, involuntary, flinging movements of the proximal upper limbs. The lesion lies in the ipsilateral *subthalamic nucleus of Luys.* Causes are:
- Vascular event (CVA) usually embolic
- Rarely, tumor, abscess multiple sclerosis can lead to it.

Q. What is athetosis? How will you differentiate it from chorea?

Ans. Athetosis means instability of posture. It is defined as slow sinuous writhing involuntary movements involving the wrist, fingers and ankle (peripheral parts of a limb). The lesion is in the putamen. Its differentiation from chorea is given in Table 1.153.

Table 1.153: Chorea vs athetosis

	Features	Chorea	Athetosis
1.	Site of lesion	Caudate nucleus	Putamen
2.	Prevalence	Common	Uncommon
3.	Tone	Decreased	Increased
4.	Movements	Rapid, continuous, uninterrupted and quasipurposive	Slow and sinuous writhing movements, i.e. extension and supination of the arm with alternating flexion and extension of fingers
5.	Effect of excitement	Increased	No effect
6.	Parts involved	Proximal more than distal	Distal parts involved more than proximal
7.	Tongue	Lizard tongue	Chewing tongue
8.	Deep tendon jerks	Pendular or hung-up	Normal

Q. What is chorea gravidarum?

Ans. It is actually rheumatic chorea manifesting during pregnancy or postpartum period.

Q. What are conditions that produce irregular, rapid jerky movements of limbs?

Ans. These are:

1. Tics. They are controlled by voluntary effort
2. Chorea
3. Hemiballismus — They are not suppressed by voluntary effort
4. Myoclonus

Q. What is myoclonus? What are its common causes?

Ans. Myoclonus is rapid, irregular jerky movements of a limb due to contraction of a single muscle or a group of muscles. They occur spontaneously at rest, in response to sensory stimuli or voluntary movements.

The common causes are:

- Cerebral hypoxia (posthypoxic intention myoclonus)
- Lipid-storage disease
- Encephalitis or Creutzfeldt-Jacob disease
- Metabolic encephalopathies, e.g. liver cell failure, renal failure, respiratory failure, electrolyte imbalance, etc.
- A feature of myoclonic epilepsy.

A young patient (Fig. 1.56) presented with unsteadiness of gait and tendency to fall on either side of the body of few months duration. The ataxia was progressive and associated with speech disturbance. Examination revealed dysarthria, nystagmus, lower limbs weakness, loss of lower limb reflexes and plantars were extensors. There was loss of joint and position sense in the lower limbs. Scoliosis and pes cavus were present. Romberg's sign was negative.

Fig. 1.56: Cerebellar ataxia. Note the unsteadiness during standing

Q. What is probable diagnosis? Give reasons in favor of your diagnosis?

Ans. Progressive ataxia in a young person with dysarthria, nystagmus, loss of lower limbs reflexes and sense of position and vibration with plantars extensor indicate cerebellar ataxia, probably Friedreich's ataxia. Negative Romberg's sign supports the diagnosis and differentiates it from sensory ataxia.

Q. What is you differential diagnosis?

Ans. Cerebella ataxia has to be differential from;

1. **Sensory ataxia:** Read the Table 1.156 for differentiation
2. **Vertiginous ataxia:** Ataxia associated with vestibular nerve or labyrinthine disease is mainly a disorder of gait associated with significant degree of dizziness, lightheadedness or the perception of movement.

3. **Proximal myopathy of lower limbs** sometimes resembles cerebellar ataxia. Weakness of proximal muscles of leg, positive Gower's sign, absent reflexes favor the diagnosis of proximal myopathy.

4. **Hysterical:** These patients are anxious and careful. They become ataxic when they are asked to walk or stand. (e.g when they are being observed) There is astasia abasia. They neither have reduced muscle power nor any sensory loss. They can move the limbs and can perform all the movements (signs of cerebellum function) very well without any incoordination but when asked to walk (tandem walking) they become ataxic.

Q. What are the symptoms and signs of ataxia?

Ans. Ataxia does not merely mean gait impairment but has following symptoms and signs

1. Gait impairment
2. Scanning speech
3. Visual disturbance due to nystagmus
4. Incoordination of hands and feet
5. Tremors

Q. What important points would you ask on the history and why?

Ans. • History of falls, wide based gait, clumsiness and difficulty with fine coordinated movements (cerebellar disease)
• H/o tremors. Intention tremors occur in cerebellar disease.
• Waxing and waning symptoms of ataxia (multiple sclerosis as the cause)
• H/o CVA (stroke) for brainstem infarction as the cause.
• Drugs toxicity e.g. phenytoin, alcohol, lead poisoning.
• History of hypothyroidism
• H/o Intracranial tumors or false localizing symptoms and signs for posterior fossa tumor
• Family history
• History of birth defect.

Q. What is Friedreich's ataxia?

Ans. It is heredofamilial ataxia (autosomal recessive) characterized by progressive degeneration of dorsal root ganglia, spinocerebellar tracts, corticospinal tracts and Purkinje cells of cerebellum.

Q. What are various cerebellar signs?

Ans. As the cerebellum maintains, tone, posture, coordination and integrates the voluntary and automatic movements, hence, the tests performed are based on these functions. A unilateral cerebellar lesion will produce these signs on the same side (ipsilateral).

247

1. *Hypotonia:* There is hypotonia on the side involved. The limbs are flaccid both at rest and on passive movements.
2. *Titubation:* Nodding of head may be present.
3. *Signs of incoordination in upper limbs:* Following signs indicating incoordination in the upper limbs will appear;
   - *Intention tremors:* The tremors appear as the patient approaches his/her target/goal. For example, ask the patient to touch his/her nose with index finger, the tremors appear as nose is approached.
   - *Finger nose test:* This is a useful test, and positive on the side involved.
   - *Finger to finger test:* In cerebellar disease, there will be pastpointing (past-pointing is positive)
   - *Dysmetria*
   - *Dyssynergia*
   - *Dysdiadochokinesia*
   - *Rebound phenomenon*
4. **Signs of incoordination in lower limbs**
   - *Knee-heel test* (positive on the side involved)
   - *Tandem walking* (heel-to-toe walking). Patient sways on the side involved
   - *Romberg's sign.* Patient sways to the side involved when he/she stands with eyes open with feet together
   - *Abnormal gait* Patient sways or tends to fall to the side involved while walking
5. *Nystagmus* with fast component to the side of lesion
6. *Speech,* e.g. dysarthria (Staccato or scanning speech).

All these signs/tests have already been described and discussed in "Clinical Methods in Medicine" by Prof. S.N. Chugh.

Q. What are the functions of cerebellum?
Ans. It maintains;
- Tone
- Posture and equilibrium
- Coordination of movements

Q. What is classical triad of cerebeller disease?
Ans. It is denoted by three 'A'
- Ataxia
- Atonia (hyptotonia)
- Asthenia

Q. What are the causes of cerebellar ataxia?
Ans. The cerebellar ataxia may be with bilateral symmetrical signs or with unilateral signs. It can be acute, subacute or chronic. The causes are given in Table 1.154.

Q. What are diagnostic criteria for Friedreich's ataxia?
Ans. The diagnostic criteria (modified from Harding) are depicted in Table 1.155.

Q. What are the causes of absent ankle jerk with extensor plantars response?
Ans. Following are the causes:
- Friedreich's ataxia
- Tabes dorsalis
- Nutritional deficiency of B1 and B12 with ataxia
- Paraneoplastic syndrome
- Motor neuron disease
- Combined conus medullaris and cauda equina syndrome (Cord-cauda) and subacute combined degeneration of spinal cord
- Peripheral neuropathy in a patient with stroke
- Hypothyroidism

Table 1.154: Causes of cerebellar ataxia

I. WITH BILATERAL SIGNS

Acute and subacute (<6 weeks)	Chronic (> 6 months)
• Acute cerebellitis, e.g. viral, bacterial (enteric)	• Hereditary ataxias, e.g. autosomal dominant (spinocerebellar) and autosomal recessive Friedreich's ataxia
• Post-infectious syndrome	• Paraneoplastic syndrome
• Toxins and drugs, e.g. alcohol, lithium, hydantoin, barbiturates	• Hypothyroidism
• Lyme disease	• Tabes dorsalis
• Nutritional (B$_1$,B$_{12}$ deficiency)	

Remember five important causes of bilateral ataxia
- *Hereditary (Friedreich's ataxia)*
- *Alcoholism and phenytoin toxicity*
- *Post-infectious*
- *Para neoplastic syndrome*
- *Hypothyroidism*

II. WITH UNILATERAL SIGNS

Acute	Chronic
• *Vascular,* e.g. cerebellar hemorrhage, infarction or subdural hematoma	• *Congenital,* e.g. Dandy-Walker syndrome, Arnold-Chiari malformation
• *Infection,* e.g. cerebellar abscess	• *Secondary gliosis* in a vascular lesion
• *Neoplasm,* e.g. glioma and metastatic tumor	• *Old demyelinating plaques* detected on MRI/CT
• *Demyelinating,* e.g. multiple sclerosis, AIDS related multifocal leukoencephalopathy	

Table 1.155: Diagnostic criteria for Friedreich's ataxia (FA)

I. **Essential criteria**
  - Progressive ataxia
  - Young age (<25 years)
  - Extensor plantar responses
  - Absent ankle and knee jerks
  - Dysarthria (after 5 years of onset of symptoms)
  - Motor nerve conduction velocity >40 m/sec in upper limbs with small or absent sensory action potential

II. **Additional criteria (present in 2/3rd patients)**
  - Pyramidal weakness in lower limbs
  - Distal loss of joint position and vibration sense in lower limbs
  - Scoliosis
  - Abnormal ECG (wide spread T wave inversion and ventricular hypertrophy)

III. **Other supportive features (present in <50% patients)**
  - Nystagmus, optic atrophy
  - Pes cavus
  - Distal weakness and wasting
  - Diabetes
  - Deafness

Q. What is lateralization of signs in cerebella ataxia?

Ans. In hemispherical cerebellar lesion, the signs are lateralized to the side of lesion. In lesion of vermis, the signs are centralized.

Q. What are neurological involvement in Friedreich's ataxia?

Ans.
  - Posterior root ganglion
  - Degeneration of peripheral sensory fibers
  - Involvement of posterior and lateral columns.

Q. What are the features of central (vermis) cerebellar lesion?

Ans. Following are the features:
  - Head nodding (titubation)
  - Truncal ataxia
  - Positive heel-to-toe gait (tandem gait)
  - Difficulty in sitting, rising from a chair, standing and walking. There is unsteadiness and swaying during these activities

Q. What is the type of tremors in cerebellar disease?

Ans. Intention tremors. An intention tremor is an involuntary movement (e.g. tremor) which becomes prominent during voluntary movement towards a target. It is absent at rest.

Q. What is genetics in Friedreich's atexia?

Ans. It is the most common inherited ataxia accounting for 50% cases of all hereditary ataxias, It is inherited in autosomal recessive manner. The chromosome involved is number 9. The mutant gene is *frataxin*, contains expanded *GAA triplet repeats*. There is point mutation of frataxin in this ataxia.

Q. Why are tendon reflexes absent even though plantars are extensor in Friedreich's ataxia.

Ans. It is due to combined involvement of pyramidal tracts and peripheral nerves (asymptomatic) in this syndrome.

Q. What are various types of ataxias?

Ans. Ataxia is a movement disorder. A movement needs coordination of cortex, cerebellum, the reflex arc and impulses from the eyes, ears (labyrinth) and cervical spine. Hence, ataxia is of following types:
  1. Cerebellar (read the causes)
  2. Sensory (e.g. peripheral neuropathy, subacute combined degeneration, tabes dorsalis)
  3. Labyrinthine or vertiginous ataxia, e.g. labyrinthitis, Meniere's disease, streptomycin - induced
  4. *Central* (lesion lies in the medulla)
  5. Miscellaneous, e.g. ataxia due to severe muscular weakness and hypotonia.

Q. If you are allowed to choose one investigation to confirm your diagnosis, which would you choose and why?

Ans. Magnetic resonance imaging (MRI) is the best test to evaluate soft tissue lesion such as plaques.

Q. Which vitamin abnormality is associated with Friedreich's ataxia?

Ans. Vitamin E (α-tocopherol)

Q. What is sensory ataxia? What are its causes? What is Romberg's sign? How will you differentiate it from cerebellar ataxia?

Ans. Sensory ataxia results from defective proprioceptive sensations (posterior column involvement), hence, does not occur with eyes open, as sense of position is compensated by open eyes. Thus, sensory ataxia manifests or gets increased when the eyes are closed.

Causes: Sense of proprioception is affected by lesions of peripheral nerves, sensory root, posterior column and postcentral gyrus in parietal lobe, hence causes are:
  1. *Lesion of peripheral nerves*, e.g. neuropathy due to any cause
  2. *Sensory root lesion*, e.g. tabes dorsalis, radiculopathy (disk prolapse)
  3. *Posterior column involvement*, e.g. multiple sclerosis, syringomyelia and intramedullary compression
  4. *Parietal lobe lesion* (sensory cortex involvement), e.g. vascular lesion or a tumor.

Sensory ataxia is differentiated from cerebellar ataxia (Table 1.156).

Features	Sensory ataxia	Cerebellar ataxia
Muscle power	Diminished	Normal
Deep tendon reflexes	Lost	Pendular or hung-up
Cerebellar signs	Absent	Present
Posterior column sensations	Lost	Preserved
Plantar reflex	Lost	Extensor response or normal
Charcoat joint and trophic changes	Present	Absent
Romberg's sign	Positive	Negative
Gait	High-steppage or stamping gait	Broad-based gait
Common causes	Tabes dorsalis and peripheral neuropathy	Friedreich's ataxia, multiple sclerosis

Romberg's Sign. It is a sign of sensory ataxia. It is said to be positive if a person can stand without swaying when eyes are open but tends to sway when eyes are closed.

It is negative in cerebellar lesions as person tends to sway with eyes open as well as closed.

NB: False positive Romberg's sign may occur in hysteria.

Q. What is vertiginous ataxia?

Ans. Vertiginous (labyrinthine) ataxia is a disorder of gait associated with vertigo, dizziness and light-headedness. The causes of labyrinthine ataxia are due to involvement of labyrinth;
• Acute labyrinthitis
• Meniere's disease
• Vestibular neuronitis
• Streptomycin-induced

Vertiginous ataxia resembles cerebellar ataxia except that vertigo and dizziness accompany the former but not the later.

Labyrinthine ataxia also occurs more when the eyes are open than when the eyes are closed. Romberg's signs is negative.

Q. Name the ataxias in which Romberg's sign is negative.

Ans. • Cerebellar ataxia
• Vertiginous ataxia
• Labyrinthine ataxia

Q. What are the signs suggestive of posterior column involvement?

Ans. Following are the signs:
1. *Sensory disturbances*
   • Girdle-like sensation at the level of compression
   • Deep sensations (sense of position, vibration), fine touch (light touch, two-point discrimination and sense of localization, stereognosis, graphesthesia etc) are lost.
   • Superficial sensations, e.g. pain, touch (crude) and temperature are preserved
   • Romberg's sign is positive
   • Lhermitte's sign is positive

2. Motor disturbances
   • Loss of coordination, e.g. sensory ataxia
   • Tone is diminished
   • Power normal
3. Reflexes
   • Deep tendon jerks absent but superficial reflexes preserved
   • Plantars are flexor
   • No bladder or bowel disturbance

Q. What is ataxia telangiectasia (Louis-Barr syndrome)?

Ans. It is an inherited ataxia due to defect in ATN gene, presents in first decade of life, is characterized by
• Cerebellar ataxia similar to Friedreich's ataxia, hence, is to be differentiated.
• Nystagmus
• Progresive telangiectatic lesion.
• Thymic hyperplasia with defective cellular and humoral immunity
• Recurrent pulmonary infections
• Sometimes, neoplasia of lymphatic and reticuloendothelial system may develop (e.g. lymphoma, leukemia)

Q. What is the treatment of ataxia?

Ans. • To identity treatable cause and remove or treat it properly.
• Ataxia with antigliadin antibodies and malabsorption may improve with gluten-free diet and steroids.
• Vitamin E deficiency must be explored and treated if co-exists.
• Drug (phenytoin) and alcohol must be stopped, if being used.
• Hypothyroidism must be explored and treated, if found.

Q. What is treatment of Friedreich's ataxia?

Ans. It is an inheritable disorder, hence, there is no definite treatment. Identification of an at-risk person's genotype, together with appropriate family and genetic counseling can reduce the incidence of these cerebellar ataxias in future generations.

CASE 57: MYOTONIA

A 50 years male (Fig. 1.57A) presented with weakness of distal groups of muscles of extremities. He also complained of frontal baldness and abnormal facial appearance and dysarthria. Examination revealed wasting of distal muscles (Fig. 1.57B), myotonia (poor hand-grip relaxation), bilateral ptosis and cataract.

Figs 1.57A and B: Myotonia dystrophica. A. Note the frontal baldness, abnormal facial appearance and dysarthria. B. Note the wasting of small muscles of hand

Q. What is the probable clinical diagnosis?

Ans. Presence of myotonia (disturbed tone) along with wasting of distal muscles in a 50-year male who presented with frontal baldness, abnormal facial expression and dysarthria suggest the diagnosis of *dystrophic myotonia*.

Q. What are the points to be asked in the history?

Ans. • Age of onset (dystrophic myotonia occurs in 3rd and 4th decade)
• Is there difficulty in releasing the grip?
• Progressive distal muscle weakness presenting difficulty in kicking the ball
• History of falls (Pseudo-drop attacks) due to proximal muscles weakness
• H/o dysphagia
• H/o impotence
• H/o Recurrent pulmonary infections

Q. How would you proceed to examine such a case?

Ans. Proceed as follows.
• Note for frontal baldness.
• Note difficulty in opening the eye after closure. Note the ptosis (bilateral), cataract or any surgery for cataract.
• Note expressionless face (hatched face) and swan neck due to thinning of neck muscles.

Examine
• Release of hand group while shaking hand. Note the slow release of handgrip.
• Note weakness of sternomastoids. Test them
• Examine for wasting of distal muscles of upper limbs.
• Elicit percussion myotonia over thenar muscles and tongue (if possible). Not the pit which slowly and slowly resolves.
• Elicit deep tendon jerks. They are depressed due to hypotonia.
• Examine the breast for gynecomastia and testes for atrophy.
• Test higher mental function for IQ

Q. What is myotonia? What are its type?

Ans. Myotonia is defined as continued muscle contraction with poor relaxation after the cessation of voluntary effort. Myotonias are inherited disorders (autosomal dominant).

The inherited rare types of myotonias are:
1. Myotonia dystrophica
2. Myotonia congenita (Thomsen's disease)
3. Proximal myotonic myopathy. It is characterized by myotonia in middle aged persons with proximal muscle weakness and cataract. It is also inherited as autosomal dominant.

Q. What is clinical significance of myotonia?

Ans. These patients of myotonia tolerate the anesthesia poorly, hence, it is essential to recognize them.

251

Q. **Name some diseases known to be associated with increased number of triplet repeats?**

Ans. • Huntington's' chorea
• Myotonic muscular dystrophy
• Spinocerebellar ataxias type 1 to 3
• Fragile syndrome
• Hereditary dentatorubral pallidoluysian atrophy (DRPLA)

Q. **What is inheritance of this condition?**

Ans. • Autosomal dominant inheritance
• Defect located on chromosome 19
• There is dynamic mutation with increased number of triplet repeats (AGC repeats)
• The repeat size typically increases from generation to generation providing a molecular basis for the clinical phenomenon of anticipation.

Q. **What are the clinical characteristics of dystrophia myotonica (mytonia dystrophica)?**

Ans. It is an autosomal dominant condition characterized by:
• Late age of onset (20-50 years)
• Progressive distal muscle weakness
• Bilateral ptosis
• *"Hatchet-face appearance"* due to atrophy of temporalis, masseter, sternomastoid and facial muscles (Fig. 1.49A)
• Dysarthria due to weakness of palatal, pharyngeal and tongue muscles
• Myotonia can be demonstrated by percusion over the tongue, thenar eminence and wrist extensor muscles. There is delayed handgrip relaxation.

Other features
• Frontal baldness
• Cataract
• Mental retardation
• Cardiomyopathy and conduction defects
• Hypogonadism and small pituitary fossa
• Glucose intolerance
• Low serum IgG leading to respiratory infections
• Somnolence
• Ocasionally external ophthalmoplegia.

Q. **What is myotonia congenita?**

Ans. This is also an autosomal dominant disorder, milder form occurs in childhood and persists throughout life. Severe form occurs in infants of affected mothers and characterised by peculiar cry, facial and bulbar muscles weakness, respiratory insufficiency and mental retardation.

This myotonia is accentuated by rest, cold and is more noticeable on starting the activity following prolonged rest. There may be diffuse hypertrophy of the muscles. Strength is well preserved. Myotonia may be apparent on shaking hands with the person.

Q. **How do you test temporalis and sternomastoids?**

Ans. Read "Clinical Methods in Medicine" by Prof.S.N. Chugh.

Q. **How will you demonstrate myotonia at the bed side?**

Ans. The methods of demonstration are:
1. *Hand grip:* There is poor relaxation of hand grip during shaking hand with the patient.
2. *Percussion:* Percussion over the thenar eminence produces a dimple which disappears (relaxes) slowly.
      Similarly percussion over the tongue produces the same above phenomenon.
3. *Slow relaxation of eye after closure.* Ask the patient to close the eyes forcibly, and now ask him to open the eyes. The patient opens the eyes slower than normal.

Q. **How will you investigate such a case?**

Ans. Investigations are:
• *Serum CK level.* It may be normal or mildly elevated
• *EMG (electromyography).* It is diagnostic, shows high frequency waxing and waning discharges and a myopathic pattern.
• *Muscle biopsy.* It shows type I fibers with increased numbers of central nuclei, ring fibers and sarcolemmal masses.

Q. **Name the drugs useful in myotonia?**

Ans. Drugs used in myotonia are:
• Phenytoin
• Quinine
• Procainamide
• Mexiletine.

Q. **Which myopathies produce distal weakness and wasting of muscles?**

Ans. • Myotonic dystrophy
• Welander's distal myopathy

Q. **What is type of cataract in dystrophic myotonia?**

Ans. Stellate cataract

Q. **What tests would you perform on patient's sister if she asks about risks to her offspring?**

Ans. • Clinical evaluation
• Slit lamp examination for cataract
• EMG

Q. **What are characteristic EMG findings in myotonia?**

Ans. Waxing and wanning of the potentials called "*dive-bomber effect*". The EMG changes can be recorded in any muscle.

Q. **What would you advise if patient had undergone major surgery?**

Ans. These patients of dystrophic myotonia tolerate the anesthesia poorly due to impaired cardiorespiratory function, hence, they need intensive postoperative observation.

Q. **How would you treat myotonia dystrophica?**

Ans. • Footdrop is controlled by caliper or moulded-foot arthroses.

• Myotonia, when disabling may respond to drugs described above

• Advanced heart block with or without syncope need pacemaker insertion.

A 6-year M (Fig. 1.58A) presented with progressive weakness of muscles of lower limbs and difficulty in walking and in climbing stairs. There was history of difficulty in running and boarding a bus. Patient has no history of mental changes. There was no history of bowel and bladder disturbances. There was no respiratory and cardiovascular complaints.

Examination revealed pseudohypertrophy of the calf muscles and Gower's sign was positive. The knee and ankle jerks were diminished. Plantars were flexor. Sensory system was normal. Respiratory and cardiovascular systems were essentially normal.

Fig. 1.58A: Duchenne muscular dystrophy

Q. What is your probable diagnosis and why?
Ans. The muscle weakness, pseudohypertrophy of calves, positive Gower's signs, loss of tendon reflexes in the lower limbs with normal plantars with no sensory involvement suggest the diagnosis of a primary muscle disorder, i.e. myopathy. In view of his age of onset and positive family history the child has Duchenne type of myopathy.

Q. What is myopathy?
Ans. Myopathy (muscular dystrophy) is defined as genetically determined primary degeneration of muscle fibers without an evidence of involvement of central or peripheral nervous system.

Q. How do you classify myopathies?
Ans. The myopathy being heredofamilial disorders are classified on the basis of inheritance (Table 1.157).

Q. Name some other X-linked myopathy?
Ans. • X-linked tubular myopathy
• Emergy-Dreifuss muscular dystrophy. It presents in early childhood and is slowly progressive. Initially it has humeral-peroneal pattern of muscle

Table 1.157: Classification of hereditary myopathies

I. **X-linked**
   • *Duchenne type* (severe type of pseudohypertrophic muscular dystrophy)
   • *Becker type* (milder form with pseudohypertrophy)
II. **Autosomal recessive**
   • Limbs girdle (e.g. scapulohumeral or pelvi-femoral)
   • Congenital muscular dystrophy
III. **Autosomal dominant**
   • Facioscapulohumeral (Landouzy-Dejerine type)
   • Scapuloperoneal
   • Oculopharnygeal or ocular
   • Distal myopathy

weakness which eventually evolves into scapulo-humero-pelvo-peroneal distribution of weakness. There is marked atrophy of humeral and peroneal muscles. Pseudohypertrophy is absent.

Q. What are the characteristic features of Duchenne type of muscular dystrophy?
Ans. Male child presents with difficulty in climbing stairs and difficulty in getting up from sitting position. Other features are:
• Positive family history
• Slow onset and progressive disease
• Mental retardation (may be present)
• Positive Gower's sign
• Pseudohypertrophy of the calves and atrophy of other limb muscles
• Jerks may be normal or diminished
• Normal sensory system and sphincter control
• No fasciculations
• Waddling gait

Q. What are similarities and dissimilarities between Duchenne and Becker muscular dystrophies?
Ans. These are given in Table 1.158.

Q. What are the differences between pseudo-hypertrophy and true hypertrophy (hypertrophic musculorum vera) of muscles?
Ans. These are given in Table 1.159.

Q. What are the causes of pseudohypertrophy of muscles?
Ans. Causes are:
• Duchenne muscular dystrophy (DMD)
• Myxoedema (hypothyroidism)
• Glycogen storage disease
• Trichinosis

Q. Which muscles are not involved in Duchenne muscle dystrophy?
Ans. Facial and small muscles of hand.

Q. What are the causes of true hypertrophy of muscle?

Table 1.158: Similarities and dissimilarities between Duchenne and Becker type of myopathy

Similarities

- Both are X-linked (mutation of dystrophin gene), progressive myopathies
- Positive family history
- Positive Gower's sign
- Presence of pseudohypertrophy
- EMG and muscle biopsy findings
- Treatment protocol similar

Dissimilarities

Feature	Duchenne type	Becker type
• Age of onset	• Infancy or childhood	• Adolescence or adult onset
• Severity	• Severe	• Mild
• Mental retardation	• Common	• Uncommon
• Cardiomyopathy and ECG abnormalities	• Common	• Uncommon
• Kyphoscoliosis	• Common	• Uncommon
• Respiratory involvement	• Early	• Late
• Prognosis	• Death occurs before second decade	• Death before second decade is rare

Table 1.159: Pseudohypertrophy vs true hypertrophy

Pseudohypertrophy	True hypertrophy
Muscle bulk is due to deposition of fibrofatty tissue	Muscle bulk is due to increase in muscle mass
Muscles are doughy to feel (elasticity is lost)	Muscles are soft and elastic
Muscles are firm and globular on contraction	Muscles are hard and globular on contraction
The muscles are weak and hypotonic in spite of bulky size	The muscles are stronger than normal
Muscles showing pseudohypertrophy are; calf muscles, glutei, quadriceps, deltoids and infraspinati. Tongue muscles may be involved	Muscles showing true hypertrophy include calf muscles or glutei and quadriceps

Ans. Causes are:
- Laborers (manual hard work)
- Athletes
- Myotonia
- Cysticercosis in the muscles
- Hypertrophic musculorum vera (a rare inherited disorder).

Q. What is limb girdle myopathy?

Ans. Limb girdle myopathy transmitted as autosomal dominant or recessive inheritance, is characterized by muscle weakness of pelvic and shoulder girdle muscles (Fig. 1.58B). It affects both males and females in the age groups of 10-30 years. Diaphragm may be involved producing respiratory insufficiency. The disease is progressive and varies from family to family. Cardiac involvement (cardiomyopathy) may lead to CHF or arrhythmias. CK levels are elevated. EMG and muscle biopsy reveal myopathic pattern.

Q. How would you proceed to examine a case with limb girdle/fascioscapulohumeral myopathy?

Ans. *History taking*
Points to be noted:
1. Age of onset (young persons between 10-40 years of age)

Fig. 1.58B: Fascioscapulohumeral myopathy. Note the wasting of shoulder girdle muscles leading to winging of scapulae

2. Onset may be either pelvic or shoulder girdle in limb girdle myopathy; while weakness begins in face and involves shoulder girdle (e.g. lower trapezzi, pectoralis, biceps and triceps) in upper limb myopathy

3. Family history may be positive in fascioscapulohumeral myopathy (H/o facial weakness in the family).

Examination
Proceed to examine the two conditions as follows:

Fascioscapulohumeral myopathy	Limb girdle myopathy
1. Face is involved e.g. ptosis, difficulty in closing the eyes, marked facial weakness leading to expressionless face with lips open. There is difficulty in whistling and puffing out the cheeks, examine all these features.	Face is not involved
2. Neck muscles including sternomastoids are weak.	No involvement of neck muscles
3. Shoulder girdle is week: • Winging of the scapula • Lower pectoralis and trapezii are wasted • Wasting of triceps and biceps • True hypertrophy of deltoids to compensate other muscles • Absent biceps and triceps jerk	3. *Upper limbs:* • Biceps brachioradialis and wrist extensors are involved. • Deltoids may show pseudohypertrophy *Lower limbs* • Initially hip flexors and glutii are weak • Wasting of quadriceps and tibialis anterior • Lateral quadriceps and calves may show hypertrophy.

Note: In both the conditions, IQ remain normal. Serum muscle enzymes are slightly elevated. EMG shows myopathic patterm.

Q. What are the causes of proximal muscle weakness?

Ans. The causes of proximal muscle weakness (myopathy) are:
- Muscular dystrophies
- Collagen vascular disorders, e.g. polymyositis
- Diabetic amyotrophy
- Endocrinal myopathy, e.g. Cushing's syndrome, thyrotoxicosis
- Metabolic myopathies, e.g. hypokalemic
- Porphyria
- Guillain-Barré syndrome
- Myasthenic-myopathic syndrome
- Drug-induced, i.e. steroid, triamcinolone
- Paraneoplastic syndrome
- Osteomalacia

Q. What are the causes of distal muscle weakness?

Ans.
- Distal myopathy of Gower
- Charcoat-Marie-Tooth disease
- Familial polyneuropathy or acquired polyneuropathy
- Myotonia dystrophica

- Guillain-Barré syndrome (postinfective)
- Chronic inflammatory demyelinating polyneuropathy (CIDP).

Q. What is Gower's sign? What are conditions in which Gower's sign is positive?

Ans. When the patient is asked to stand from lying down, he adopts a peculiar manner of rising – called Gower's rising sign or Gower's sign. To demonstrate this sign, the patient (child) is asked to sit on the floor and then rise. In rising from the floor, the affected child gets up first on his hands and knees (see Fig. 1.50A), brings the legs close to the arms, then "climbs up" the legs to the erect position.

Significance: This sign indicates just the proximal (pelvic girdle) muscle weakness, hence, is not specific for Duchenne muscular dystrophy (DMD). It may be present in following conditions:
- Proximal myopathy involving legs (pelvic girdle) due to any cause
- Myasthenia gravis with proximal limb muscles involvement
- Polymyositis
- Spinal muscular dystrophy
- Endocrinal myopathy

Q. What is Waddling gait?

Ans. It is akin to the "gait of a duck". In this type of gait, patient walks on a wide base and sways from side to side during walking. The heels and toes are brought down simultaneously. There is increase in lumbar lordosis. It indicates the proximal muscle weakness and is seen in proximal myopathy. The other causes are:
- Duchenne muscular dystrophy
- Advanced pregnancy
- Bilateral dislocation of hips
- Osteomalacia
- Sometimes huge ascites.

Q. What is winging of scapulae? What are its causes?

Ans. This is lifting off the scapula from the chest when patient attempts abduction and forward movement, e.g. pressing against a wall in standing position. This is due to weakness of scapular stabilizer muscles, is seen in facioscapulohumeral myopathy (Fig. 1.50), palsy of long thoracic nerves (C5-C7) and brachial neuritis.

Q. Which muscles are weak to produce winging of scapulae?

Ans.
- Serratus anterior
- Trapezius

Q. How would you differentiate winging of the scapulae caused by serratus anterior palsy from that of trapezius palsy?

Ans. In serratus anterior palsy, abduction of the arm laterally produces little winging whereas winging is intensified due to weakness of trapezius on abduction of arm against resistance.

Q. What is oculopharyngeal myopathy?

Ans. It is an autosomal dominant disorder, characterised by:
- Late onset (5th or 6th decade)
- Ptosis (bilateral), external ophthalmoplegia (limitation of eye movements with sparing of pupillary reaction for light and accommodation).
- Diplopia is not a feature
- Dysphagia resulting in pooling of secretions and repeated episodes of aspiration
- There may be involvement of facial, neck and limb muscles (occasional).

Q. What are the causes of muscle wasting?

Ans.
- LMN lesion
- UMN lesion with disuse atrophy
- Muscular dystrophies
- Disseminated malignancy (malignant cachexia)
- Diabetes mellitus
- Thyrotoxicosis
- Advanced malnutrition or debility
- Anorexia nervosa

Q. What do you know about brachial neuritis?

Ans. Brachial neuritis (neuralgic amyotrophy) often follows an infection or surgery. Initially, patient has pain around the shoulder followed by muscular weakness affecting the shoulder girdle especially deltoid and serratus anterior producing winging of the scapula. Atrophy around the shoulder is prominent feature.

In this syndrome, more than one nerve lesion is involved Recovery occurs over a period of a year but may not be complete.

Q. How will you investigate a case of myopathy?

Ans. Following investigations are helpful;
- *CK (creatinine kinase) enzyme serial estimation.* The levels are increased
- *EMG* shows myopathic pattern
- *Muscle biopsy confirms the diagnosis* by showing changes of muscle degeneration and regeneration without any cellular infiltration. There is decreased level of dystrophin in the muscles demonstrated by immunochemical staining (Western blot)
- *ECG changes* are present if cardiac muscle is involved (cardiomyopathy). These include tall R waves in V1 and V2, deep Q waves in V5-V6 and RBBB.

Note: Read testing of individual muscle in clinical methods in medicine by Prof SN Chugh.

Q. What is myasthenia gravis? How does it differ from oculopharyngeal myopathy?

Ans. Myasthenia gravis is an autoimmune disorder of neuromuscular junctions characterized by weakness and fatiguability of muscles worsened by repetitive use with a tendency to recover with rest and anticholinergic drugs. The underlying defect is a decrease in the number of acetycholine receptors (AchRs) at neuromuscular junctions due to antibody-mediated autoimmune attack.

The differences between myopathy and myasthesia gravis are given in Table 1.160.

Table 1.160: Myasthenia vs oculopharyngeal myopathy

Myasthenia	Oculopharyngeal myopathy
1. An autoimmune disorder (anticholinergic receptors antibodies present)	• Heredofamilial disorder
2. Can occur in any age group	• More common in younger age
3. Common in females	• Occurs in both sexes
4. Defect lies in neurotransmission at neuromuscular junction	• Defect lies in the muscles (intrinsic muscle disease)
5. Muscle weakness is intermittent, worsened by repetitive use and relieved by rest and anticholinergics	• Weakness is stationary and progressive
6. Bilateral ptosis with diplopia	• Bilateral ptosis without diplopia. Progressive external ophthalmoplegia is presenting feature
7. Exacerbations and remissions common	• Slowly progressive disease
8. Facial muscles and muscles of mastication are commonly involved. Limb muscles are also involved	• They are rarely or occasionally involved. Involvement of limb muscles is uncommon
9. Thymoma may be associated	• No link with thymoma
10. Repetitive nerve stimulation (reduction in the amplitude of evoked response) and anticholinergic receptors antibodies tests are positive and diagnostic	• EMG and muscle biopsy are specific but anticholinergic receptor antibodies are absent
11. Steroids, immunosuppressive drugs, thymomectomy, plasmapheresis and I.V immunoglobulins are therapeutic options	• No treatment, hence, no therapeutic option

CASE 59: WASTING OF SMALL MUSCLES OF HAND AND CLAW HANDS

The patient 30 years M (Fig 1.59) presented with thinning of palms of the hands without pain, paresthesias or numbness along with weakness of both the lower limbs. There was history of widespread twitchings of the muscles. There was no history of bowel and bladder disturbance. Examination revealed wasting of thenar and hypothenar eminence with clawing of hands. The knuckles and bony prominences of hands were prominent. There was hollowing of dorsal interosseous spaces. No trophic changes or sensory loss. Upper limb reflexes were exaggerated despite wasting. In the lower limbs there were exaggerated deep tendon reflexes with ankle clonus. Plantars were bilateral extensors.

Fig. 1.59: Wasting of small muscles of hands

Q. What is the probable diagnosis and why?

Ans. The probable diagnosis is motor neuron disease. The points in favor of the diagnosis are:
1. Wasting of small muscles of hands with exaggerated reflexes in upper limbs despite wasting
2. Diffuse widespread twitchings (fasciculations)
3. UMN type of quadriplegia (spastic quadriplegia)
4. No sensory loss or trophic changes.

Q. How would you proceed to examine such a case with atrophy of small muscles of hands?

Ans. *History*
Points to be noted on history:
1. H/o joint pains (small joints of hands and evidence of deformity for rheumatoid arthritis).

2. H/o shoulder pain or painful neck movements (cervical spondylosis)
3. H/o of twitchings of muscles and weakness (motor neuron disease)
4. Associated dissociated sensory loss or marks of burns or injury on hands or trophic changes (syringomyelia)
5. Family history (Charcot-Marie Tooth disease)
6. Ascending weakness (Guillain-Barre syndrome)
7. H/o trauma to upper limbs (bilateral median and ulnar nerves lesion)

Examination
Proceed as follows:
- Look for fasciculations all over the body especially hands or upper limbs or elicit fasciculations by tapping the muscles.
- Looks for any deformity and swelling
- Check sensations over the hands especially index and little fingers
- Look for atrophy of thenar and hypothenar eminences
- Test handgrip
- Test muscles of thenar and hypothenar eminences.
- Test for median and ulnar nerver compression
- Ask the patient to perform some movements such as unbutton clothes or to write to confirm weakness of small muscles
- Palpate for the cervical ribs and compare radial pulses
- Look for Horner's syndrome
- Examine the neck for lymph nodes and neck movements.

Q. What are the causes of wasting of small muscles of hands?

Ans. The involvement of lower motor neuron in the upper limbs from its origin (anterior horn cells) to its end (muscle) can produce wasting of small muscles of the hand. Depending on the site of involvement, the causes are divided into various groups:
 I. *Diseases involving the anterior horn cells (AHC)*
 - Poliomyelitis
 - Motor neuron disease (amyotrophic lateral sclerosis)
 - Syringomyelia
 - Intramedullary tumors (gliomas, ependymoma)
 II. *Diseases involving motor (anterior) nerve roots (radiculopathy)*
 - Leptomeningitis
 - Arachnoiditis (patchy)
 - Cervical spondylosis
 - Neuralgic amyotrophy

III. Lesions in brachial plexus
- Birth injury (Klumpke's paralysis – C_8-T_1)
- Cervical rib
- Thoracic inlet-syndrome

IV. Peripheral nerve lesions
- Peripheral neuropathy
- Peroneal muscular atrophy involving the upper limbs also
- Carpal tunnel syndrome
- Median and ulnar nerve palsy due to injuries

V. Diseases of the muscles
- Distal myopathy (early and late onset)
- Myotonia dystrophica
- Volkmann's ischemic contractures
- Muscular ischemia due to peripheral vascular disease

VI. Disuse atrophy (reflex wasting, Sudeck's atrophy)
- Rheumatoid arthritis
- Postparalytic (UMN paralysis)
- Post-fracture

VII. As a part and parcel of systemic wasting
- Malignancy, diabetes, thyrotoxicosis, tuberculosis and nutritional
- Paraneoplastic.

Remember:
Some common causes of wasting of small muscles of hands bilaterally
- Motor neurone disease
- Syringmyelia
- Bilateral cervical ribs
- Bilateral median and ulnar nerve palsy
- Distal myopathy
- Myotonia dystrophica
- Charcot-Marie-Tooth disease
- Cervical spondylosis
- Guillain-Barre syndrome

Q. Which nerve roots supply small muscles of hands?
Ans. C_8 and T_1 nerve roots

Q. How will you test small muscles of hands?
Ans. Read Clinical Methods in Medicine by Dr SN Chugh.

Q. What are the causes of fasciculations?
Ans. Read Clinical Methods in Medicine by Dr SN Chugh.

Q. How do you diagnose a cervical rib clinically?
Ans. The cervical rib is suspected clinically when the patient complains of pain along the ulnar border of the hand and forearm. Examination reveals sensory loss in the distribution of T1 with wasting of the thenar muscles. Horner's syndrome may occur. The Adson's test is positive.

Adson's test: This is positive in cervical rib and thoracic outlet syndrome. The examiner feels the pulse of sitting patient by standing behind the patient. Now patient is instructed to turn the head on the affected side and asked to take deep breath. The pulse either get diminished or obliterated on the side affected during this maneuver.

Q. Name the muscles of thenar and hypothenar eminence.
Ans. Following are the muscles:

Muscles of thenar eminence	Muscles of hypothenar eminence
• Abductor pollicis brevis	• Abductor digiti minimi
• Flexor pollicis brevis	• Flexor digiti minimi
• Opponens pollicis	• Opponens digiti minimi

Q. What is claw hand? What are its causes?
Ans. Read case discussion on peripheral neuropathy.

Paralysis of interossi and lumbricals produce *claw hand*.

Q. What is wrist drop?
Ans. Read case discussion on peripheral neuropathy.

Q. What are trophic changes? Name the trophic changes in skin?
Ans. Trophic changes are neurogenic in origin, involve skin, its appendages and joints (charcot joint), occur due to repeated trauma in the region of anesthesia.

The trophic changes in the skin include;
- Dry and rough skin with lack of sweating
- Pigmentation
- Fall of hairs (hypotrichosis)
- Local cyanosis or edema
- Nails are brittle
- Trophic ulcers.

Q. What are sites of trophic changes? What are its causes?
Ans. Trophic changes are common at pressure points such as:
- On the lateral malleolus
- Back of heel of the foot/feet
- Over the sacrum (classical site for bedsore)
- Back of shoulder girdle.

The causes are same as that of Charcot joint.

Q. What is Charcot joint? What are its causes?
Ans. It is a neuropathic joint characterized by:
- Painless joint swelling (e.g. knee, hip, shoulder joint)
- Hypermobile joint
- Disorganized and destroyed joint
- Loose bodies or osteophytes in the joint cavity
- Palpable crepitus

The causes of Charcot's joint are:
- Peripheral neuropathies, commonly due to leprosy, diabetes and hereditary sensory neuropathy
- Syringomyelia (upper limb joints are commonly involved)
- Tabes dorsalis (lower limb joints are commonly involved)

For Charcot joint, always test for the sensations.

Q. How will you arrive at the etiological diagnosis of wasting of small muscles of hands?

Ans. History and physical examination will help to find out the cause of wasting of small muscles of hand.

1. *History:* Wasting since childhood is common with poliomyelitis and birth injury (Klumpke's paralysis)
2. *Neck pain* indicates cervical spondylosis, cervical rib and intra- or extramedullary tumor
3. Fasciculations with brisk tendon reflexes in the case described above indicate amyotrophy lateral sclerosis
4. Symmetrical joint involvement suggests rheumatoid arthritis
5. Trophic changes in hands occur leprosy, syringomyelia, cervical rib
6. Thickened ulnar nerve points towards leprosy
7. No sensory loss indicates motor neuron disease while dissociated sensory loss indicates syringomyelia.

Patient (Fig. 1.60) complained of easy fatiguability and muscle weakness. The muscle weakness was marked in the evening and increases with exercise. There was difficulty in chewing and speaking. The patient also complained of drooping of upper eyelids in the evening.

Fig. 1.60

Q. What is your probable diagnosis? Give points in favor of your diagnosis.

Ans. After history and examination, my provisional diagnosis is myasthenia gravis.

Points in favor of my diagnosis are:

- H/o easy fatiguability and weakness, more marked in the evening. There is difficulty in chewing.
- Presence of bilateral ptosis, snarling smile and nasal speech.
- Proximal muscle weakness without wasting and deep tendon jerks are preserved.
- There is no sensory disturbance.

Q. What would you ask from such a case in history?

Ans. *Points to be noted on history*

- Obtain history of weakness and diplopia at the end of the day.
- Is muscle weakness painless and transient? Does it improve with rest and sleep?
- Obtain history in details regarding the muscles affected, i.e. difficulty in smiling, difficulty in chewing, speaking, difficulty in holding the neck for long period, difficulty in walking.
- Obtain history of thyrotoxicosis, diabetes mellitus, rheumatoid arthritis, SLE and thymoma (mediastinal compression).
- H/o drug e.g. d-penicillamine.

Q. How would you proceed to examine such a case?

Ans. *Examination*

- Examine the eyes for ptosis

- Check the worsening of ptosis after sustained upward gaze for one minute.
- Check extraocular muscles for diplopia or squint
- Ask the patient to smile; note the characteristic snarling smile
- Speech is nasal (nasal twang)
- Ask the patient to sip some amount of water, note any nasal regurgitation
- Examine the limbs for weakness, hypotonia, decreased power and reflexes. The limb weakness is proximal and symmetric. Deep tendon reflexes are preserved.
- Examine the neck muscles. Neck extensors may be weak.
- Test for sensations and coordination.

Q. What is your differential diagnosis?

Ans. Other conditions that can mimic myasthenia gravis are:

- Botulism
- Drug-induced myasthenia
- Myasthenia-myopathic syndrome (Eaton-Lambert syndrome)
- Hyperthyroidism
- Neuroasthenia
- Oculopharyngeal myopathy

Q. What is peak age for myasthenia gravis?

Ans. The peak age in women is 20-30 years and in men is 50-60 years, hence, incidence has two age peaks.

Q. What groups of muscles are commonly affected in myasthenia?

Ans. The muscles involved in order of likelihood are:

- Extraocular
- Bulbar
- Neck
- Limb girdle
- Distal limbs
- Trunk

Q. What is neuroasthenia?

Ans. It is a historic term used for myasthenia-like fatigue syndrome without an organic basis. These patients may present with subjective symptoms of weakness and fatigue. Muscle testing reveal "jerky release" or "give-away weakness" characteristic of nonorganic disorders. The complaint of fatigue in these patients means tiredness or apathy rather than decreasing muscle power on repeated effort.

Q. Name the disorders associated with myasthenia gravis?

Ans. Myastheria gravis is an autoimmune disorder, hence other autoimmune diseases may be associated with it. These include Hashimoto's thyroiditis, Graves' disease, rhenumatoid arthritis and SLE.

Disorders of thymus, i.e. thymoma or hyperplasia may also be associated.

Q. Which drug causes myasthenia?

Ans. Penicillamine used for treatment of rheumatoid arthritis and scleroderma may result in true myasthenia gravis, but weakness is mild and transient, recovery occurs within weeks or months after discontinuing its use.

Q. Name the drug or disorders that may exacerbate myasthenia gravis?

Ans.
- Fatique, exercise, emotion, change of climate
- Pregnacy
- Thyroid disorders, i.e. both hyper- and hypothyroidism
- Occult infection
- Drugs, e.g. aminoglycosides, quinine, antiarrhythmics (procainamide)
- Magnesium enemas.

Q. Name the disorders that interfere with therapy?

Ans.
- Tuberculosis
- Peptic ulcer
- Retinal disease
- Asthma
- Obesity
- Diabetes
- GI bleed
- Hypertension
- Osteoprosis

Q. How does myasthenia differ from oculopharyngeal myopathy?

Ans. Read the table 1.160 in case discussion of myopathy

Q. How is myasthenia graded clinically?

Ans. Osserman's grading of severity is

Grade I: Ocular myasthenia

Grade IIA: Mild generalized myasthenia with slow progression; no crises; drug responsive

Grade IIB: Moderate generalized myasthenia, severe skeletal and bulbar involvement but no crises, drug response is less satisfactory.

Grade III: Acute fulminant myasthenia, rapid progession of severe symptoms of respiratory crises and poor drug response, high incidence of thymoma; high mortaly rate

Grade IV: Late severe myasthenia; same as grade III but takes two years to progress from class I to II crises; high mortality rate.

Q. What investigation would you like to perform in this patient?

Ans.
- *Serum acetylcholine receptors (AChR) antibodies* positive in > 85% cases of generalized myasthenia and 50% in ocular myasthenia
- *Eudrophonium chloride (tensilon) test*; An initial test dose of 2mg I.V. is given, if definite improvement in weakness and muscle strength occurs, test is said to be positive and is terminated. It there is no change, an additional dose of 8 mg I.V. is given and test the response again.

- *Vital capacity* may be reduced.
- *CT and MRI of chest* for thymoma/mediastinal growth
- *Plasma thyroxine levels* to rule out associated thyroid disease
- *Detection of antibodies such as*
  - Antistriated muscle antibodies (seen in association with thymoma)
  - Antinuclear antibodies, rheumatoid factors, antithyroid antibodies for associated other autoimmune disorders
  - Tuberculin test if immunosuppressive therapy is contemplated
- *EMG abnormalities*
  - Repetitive nerve stimulation for decremental response; decrement of >15% indicates highly probable diagnosis.
  - Single fiber electromyography; an evidence of neuromuscular blockade in the form of jitter and blocking of motor action potential, with normal fiber density, is confirmatory.

Q. What treatment modalities are available?

Ans. Symptomatic treatment with an anticholinesterase drug e.g. pyridostigmine (60 mg orally 3 to 5 times a day). For definite treatment, following drugs are used;

- Corticosteroids
- Immunosuppressive, e.g. azathioprine, cyclosporine, mycophenolate mofetil
- Plasmapheresis
- Intravenous immunoglobulins as immunomodulator
- Thymectomy

Q. What is myasthenic crisis?

Ans. Myasthenic crisis is defined as an exacerbation of weakness sufficient to endanger life; usually consists of respiratory failure caused by bulbar, diaphragmatic and intercostal muscle weakness which predispose to respiratory infection.

Thus, crisis can be precipitated by respiratory infection and surgery. Such patients with bulbar and respiratory involvement must be closely monitored for pulmonary function. Treatment includes respiratory support, treatment of respiratory infection and fluid and electrolyte therapy.

Q. What is cholinergic crisis? How does it manifest?

Ans. It is defined as excessive anticholinesterase medication in a patient of myasthenia.

Excessive salivation, lacrimation, confusion, miosis, pallor and collapse are its manifestations.

Treatment is stop anticholinesterase drug therapy.

Q. What is role of thymectomy in myasthenia?

Ans. Thymoma is commonly associated with myasthenia, hence in the case of thymoma, thymectomy is necessary to prevent tumor spread though it is benign. In the absence of thymoma, thymectomy has also been found useful in 85% of patients.

Q. What are the differences between myasthenia gravis and myasthenia-myopathic syndrome?

Ans.

Myasthenia gravis	Myasthenia-myopathic syndrome
• An autoimmune disorder involving AchR i.e. there is deficiency of acetylcholine receptors	• Presynaptic disorder of neuromuscular junction. AChR are not involved
• More common in females	• Common in males
• Other autoimmune disease may be associated	• No such association
• Deep tendor jerks are preserved	• Tendon jerks are lost

Contd...

Contd...

Myasthenia gravis	Myasthenia-myopathic syndrome
• Muscle weekness is proximal as well as distal	• Muscle weakness is proximal
• Autonomic changes uncommon	• Autonomic changes, e.g. dry mouth, impotence common
• EMG shows decremental response on repetitive nerve stimulation	• Incremental rather decremental response is seen on EMG on repetitive nerve stimulation.
• It is caused by antibodies directed against acetylcholine receptors (AChR) which can be assayed	• It is caused by auto-antibodies directed against P/Q type calcium channels at the motor nerve terminals. These antibodies can be detected on radioimmunoassay
• Thymoma or thymic hyperplasia is common	• It is associated with malignancy commonly small cell carcinoma of lung

Examine the Lower Limbs

The patient (Fig 1.61) presented with weakness of both lower limbs, left more than right since childhood. This weakness was stable but caused difficultly in walking. Patient used callipers for walking. There was no history of fasciculations, bowel or bladder disturbance.

Fig. 1.61A: Postpolio paralysis of leg

Q. What is your provisional diagnosis and why?

Ans. In view of selective weakness of lower limbs (Left > Right) with thinning of legs since childhood, the provisional diagnosis is postpolio paralysis of lower limbs.

The points in favor of diagnosis are:
1. Weakness since childhood.
2. Asymmetric paralysis of lower limbs (left > Right)
3. Thinning of left lower limb more than right
4. Areflexia of lower limbs with other signs of LMN paralysis.
5. No bowel and bladder involvement
6. Weakness is stationary and nonprogressive.

Q. What would be your differential diagnosis?

Ans. All the conditions that produce lower motor neuron paralysis of lower limbs will come into differential diagnosis.

1. *Peripheral neuropathy.* The characteristic features are:
   • Gloves-stocking sensory symptoms and sensory loss of all modalites.
   • Symmetric weakness of peripheral part of lower limbs
   • LMN paralysis of lower limbs (legs)

• No bladder and bowel involvement
   • Nerve conduction velocities show delayed conduction and delayed terminal latency.
   • Trophic changes may be present.

2. *Guillain-Barre syndrome.* The characteristic features are:
   • Acute or subacute onset of paralysis of legs following sore throat or viral infection or vaccination etc.
   • Symmetric weakness of lower limbs (legs are more involved than thighs).
   • Paresthesias
   • Urinary symptoms.
   • Lower motor neuron paralysis (areflexia, hypotonia).
   • Paralysis may ascend to thorax and cause dyspnea due to diaphragmatic and intercostal muscles paralysis
   • Cranial nerves may also get involved.

3. *Motor neuron disease* (Progressive muscular atrophy). The features are:
   • Late onset and progressive muscular weakness
   • Distal weakness is more marked than proximal
   • Weakness is symmetrical
   • Jerks may be retained inspite of severe muscular weakness.
   • Fasciculations are present and marked in lower limbs

4. *Cauda equina syndrome.* The features are:
   • Pain in the anterior thighs and weakness and wasting of proximal muscles more than distal muscles of lower limbs (thigh > legs).
   • Flaccid, asymmetric paraparesis (LMN paralysis)
   • Saddle- shaped sensory loss upto level of L_1.
   • Bladder and bowel involvement common
   • History of neural claudication or history of trauma to spine.

5. *Postparalysis* (postpolio muscular atrophy, postpolio syndrome) atrophy.
   • History of fever followed by weakness of one limb or more than one limb during childhood. This develops 20-30 years after initial attack of poliomyelitis.
   • The weakness/atrophy is selective, involves one or more groups of muscles, usually of legs. weakness is more proximal than distal.
   • Flaccid, asymmetric paralysis involving one limb or both limbs (in my case both limbs are involved)
   • There is thinning of legs/lower limbs. Weakness is nonprogressive.

- There is lower motor neuron paralysis, deep tendon jerks are absent but tone may be normal in the atrophic muscles.
- Fasciculations may be present

6. **Closed Spina bifida**
- Usually asymptomatic and unilateral involvement
- Bilateral involvement is uncommon, may produce shortening of limbs with atrophy of muscles below the knee.
- There is dermatomal sensory loss. Ankle jerk is absent.
- Neuropathic bladder and enuresis
- There may be a tulf of hair, or a cutaneous lipoma or a dimple or naevus above the sacrum
- Radiology is diagnostic, shows failure of closure of one or several vertebral arches, scoliosis, pedicle erosion and bony spur.

7. *Lumbar spondylosis (lumbar disk disease)*
- Occurs in old age
- There is low back pain or foot pain which increases with coughing, sneezing and during straining.
- The disease is commonly unilateral but central disk prolapse may produce bilateral symptoms. Bilateral symptoms are common in spinal canal stenosis with degenerative disk disease.
- Sensory symptoms include radicular pain and dermational sensory loss.
- Motor symptoms include, abnormal posture, limitation of spinal involvement, focal weakness, muscle atrophy of leg/legs, fasciculations and loss of jerks (ankle).

8. *Spinal muscular atrophy*

Fig. 1.61B: Spinal muscular atrophy

- It is an autosomal recessive neurodegenerative disorder primarily affecting anterior horn cells in spinal cord and bulbar motor nuclei.
- It produces asymmetric weakness and wasting of proximal muscles of limbs in children and adults (type 3), first involves lower limbs and later upper limbs.
- Neck, trunk muscles may be involved. Bulbar nuclei may be affected.
- Lumbar lordosis and calf hypertophy may be seen in most of cases.
- All the tendon reflexes are diminished but ankle reflexes are preserved till late.

Q. What are the causes of unilateral leg wasting?
Ans. 1. Poliomyelitis
2. Lumbar disk prolapse.
3. Radiculopathy.
4. Wasted leg syndrome, seen in farmers, reported from punjab, occurs due to compression of sciatic nerve during ploughing of field when farmer keeps one leg over the 'Hal' during ploughing. It is reversible but repeated trauma may result in atrophy.
5. Sciatica syndrome

Q. What is fasciculation? What are its causes?
Ans. Read 'Clinical Methods in Medicine' by Prof SN Chugh.

Q. Where is the site of lesion in poliomyelitis?
Ans. In the anterior horn cells of the spinal cord

Q. Is muscular atrophy in poliomyelitis stationary or progressive?
Ans. Paralytic poliomyelitis usually remains stable after the initial attack. However in some cases, new muscle weakness and atrophy involving previously affected muscles or even unaffected muscles occurs and this deterioration can continue as long as 30 years after first attack called postpolio muscular atrophy or postpolio syndrome. This progression is slow but distinct from motor neuron disease. It is not clear why it occurs in some patients not in all. It has been reported to occur in those cases who have widespread paralysis and poor immune status.

Q. What is prevention of poliomyelitis?
Ans. Poliomyelitis is preventable disease caused by polio virus. Three types of polio vaccine are available (each containing all three strains of the virus)
1. *Oral polio vaccine of sabin.* It consists of live attenuated virus.
2. *Salk vaccine.* It consists of killed or inactivated virus.
3. *Enhanced potency vaccine of vanwezel.*

Q. Which vaccine has been associated with paralytic poliomyelitis?

Ans. Oral polio vaccine particularly in immunodeficient persons has been associated with vaccine-associated paralytic polio (VAPP). Such individuals and their household contacts should be given inactivated vaccine.

Q. What is pulse polio immunization program (Fig. 1.61C)?

Ans. This is WHO recommended program in countries where poliovirus transmission is widespread or APP surveillance is unreliable or both.

In this program, all children less than 5 years of age are immunized on national immunization days (NIDs) with two doses of oral polio vaccine (OPV) spaced about 1 month apart regardless of their previous immunization status. These mass compaigns aim to colonize the guts of children with vaccine virus so that child to child spread of wild poliovirus is hampered and circulation of virus stops. Population immunity resulting from NIDs appears to be superior to that produced by routine immunization.

Q. What do you understand by "provocation poliomyelitis"?

Ans. Provocation poliomyelitis is caused by the administration of intramuscular injection during the incubation period of wild type poliomyelitis or shortly after exposure to oral polio vaccine.

Q. What are complications of paralytic poliomyelitis?

Ans. 1. Gastric dilatation
2. Intestinal erosions

Fig. 1.61C: Despite pulsepolio program in India, polio still persists in UP, Bihar and certain other states in India

3. Hypertension
4. Myocarditis
5. Skeletal decalcification.

Q. How does polio spread in human?

Ans. By feco-oral route from infected to healthy child

Q. How does polio virus reach the nervous system?

Ans. Two routes of viral entry have been proposed, i.e. via bloodstream or via. peripheral nerves. Since viremia precedes the onset of neurologic disease in humans, it has been assumed that virus enters the CNS via bloodstream. Through the bloodstream, it reaches the muscles where poliovirus receptors are present in the motor end plate region of neuromuscular junction. It travels across the neuromuscular junctions up the axon to the anterior horm cells where it settles down to cause the disease.

Q. What are important clinical stages of poliomyelitis?

Ans. 1. *Asymptomatic stage*
2. *Abortive poliomyelitis.* After incubation period of 3-6 days, 5% individuals have minor illness, fever, myalgia, sore throat, headaches. This resolves within 3 days.
3. *Nonparalytic poliomyelitis.* About 1% individuals with abortive poliomyelitis, donot resolve, pass on to develop aseptic meningitis (nonparalytic poliomyelitis) which is diagnosed on CSF examination by lymphocytosis. The symptoms of abortive poliomyelitis are present during this phase.
4. *Paralytic poliomyelitis* After one to several days, signs of aseptic meningitis in some patients are followed by back, neck and muscle pain followed by motor paralysis. Weakness is generally asymmetric, is proximal more than distal.

Q. What is bulbar poliomyelitis?

Ans. Involvement of bulbar nuclei due to polio virus is called *bulbar poliomyelitis.* It is characterised by dysphagia, difficulty in handling secretions, or dysphonia, respiratory paralysis and circulatory collapse due to medullary paralysis.Most patients with paralysis recover some function weeks to months after infection, about two thirds of patients have residual disease.

Q. Which muscles are paralyzed in polio?

Ans. • Limb muscles (proximal>distal)
• Thoracic and abdominal muscles.
• Bulbar muscles

Complex Partial Seizures with Generalization

The patient in picture (Fig.1.62) presented with history of a fit (seizure) in the morning while doing some work. During an attack, attendant noticed jerking of all the limbs with frothing at the mouth. There was passage of urine in the underwear. Patient became unconscious and sustained forehead injury and biting of tongue and loss of an incisor.

Fig. 1.62: A patient with complex partial seizure

Q. What is your clinical diagnosis?

Ans. The patient has grand mal (complex partial seizure) epilepsy, the cause of which has to be found out.

Q. How would you proceed to examine such a case?

Ans. History

Points to be noted
- Take a detailed history regarding description of fit/fits from the attendant(s) or from a person(s) who has/have observed the fit/seizure.

Specific enquiries about fit/fits
- Timing and duration of an attack.
- Presence of an aura, its duration and symptoms.
- Precipitating event leading to an attack.
- Abnormal movements, i.e. jerking limb, stiffening or automatism.
- Salivation or frothing at the mouth.
- Biting of the tongue.
- Incontinence of urine and faeces.
- Postictal phenomenon, i.e. headache, drowsiness or aches and pain, weakness of a limb or me half of the body (Todd's paralysis)
- Cyanosis
- Past history of head injury, diabetes, hypertension etc.

- Family history of seizure
- Habits, e.g. vegetarian/non-vegetarian

Physical signs
- Examination of pulse, BP and heart.
- Palpation of carotid arteries and ausculation over them for a bruit or a murmur
- Examination of head for trauma.
- Any paralysis of limb/limbs.
- Skin for epiloia, neurofibromatosis or pigmentation.
- Visual fields examination.
- Optic fundi examination.

Q. What is Todd's paralysis?

Ans. Paralysis of a limb or hemiplegia occurring after an epileptic attack is called *Todd's paralysis*. It occurs due to exhaustion of neurons in precentral gyrus. The paralysis is transient and may last few days (1-3 days)

Q. What is Jacksonian epilepsy?

Ans. It is a simple partial seizure of focal onset arising in one portion of the precentral gyrus resulting in a fit involving one part of the body (e.g. thumb) and then spreads to involve that side of the body or the whole body. It suggests usually an intracranial space occupying lesion.

Q. What is the major difference between complex partial and simple partial seizure?

Ans. In simple partial of seizure, awareness is preserved while it is lost in complex partial seizure.

Q. Why does consciousness lost in Grand mal seizure?

Ans. The generalized spread of discharge involving both the cerebral hemispheres produces unconscious due to involvement of reticular activating system (RAS) bilaterally.

Q. What are various phases of grand mal seizure?

Ans.
- *Prodromal Phase.* Patient feels uneasiness or irritability.
- *Aura.* It precedes tonic-clonic phase characterized by hallucinations (e.g. visual, deja vu phenomenon), Jerking of a limb, GI symptoms
- *Tonic-clonic phase* characterized by jerking of a limb or one half of the body, frothing from the mouth, biting of tongue, incontinence of sphincters etc.
- *Unconciousness,* i.e. there is loss of conciousness
- *Postictal phenomenon* e.g. confusion, headache and automatic behavior

Q. What are common causes of seizures in an adult?

Ans.
- Idiopathic
- Space occupying lesion (e.g. brain tumor, neurocysticercosis)
- CVA (Cerebrovascular accidents)
- Hypertensive encephalopathy

267

- Head Injury
- Infections, e.g. meningitis, encephalitis, brain abscess
- Alcohol withdrawl
- Metabolic e.g. Hepatic failure, renal failure, hypoglycemia
- Electrolyte disturbance (hyponatremia)
- Alzheimer's disease

Q. What are precipitating factors?

Ans.
- Insomnia
- Physical or mental fatigue
- Drugs
- Flashes of bright light (photosensitivity)
- Loud noise or music
- Stress
- Pyrexia
- Infection
- Alcohol ingestion or withdrawal
- Reading or writing

Q. What are differences between a hysterical fit and an epileptic fit?

Ans. The difference are given below:

Grand mal fits	Hysterical conversion fits
• The fits occur in a coordinated fashion due to hypersynchro-nous discharge of neurons.	• The fits may from simple falling to the ground to bizarre attacks
• Stereotyped movements of limbs (tonic and clonic) occur.	• There is wild bizarre movements (shaking twitching) of all the four limbs simultaneously. There is usually no tonic phase.
• Attacks can occur during any time of the day	• Attacks occur when patient is being observed or somebody is present.
• Patient may injure himself or herself during an attack	• Patient does not hurt himself during an attack
• These are unprovoked fits. There is no purpose behind these fits. These are true seizures	• Attacks occur with some purpose, i.e. to draw the attention to hears and dears or to seek compensation or sympathy. These are seizurespseudo.
• There may be biting of tongue during seizure.	• There is no biting of tongue during fit.
• There is urine and faecal incontinence	• There is no urine or faecal incontinence.
• The seizures may be precipitated by some known factors	• There are no known precipitating factors.
• Pattern of the fits is fixed.	• Frequent change in the pattern of fits. There may

Contd...

Grand mal fits	Hysterical conversion fits
	either be an additon or deletion of some symptoms during the fit.
• EEG is often abnormal	• EEG is normal
• Serum prolactin levels high during or after seizure	• Serum prolactin level normal

Q. How would you investigate such a case?

Ans.
- Complete hemogram
- Blood biochemistry, e.g. urea, creatinine, magnesium, glucose
- Liver function fests
- Serological tests for syphilis and HIV
- X-rays chest and skull
- EEG
- CT scan
- MRI scan

Q. What does serial seizuess mean? How does it differ from status epilepticus?

Ans. Serial epilepsy means fits occur in succession but patient is conscious in between seizures.

Status epilepticus means seizures follow each others in succession without recovery of consciousness in between seizures.

Q. How would you treat a patients with epilepsy?

Ans.
- *General advice* regarding Do's and Don'ts in epilepsy
- *Drug therapy.* The first line drugs in grand mal epilepsy include phenytoin, sodium valproate, carbamazepine, lamotrigine as monotherapy. Several new add-on-drugs have been developed for combination therapy. The main aim of treatment is to control seizure. When seizures are controlled, the drug (s) can be continued for 3 years to produce seizure free period, after which the drug may be withdrawn slowly. If seizure occurs during this period, the drug(s) should be reinstituted and continued throughout life.
- *Advice* about arriving.

Q. What are do's and dont's in epilepsy?

Ans.

Do's (to be done)	Don't (not to be done)
A. During an epileptic fit	During an attack of fit
• Move the patient to safer place	• Neither put your finger, nor allow any one to put the finger into the mouth

Contd...

Contd...

Contd...

Do's (to be done)	Don't (not to be done)
• Loosen the clothes around neck • Make the patient to breath fresh air and comfortable • Try to prevent the tongue biting by putting tighly packed handkerchief or a piece of cloth in the mouth • Remove the artificial denture if any B. After the convulsion ceases • Turn the patient to semiprone position • Make the air passage clear Advise the patient to consult doctor	• Do not put any thing (liquid) into the mouth

Q. What precautions an epileptic patient should observe?

Ans. Following precautions should be observed before a good control of seizures is achieved.

- Avoid working or recreation near open fires
- Not to operate dangerous machinery.
- Not to lock bathroom door while taking bath
- They should take shallow bath in a pond or a canal, that too in the presence of someone.
- Cycling, swimming, mountaineering should be discouraged until 6 months seizure free interval is achieved. Driving is prohibited unless one year symptom, free period is achieved.

Q. How would you classify epilepsy?

Ans. They are classified into 3 groups

   I. **Generalized seizures**
- Tonic-clonic seizures (Grand mal type)
- Tonic seizure
- Absence seizures
- Akinetic seizures
- Myoclonic seizures

   II. **Partial seizures**
- Simple partial (Jacksonian type)
- Complex partial
- Partial seizures with secondary generalization (tonic-clonic evolution)
- Generalized tonic-clonic seizures with an evidence of focal onset.

   III. **Unclassified seizure**

Skin Diseases

CASE 63: ALOPECIA

A female patient (Fig. 1.63) presented with loss of hair on the scalp. Examination showed patchy loss of hair on the scalp.

Fig. 1.63: Alopecia areata. A young female with non-scarring loss of scalp hair

Perform General Physical Examination

Q. What is the most likely diagnosis and why?

Ans. • *Alopecia areata* is probable diagnosis. Sudden onset of patchy hair loss with regrowing of hair as fine depigmented downy growth in an adult suggests alopecia areata. There is no scarring

Q. What is alopecia areata?

Ans. It is probable an autoimmune disorder involving, skin, hair, and nails causing patchy nonscarring alopecia with pitting, ridging and furrowing of nails.

Q. How would you proceed to examine such a case?

Ans. History

Point to be asked
- H/o atopy
- H/o family occurrence
- H/o any local symptoms
- H/o drugs
- H/o any systemic illness such as SLE, thyroid disease, HIV and syphilis or autoimmune disease

Examination
- Look at the patch of hair loss carefully and note whether hair loss is well defined and there is regrowing of hair in the patch as depigmented downy growth.
- Look at the other sites, e.g. eyebrows and beard area for hair loss.
- Note whether alopecia is scarring or nonscarring.
- Examine the nails for fine pitting, transverse lines dystrophy, fragmentation (anonychorrhexis) and ridging and nail dystrophy (roughened nail surface and brittle free nail edge)
- Look for any evidence of vitiligo.

Q. What is differential diagnosis of alopecia areata?

Ans. All the causes of nonscarring alopecia (primary cutaneous disorders) that come into the differential diagnosis are tabulated (Table 1.162).

Q. Is scarring present in alopecia areata?

Ans. No. Read the causes of nonscarring alopecia in Table 1.161.

Q. What is alopecia totalis and alopecia universalis?

Ans. If all the hair on the scalp are lost, it is called *alopecia totalis*, and if there is complete loss of body hair from all sites, it is called *alopecia universalis*.

Q. What are the causes of alopecia?

Ans. These are given in Table 1.161.

Table 1.161: Causes of alopecia

1. **Nonscarring alopecia**
   A. *Primary cutaneous disorders*
      - Telogen effluvium
      - Androgenic alopecia
      - Alopecia areata
      - Taenia capitis
      - Traumatic alopecia
   B. *Drugs*, e.g. Thallium, heparin, antimetabolites, antithyroid, hypervitaminosis, retinoids, oral contraceptives
   C. *Systemic diseases*
      - SLE
      - Secondary syphilis
      - Hypo- and hyperthyroidism
      - Deficiency of proteins, biotin and Zn
      - HIV infection

II. **Scarring alopecia**
   A. *Primary cutaneous disorders*
      - Cutaneous lupus
      - Lichen planus
      - Folliculitis decalvans
      - Linear scleroderma (morphea)
   B. *Systemic diseases*
      - SLE
      - Sarcoidosis
      - Cutaneous metastases

Q. What are the sites of alopecia areata?

Ans. The sites are:
   1. Scalp

Table 1.162: Diagnosis and differential diagnosis, pathogenesis and treatment of various nonscarring alopecia including alopecia areata

Condition	Clinical features	Pathogenesis	Treatment
Alopecia areata	• Well-circumscribed patchy areas of hair loss, 2-5 cm in diameter • Extensive involvement may lead to hair loss on other hair-bearing surfaces of the body • Nail pitting, ridges, and furrows can be seen	• The germinal zones of the hair follicles are surrounded by T-lymphocytes leading to cessation of hair growth and club-hair formation • Hereditary (Down's syndrome), stress, endocrinal and other autoimmune disorders like Addison's disease, hyper- and hypothyroidism, vitiligo, pernicious anemia may be associated	• Topical anthraline, intralesional and systemic steroids, topical contact sensitizer
Telogen effluvium (It is transitory) increase in the number of hair entering into dying phase (telogen phase-resting phase) of hair growth cycle.	• Sudden diffuse shedding off normal hairs • Causes include certain major stresses, e.g. pregnancy, postpartum, acute severe infection, acute psychiatric illness, emotional or physical trauma, surgery, oral contraceptives • Reversible without treatment	Stresses cause the normally asynchronous growth cycles of individual hair to become synchronous, therefore large number of growing hairs (anagen) simultaneously enter the dying (telogen) phase	• No treatment required • Only observation • Discontinue the offending drug • Check thyroid functions • Prognosis is good
Androgenic alopecia (common male baldness)	• Symmetric diffuse hair loss in fronto-central (midline) area of the scalp • Recession of anterior, posterior and lateral hair lines in all men and some women	• Increased sensitivity of affected hairs to testosterone • Increased levels of circulating androgens (ovarian and adrenal source in women)	If no evidence of hyper-androgen state then topical minoxidil ± tretinoin; hair transplant or wig wearing on the scalp is last option.
Tinea capitis	Hair loss varies from scaling with minimal hair loss to discrete patches with black dots (broken hairs) to boggy plaque with pustules (kerion)	Invasion of hairs by dermatophytes	• Oral griesofulvin plus 2.5% selenium sulphide or ketoconazole shampoo • Examine other family members
Traumatic alopecia	• Broken hairs • Irregular outline	• Traction with curlers, rubber bands, braiding • Exposure to heat or chemicals • Mechanical pulling (trichotillomania)	• Discontinue the offending hair style or chemical treatment • Hair clipping and psychotherapy for trichotillomania

2. Beard, eyebrows and eyelashes
3. Moustache.

Q. What is pathognomonic sign of alopecia areata?

Ans. The presence of *"exclamation mark hair"* at the periphery of lesion is the pathognomonic sign of disease activity. These hair are short that taper and become depigmented as the scalp is approached. Plucking reveals that the hair are in telogen phase.

Q. Which systemic disorders are associated with alopecia areata?

Ans. Alopecia areata being an immune-mediated non-inflammatory disorder is associated with other autoimmune disorders such as:
  • Autoimmune thyroid disorders, Addison's disease
  • Vitiligo

  • Pernicious anemia
  • Atopy

Q. Name the drugs causing alopecia?

Ans. Read the Table 1.161.

Q. What is the commonest cause of alopecia.

Ans. Alopecia areata.

Q. Name the commonest systemic disorder producing alopecia.

Ans. SLE

Q. What is treatment of alopecia areata?

Ans. • Steroids (topical and systemic)
  • PUVA therapy but alopecia returns after stoppage of therapy
  • Dithranol is left on the scalp for 20-30 minutes
  • Topical minoxidil

271

Q. What is trichotillomania?

Ans. It is mechanical pulling of hair leading to broken hair. Hair loss is irregular and there is always hair growing as they are not long enough to be pulled out. The patch of hair loss is unilateral and occurs on the same side as the patient's dominant hand. The patient may be unaware of this habit.

Q. What is telogen effluvium?

Ans. Read the differential diagnosis in Table 1.162.

Q. What do you understand by male pattern baldness?

Ans. In some men who are predisposed to this pattern of baldness, androgens cause a switch from terminal to vellus or vellus like follicles on the scalp hair of men and a reduction in the duration of an anagen phase. These individuals have increased androgens receptors and 5α-reductase (converts testosterone to 5-dehydrotestosterone) activities in frontal hair follicle is greater than in occipital follicles. This is an explanation of frontal baldness in men. Based on this concept, finasteride - 5α-reductase inhibitor is useful for treatment as it causes regrowth of hair in 70% men after 2 years of continuous use.

CASE 64: ERYTHEMA NODOSUM

The patient presented with bilateral painful small nodules over the skin after taking some drug. There was associated history of fever and arthralgia. The nodules were tender and palpable (Fig. 1.64).

Fig. 1.64: Erythema nodosum over the skin

Q. Describe the skin lesions. What is your clinical diagnosis?

Ans. • The lesions are multiple, red erythematous nodules which are non-itchy but painful and tender
• They are bilateral and symmetrical (only one side is shown)
• They are present on the shin

The probable clinical diagnosis is Erythema Nodosum.

Q. What would you like to ask on history from the patient?

Ans. Following points are to be asked:
• Ask history of fever preceding lesion.
• H/O arthralgias
• Sore throat (β-hemolyticus streptococcal infection)
• Drugs (oral contraceptives, penicillins, sulpho-namides)
• Gastrointestinal symptoms (*Yersinia enterocolitica infection*)
• Infections e.g. tuberculosis, leprosy, coccidioido-mycosis, histoplasmosis
• Sarcoidosis

Q. What is erythema nodosum? What is common site of this lesion?

Ans. Erythema nodosum is a panniculitis (inflammation of fat) characterized by painful, tender, subcutaneous,

red (erythematous) nodules. The lesions are present on the extensor surfaces, e.g. anterior portion of leg (over the shin), thigh, upper arm or forearm. The lesions appear in crops, therefore, lesions in different stages of evolution may be seen. Shin is the commonest site.

Q. What are the common causes of erythema nodosum?

Ans. Common causes are:
• Primary pulmonary tuberculosis
• Infections, e.g. β-*hemolyticus streptococci, yersinia, salmonella and chlamydia*
• Lepromatous leprosy
• Inflammatory bowel disease, e.g. ulcerative colitis or Crohn's disease
• Sarcoidosis
• Drug hypersensitivity, e.g. sulphonamides, penicillins, oral contraceptives and barbiturates
• Fungal infections, e.g. *histoplasmosis or coccidiodomycosis*
• Behcet's syndrome
• Brucellosis
• Rarely in rheumatic fever.

Q. What is basic pathology of the lesion?

Ans. This is type III (immune complex) hypersensitivity reaction, involves the fat (panniculitis) and the blood vessels (vasculitis).

The shin is the most common site of involvement because foreign proteins and bacteria are slowly removed from the "front of the legs" due to poor lymphatic drainage.

Q. How would you confirm the diagnosis?

Ans. By a deep wedge biopsy of the tissue which shows inflammatory reaction in the subcutaneous fat, i.e. edema, widening of connective tissue septae, fibrin, exudation and neutrophil infiltration followed by infiltration of lymphocytes, histiocytes and giant cells in later stages.

Q. What are other common skin lesions over the shin?

Ans. In additon to erythema nodosum, other lesions are:
• Pretibial myxoedema (a feature of Graves' dermopathy)
• Necrobiosis lipoidica diabeticorum (seen in diabetes)
• Lichen amyloidosis.

Q. What is erythema nodosum leprosum?

Ans. Read the question on lepra reactions in leprosy.

Q. What are the causes of red (erythematous), subcutaneous nodules?

Ans. Causes are:
1. Inflamed epidermal inclusion cysts, acne cysts and furuncles

2. Panniculitis due to any cause.
3. Cutaneous/systemic vasculitis e.g.
   - Polyarteritis nodosa
   - Allergic granulomatosis
   - Wegener's granulomatosis
4. Cutaneous metastases

Q. How would you treat such a patient?

Ans. Local: Hot and cold compresses
Systemic: NSAIDs, salicylates, steroids or potassium iodide.

Q. What is Panniculitis?

Ans. It is inflammation of subcutaneous fat, characterized by tender nodules either singly or in multiple crops.

Causes
- Collagen vascular disorders
- Factitious
- Lymphoma
- Weber Christian disease
- Pancreatitis
- α_1 antitrypsin deficiency
- **N.B.** Erythema nodosum is a common example of panniculitis

Q. What is vasculitis? What are its causes?

Ans. Vasculitis is inflammation of the blood vessels, can be due to:
1. Infections
2. Drugs
3. Immunological diseases, e.g. SLE, dermato-myositis, systemic sclerosis, rheumatoid arthritis, polyarteritis nodosa, Wegener's granulomatosis
4. Malignant diseases.

Q. What are cutaneous manifestations of vasculitis?

Ans. The cutaneous features are:
1. *Erythema*, e.g. generalized rash, palmar erythema, erythema multiforme, erythema nodosum
2. *Purpura*, e.g. purpuric spots, palpable purpura
3. *Dactylitis, digital ulceration, gangrene.*

Q. What is small vessel vasculitis? Name various conditions associated with small vessel vasculitis.

Ans. Involvement of small vessels in vasculitic process is called *small vessel vasculitis.* It is commonly ANCA associated vasculitis. The conditions are:
1. Churg-Strauss syndrome
2. Microscopic polyangiitis
3. Wegener's granulomatosis
4. Anaphylactoid purpura
5. Hypersensitivity (cutaneous) vasculitis
6. Essential cryoglobulinemic vasculitis.

Q. What is erythema multiforme? What are its causes? What is Stevens-Johnson's syndrome?

Ans. Erythema multiforme is an abnormal cutaneous vascular cell-mediated hypersensitivity reaction to a number of stimuli.

The causes are:
1. Herpes simplex viral infection
2. Bacterial (streptococcus, mycoplasma) infection
3. Fungal infection, e.g. histoplasmosis
4. Parasitic infestations
5. Drugs, e.g. sulphonamides, barbiturates, penicillins, antimalarials
6. Systemic diseases, e.g. SLE, lymphoreticular malignancies (lymphomas), multiple myeloma
7. Pregnancy.
8. Idiopathic. In 50% cases, no cause is found out.

Stevens-Johnson's syndrome is severe or major form of erythema multiforme characterized by erosions of skin and mucous membrane with hemorrhagic crusting, may lead to shock or hypotension creating an emergency situation in dermatology.

Q. What is erythema marginatum?

Ans. It is erythematous lesion (rash) seen in patients with acute rheumatic fever. It is a type of erythema multiforme, characterized by red/pink macules with pallor centre and irregular, red spreading margins. It is migratory lesion, i.e. appears and disappears before the examiner's eyes.

It is nowadays rare lesion and usually not appreciated in the dark-complexion patients.

Q. What is Behcet's syndrome?

Ans. It is a syndrome of recurrent orogenital mucocutaneous ulceration of unknown etiology. Systemic manifestations involving the eyes, joints, brain may also occur. The mucocutaneous lesions are treated by colchicine or thalidomide while systemic manifestations require steroids or anti-mitotic drugs.

Q. What is erythema ab Igne?

Ans. It is dusky discoloration of the skin due to repeated exposure to heat. The heat (<45°) which is not painful and does not burn the skin but produces reticulated net-like pigmentation over the exposed part (front of the legs in old person who sit in front of open fireplaces or abdomen or back of patients who use hot water bottles or heating pads for relief of pain in chronic painful conditions)

This type of rash can be seen over abdomen in intra-abdominal malignancy or chronic pancreatitis from which it has to be differentiated.

CASE 65: HYPERPIGMENTATION

A male 25 years presented with diffuse hyperpigmentation (Fig. 1.65). There was no history of loose motion and weakness. Examination revealed normal BP with pigmentation of hands and tongue. There were no signs of nutrients or vitamins deficiency.

Fig. 1.65: Hyperpigmentation. Note the black pigmentation of face, tongue and hands

Q. What is your diagnosis?

Ans. Hyperpigmentation, probably idiopathic.

Q. What is hyperpigmentation? What are its causes?

Ans. Abnormal increased pigmentation is called *hyperpigmentation* which may be localized (due to skin disorders) or generalized (due to systemic disorders).

The localized forms are due to increased epidermal alteration, melanocytes proliferation, or an increased melanin production. The generalized forms occur due to darkening of the skin usually of equal intensity over the entire body or pigmentation may be accentuated in the sun-exposed areas. The causes of hyperpigmentation are tabulated (Table 1.163).

Q. What are the sites to be seen for hyperpigmentation?

Ans. Sites are:
- Face
- Inside the buccal cavity especially inner sides of cheeks (commonly for Addison's disease, malabsorption, Peutz-Jegher's syndrome) and palate
- Palmar creases (Addison's disease)
- General skin over pressure points, scar, palms and soles

Q. What is kala-azar? What is the type and site of pigmentation?

Table 1.163: Causes of hyperpigmentation

I. *Localized*

(i) *Epidermal alteration*
- Seborrhoeic keratosis
- Acanthosis nigricans

(ii) *Proliferation of melanocytes*
- Lentigo, systemic diseases, e.g. Peutz-Jeghers, LEOPARD syndromes, xeroderma pigmentosa
- Melanoma
- Nevus, NAME and LAMB syndromes

(iii) *Increased melanin production*
- Ephelides (freckles)
- Café-au-lait spots

II. *Generalized*

(i) *Endocrinopathies*
- Addison's disease. Nelson's syndrome
- Ectopic ACTH production. Cushing's syndrome

(ii) *Metabolic*
- Porphyria cutanea tarda
- Hemochromatosis
- Vit B_{12} and folate deficiency
- Pellagra
- Malabsorption, Whipple disease

(iii) *Autoimmune*
- Primary biliary cirrhosis
- Scleroderma, SLE
- POEM syndrome

(iv) *Melanosis secondary to metastatic melanoma*

(v) *Drugs and metals*
- Minocycline, cancer chemotherapy, clofazimine, psoralens, bleomycin
- Heavy metals, e.g. gold, arsenic, silver and lead

Ans. Kala-azar (Hindi version of "black fever") is caused by Leishmania, hence called *leishmaniasis*.

The skin lesions including hyperpigmentation develop in some patients during or within a few months of therapy (e.g. in East Africa) or years after therapy (e.g. in India). The lesions are pigmented macules, papules, nodules or patches typically seen over the face around the mouth, on the temple and forehead. Persons with skin lesions act as reservoirs of infections.

Q. What is Addison's disease?

Ans. Read Addison's disease as a separate case.

Q. What are the sites of pigmentation in Addison's disease?

Ans. Sites are:
1. Pressure points (elbow)
2. Normally pigmented areas (areola, genitalia, knuckles, palmar creases and scars)
3. Mucous membranes (mouth).

Q. What do you understand by hemochromatosis? What is the site and type of pigmentation in this disease?

Ans. *Hemochromatosis* is a common disorder of iron storage in which inappropriate increase in iron absorption from the intestine results in excessive iron deposition into the parenchymal cells of liver, pancreas, heart and pituitary leading to their dysfunction. The characteristic features of the disease are:

- An autosomal recessive disorder
- Excessive skin pigmentation, e.g. bronze pigmentation
- Diabetes mellitus (bronze diabetes)
- Cardiac involvement, e.g. cardiomyopathy, CHF
- Hepatic enlargement (cirrhosis of liver, hepatocellular carcinoma in advanced disease)
- Arthropathy
- Hypogonadism, e.g. loss of libido, testicular atrophy

  Skin pigmentation is called *bronze pigmentation*, occurs due to excessive deposition of melanin and iron, gives a metallic or slate gray hue to the skin. The pigmentation is diffuse and generalized but may be more pronounced on the face, neck, extensor surfaces of lower forearms, dorsum of the hand, lower legs, genitalia and in scars.

Q. What is Peutz-Jegher's syndrome?

Ans. It is heritable (autosomal dominant) disorder characterized by polyposis of small intestine and colon with mucocutaneous (circumoral) pigmentation and tumors of the ovary, breast, pancreas and endometrium. The chances of malignant transformation of polyposis are rare.

Q. What is chloasma or melasma?

Ans. This is symmetrical hyperpigmentation seen on malar prominences and bridge of the nose mostly in young females (very rare in males) precipitated by pregnancy (chloasma gravidarum) or following prolonged use of oral contraceptives – called *mask of pregnancy*.

Q. What is malar flush? What is plethoric face?

Ans. • Read malar flush in mitral stenosis (mitral facies).
- The plethoric or suffused or congested face is discussed in Cushing's syndrome and SVC obstruction.

Q. Name the syndromes associated with localized hyperpigmentation (lentigines)?

Ans. 1. LEOPARD syndrome
- L stands for lentigines (localized multiple hyperpigmentation)
- E stands for ECG abnormalities (conduction defects)
- O for ocular hypertelorism
- P stands for pulmonary stenosis and aortic stenosis
- A stands for abnormal genitalia (cryptorchidism, hypospadias)
- R stands for retardation of growth
- D stands for deafness – sensorineural

2. *NAME and LAMB syndromes*
   Localized pigmentation, e.g. lentigines are associated with atrial myxomas in two syndromes, i.e. NAME (Naevus, Atrial myxoma, Myxoid neurofibroma and Ephelides) and LAMB (Lentigines, Atrial myxoma, Mucocutaneous myxomas and Blue naevi). These patients can have endocrinopathies in the form of Cushing's syndrome, acromegaly or sexual precocity.

Q. What is lentigines? How do they differ from freckles?

Ans. Lentigines are light brown or dark brown macules of varying sizes (1-10 mm), discrete and present on any part of the body. The differences between freckles and lentigines are given in the Box 65.1.

BOX 65.1: FRECKLES VS LENTIGINES	
Freckles	*Lentigines*
• Individuals are fair-skined	Any skin color
• Located to photoexposed areas	Any part of the skin and even mucosa
• Variable in color, e.g. light to dark	Each lesion is of uniform color
• Darken on exposure to sunlight	No change in colour

Q. What are endocrinal causes of pigmentation?
Ans. See the Table 1.163.

Q. Name the drugs producing pigmentation.
Ans. See the Table 1.163.

A patient presented with few hypopigmented dry anesthetic macules (Fig. 1.66A) with loss of hair. On examination, ulnar nerves were palpable and firm to feel. No other organomegaly.

Fig. 1.66A: Maculoanesthetic area due to leprosy

Q. What is probable clinical diagnosis and why?

Ans. Tuberculoid leprosy. The palpable nerves with hypopigmented anesthetic patches are characteristic features of T. leprosy.

Q. What is differential diagnosis of leprosy?

Ans. *The skin lesion in leprosy* has to be differentiated from other conditions given below. The hypoaesthetic lesion and involvement of peripheral nerve trunks in the areas involved are characteristics of leprosy.

Differential diagnosis of leprosy

SLE: An early diffuse maculopapular lesion or circular lesion (discoid lupus) with erythematous rim may be seen over the face with depigmentation and follicular plugging. Diagnosis is established by skin bropsy which is sent for histopathology and immunopathology.

Lupus Vulgaris: Well defined annular/arcuate plaques with erythematous periphery is characteristic. Centre is depigmented and atrophic hence resembles leprosy. Sensations over the lesion are normal. Nerves are not palpable. The site of lesion is face and buttocks. Diagnosis is confirmed by biopsy.

Sarcoidosis: Maculopapular rash with pruritus are common cutaneous lesion in sarcoidosis. Lupus pernio is common in black patients. Other features of the disease are cough, fever, arthralgia lymphadenopathy, hepatosplenomegaly, ocular and cardiac features. The diagnosis is established by negative tuberculin and positive Kveim test and raised serum ACE levels. Confirmation is done by biopsy of the lesion.

Yaws: It is a chronic relapsing, nonveneral treponematosis characterised by early maculopapular lesions which can be confused with leprosy, These lesions are not anesthetic. Rheumatic like pains and palmar and plantar hyperkeratosis usually accompany these lesions. In late yaws, bones, cartilage, CNS, eyes, aorta or other organs are involved. Diagnosis is confirmed by dark-field microscopy and serology.

Post kala-azar dermal leishmaniasis: Even after successful treatment about 10% patients in India develop post kala-azar dermal leishmaniasis characterized by depigmented macules or pinkish papules and nodules. These macules are not anesthetic and LD bodies can be demonstrated in >60% cases in macules and >90% cases with nodules/papules. It may disappear after several weeks (in African cases) but may persist for years or life long in Indian cases constituting a persistent reservoir of infection.

Q. How is it caused? What is mode of transmission?

Ans. It is caused by *Mycobacterium leprae* – a gram-positive acid-fast and alcohol – fast bacillus-called *Hansen's bacillus.*

Mode of Transmission

Man is only reservoir of infection, hence, untreated patients with extensive disease (smear positive) are potential source of transmission to healthy persons. The routes of transmission are; nasal (aerosol) and oral while skin contact may also be a mode if lesion is ulcerated. Foamites and vectors do not play any role in its transmission.

Q. How do you classify leprosy? What are its different clinical types?

Ans. Depending on the cell-mediated immunity (CMI), the leprosy is classified into two polar forms and a borderline form (Fig. 1.66B).

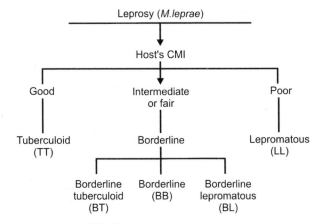

Fig. 1.66B: Clinical types of leprosy depending on host immune status/CMI

Note: Lepromatous leprosy means multibacillary (highly bacillated), low resistance with systemic disease; while tuberculoid leprosy means paucibacillary, high resistance with localized disease.

Q. What are the clinical features of leprosy?

Ans. Three common clinical types are compared in Table 1.164. Incubation period is 3-5 years.

Q. What are systemic manifestations of leprosy?

Ans. The systemic manifestations are common only in lepromatous leprosy due to low resistance/CMI. The manifestations are:

1. Hepatosplenomegaly/lymphadenopathy
2. Nephrotic syndrome
3. Symmetric peripheral neuropathy with gloves and stocking type of anesthesia
4. Granulomatous uveitis and keratitis
5. *Leonine facies (Fig. 1.66C)*
6. Testicular atrophy/Gynecomastia

Fig. 1.66C: Lepromatous leprosy. Note the typical leonine face in this type of leprosy

7. Anemia (hemolytic, megaloblastic or iron deficiency)

Q. What is leonine facies?

Ans. It includes:

- Lines on the forehead become deeper as well as upper central incisor teeth loosen or may fall. There is hoarse voice.
- Loss of hair on lateral thirds of eyebrows and thickened eyebrows.
- Saddle deformity of nose
- Perforation of nasal septum
- Thickened skin of face due to massive infiltration especially earlobes.

Q. What are causes of thickened peripheral nerves?

Ans. Causes are:

- Leprosy
- Amyloidosis
- Diabetic neuropathy
- Sarcoidosis
- Charcoat-Marie-Tooth disease
- Idiopathic hypertrophic neuropathy
- Neurofibromatosis
- Acromegaly
- Post-Guillain-Barre syndrome
- Dejerine–Sottas type neuropathy or Refsum's disease

Q. What are conditions that produce leonine-like face?

Ans. Causes are:

- Albright's disease

Table 1.164: Clinical features of three common types of leprosy

Feature	Tuberculoid (TT)	Borderline (BB)	Lepromatous (LL)
• No. of lesion	One to three	Many	Numerous
• Distribution	Localized	Widespread, asymmetrical	Generalized, symmetrical
• Size of lesion	Large	All sizes	Small lesions
• Margin/edge	Well defined	Ring lesions	Vague
• Surface	Dry and hair loss present	Some dry, some smooth	—
• Sensation over lesion	Impaired	Larger lesion may have impaired sensation	Impaired sensation over periphery
• Type of sensory loss	Localized	Localized	Glove and stocking type of anesthesia (peripheral neuropathy)
• Nerves (nerve twigs or peripheral nerves)	Limited, thickened and may be palpable	Many regional nerves thickened	Symmetrical peripheral neuropathy with trophic changes
• Hepatosplenomegaly/ lymphadenopathy	Absent	May or may not be present	Present usually
• Skin smear	Negative	Negative /positive	Positive
• Lepromin test	Highly positive	Just positive	Negative

- Carcinoid syndrome
- Amyloidosis
- Cleidocranial dysostosis
- Primary hypertrophic osteoarthropathy
- B-cell lymphoma

Q. What are complications of leprosy?

Ans. Complications are:
- Crippling deformities, e.g. claw hand
- Blindness
- Tuberculosis
- Secondary amyloidosis
- Social stigma

Q. What is lepromin test? What is its significance?

Ans. Lepromin is suspension of autoclaved *M. leprae* obtained from human or armadillos. 0.1 ml is injected intradermally and test result is read after 48-72 hours (*Fernandez reaction*) and 4 weeks (*Mitsuda reaction*). Fernandez reaction represents the delayed hypersensitivity while *Mitsuda reaction* represents cell-mediated immunity (CMI).

The test is strongly positive in tuberculoid leprosy, just positive in borderline tuberculoid and negative in lepromatous. In borderline it is weakly positive and negative in borderline lepromatous.

Q. What is borderline leprosy?

Ans. The borderline portion of the leprosy spectrum (Fig. 1.66B) lies between the tuberculoid and lepromatous poles and is further subdivided into:
- Borderline tuberculoid (BT)
- Borderline or dimorphous (BB)
- Borderline lepromatous (BL)

Classification within the borderline region is less precise than at the poles. Lesions tend to increase in number and heterogeneity but decrease in individual size as the lepromatous pole is reached. The skin lesions of borderline tuberculoid leprosy generally resemble those of tuberculoid disease but are more numerous and less well defined. Involvement of multiple peripheral nerve trunks are more common than in polar tuberculoid leprosy.

The borderline disease states are unstable and may shift towards lepromatous form in untreated patient or toward the tuberculolid pole during treatment. Change of one polar type to other is rare.

Q. What are various reactions in leprosy?

Ans. 1. *Type I lepra reaction (reversal reaction).* It can complicate all the three borderline (BB, BT, BL) types, existing skin lesions develop erythema and swelling, new lesions may appear and the nerves become tender. It is managed by aspirin, corticosteroid and chloroquine.

2. *Type II Lepra reaction or erythema nodosum leprosum (ENL).*

It occurs in lepromatous (LL) or borderline lepromatous (BL) patients. It occurs in patients in their second year of treatment. Tender, inflamed subcutaneous nodules develop in crops with pain in the nerves. Fever, arthritis, lymphadenopathy may accompany severe ENL. Each nodule lasts for a week or two but new crops may continue to appear.

It is treated by analgesics, antipyretics, thalidomide (contraindicated in pregnancy) or steroid and increasing the dose of clofazimine.

ENL develops due to immune–mediated (immune complex) reaction.

3. *Lucio phenomenon.* It is characterized by arteritis, is limited to patients with diffuse infiltrative non-nodular lepromatous leprosy. The patients develop angular ulcers. It is a complication rather than reaction.

Q. What are disabilities/deformities in leprosy?

Ans. These are given in Table 1.165.

Q. What is claw hand? What are its causes?

Ans. *Claw hand (main-en-griff):* is a condition where the metacarpophalangeal (MCP) joints are hyper-extended and the PIP and DIP joints are flexed.

Claw hand is produced by paralysis of interossei and lumbricals (small muscles of hand)

The causes and differential diagnosis of claw-hand include:

1. Combined lesion of ulnar and median nerve by injury or leprosy
2. Cervical rib or thoracic inlet syndrome involving lower trunk of brachial plexus
3. Klumpke's paralysis
4. Motor neuron disease (amyotrophic lateral sclessosis)
5. Syringomyelia and intramedullary tumors.
6. Polyneuropathy, Anterior poliomyelitis

Q. How would you grade disabilities in leprosy?

Ans. Read Table 1.166

Q. What is differential diagnosis of peripheral neuropathy?

Ans. Read case discussion on peripheral neuropathy.

Q. How do you diagnoses leprosy?

Ans. Diagnosis is based on clinical examination and investigations such as:

1. *Slit skin smear stained with modified Ziehl-Neelsen method* to detect the lepra bacillus at a

Table 1.165: Disabilities/deformities in leprosy

Site	Nerve	Disability	Deformities if any
Face	Facial nerve	Lag ophthalmos or inability to close the eyes	Exposure keratitis
	Trigeminal	Corneal anesthesia	Exposure keratitis and blindness
Hand	Ulnar	Clawing of 4th and 5th fingers	Deformities of these fingers
		Anesthesia over the little and inner half of ring fingers	
	Median nerve	Loss of abduction and apposition of thumb	Deformities of these fingers
		Anesthesia over the thumb, index, middle fingers and outer half of ring finger	
	Ulnar and median	Claw hand	Claw hand deformity and contracture
		Loss of sensations over the whole palm	Contractures
	Radial	Wrist drop	Ulceration
		Loss of sensations and sweat over the back of hand	
Foot	Common peroneal and lateral popliteal	Footdrop	Contractures
		Anesthesia over lower leg and dorsum of foot	Trophic ulcers on the leg
	Posterior tibial	Claw toes	Contractures of toes
		Anesthesia and loss of sweat over the sole of foot	Trophic ulceration

Table 1.166: WHO grading of deformities/disabilities in leprosy

Grade	Hands and feet	Eye
Grade 0	No anesthesia. No visible deformity or damage	No eye problem due to leprosy. No Visual impairment
Grade 1	Anesthesia present. No visible deformity or damage	Eye problems due to leprosy are present Vision 6/60 or better, the patient can count fingers at 6 meters
Grade 2	Visible deformity or damage present	Severe visual impairment (vision less than) 6/60, the patient is unable to count fingers at 6 meters

concentration >104 /g of tissue. Bacteriological index (number of bacilli living or dead) is calculated on 6 points logarithmic scale.

Bacteriological Index in LL is 5-6
Bacteriological index in TT is 0

The morphological index (MI) of smear (% of all bacilli that stain solidly indicating living bacilli) is also calculated. This confirms the diagnosis.

2. *Skin biopsy:* It is done where diagnosis is in doubt and to classify the disease accurately.
3. *Nerve biopsy:* It is done in pure neuritic leprosy.
4. *Lepromin test* (positive in LL)
5. *Sweat function test* by pilocarpine or acetylcholine. Loss of sweat indicate leprosy.
6. *Fluorescent leprosy antibody absorption* (FLA- ABS) test to detect *M. lepra* specific antibody.
7. *ELISA* for antibody.
8. *Polymerase chain reaction* (PCR).

Q. How do you treat leprosy?

Ans. The WHO and NLEP regimens for treatment of paucibacillary (tuberculoid, borderline tuberculoid and indeterminate classes) and multibacillary (borderline lepromatous, lepromatous leprosy and indeterminate classes) leprosy are tabulated (Table 1.167).

Side Effects of Anti-leprosy Drug:

1. Clofazimine – red coloration of skin, urine and body secretions, abdominal pain, anorexia, nausea, vomiting, pruritus
2. Dapsone – exfoliative dermatitis, hemolytic anemia, agranulocytosis, hepatitis, psychosis and hypoproteinemia.

Q. What are uses of rifampicin (bactericidal drug)?

Ans. • Tuberculosis and other atypical mycobacterial infection
• Leprosy
• For prophylaxis of meningococcal meningitis
• Legionnaires' disease
• Brucellosis (given alongwith other drugs)
• Eradication of carrier state of typhoid (along with co-trimoxazole)
• Endocarditis (*Staph. aureus*, *Corynebacterium*). It is given along with vancomycin.

Q. Name the other drugs used in leprosy. What is the possibility of vaccine in leprosy?

Ans. Other drugs used are:
• Acedapson (DADDS)
• Ethionamide
• Thiocetazone
• Thiobutosine
• Minocycline
• Ofloxacin

Vaccine: Attempts have been made to achieve quicker control of leprosy after the drugs have killed the lepra bacilli. For this various agents like BCG and mycobacterial vaccine (BCG + killed M. lepra, killed ICRC vaccine and killed M.W.) are being tried.

Table 1.167: WHO and NLEP regimens for leprosy

Group	Drugs	Adult dose (mg)	Regimen	Duration
1. Paucibacillary (PB), i.e. BT, BB and TT	• Rifampicin • DDS	600 100	One monthly supervised Daily self-administered	6 monthly pulses to maximum of 9 month
2. Multibacillary (MB), i.e. BL, LL	• Rifampicin • Clofazimine • Dapsone • Clofazimine	600 300 100 50	Once monthly supervised Daily self-administered	12 monthly pulses to maximum of 18 months

CASE 67: RAYNAUD'S PHENOMENON

Do General Physical Examination of the Patient

The patient presented with episodes of pain and paresthesias of the fingertips followed by changes in the color of the skin (Fig. 1.67). Examination revealed cyanosis of the fingers without clubbing. On symptomatic enquiries, patient admitted paleness before bluishness of fingers and after sometimes there was return of normal skin color on rubbing the fingers. There was no evidence of digital gangrene.

Fig. 1.67A: Raynaud's phenomenon. Note the bluish fingers of left hand. Pulse was normal. This was the second phase of tricolor response of Raynaud's phenomenon

Q. What is your clinical diagnosis?

Ans. The episodic nature of change in color of the skin from pale to blue (cyanosis) and then red (rubor) without any digital gangrene indicates vasospastic disorder probably Raynaud's phenomenon.

Q. What is Raynaud's phenomenon?

Ans. Raynaud's phenomenon is characterized by episodic vasospasms of digital arteries leading to sequential development of tricolor response (digital blanching, cyanosis and rubor) of the fingers or toes following cold exposure and subsequent return on rewarming. In this phenomenon, patient experiences pallor or whiteness of fingers or toes when exposed to cold environment or touching a cold object. Emotional stress precipitates this phenomenon.

Q. What important points have you asked or would you like to ask from the patient?

Ans. • Whether the condition is precipitated by cold, emotion and relieved by heat?
   • Whether episodes of skin change is painful or not?

• It there any sensory disturbance in hands (e.g. numbness), stiffness, aching pain?
• What is occupation of patient?
• Is there any dysphagia (ask for CREST syndrome)?
• H/o use of electrically heated gloves.
• H/o SLE or other collagen vascular disease (butterfly rash, arthralgia, dry mouth, etc.)

Q. How would you proceed to examine and what would you examine in this patient?

Ans. • Examine the face for signs of scleroderma, i.e. mask-like face, thickening and tightening of skin over face and mouth, inability of open the mouth, telangiectesia of face, lip, tongue etc.
• Look for butterfly rash, polyarthritis.
• Examine the hands. The hands and fingers are painful, tender, cyanosed and cold or may be warm or red or blue. The thumbs are rarely affected.
• Examine upper limb pulses.
• Blood pressure in both the upper limbs for cervical rib.

Q. What is differential diagnosis of Raynaud's phenomenon?

Ans. The differential diagnosis lies within the causes of Raynaud's phenomenon, i.e.
   1. Raynaud's disease
   2. Scleroderma (systemic sclerosis)
   3. Vasculitis (connective tissue disease)
   4. Thoracic outlet syndrome or cervical rib.

Q. What is pathophysiology of Raynaud's phenomenon?

Ans. Raynaud's phenomenon is cold-induced episodic digital ischemia secondary to reflex sympathetic vasoconstriction or an enhanced vascular responsiveness to cold or normal sympathetic stimuli.

   The tricolor response and its pathogenesis is described in Table 1.168.

Q. How do you classify Raynaud's phenomenon?

Ans. It is divided into two categories:
   1. *Raynaud's disease.* It is idiopathic where no cause is known.
   2. *Secondary Raynaud's phenomenon.* It is secondary to some identifiable or known cause.

Q. Can Raynaud's phenomenon lead to gangrene?

Ans. Yes, though Raynaud's phenomenon is reversible on rewarming but in severe disease, prolonged vasospasm can result in loss of digital pulp, stellate digital ulcer and eventually gangrene.

Table 1.168: Tricolor response in Raynaud's phenomenon

Color	Mechanism
Pallor or whiteness	Digital ischemia due to vasoconstriction
Bluishness (cyanosis)	Local capillaries and venules dilate and cyanosis results from deoxygenated blood present in these vessels
Redness (Rubor)	Resolution of vasospasm and reactive hyperemia due to vasodilatation and return of blood flow imparts a bright red color to the digits

Note: Although tricolor response is characteristic of Raynaud's phenomenon but some patients may experience only pallor and cyanosis or only cyanosis

Q. **What is Raynaud's disease?**

Ans. It is primary idiopathic Raynaud's phenomenon. The term is used when the secondary causes of Raynaud's phenomenon have been excluded, hence, it is diagnosed by exclusion.

It affects young females (20-40 years); and is confined to fingers more frequently than toes. Examination is entirely normal. Peripheral (radial, ulnar and pedal) pulses are normal.

The patients tend to have attacks of pain and paresthesias with tricolor response which resolves completely in most of the cases or may improve spontaneously in about 15 percent cases; while in 30 percent cases it may progress.

Q. **What are common causes of Raynaud's phenomenon?**

Ans. 1. Raynaud's disease (idiopathic)
2. Collagen vascular diseases, e.g. SLE, scleroderma
3. Primary pulmonary hypertension
4. Cold injury or mechanical injury.
5. Myeloproliferative disorders, e.g. leukemias, lymphomas
6. Thoracic outlet syndrome.
7. Drugs, e.g. ergot alkaloids, betablockers, methysergide.

Q. **What is signification of occupational history in Raynaud's phenomenon?**

Ans. Mechanical injury in certain occupation (i.e. polishing tools, vibrating tools, typing, drilling piano-playing) can lead to vasospastic (Raynaud's) phenomenon.

Q. **Name some vasospastic conditions.**

Ans. • White finger syndrome
• Livedo reticularis
• Erythromelalgia
• Chilblain

Q. **How would you investigate a case of Raynaud's phenomenon?**

Ans. • Complete hemogram, ESR
• Total immunoglobulin and immunoglobulin electrophoresis
• Urine exam

• Chest X-ray
• Renal and liver function test.
• Test for antinuclear antibody
• Hand radiography
• Nail-fold capillaroscopy.

Q. **What is treatment of Raynaud's phenomenon?**

Ans. Most of the patients have mild attacks, do not need treatment except reassurance and protection of the body from exposure to cold by warm clothings, gloves and socks.

• *Drug treatment:* It is indicated in severe cases. The calcium channel blockers, e.g. nifedipine (10-30 mg tds) and diltiazem (30-90 mg tds) or nitrates decrease the frequency and severity of attacks. Postsynaptic alpha blockers, e.g. prazosin (1-5 mg tds), doxazosin and tetrazosin may be effective. Long-term use of reserpine (0.25-0.5 mg q.i.d.) therapy is not recommended due to adverse effects.

Treatment with vasodilator prostaglandins 12 is under investigation.

• *Surgical sympathectomy* is helpful in those cases who are resistant to medical therapy and trophic changes interfere with work.

Q. **What is scleroderma? What are its type and manifestations?**

Ans. *Scleroderma* – also called *systemic sclerosis* is a multisystem disorder of unknown etiology characterized by inflammatory, vascular and fibrotic changes in the skin, blood vessels and internal organs (chiefly GI tract, heart, lungs, and kidneys). Immunological mechanism leading to vascular damage and stimulation of fibroblasts are considered responsible for it.

Q. **What important points would you likely to ask in scleroderma?**

Ans. • H/o of tightness of fingers and face
• H/o Raynaud's phenomenon
• Puffy hands (fingers) and feet (toes)
• Fatigue, weakness
• H/o dyspnea, dry cough (lung involvement)

- H/o dysphagia, diarrhea, bloating and indigestion (GI involvement)
- Dryness of eyes
- H/o joint pain/polyarthritis or muscular weakness (proximal myopathy)
- H/o hypertension or renal failure or CHF.

Q. How would you proceed to examine such a case?

Ans. I will do general physical examinaion specifically face and hands (Read Table 1.171 and proceed according to it)

- Examine the system likely to be involved, i.e.
  - CVS
  - Respiratory
  - Abdomen, e.g.liver for primary biliary cirrhosis

Q. What are types of scleroderma?

Ans. Types/Subsets of Scleroderma

1. *Diffuse cutaneous scleroderma*. It involves skin of proximal and distal extremities, face and trunk. Visceral involvement occurs in early course of the disease.
2. *Limited cutaneous scleroderma or CREST syndrome*. It is characterized by **C**alcinosis, **R**aynaud's phenomenon, **E**sophageal dysmotility, **S**clerodactyly and **T**elangiectasia. Skin involvement is limited to face and extremities distal to elbows. It has better prognosis.
3. *Systemic sclerosis* in which there is visceral involvement only without Raynaud's phenomenon or other skin manifestations is called *systemic sclerosis sine scleroderma, scleroderma sine scleroderma*.

Q. How would you diagnose scleroderma?

Ans. Diagnosis is based on clinical manifestations (Table 1.170), physical examination (especially of face and extremities, Table 1.171) and confirmation is done by skin biopsy.

Q. Name the localized form of scleroderma.

Ans. Localized forms are:

- *CREST syndrome* Read as discussed above
- *Morphea* (single or multiple plaques of skin induration)
- *En coup de-sabre* (e.g. linear scleroderma of one side of face. It may be associated with facial hemiatrophy).

Q. What is mixed connective tissue disease (MCTD)?

Ans. It is an *overlap syndrome* comprising of features of SLE, scleroderma, polymyositis and rheumatoid arthritis. It is accompanied by high titers of circulating antibodies to nuclear ribonucleoprotein (NRNP) antigen.

Table 1.169: Causes of Raynaud's phenomenon

1. **Collagen vascular disorders**
   - Scleroderma
   - SLE
   - Rheumatoid arthritis
   - Dermatomyositis and polymyositis
   - Mixed connective tissue disorders (MCTD)
2. **Occlusive arterial disease**
   - Atherosclerosis of peripheral vessels
   - Thromboangiitis obliterans (Buerger's disease)
   - Thoracic outlet syndrome, cervical rib
3. **Primary pulmonary hypertension**
4. **Neurological disorders**
   - Intervertebral disk disease
   - Syringomyelia
   - Spinal tumors
   - Poliomyelitis
   - Stroke
   - Carpal tunnel syndrome
5. **Blood dyscrasias**
   - Myeloproliferative disorders
   - Cryoglobulinemia
   - Waldenström's macroglobulinemia
   - Cold agglutinins
6. **Trauma**
   - Mechanical injury, e.g. typing, piano-playing, vibrating, machines, drills etc.
   - Cold injury
   - Hammer hand syndrome
   - Electric shock
7. **Drug-induced**
   - Ergot derivatives, methysergide, beta blockers, bleomycin, vinblastine, cisplatin, bromocriptine.
8. **Idiopathic**

Q. What is differential diagnosis of scleroderma?

Ans. 1. Read the differential diagnosis of Raynaud's phenomenon
2. Read vasculitis in case discussion on erythema nodosum.

Q. What are cutaneous manifestations of scleroderma?

Ans. Read Tables 1.170 and 1.171.

Q. What are pulmonary manifestations of scleroderma?

Ans. Read Table 1.170.

Q. What are cardiac manifestations of scleroderma?

Ans. Read Table 1.170.

Q. What are diagnostic criteria for scleroderma?

Ans. I. Major criteria
- Proximal scleroderma affecting metacarpo-phalangeal and metatarsophalangeal joints.

II. Minor Criteria
- Sclerodactyly

Table 1.170: Clinical manifestations of scleroderma

1. **Cutaneous**
   - Raynaud's phenomenon with puffy fingers (90% cases) is the presenting manifestation
   - Thickening of skin which is tightly bound to underlying subcutaneous tissues, e.g. extremities, face and trunk
   - Mat-like telangiectasia
   - Calcinosis cutis on pressure points
   Some of these features are included in CREST syndrome.

2. **Musculoskeletal**
   - Symmetrical polyarthritis
   - Carpal tunnel syndrome
   - Proximal muscle weakness or myopathy

3. **GI tract/ Liver**
   - Esophageal hypomotility (e.g. heart burn, GERD, dysphagia)
   - Intestinal hypofunction, e.g. pseudo-obstruction, malabsorption, chronic constipation
   - Primary biliary cirrhosis.

4. **Pulmonary**
   - Aspiration pneumonia/alveolitis
   - Fibrosis or interstitial lung disease
   - Restriction of chest movements (hidebound chest)

5. **Cardiac**
   - Pericarditis
   - Cardiomyopathy (restrictive)
   - Conduction defects /arrhythmias
   - Hypertension and left vetricular failure

6. **Renal**
   - Hypertension
   - Renal failure

- Digital tip pitting or loss of distal fingers pads
- Bilateral basal pulmonary fibrosis
  Note: The major criteria plus two or more minor criteria clinch the diagnosis.

Q. What is treatment of systemic sclerosis (scleroderma)?

Ans. The treatment is as follows:

1. Regular exercises to maintain flexibility of the limbs
2. *Drug treatment*
   - D-penicillamine (diminishes cross-linkage collagen)
   - Colchicine (inhibits procollagen conversion to collagen)
   - PABA
   - Vitamin E
   - Dimethyl sulphoxide
3. *Symptomatic treatment*
   - For reflux esophagitis (use mosapride or itopride)
   - For myositis – use steroids
   - For articular symptoms – use NSAIDs
   - Antibiotics for infection
   - ACE inhibitors for hypertension
4. *Treatment of Raynaud's phenomenon-* already described.

Q. What are the causes of anemia in scleroderma?

Ans.
- Iron deficiency combined with folate and vit. B_{12} deficiency due to GI tract involvement.
- Anemia due to chronic disease
- Microangiopathic hemolytic anemia

Table 1.171: Physical sign in scleroderma

Face in scleroderma
- Expressionless (mask-like) face
- Absence of normal skin wrinkling
- Pinched out nose or beaking of nose
- Microstomia
- Telangiectasia of fingers, face, lips, tongue etc.
- Inability to open the mouth
- Skin is glossy and shiny
- Pigmentation and depigmentation

Hands in scleroderma
- Sclerodactyly, e.g. skin is thick and tight bound on the fingers and cannot be lifted (Fig. 1.56B)
- Symmetrical puffy fingers
- Limitation of movements (extension and flexion of fingers) leading to contractures
- The fingertips may lose soft tissue (pulp atrophy) due to sclevodactyly and develop digital ulcers (Fig. 1.56B) and scars
- Skin is dry, coarse but shiny with loss of hairs
- Nail fold changes include thrombi, blotchy telangiectasia
- Digital infarcts and gangrene
- Pseudoclubbing (beaking of nails) may be present due to bone resorption of terminal phalanx

Fig. 1.67B: Systemic sclerosis. Sclerodactyly with stellate fingertip ulcers

Q. What are early and late skin changes in scleroderma?

Ans. *I. Early change*
- Pitting edema of hands, fingers, toes, feet, face and extremities.
- Tightening of skin over the fingers and face etc.

II. Late changes
- Atrophy of pulps of fingers, hands, toes and feet leading to contractures/fibrosis.
- Depigmentation

Q. What are the uses of Colchicine?

Ans. Uses are:
- Acute gout
- Scleroderma
- Familial Mediterranean fever
- Chromosomal study

- Primary biliary cirrhosis
- Amyloidosis
- Behcet's syndrome
- Psoriasis
- Myelofibrosis

Q. Name the drugs that produce scleroderma like illness.

Ans. Drugs are:
- Bleomycin
- Vinylchloride
- Pentazocine

Q. What are causes of death in scleroderma?

Ans. The fatal events in scleroderma are:
1. Cardiac failure
2. Renal failure
3. Respiratory failure

Perform General Physical Examination

A patient (Fig. 1.68) presented with subcutaneous swellings (arrows), nontender which are present diffusely on the body. Examination revealed rubbery multiple swellings located along the distribution of peripheral nerves under the skin which can be moved from side to side but not from above downwards. There was no evidence of pigmentation, hypertension or deafness. There was positive family history. The patient even brought his son for the examination and treatment of these swellings.

Fig. 1.68: Neurofibromatosis. Note the multiple subcutaneous swellings. Family history was positive in this case

Q. What is the clinical diagnosis in this case and why?

Ans. The multiple subcutaneous swellings along the peripheral nerves, soft in consistency, nontender, moving from side to side only, indicate subcutaneous neurofibromas.

Q. What are the causes of subcutaneous swellings?

Ans. The causes are:

- Neurofibromatosis
- Cysticercosis
- Rheumatoid nodules
- Xanthomas
- Rheumatic nodules
- Lipomas, fibromas
- Leprosy
- Calcinosis
- Osler's nodes
- Gouty tophi
- Skin metastases from carcinomas
- Panniculitis (erythema nodosum)

Q. How would differentiate among common conditions producing subcutaneous nodules?

Ans. Read Table 1.172 for differential diagnosis of subcutaneous nodules.

Q. What do you understand by neurofibromas?

Ans. Neurofibromas are multiple benign tumors of the peripheral nerves, comprising of Schwann cells and fibroblasts. They are fixed to the nerves from which they arise, hence, can only be moved from side to side. They are soft, usually nontender (sometimes painful and tender) and exhibit the "*button–hole*" *sign*, i.e. they invaginate into the skin with pressure.

Q. What is neurofibromatosis? What are its types?

Ans. Neurofibromatosis is an inherited autosomal dominant condition characterized by neurofibromas and pigmented lesions of the skin, e.g. *cafe-au-lait spots* and phakomatosis (collection of neuroglial tissue) of retina.

Types

1. *Neurofibromatosis type I (von Recklinghausen's disease)* is peripheral type of neurofibromatosis. Mutation of the neurofibromatosis gene I (NF1) causes it. The gene is situated on chromsome 17 that encodes a protein called *neurofibromin*. The features of the disease are:
   1. Multiple cutaneous or subcutaneous neuro-fibromas
   2. Compressive radioculopathy or neuropathy
   3. Café-au-lait spots (> 6 in number and > 1.5 cm in diameter)
   4. Hamartomas of iris (*Lisch nodules*)
   5. Axillary freckling
   6. Pseudoarthrosis of tibia
   7. Hydrocephalus, sclerosis, short stature, hypertension (pheochromocytomas), epilepsy and mental retardation may occur.

2. *Neurofibromatosis type 2*. It is central type of neurofibromatosis. Mutation of gene NF2 causes it. The gene is situated over the chromosome 22 that encodes a protein called *neurofibromin 2, Schwannomin* or *merlin*. The features of this type of disease are:
   1. Bilateral acoustic Schwannomas
   2. Predisposition to development of meningiomas, gliomas and Schwannomas
   3. Cataract (juvenile posterior subcapsular lenticular opacity)
   4. Multiple café-au-lait spots
   5. Peripheral neurofibromas.

Q. What is the diagnostic triad iof neurofibromatosis?

Ans. The diagnostic triad of neurofibromatosis I include neurofibromas, cafe au- lait spots and Lisch nodules in iris.

Type	Site	Characteristics	Associated features
Cutaneous neurofibromas (molluscum fusrosum)	• Side of neck • Extremities • Trunk	Small, superficial, soft palpable, skin colored or darker color dome-shaped nodules which can be pushed through a defect (*button-hole sign*) or diffuse plaques with knotty or wormy feel (plexiform neuro-fibromas)	• Cafe-au-lait macules (CALMS). These are light brown oral macules with were defined margins. More than 6 (>1.5 cmin diameter) are diagnostic of neurofibromatosis. • Freckling of axillary and inguinal region • Lisch nodules on iris (slit lamp examination). Two or more are diagnostic • A parent, sibling or child with neurofibromatosis
Rheumatoid nodules	Flexor and extensor tendons of hands, elbow, sacrum and Achilles tendon	These are periarticular, marble like nodules seen in seropositive patients of rhenumatoid arthritis	• Rheumatoid nodules may be seen in viscera e.g. lungs, sclera and myocardium. • Other skin lesions of rheumatoid arthritis i.e. Vasculitis, nail-fold infarct, palmar erythema may be present
Rheumatic nodules	Situated over the bony prominences or pressure points	They are small often tender nodules which are freely mobile	• Subcutaneous rheumatic nodule is a Jone's major criteria, is uncommonly seen. • Other John's major criteria e.g. carditis, polyarthritis, chorea, erythema marginatum may be present
Xanthomas	• Tendon xanthomas over extensor tendons • Eruptive xanthoma over the extensor surfaces, i.e. buttocks back, knee and elbows • Palmar xanthomas over the palmar and digital creases	They are yellowish orange small or large (eruptive) subcutaneous swelling which may be itchy They are mobile	• They are present in children with familial hypertrigly-ceridemia/hypercholestremia • Xanthelasma over the eyelids may be present • Serum lipids are high. • Family history is positive
Gouty tophi	• Around the joints of hands/feet, pressure points • Helix of ear • Olecranon bursa • Achillies tendon • Forearm	They are yellow colored small, firm swellings which are tender and mobile	• Asymmetric polyarthritis involving small joints i.e. feet (common) • Painful arthritis, worst at night, often occurs with redness (acute attack) • Systemic symptoms e.g. fever • Serum uric accid high.
Cutaneous or Muscular Cysticercosis	• In muscle/skin any where in the body	Small from nodules, non tender mobile from side to side not above downward/ muscular mobilities	• Patient of pork-eater • Other features of neurocysticercosis present.
Skin metast-ases	• Any where	They are firm, skin coloured subcutaneous nodules or firm, red to red-brown nodules.	• They occur due to haematogenous/lymphatic spread from internal malignancy i.e. lung, colon, melanoma and oral cavity in men, breast, colon, lung in women.
Panniculitis (erythema nodosum, erythema induratum	• Shin is common site for erythema nodosum • Calf is common site for erythema induratum.	Initially these nodules are red (erythematous) become blue as they resolve	• Patients have symptoms of systemicillness, i.e. fever, malaise, arthralgia or arthritis.
Calcinosis	• Extremities and trunk	Wide spread cutaneous or subcutaneous nodules or plaques, firm, small	• Symptoms or signs of collagen vascular disease or CREST syndrome • Hypercalcemia/hyperphosphatemia

Q. What are diagnostic criteria for neurofibromatosis Type 2?

Ans. • Bilateral 8th cranial nerve palsy confirmed by CT or MRI
• A parent, sibling or child with neurofibromatosis type 2 and either unilateral 8th nerve mass or any two of the followings, i.e. neurofibroma, meningioma, schewannoma or juvenile posterior subscapsular cataract.

Q. What are the common causes of café-au-lait spots?

Ans. • Neurofibromatosis
• Albright's disease (polyostotic fibrous dysplasia)
• Tuberous sclerosis
• Ataxia telangiectasia
• Multiple endocrine adenomatosis type III
• Occasionally occur normally usually <3 in number
• Watson's syndrome (neurofibromatosis with pulmonary stenosis)

Café-au-lait spots are commonly seen on the trunk.

Q. What are the common sites of cutaneous neurofibromas? What is plexiform neurofibromatosis?

Ans. Sites of cutaneous neurofibromatosis are:
• Sides of the neck
• Extremities
Plexiform neurofibromatosis refers to diffuse overgrowth of the skin and subcutaneous nerve trunks leading to a boggy swelling. The common sites are temple, upper eyelids and back of the neck. *Elephantiasis neurofibromatosa* is severe form of this variety involving the lower limbs.

Q. Is biopsy necessary to make diagnosis of neurofibroma?

Ans. No. The diagnosis is made purely on clinical grounds.

Q. What is pachydermocele?

Ans. It is a variety of neurofibromatosis on which coils of soft tissue hang around the neck.

Q. What are Lisch nodules? What is their significance?

Ans. These are melanocytic hamartomas that appear as well defined dome-shaped swellings projecting from the iris and are clear or yellow, brown in color. They are seen on slit lamp examination. Their presence establishes the diagnosis of type I neurofibromatosis.

Q. What is phakomatoses? What are conditions associated with it?

Ans. Phakomatoses include a group of genetic disorders in which a variety of developmental abnormalities involve the skin, nervous system, retina and other organs. The causes are:
1. von Recklinghausen's disease
2. Von Hippel-Lindau syndrome
3. Multiple endocrine neoplasia 1 (Werner's syndrome)
4. Retinoblastoma
5. Tuberous sclerosis
6. Sturge-Weber disease
7. Turcot's syndrome

These are also called congenital or hereditary neuro-cutaneous syndromes.

N.B. Phakoma is seen as a grayish circular mass about the size of the half of the disk in the retina and is produced by collection of abnormal glial tissue.

Q. What is xanthomas and xanthelasma? What are their causes?

Ans. Xanthomas are yellow-colored cutaneous papules/nodules or plaques, commonly associated with hyperlipidemia (hypertriglyceridemia), occur mainly on the extensor surfaces of the extremities and buttocks.

Types of Xanthomas

I. *Planus xanthomas*
• Xanthelasma on the eyelids
• Tendinous xanthomas seen on Achilles and extensor finger tendons
• Plane xanthomas seen on palmar creases, face, upper trunk and scars.

II. *Tuberous xanthomas.* They are seen over the large joints (elbow, wrist, knee, ankle) and buttocks. They are seen in patient's with hypercholestrolemia due to prolonged cholestasis.

Common causes of xanthomas
• Familial hyperlipidemia and hypercholesterolemia
• Biliary cirrhosis or prolonged cholestasis
• Uncontrolled diabetes mellitus
• Multiple myeloma or monoclonal gammopathy
• Hypothyroidism
• Nephrotic syndrome or chronic renal failure
• Obesity
• Drug induced hyperlipidemia

Q. What do you understand about gouty tophi?

Ans. Tophi are yellow-colored, firm, small swellings that, occur in gout due to deposition of crystals of monosodium urate in the skin around the joints particularly of the hands and feet. Other sites of tophi are:
• Helix of the ear
• Olecranon and prepatellar bursae
• Achilles tendon
• Ulnar surface of forearm
• Other pressure points.
Diagnosis is confirmed by demonstration of urate crystals in the aspirated contents of a lesion under polarized light. Urate crystals are needle-shaped and negatively birefringent.

Q. What is calcinosis? What are its causes?

Ans. *Calcinosis cutis* is a condition in which insoluble calcium salts are deposited in the dermis. Widespread calcinosis affecting the skin, subcutaneous tissue and the muscles is called *calcinosis universalis*.

In calcinosis, nodule/plaques are distributed symmetrically over the extremities and trunk. Read Table 1.173.

Causes of calcinosis

1. Collagen vascular diseases, e.g. scleroderma, CREST syndrome, dermatomyositis
2. Trauma
3. Post-inflammatory/postinfective
4. Neoplasia.

Q. How will you differentiate rheumatoid nodules from rheumatic nodules?

Ans. The differences are tabulated (Table 1.172).

Q. What is cutaneous cysticercosis?

Ans. Cutaneous or muscular cysticercosis produces small, firm nodules in the voluntary muscles anywhere in the body. These nodules are palpable and contain the calcified cyst of *Taenia solium*. Patients are usually pork-eaters and may have features of neuro-cysticercosis (epilepsy, hydrocephalus, behavioral or mental changes and fluctuating neurological signs).

A patient (Fig. 1.69) presented with intense itching of upper limbs, e.g. hands, fingers, forearms, scrotum and groin, worst at night or after a hot bath. Examination revealed, scratch marks over the fingers, arm, forearms, scrotum and groin. Papulo-vesicular lesions were also seen between fingers, axillae, belt line, buttocks, thighs and scrotum.

Fig. 1.69: Scabies

Q. What is probable clinical diagnosis?

Ans. Scabies

Q. Describe the skin lesions.

Ans. Papulovesicular lesions are seen between fingers and axillae. These lesions are itchy. Burrows/tunnels are also seen between the fingers which indicate the entry point of the parasite.

Q. How is scabies caused? How does it get transmitted?

Ans. The scabies is caused by infestation by an ectoparasite – *Sarcoptes scabiei,* a human itch mite. Gravid female mites burrow beneath the skin (stratum corneum) for a month, depositing the eggs. Nymphs hatch out from these eggs and mature into adults on the surface of the skin, where they mate and subsequently reinvade the skin of the same or another person.

Transfer of newly fertilized female mites from person to person by intimate personal contact is the mode of transmission of scabies. Medical practitioners are, therefore, at particular risk of infestation.

The crowding, uncleanliness, promiscuity are the precipitating factors. Transmission via sharing of the contaminated bedding, clothing, towel, is infrequent because these mites cannot survive more than a day without host contact.

Outbreaks occur in nursing homes, mental institutions and hospitals.

Q. What is pathognomonic lesion of scabies? What is its characteristic distribution? Which areas are spared?

Ans. *Burrow or tunnel* is the pathognomonic lesion. Burrows appear as dark wavy lines in the epidermis caused by tunnelling of the mite in the skin and end in a small pearly bleb that contains the female mite.

The Characteristic Distribution of Burrows:

The areas involved are:

- Webs of the fingers, volar aspect of wrist, ulnar border of forearm and arms, anterior axillary folds
- Scrotum, penis, vulva, groin and medial aspects of thigh and webs of toes

Areas spared are:

Face, scalp, neck, palms and soles.

Q. Name the various lesions in scabies.

Ans. Various lesions are:

- Typical burrows seen as wavy lines
- Small papules and pustules often accompanied by eczematous plaques
- Pustules or nodules
- Crusted scabies and prominent fissuring can occur due to bacteremia in AIDS patients.

Q. What is non-itchy (Norwegian) scabies?

Ans. Features of non-itchy scabies are:

- *Crusted (or Norwegian) scabies* is a non-itchy scabies. It results from hyperinfestation with thousands or millions of mites; the predisposing conditions being steroids use, immuno-compromised state and neurological or psychiatric illness (mentally retarded patients).

Q. Why is the itch nocturnal in scabies?

Ans. The mites need a warm environment to move, hence, when patient retires in a warm bed at night, the mites start moving within the burrows and cause itch.

Q. How do you diagnose scabies?

Ans. The diagnostic clues are:

- Pruritus and polymorphic skin lesions at characteristic locations
- Burrows or comedones
- Itching either nocturnal or occur after a hot bath
- History of involvement of several members of the family due to household contact
- Biopsy or scrappings of papulovesicular lesions for mite, its eggs or fecal matter may also be confirmative.
- Burrows unroofed with a sterile needle or scalpel blade and scrapings taken and transferred to a glass slide on which 10% potassium hydroxide is kept. The slide is then examined under microscope for mite, its eggs or its fecal pellets which confirm the diagnosis.

Q. Which skin conditions lead to itching?

Ans. The conditions are:

- Scabies
- Urticaria
- Lichan planus
- Ringworm
- Psoriasis
- Dermatitis herpetiformis
- Eczematous dermatitis
- Insect bite
- Pediculosis

Q. What are the medical causes of generalized pruritus?

Ans. Medical causes are:

- Cholestasis (obstructive jaundice)
- Thyrotoxicosis
- Diabetes mellitus
- Chronic renal failure (CRF)
- Polycythemia rubra vera
- Drug-induced
- Systemic anaphylaxis
- Psychogenic
- Carcinoid syndrome
- Pregnancy
- Systemic mastocytosis

Q. What are complications of scabies?

Ans. Common complications of scabies are:

- *Superinfection*, e.g. pyoderma
- *Acute glomerulonephritis* due to sensitization to nephrogenic strains of streptococci (super-infection)
- *Eczematous dermatitis* due to prolonged itching or sensitization from parasite
- Complication due to treatment, e.g. sulphur dermatitis.

Q. How do you treat scabies?

- Family contacts to be screened and treated simultaneously
- Secondary infection is treated by antibiotics
- Medicine used and instructions given to the patient are:

Medicines used:

1. Twenty-five percent benzylbenzoate
2. Unguentum sulphur
3. Gamma benzene hexachloride (1%) – not to be used in pregnant women and infant
4. Monosulfiram used as soap
5. Topical thiabendazole
6. Permethrin (5% cream)
7. Malathione (0.5%)
8. Ivermectin (200 mg/kg/orally as a single dose). Patients with crusted scabies (Norwegian variety) require two or more doses of ivermectin.

Method of use

Patient is advised to take bath with soap and H_2O. During bath, patient must scrub his body to open the burrows and then allow the skin to dry. Now apply the specific medicine from neck to foot for 3 consecutive days. Patient should take bath daily and wear fresh garments. Clean or autoclave the bed-sheets and used garments.

- Antihistamines and calamine lotion may be used to relieve itching
- Patient's nail should be cut properly. His daily used articles (towel, pillow, bedsheet) to be kept separately.

The patient (Fig. 1.70) presented with itching and silvery scaly lesion mainly on the extensor surfaces. Scraping or removal of the scales left behind bleeding spots.

Fig. 1.70: Psoriasis. Note dry, scaly plaques on the extensor surfaces of extremites and trunk

Q. What is your probable spot diagnosis?

Ans. Psoriasis

Q. Describe the skin lesions

Ans. 1. The patient has well-demarcated salmon pink plaques with silvery white scales over extensor surfaces, scalp, navel and natal cleft. The skin lesions are itchy.
2. There is moist red surface on removal of scales (*bulkeley's membrane*)
3. *Auspitz's sign* is positive, i.e. there is bleeding on removal of silvery scales from the plaques.
4. New skin lesion present at the site of trauma (*Koebner's phenomenon*).

Q. What is its incidence?

Ans. It affects 1–2% of the population.

Q. What is differential diagnosis?

Ans. Psoriasis has to be differentiated from mycosis fungoides (read it in this chapter).

Q. What do you understand by psoriasis?

Ans. It is a common chronic inflammatory skin disorder clinically characterised by red erythematous plaques covered with silvery white scales.

Q. What are the characteristics of psoriatic lesion?

Ans. The characteristics of psoriatic lesions are:
1. Classic lesion is a well defined erythematous plaque covered with silvery–white adherent scales

2. The lesions are distributed over the extensor surfaces (e.g. knees, elbows, buttocks), may also involve scalp, hands, palms and soles.
3. The skin lesions are pruritic.
4. Traumatized areas often develop lesions of psoriasis by local spread (*Koebner's phenomenon*)
5. On grattage, characteristic coherence of scales can be seen as if one scratches a wax candle (*signe de la tache de bougie*)
6. Scrapping or removal of scales leaves behind punctate bleeding spots (*Auspitz's sign*) is diagnostic
7. Associated findings include psoriatic arthritis and nail changes (onycholysis, pitting or thickening of nail plate with accumulation of subungal debris).

Q. What is its etiology?

Ans. Following are causes:
1. *Genetic basis.* Psoriasis occurs in families (50% patients with psoriasis have positive family history). HLA studies have shown increased frequency of HLA – B13, HLA – B17 and HLA-BW16 in the affected patients. Twin studies report 70% concordance rate among monozygotic twins.
2. *Immunological basis.* Evidence has accumulated indicating a role of T cells in pathophysiology of psoriasis. There is persistent activation of T cells by the antigen as a result of autoreactivity or by the cytokines such as interleukin 2 released from keratinocytes during chemical/physical or UV injury.
3. *Precipitating factors.* Skin trauma, winter season, emotional stress, depression, infection (streptococcal/HIV), pregnancy and upper respiratory infection precipitate it.
4. *Drugs.* Beta blockers, NSAIDs, lithium, calcium channel blockers, chloroquine, valproate, carbamazepine, clonidine, penicillin, tetracyclines, glibenclamide and topical coal tar precipitate psoriasis.

Q. What are clinical forms or types of psoriasis?

Ans. The forms are explained in Table 1.173.

Q. What is psoriatic arthropathy (PA)?

Ans. It is an inflammatory arthritis that occurs in 5 to 10 percent of patients with psoriasis with negative rheumatoid factor (seronegative arthritis). It is commonly associated with HLA-B 27. Five distinct types recognized are:
1. *Oligoarticular PA.* It is asymmetrical involvement of single or few small joints of fingers. This is commonest type (38%)
2. *Rheumatoid type.* It is symmetrical seronegative arthritis involving the small joints (30%).

Table 1.173: Clinical forms of psoriasis

Forms	Clinical characteristics of lesions
Numular/Chronic plaque psoriasis	Discoid, coin-shaped lesion (commonest form)
Guttate	Drop-like, small sized lesions
Exfoliative/erythrodermic	Erythrodermic scaly dermatitis
Pustular (palmoplantar type)	Superficial pustules containing sterile pus are seen on palms and soles
Generalized pustular (Von Zumbusch psoriasis)	Rare. Generalised pustules with signs of toxemia, e.g. fever, headache, myalgia are evident
Genital type	Penis and vulva are the sites of lesion
Flexural (intertriginous)	Instead of extensor surfaces, flexural sites are affected
Scalp psoriasis	Fairly common, not associated with alopecia
Psoriasis unguis (nail psoriasis)	Onycholysis separation of nail plate from the bed, pitting of nail plates, subungal hyperkeratosis, yellow discoloration, etc.

3. *Classical psoriatic arthropathy.* This is arthritis involving the distal interphalangeal joints (16%)
4. *Psoriatic spondylitis* (*Sacroilitis* and/or *spondylitis*). This constitues 15% cases of PA.
5. *Arthritis mutilans.* Severe destructive arthritis (5%) producing gross deformities of joints of hands and feet.

Q. What are the dermatological causes of pitting nails?

Ans. Dermatological causes are:
- Psoriasis unguis
- Eczema
- Alopecia areata

Q. Name the skin diseases precipitated by trauma (positive Koebner's phenomenon).

Ans. These are as follows:
- Psoriasis
- Lichan planus
- Viral warts

Q. What are histological changes in psoriasis?

Ans. Following are the changes:
- Hyperkeratosis and parakeratosis
- Absence of granular layer
- Hyperplasia of stratum malpighii
- Dilated and tortuous blood vessels in dermal papillae
- Microabscesses of *Munro* in the horny layer

Q. What is mycosis fungoides? What is Sezary's syndrome?

Ans. *Mycosis fungoides* is cutaneous T cell lymphoma characterized by reddigh-brown itchy plaques with or without lymph nodes enlargement. In early stages, these erythematous plaques resemble erythematous lesion of psoriasis. *Sezary's syndrome* is erythrodermic variant of mycosis fungoides (cutaneous T cell lymphoma) characterized by lymphadenopathy and large mononuclear cells (Sezary cells) in the skin and blood: It is often resistant to treatment and carries poor prognosis.

Q. How will you investigate a case with psoriasis?

Ans. Following are the investigations:
- TLC, DLC for an evidence of infection
- Rheumatoid factor
- Skin scrappings and nail clippings may be examined for tinea (fungal infection has to be differentiated from psoriasis)
- Skin biopsy. It is rarely required.
- X-rays of hands and feet may show fish tail or "pencil-in-cup" deformity if joints are involved. Subarticular erosions and later cystic destruction of bones may occur. Sacroilitis may occur.

Q. What will you treat such a case?

Ans.
- Triggering factors should be found out and eliminated
- Good diet with supplementation of iron and folate
- Any focus of infection may be treated with antibiotics

A. *Topical treatment:* It consists of:
1. Dithranol (anthralin). It inhibits keratinocytes proliferation by activated T cells and inhibits formation of interleukins.

   Ingram regimen consists of coal tar bath, exposure to UV rays and application of anthralin (0.1 to 0.8%) in Lassar's paste to psoriatic plaques.
2. Crude coal tar preparation with keratolytic salicylic acid is used as ointment. It may be combined with UV light or anthralin as described above.
3. *Local steroid ointments*
4. *Vitamin D analogue (calcipotriol)* is used locally
5. *Topical preparation* of retinoic acid derivatives (0.1%)
6. Systemic therapy plus/*Tazarotene-a retinoid is used as 0.1% gel.*

B. *Systemic therapy*

Indications for systemic therapy
- Failure of tropical therapy
- Extensive plaque psoriasis in the elderly
- Generalized pustular or erythrodermic psoriasis
- Servere psoriatic arthropathy.

PUVA therapy. Administration of psoralens (p stands for Psoralens) and subsequent long wave UVA radiation is called PUVA therapy. Oral psoralens (8 - methoxy psolarens) is followed 2 hours later by UVA therapy. Two to four sittings per week are necessary (total 10-20 sittings). UVB is useful in winter season. *Other drugs used are:*

1. Methotrexate (2.5-5 mg orally at 12 hours interval, 3 consecutive doses in a week). *Cycloporine A* may be given 3-5 mg/kg.

2. Mycophenolate Mofetil – an immunosuppressant is used in the dose of 2-3 mg/day

3. Oral Retinoids (etretinate, treatinoin) are used as immuno-modulators in psoriasis. Dose is 0.5-1 mg/kg daily for 4-20 weeks.

4. Oral corticosteroids may be used judiciously in refractory psoriasis, psoriatic arthropathy and in erythrodermic form of psoriasis.

5. NSAIDs are used for arthropathy.
   Novel approach: Anti-CD4 monoclonal antibody. It is a novel approach

Q. Name the common scaly lesions of skin.

Ans. Common scaly lesions are:

- Psoriasis
- Seborrheic dermatitis
- Eczema
- Ringworm
- Pityriasis (all the varieties)
- Lichen planus
- Exfoliative dermatitis.

CASE 71: PITYRIASIS VERSICOLOR (TINEA VERSICOLOR)

The patient (Fig. 1.71) presented with non-itchy depigmented scaly skin lesions on the back of the chest and side of the neck.

Fig. 1.71: Pityriasis versicolor

Q. **What is your diagnosis? Describe the skin lesions. How is it caused?**

Ans. The diagnosis is:
- Pityriasis versicolor
  The lesions are well defined hypopigmented macules with fine branny scales of different shapes and sizes. These are non-itchy.
  Sites involved are:
- Front and back of the chest, side of neck, upper arm and face.
  It is caused by *M furfur* – a parasitic form of saprophytic yeast often called *pityrosporum orbiculare*.

Q. **What are its precipitating factors?**

Ans. These are as follows:
- Profuse sweating
- Diabetes mellitus
- Pregnancy.

Q. **How do you confirm the diagnosis?**

Ans. The diagnosis is confirmed by demonstration of fungal hyphe in the scraped scales treated with KOH (10% solution) taken on a slide and examined under microscope.

Q. **What are the causes of hypopigmented macules?**

Ans. Following are the causes:
1. *Tuberculoid leprosy* (the hypopigmented macules are anesthetic)
2. *Vitiligo* (idiopathic or associated with other autoimmune disease)
3. *Pityriasis alba* and *pityriasis versicolor*
4. *Following burn* (H/o burn)
5. *Tuberous sclerosis* (Shagreen patch). There is history of epilepsy, low intelligence and sebaceous adenoma. It may be familial.
6. *Prolonged use of chloroquine* in rheumatoid arthritis and SLE
7. *Psoriasis*
8. *Albinism*

Q. **What is ringworm? What are characteristics of its lesions? How do you diagnose it? Describe the treatment.**

Ans. Ringworm (*Tinea corporis*) is a fungal skin infection caused by fungi like *Trichophyton*, *Epidermophyton* or *Microsporum*. The characteristic lesions are:
- Single or multiple, small or large, usually circular having a ring of active margin made up of erythematous papules or tiny vessels (papulovesicular scaly with active border).
- Lesions resolve centrally and progress peripherally to produce ring-like configuration, hence, the name ringworm.
- The lesion may fluoresce bluish green under Wood's lamp.

Diagnosis: It is diagnosed by demonstration of fungi (hyphe and spores) when skin scales, hair or nails are mounted in KOH for several hours and examined under microscope.

Q. **What are various sites and types of tineasis?**

Ans. These are given in Table 1.174.

Table 1.174: Various sites and types of tineasis

Name	Site of involvement
• Tinea corporis	• The whole body
• T. cruris ("Dhobi" itch)	• Thighs and buttocks
• T. capitis	• Scalp
• T. pedis	• Foot
• T. manuum	• Hand
• T. Barbae	• Beard
• T. unguium	• Nail

Q. **What is treatment of ringworm?**

Ans. Following are treatments
1. *General measures*
   - Correction of contributory factor, e.g. diabetes, HIV, hot humid environment, occlusive clothings and footwear
2. *Topical antifungals*
   - Clotrimazole, miconazole, ketoconazole, terbinafin, are used in lotion, cream or powder. Lotions and powders are desirable for intertriginous area and hairy area (scalp)

3. *Systemic antifungals*
   - Griseofulvin (micronized) 250 mg twice a day (10 mg/kg/day in children) was till recently the standard treatment for dermatophytosis. The duration of treatment varies from 4 weeks (Tinea cruris) to 1-2 years (Tinea unguium) depending on the site involved. Now other safe and effective drugs are available as described below
   - Ketoconazole is effective in dose of 200 mg once a day, itraconazole is safer and effective (100-200 mg/day) or fluconazole (150 mg/week orally) or terbinafine 250 mg/day is highly effective against all dermatophytes.

     Indications for systemic therapy include Tinea unguium, Tinea pedis, tinea manuum, tinea capitis; widespread or unresponsive or recurring infections of any site in presence of diabetes, immunodeficiency and obesity.

Q. Name the various fungal infections of the skin.

Ans. These are divided into superficial and deep infections.

1. *Superficial fungal infections:*
   - P. versicolor
   - Tinea infection
   - Candidiasis

2. *Deep fungal infections*
   - Mycotic mycetoma
   - Sporotrichosis
   - Chromomycosis.

Q. Name the opportunistic fungal infections in HIV.

Ans. These are as follows:
   - Cryptococcosis
   - Mucormycosis
   - Aspergillosis
   - Candidiasis.

Q. What is the treatment of P. versicolor?

Ans. The treatment includes:
   - Maintain good personal hygiene
   - Topical sodium thiosulphate (25-40% solution) locally is inexpensive therapy used daily for 3 weeks
   - Selenium sulphide 2.5% locally at night and wash off in the following morning; 2-3 applications are adequate, weekly shampoo for 3-4 weeks should accompany
   - Topical antifungal solutions such as 1% clotrimazole, 2% miconazole, 1% tolnafitate and 2% ketoconazole are effective
   - For recurrence, weekly use of selenium sulphide or zinc pyrithionate shampoo are useful.

A 20-year female (Fig. 1.72) presented with malar rash, edema face, alopecia, fever, polyarthritis and fatigue. Examination showed hypertension (BP 180/100 mm Hg). There was no positive finding on systemic examination.

Fig. 1.72: Systemic lupus erythematosus. Note the butterfly (heliotrophic) rash

Q. What is your probable clinical diagnosis?

Ans. The malar rash (butterfly rash) with alopecia, hypertension and polyarthritis in a female patient suggest the diagnosis of systemic lupus erythematosus (SLE).

Q. Describe the face of the patient.

Ans. The patient has typical lupus face consisting of;
- Classical photosensitive 'butterfly' rash over the nose extending over the malar areas
- Patchy alopecia
- Lupus hairs – short broken hair seen above the forehead
- Oral ulcers seen on opening the mouth.

Q. How would you proceed to examine such a case?

Ans. *History*

Ask about
- Tiredness and fatiguability
- Polyarthritis (Small joints involvement)
- Digital gangrene (vasculitis)
- Skin rash, alopecia, Raynaud's phenomenon
- Mouth ulcer
- Puffiness of face, edema (hypertension)

- Fever and lymphadenopathy
- Bleeding from gums, nose or menstrual bleeding
- History of seizures
- History of drug relapses and remission

Examination
- *Face* for butterfly rash, edema and cushingoid features
- *Conjunctiva* for anemia
- *Mouth* for oral ulcers
- *Scalp* for alopecia
- *Blood pressure*
- *Neck* for JVP and lymphadenopathy
- Look for subcutaneous nodules and vasculitic rash over sun exposed areas
- *Nails* for splinter hemorrhages, finger infarcts and digital gangrene
- *Hands* for palmar erythema, Raynaud's phenomenon
- *Joints* for arthritis
- *Feet* for pitting edema
- *Urine* for proteinuria
- *Abdomen* for hepatosplenomegaly.

Q. What do you understand by the term SLE?

Ans. Systemic lupus erythematosus is a inflammatory disease of unknown etiology, characterized by inflammation and damage to different tissues and cells by pathogenic autoantibodies and immune complexes.

Q. What are skin manifestations of SLE?

Ans. The cutaneous manifestations of SLE can be divided into acute, subacute and chronic (i.e. discoid LE). In addition to 'butterfly rash', the other lesions are:
- Ill-defined, discrete erythematous papules (papulosquamous form) on the back, chest, shoulders and extensor surfaces of arms and hands. There is associated scaling
- Sometimes annular lesions resembling erythema multiforme may appear as an oral or circular erythematous papules
- Purpura
- Bullous lesion
- Panniculitis
- Digital infarcts
- Livedo reticularis
- Raynaud's phenomenon
- Angioneurotic edema
- Pigmentation and patchy alopecia.

Q. What is discoid lupus?

Ans. Discoid lupus is a chronic skin lesion in SLE characterized by:
- Circular lesions with an erythematous rim over the face, scalp or external ears

- Follicular plugging (thick scales occlude the hair follicles). When scales are removed, its underside will show small excrescences that correlate with the openings of hair follicles and is termed as *"carpet track appearance"*. This finding is specific for DLE
- Longstanding lesions develop scarring and atrophy
- Hypopigmentation
- Telangiectasia.

Note: Only 5 to 10% patients with DLE develop systemic involvement (i.e. turn into SLE). On the other hand, DLE occurs in 20% patients of SLE. DLE is associated with positive antinuclear factor (ANF) and normal complement. Direct immunofluorescence microscopy shows deposits of immunoglobulin and complement at the basement membrane in 90% cases.

Q. What are the causes of SLE?

Ans. Etiological factors incriminated in SLE are:
1. *Genetic*
   HLA B8, DR3, DR2
   Inherited complement deficiencies, C4 null allele
2. *Environmental*
   - UV light
   - Physical and emotional stress
   - Infection
   - Female sex hormones
   - Drugs, e.g. procainamide, quinidine, hydralazine, methyldopa, isoniazide, chlorpromazine.

Q. What are clinical manifestations of SLE?

Ans. They are tabulated (Table 1.175) according to frequency of occurrence.

Table 1.175: Frequency-wise clinical manifestations of SLE

I. *General systemic (95%)*
Fatigue, fever, malaise, anorexia, weight loss
II. *Musculoskeletal (95%)*
• Arthralgia /arthritis   • Myositis/myopathy
III. *Cutaneous (80%)*
• Malar rash   • Alopecia
• Photosensitivity   • Vasculitis
• Oral ulcers   • Panniculitis
• Discoid rash
IV. *Hematological (70%)*
• Anemia, leukopenia, thrombocytopenia
• Lupus anticoagulant (anti-phospholipid syndrome)
• Splenomegaly and lymphadenopathy
V. *Neurological (50%)*
• Headache, migraine
• Cognitive dysfunction
• Organic brain syndromes (e.g. psychosis, seizures)
• Cranial nerve involvement, hemiplegia
• Transverse myelitis
• Peripheral neuropathy
• Extrapyramidal disorders (chorea) and cerebellar dysfunction

Contd...

Contd...

VI. *Cardiopulmonary (50%)*
• Pleurisy   • Pneumonitis
• Pericarditis/ myocarditis   • Pleural effusion
• Endocarditis (Libman-Sachs)   • ARDS
• Interstitial fibrosis/fibrosing alveolitis
• Heart blocks and arrhythmias
VII. *Renal (50%)*
• Proteinuria, hematuria   • Renal failure
• Nephrotic/Nephritic syndrome   • Urinary tract infection
VIII. *Ocular (50%)*
• Conjunctivitis /episcleritis   • Sicca syndrome
• Retinal vasculitis
IX. *GI tract (30%)*
• Nausea, anorexia, diarrhea   • Vasculitis with bleeding
• Abnormal liver enzymes   • Arterial/venous thrombosis
X. *Fetal loss (30% of pregnancies)*

Q. What are the criteria for diagnosis of SLE?

Ans. Following are the criteria for diagnosis:
1. Malar rash
2. Discoid rash
3. Photosensitivity
4. Oral ulcers
5. Arthritis (nonerosive polyarthritis)
6. Serositis (pleuritis or pericarditis)
7. Renal involvement, e.g.
   i. Proteinuria >0.5 g /d **or**
   ii. > 3+ **or**
   iii. Cellular casts
8. *Neurological, e.g.*
   Seizure or psychosis without any other cause
9. *Hematological*
   - Hemolytic anemia or leukopenia (<4000/ml) **or**
   - Lymphopenia (<1500/ml) **or**
   - Thrombocytopenia (<1 lac/ml) in the absence of an offending drug
10. *Immunological evidence*
    - Positive LE cells **or**
    - Anti-ds DNA or anti-Sm antibodies **or** false positive VDRL.
11. *Antinuclear antibodies*
    An abnormal titer of ANAs (positive ANA) in the absence of drugs known to induce it.

N.B.: If four of these eleven criteria are met at any time during the course of the disease, a diagnosis of SLE can be made with 98 percent specificity and 97 percent sensitivity.

Q. Name the autoantibodies in SLE.

Ans. The autoantibodies in SLE are:
1. *Antinuclear antibodies* against multiple nuclear antigens. These are sensitive but not specific autoantibodies.
2. *Anti-ds DNA* is more specific than anti-s DNA.

3. *Anti-Sm* (specific for SLE).
4. *Anti-RNP* – present in mixed connective tissue disease.
5. *Anti-RO (SS-A)* is associated with ANA negative lupus.
6. *Anti-LA (SS-B)* occurs in neonatal lupus, in elderly Sjögren's syndrome.
7. *Anti-histone*, e.g. drug–induced lupus.
8. *Antiphospholipid, antibodies* (e.g. three types are recognized such as lupus anticoagulant, anti-cardiolipin and false positive serology for syphilis).
9. *Anti-erythrocytes* antibodies.
10. *Anti-platelet*, anti-lymphocyte antibodies.
11. *Anti-neuronal*, e.g. in diffuse CNS lupus.
12. *Anti-ribosomal* P, e.g. in psychosis, CNS lupus.

Q. What is an autoantibody? Which antibody is more sensitive and which one is more specific for SLE?

Ans. Autoantibody means antibody produced against own (self) antigen. Antinuclear antibodies (ANAs) mean antibodies produced against nuclear components of a cell.

Antinuclear antibodies are the best screening test as they are more sensitive. A positive ANA test is not specific for SLE as it is produced by:
- Normal individual (low titer)
- Other autoimmune diseases
- Viral infections
- Chronic inflammatory diseases
- Several drugs-induced ANA

N.B. Anti-Sm is specific for SLE.

Q. What are antiphospholipid antibodies and what is their significance in SLE?

Ans. A syndrome resulting from the production of antiphospholipid antibodies (e.g. lupus anticoagulant, anticardiolipin and false-positive VDRL) is called *antiphospholipid syndrome*, commonly seen in SLE and other autoimmune disorders.

The presence of these antibodies is associated with:
- Increased coagulopathy (arterial, venous thrombosis)
- Fetal loss
- Thrombocytopenia
- Valvular heart disease.

Q. What is antiphospholipid antibody syndrome (APS)? How do you classify it? What are its clinical presentation and treatment?

Ans. The antiphospholipid antibody syndrome (APS) is said to be present if the patient has persistently elevated (twice at least 3 months apart) levels of anti-phospholipid antibody and/or positive lupus anticoagulant test, and the presence of one of the following, i.e. arterial or venous thrombosis, fetal loss, thrombocytopenia.

Causes of APS
1. *Primary* – no definite cause is known.
2. *Secondary*
   - SLE
   - Drug-induced lupus
   - Infections
   - Malignancy.

Clinical features of APS
- Recurrent thromboembolism
- Recurrent fetal loss (2 or more)
- Livedo reticularis
- Nonstroke neurological manifestations
- Valvular heart disease
- Thrombocytopenia
- Catastrophic vascular occlusion.

Classification of APS

Type 1 : DVT with pulmonary embolism
Type 2 : Coronary and peripheral artery thrombosis
Type 3 : Cerebrovascular or retinal artery thrombosis
Type 4 : Mixed type

Treatment
- Anticoagulants, e.g. heparin including low molecular weight (LMWH)
- Antiplatelets, e.g. aspirin
- Intravenous immunoglobulins (IgG)
- Immunosuppressants and steroids.

Q. How will you investigate a case of SLE?

Ans. The investigations done are:
- *Hemoglobin* for anemia. ESR will be raised
- *Total leukocyte and differential leukocyte count* for leukopenia, lymphopenia and thrombocytopenia
- *Urine* for hematuria and proteinuria and casts
- *Serological tests for syphilis* – may be positive
- *Autoantibodies detection.* The ANA, anti-Sm, anti-DNA and antiphospholipids antibodies are done commonly
- *Coombs' test* – Direct test may be positive
- *Serum complement* - low
- *Other tests* depending on the organ/system involvement.

Q. What is the treatment of SLE?

Ans. Treatment according to severity is as follows:
I. *Therapy for mild to moderate disease*
- Bed rest
- NSAIDs and Cox-2 inhibitors
- Antimalarials, e.g. hydroxy-chloroquine, chloroquine for treating lupus rashes and arthritis that do not respond to NSAIDs. Chloroquine 200 mg/day is given. Patient is advised eye check-up after every 6 months.

II. *Therapy for SLE with life-threatening manifestations*

- Topical steroids are used for skin lesions.
- Systemic steroids are used in SLE with life-threatening manifestations such as glomerulonephritis, hemolytic anemia, myopericarditis, CNS involvement and thrombotic thrombocytopenic purpura. The initial dose is 0.5 to 2 mg/kg (average 40-60 mg) orally/ daily for 4-6 weeks, followed by tapered dose 5-10 mg/week to sustain remission.
- Methyl prednisolone can also be used in the dose of 1 g daily for 3 days followed 0.5 to 1 mg/kg/day of oral prednisolone.
- Lupus nephritis needs renal biopsy for confirmation. Focal renal lesions respond to steroids. However, diffuse proliferative or membranoproliferative forms of nephritis (WHO grades III, IV, V) need cyclophosphamide or azathioprine along with steroids. Dialysis is indicated in renal failure.
- Antiphospholipid syndrome is treated with aspirin and anticoagulation.
- Infection is treated with appropriate antibiotics
- *Pregnancy with lupus.* SLE is controlled with the lowest dose of prednisolone for the shortest period. Pregnancy with recurrent fetal loss and antiphospholipid antibodies is treated with aspirin and low molecular heparin.
- SLE with thrombotic thrombocytopenic purpura or hemolytic uremic syndrome is treated by plasmapheresis.

Blood Disorders

CASE 73: THROMBOCYTOPENIA

A female patient (Fig. 1.73) presented with reddish bluish spots on the upper limbs, trunk and legs. There was no history of itching, fever, joint pains or drug intake. Examination revealed that spots were not elevated from the surface of skin and did not blanch with pressure. They were distributed all over the body.

Fig. 1.73: Thrombocytopenic purpura. Note the generalized purpuric spots

Q. Describe these spots and what is your clinical diagnosis?

Ans. These spots are hemorrhagic (bluish red), not elevated from the surface and do not blanch with pressure. They are present on the extremities and front and back of the chest.

The diagnosis is nonpalpable purpura.

Q. How would you proceed to examine such a case?

Ans. Proceed as follows

1. **History**

   Ask for the followings:
   - Age for senile purpura
   - Drugs, e.g. steroids, anticoagulants, phenylbutazone, carbimazole, chloramphenicol, gold salts, etc. for drug-induced purpura.
   - History of chronic liver and renal disease.
   - H/o joint pains, abdominal pains, etc. for Henoch-Schönlein purpura.

- H/o mouth ulcers or necrotising mouth lesions, etc. for neutropenia or pancytopenia.

II. **Examination**

Look for the following signs
- Mouth examination for ulceration and infection (for pancytopenia)
- Signs or stigmata of chronic liver disease or chronic renal failure
- Anemia for marrow aplasia, leukemia and marrow infiltration
- Consider the age of the patient, e.g. young and old
- Signs/deformities of rheumatoid arthritis and drugs-induced purpura
- Symptoms/signs of scurvy, e.g. bleeding gums, corkscrew hair, perifollicular hemorrhage
- Cutis laxa and hyperextensibility of the joints (Ehlers-Danlos syndrome)
- Bleeding from punctured sites, e.g. for DIC.
- Examine the patient for lymph nodes, spleen and liver enlargement.

Q. What is purpura? How does it differ from petechiae and ecchymosis? What is its characteristic feature?

Ans. *Purpura* is defined as hemorrhagic spots of pin-head size, occurs due to extravasation of blood (RBCs) into the dermis.

Petechiae are smaller hemorrhagic spots (≥ 2 mm) while purpuric spots are larger (≥ 3 mm). The *ecchymosis or bruises* are still larger purpuric spots/lesions. *Hematoma* is a large collection of blood in the skin producing swelling with fluctuation sign positive.

The *characteristic feature* of purpuric spots is that they do not blanch with pressure by a pin head or glass slide. This feature differentiates it from vasculitis produced by vasodilatation that blanches with pressure. The telangiectasia, mosquito bite marks, spider nevi blanch on pressure, hence, can easily be differentiated.

Q. What are the causes of bruising?

Ans.
1. Thrombocytopenia (e.g. ITP, marrow infiltration by leukemic cells).
2. Vascular defects (e.g. Henoch-Schönlein purpura, scurvy, von Willebrand's disease, uremia, senility, drug induced).
3. Coagulation disorders (hemophilia A and B, anticoagulants).
4. Drugs.

Q. What are the causes of purpura?

Ans. Purpura may be elevated from the surface (palpable) or may be in line with the surface of the skin (nonpalpable). Primary cutaneous disorders and some systemic diseases produce nonpalpable purpura. *Palpable purpura* is seen in leukocytoclastic vasculitis or allergic vasculitis (Henoch-Schönlein purpura), polyarteritis nodosa and can occur due to infective emboli (e.g. meningococcemia, disseminated gonococcal infection, Rocky Mountain spotted fever). The causes are tabulated (Table 1.176). Purpuric spots occur either due to platelet defect (qualitative and quantitative) or vessels wall abnormalities, e.g. vasculitis.

Table 1.176: Causes of purpura

I. Primary skin disorders
  a. Non-palpable purpura
    – Trauma
    – Solar purpura
    – Steroid (Cushing's) purpura
    – Capillaritis
    – Livedo vasculitis

II. Systemic disorders
  a. Non-palpable
    i. *Platelet defect*
      • Thrombocytopenia, e.g. idiopathic thrombocytopenic purpura (ITP)
      • Abnormal platelet function
    ii. *Vascular fragility*
      • Amyloidosis
      • Scurvy
      • Connective tissue disease, e.g. Ehlers-Danlos syndrome
    iii. *Thrombosis*
      • Disseminated intravascular coagulation (DIC)
      • Cryoglobulinemia
      • Thrombotic thrombocytopenic purpura
      • Warfarin reaction
    iv. *Emboli*
      • Cholesterol
      • Fat
    v. *Immune-complex*
      • Gardner-Diamond syndrome
      • Waldenstrom's hypergammaglobulinemic purpura
  b. *Palpable*
    i. *Vasculitis*
      • Allergic purpura (Henoch – Schönlein)
      • PAN (polyarteritis nodosa)
    ii. *Infectious emboli*
      • Meningococcemia
      • Disseminated gonococal infection
      • Rocky Mountain spotted fever
      • Ecthyma gangrenosum

Q. What are the causes of non-thrombocytopenic purpura?

Ans. Causes are as follows:
- Infections, e.g. meningococcal, gonococcal, rickettsial and viral
- Allergic purpura (Henoch-Schönlein)
- Hereditary telangiectasia
- Drug-induced
- Senile purpura
- Purpura simplex (Devil's pinches)
- Steroid-induced (Cushing's syndrome)
- Paraproteinemia
- Vasculitis
- Uremia.

Q. What are the causes of thrombocytopenic purpura?

Ans. Thrombocytopenia is caused by one of the three mechanisms:
1. Decreased bone marrow production
2. Increased splenic sequestration
3. Increased/accelerated destruction

Depending on these mechanisms, the causes of thrombocytopenia are summarized in Table 1.177.

Table 1.177: Causes of thrombocytopenia

I. Decreased bone marrow production
  • Aplasia/hypoplasia of marrow
  • Fanconi syndrome
  • Myelophthisic process (malignant infiltration of marrow)
  • Deficiency states, e.g folic acid, vit. B_{12}
  • Paroxysmal noctural
  • Hemoglobinuria
  • Drugs/physical
  • Myelofibrosis

II. Increased splenic sequestration
  • Infective
  • Congestive
  • Neoplastic

III. Increased/Accelerated destruction of platelets
  A. *Immune*
    • Idiopathic (immune) thrombocytopenic purpura (ITP)
    • SLE
    • Lymphoreticular disorders
    • Hypothyroidism
    • Drugs
  B. *Non-immune*
    • Thrombotic thrombocytopenic purpura
    • Disseminated intravascular coagulation (comsumptive coagulopathy)
    • Valvular disorders (microangiopathic)

Remember few common causes of thrombocytopenia

- ITP (Idiopathic Thrombocytopenic Purpura)
- SLE
- Hypoplasia of marrow/myelofibrosis
- Drug-induced
- Thrombotic thrombocytopenic purpura
- DIC
- Infections, e.g. Dengue hemorrhagic fever

Q. What are clinical characteristic of ITP?

Ans. The three clinical characteristics are:

1. Bleeding is the characteristic feature of ITP which occurs at the following sites:
   - Skin, e.g. petechiae, purpura, ecchymosis
   - Mucous membrane and gum bleeding
   - Nasal bleeding (epistaxis)
   - Genitourinary tract bleeding (hematuria, menorrhagia)
   - Intracranial and intra-abdominal bleeding
2. Reduced platelet count
3. Hypercellular marrow with megakaryocytosis.

Q. What are the causes of palpable purpura?

Ans. Read Table 1.176

Q. What is disseminated intravascular coagulation (DIC)?

Ans. It is defined as bleeding disorder characterized by consumptive coagulopathy (consumption of thrombocytes and coagulation factors) leading to thrombocytopenia, infarction and gangrene. It may be acute or chronic. It is caused by a variety of triggering factors.

Q. Name the drugs that cause thrombocytopenic purpura.

Ans. The drugs either suppress platelet production in marrow or cause accelerated platelet destruction. The causes are:

I. Drugs causing suppression of platelets production
   - Myelosuppressive drugs, e.g. cytosine arabinoside, daunorubicin, cyclophosphamide, busulfan, methotrexate, 6-MP, Vinca alkaloids
   - Thiazide diuretics
   - Ethanol (binge drinker)
   - Estrogen.

II. Drugs producing immunological destruction of platelets
   - Antibiotics, e.g. sulphonamide, tetracyclines, novobiocin, PAS, rifampicin, chloramphenicol
   - Cinchona alkaloids, e.g. quinine, quinidine
   - Sedatives, hypnotic, and anticonvulsants (carbamazepine)
   - Digoxin
   - Alpha-methyldopa
   - Anti-inflammatory, e.g. aspirin, phenylbutazone
   - Chloroquine, gold salts, arsenicals
   - Insecticides

Q. What are causes of splenomegaly with purpura?

Ans. Following are the causes:

1. Lymphoreticular malignancy, e.g. leukemia and lymphoma, acute blastic crisis of CML and CLL

2. Infections, e.g. subacute infective endocarditis, septicemia
3. Connective tissue disorders, e.g. SLE
4. Myelofibrosis
5. *Hypersplenism:* Though hypersplenism means hyperfunction of the spleen. The term has nothing to do with the size, but hypersplenism is usually associated with splenomegaly. The causes are:
   - Portal hypertension
   - Myeloproliferative disease
   - Lymphoma.

Q. What is Henoch-Schönlein purpura (Anaphylactoid purpura)?

Ans. It is self-limiting type of vasculitis, occurs in children and young adults, characterized by purpuric spots or urticarial rash on the extensor surfaces of the arms and legs, polyarthralgia or arthritis, abdominal colic and hematuria (focal glomerulonephritis). The syndrome follows an episode of URI or streptococcal pharyngitis. All the coagulation tests are normal despite purpura. Bleeding time is normal.

Q. What is thrombotic thrombocytopenic purpura (Moschcowitz's syndrome)?

Ans. Thrombotic thrombocytopenic purpura is an acute disorder characterized by thrombocytopenic purpura, microangiopathic hemolytic anemia, transient or fluctuating neurological features, fever and renal involvement (read Emergency Medicine by Prof SN Chugh).

Q. How will you investigate a case with purpura?

Ans. The **investigations** are as follows:
   - Hemoglobin – may be low
   - Urine for hematuria, proteinuria
   - Platelet count – low in thrombocytopenic purpura, normal in non-thrombocytopenic purpura
   - Bleeding time is prolonged. Clotting time is normal.
   - PTTK and PT (prothrombin time) are normal
   - Antiplatelets antibodies. They are present in immune thrombocytopenic purpura
   - Serological tests for hepatitis, cytomegalovirus, Epstein-Barr virus and HIV
   - Bone marrow examination. It should be done when platelet count is >50,000/μl and there is no bleeding
   - Antinuclear antibodies (ANAs) for SLE
   - USG for spleen enlargement
   - Radiolabeled platelets and their destruction in the spleen will confirm hypersplenism.

Q. What is treatment of ITP?

Ans. This is as follows:

- Specific therapy is not necessary unless platelet count is <20,000/ml. Analgesic (codeine and paracetamol) may be used for pain or fever
- *Corticosteroids* are used to control bleeding in acute ITP. Oral prednisolone is given in dose of 40-60 mg/day for few weeks followed by tapering of the dose to maintenance dose of 5-10 mg/day
- *IV immunoglobulin (IVIG)* is reserved for patients with severe thrombocytopenia and clinical bleeding who fail to respond to steroids and other measures
- *Plasmapheresis means removal of immune complexes is as useful as IV immunoglobulin in ITP*
- Blood transfusions/platelets transfusion is given to raise the platelet count in severe thrombocytopenia
- *Splenectomy*. It is indicated in patients with ITP who are resistant to other measures
- *Immunosuppressive therapy*. Patients who remain thrombocytopenic after steroid therapy or splenectomy or who relapse within months to years after initial therapy are candidates for immunosuppression with azathioprine, cyclophosphamide or vincristine/vinblastine.

Q. How do you diagnose asplenia or hyposplenia?

Ans. The diagnostic signs are:

1. Presence of Howell-Jolly bodies, Heinz bodies and basophilic stippling in RBCs. There is marked anisocytosis and poikilocytosis.
2. USG will show absence of spleen.
3. Radionuclide scan for spleen will confirm its absence.

Q. What are the risks of splenectomy?

Ans. The risks are:

1. Increased susceptibility to bacterial infection by capsular organisms, e.g. *S. pneumoniae, H. influenzae* and some *gram-negative organisms*. Immunization against these may be done before splenectomy.

2. There is increased susceptibility to parasitic disease, e.g. babesiosis in certain endemic areas.

The vaccination schedule before and after splenectomy has already been discussed in case discussion on splenomegaly.

Q. What is Dengue Hemorrhagic Fever? What is Hess capillary test?

Ans. Dengue is a mosquito-borne (Aedes aegypti) viral infection caused by one of the 4 types of *flavi viruses* (dengue 1 to 4), occurs in epidemics, and is characterized by febrile illness (classic dengue), bleeding manifestations (dengue hemorrhagic fever) and shock (dengue shock syndrome).

Dengue hemorrhagic fever is characterised by all manifestations of classic dengue fever, thrombocytopenia (platelet count < 1 lac/cumm), vascular instability and increased permeability and local hemorrhage (spontaneous petechiae and/or purpura) with positive tourniquet test called *Hess capillary test*. The hemorrhage in dengue is due to combined effect of vascular damage and thrombocytopenia.

Hess capillary test (Tourniquet test)

It is positive in dengue fever and severe thrombocytopenia (ITP). It indicates vascular instability.

It is performed by blood pressure cuff wrapped in upper arm and BP is raised and maintained between systolic or diastolic (usually around 100 mmHg) for 5 minutes. The hemorrhagic spots are counted in a circle marked on the mid-forearm with a diameter of one inch. The hemorrhagic spots more than 10 are abnormal, indicate positive test.

Q. What is critical platelet count?

Ans. Critical platelet count means the lowest platelet count at which spontaneous bleeding into the skin, brain or internal organs may occur and may be fatal. The critical count is <20,000/μl. The count between 20,000/μl and 50,000/μl leads to bleeding only after minor trauma or stress.

Q. What is difference between bleeding and clotting disorder?

Ans. Read Clinical Methods in Medicine by Prof SN Chugh.

Cardiovascular Disorders

CASE 74: CYANOTIC CONGENITAL HEART DISEASE

A 14-year female presented with cyanotic spells (bluishness during exertion), syncope and tachypnea. On symptomatic equiry, it was found that she had bluishness of tongue and nails since infancy and childhood which increased during crying or on waking up from sleep. The parents admitted that child used to sit in squatting position after playing. The examination revealed cyanosis, clubbing (Fig. 1.74) and an ejection systolic murmur in 2nd left intercostal space with loud single second heart sound.

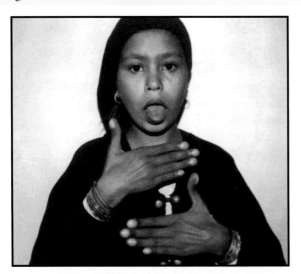

Fig. 1.74: Congenital cyanotic heart disease. A young female with Fallot's tetralogy. Note the drum-stick clubbing and central cyanosis

Q. **What is the clinical provisional diagnosis?**
Ans. The patient has cyanotic congenital heart disease–Fallot's tetralogy.
Q. **What are the components of Fallot's tetralogy, triology and pentalogy?**
Ans. Table 1.178 describes all the components of Fallot's.
Q. **What is the cause of cyanosis in Fallot's tetralogy?**
Ans. This is due to mixing of the unoxygenated blood from right ventricle to left ventricle through VSD as the shunt between two ventricles is either bidirectional (blood flows from either ventricles depending on the pressure) or from right to left and the over-rided aorta gets mixed blood from both the ventricles leading to cyanosis.

Note: Right to left shunt produces cyanosis; left to right shunt does not.

Q. **Name few common cyanotic and acyanotic congenital heart disease.**
Ans. These are as follows:
Cyanotic congenital heart disease
- Fallot's tetralogy
- Transposition of great vessels
- Total anomalous pulmonary venous drainage
- Single ventricle
- Truncus arteriosus
- Tricuspid atresia
- Ebstein's anomaly (some cases are cyanotic)
- Eisenmenger's complex and syndrome.
  Acyanotic congenital heart disease. These are either with left to right shunt or with outflow tract obstruction.
  1. *Left to right shunt*
     - ASD, VSD, PDA
     - Endocardial cushion defects
     - Rupture of sinus of Valsalva
     - Coronary arteriovenous fistula
  II. Obstructive lesions
     - Coarctation of aorta
     - Congenital aortic stenosis
     - Congenital pulmonary stenosis.

Q. **What is the cause of ejection systolic murmur in this case?**
Ans. In Fallot's tetralogy, there is pulmonary stenosis which produces an ejection systolic murmur and single second heart sound. The pulmonary stenosis in Fallot's tetralogy may be infundibular (common) or valvular (uncommon).

Table 1.178: Components of Fallot's tetralogy, triology and pentalogy

Fallot's tetralogy	Fallot's triology	Fallot's pentalogy
• VSD • Pulmonary stenosis • Right ventricular hypertrophy • Over-riding of aorta	• VSD • ASD • Pulmonary stenosis	• ASD is added to Fallot's tetralogy to make it pentalogy

Q. Why VSD in Fallot's does not produce murmur?

Ans. Murmur is produced due to presence of a flow gradient across a congenital defect or a valve. In Fallot's tetralogy, the shunt at VSD level is more or less balanced without much flow gradient across the defect, hence, murmur is not produced.

Q. What is Eisenmenger's complex and Eisenmenger's syndrome?

Ans. In VSD, there is usually left to right shunt.
Eisenmenger's complex means a VSD with reversal of shunt (right to left).
Eisenmenger's syndrome means reversal of any left to right shunt (e.g. ASD, PDA) except VSD.

Q. How does squatting position helps in Fallot's tetralogy?

Ans. Squatting is the posture adopted by children with Fallot's tetralogy in which child sits with flexed hips and knees. It helps to reduce venous return of desaturated blood and an increase in peripheral vascular resistance, thus, reduces right to left shunting and improves cerebral oxygenation. This posture reduces cyanotic spells.

Q. What are genetic and environmental factors implicated in congenital heart diseases?

The various factors associated with congenital heart disease are tabulated (Table 1.179).

Q. What is ASD? What are its type and physical signs?

Ans. Atrial septal defect (ASD) is a common cardiac anomaly manifestating in adults more commonly in women. In this condition, there is defect in atrial septum leading to shunting of blood from left atrium to right atrium (LA to RA). It is acyanotic congenital heart disease.

Types and defects are given in Table 1.180.

Table 1.180: Classification of ASD

Types	Defects
Ostium secundum (commonest)	At the level of fossa ovalis
Sinus venosus	Posterior to foramen ovale
Coronary sinus	Inferior and anterior to foramen ovale
Ostium primum (rare)	Anterior and inferior to foramen ovale and cleft mitral and tricuspid valves

Physical signs in ASD are:

1. ***Sternal impulse (heave).*** There is right ventricular impulse or heave
2. ***Sounds.*** Ist sound is loud. The second heart sound is loud, fixed and widely split.

Table 1.179: Genetic and environmental factors and associated congenital heart disease

I. Genetic factors	
A. *Chromosomal defects*	*Associated Cardiac defects*
• Trisomy 21 (Down's syndrome)	VSD, ASD, PDA, Fallot's tetralogy
• Trisomy 13 (Patau's syndrome)	VSD, ASD, PDA
• Trisomy 18 (Edward's syndrome)	VSD, PDA
• Turner's syndrome (45X0)	Coarctation of aorta
• Cri-du-chat syndrome (Short arm deletion –5)	VSD
• XXXY and XXXXX	PDA
B. Single gene defect	
• Ellis-Van Crevald syndrome (R)	ASD, single atrium
• Carpenter' syndrome (R)	PDA, ASD
• Holt-Oram (D)	ASD, VSD
• Noonan syndrome (D)	Pulmonary stenosis, aortic stenosis, ASD
II. *Environmental factors*	
• Maternal rubella	PDA, peripheral pulmonary stenosis
• Maternal alcohol abuse	Septal defects (ASD, VSD)
• Coxsackie virus	PDA, VSD
• Thalidomide	ASD, VSD, truncus arteriosus
• Maternal SLE	Congenital complete heart block
• Maternal DM	VSD, transposition of great vessels, coarctation of aorta

Abbrev. ASD – atrial septal defect
VSD – ventricular septal defect
PDA – patent ductus arteriosus

3. *Murmurs*
   - A grade 2 or 3 pulmonary ejection or midsystolic murmur best heard at 2nd or 3rd left interspace
   - A short diastolic flow murmur in tricuspid area (e.g. at lower left sternal border).

   Both these murmurs are flow murmurs. There is no murmur due to left to right shunt across the defect because of low pressure gradient between two atria.

Q. **What is PDA? What are its characteristics?**

Ans. The ductus arteriosus is normally present in the fetus and allows the right ventricular output to enter the descending aorta as the lungs are non-functioning and the pulmonary circulation is not essential in fetal life.

It closes within 24-48 hours after birth as the lungs expands and pulmonary circulation established. Premature babies commonly have PDA (patent ductus arteriosus) which closes spontaneously when the baby reaches the full term.

PDA means persistence of ductus arteriosus after birth leading to shunting of blood from aorta to pulmonary artery (L to R shunt).

This is the commonest lesion in babies with rubella syndrome, prematue baby and babies born at high altitude. Hemodynamics include a continuous flow of blood from the aorta to pulmonary artery during systole leading to overloading of the lungs (pulmonary plethora) and left atrium and left ventricle.

Physical Signs

Signs of hyperdynamic circulation, e.g. bounding peripheral pulses, tachycardia, pulsations in suprasternal notch and carotid pulsations, wide pulse pressure.

Apex beat – hyperkinetic /forceful but ill sustained

Thrill – A systolic or continuous thrill may be palpable rarely at the 2nd left intersapce.

Sounds
- The first sound is loud
- The second sound is loud with narrow split in small shunts but paradoxically split in large shunt.
- A third heart sound at the apex is common.

Murmurs
- A continuous '*machinery*' murmur (Gibson's murmur) is heard at 2nd left intercostal space below clavicle
- A mid-diastolic murmur (flow murmur) at apex due to left to right shunt.

Q. **What is a continuous murmur? What are its causes?**

Ans. A continuous murmur is defined as a murmur which starts with the first heart sound (S1), continues throughout the systole and peaks at the second heart sound (S2) and spills into diastole after the sound (waning character).

Causes
- PDA
- Aortopulmonary window
- Rupture of sinus of valsalva into right atrium or ventricle
- Coronary arteriovenous fistula
- Pulmonary arteriovenous fistula
- Heard over the collateral vessels
- Peripheral pulmonary artery stenosis.

Q. **What are radiological characteristics of left to right shunts? (Read the radiological section 4)**

Ans. Chest X-ray (PA view) shows:
- Prominent heart shadow or cardiomegaly with left ventricular configuration
- The pulmonary conus is prominent
- Pulmonary plethora (increased bronchovascular marking from hilum to periphery) present
- The aortic knuckle is also prominent.

Q. **What are clinical hallmarks of a large left to right shunt?**

Ans. The clinical hallmarks are due to hyperkinetic circulation with systemic overloading. The various signs are:
- Bounding pulses, may be *water-hammer*
- Prominent carotid and suprasternal pulsations
- Palpable parasternal heave
- Hyperkinetic apical impulse
- Loud sounds (1st and 2nd) and presence of 3rd heart sound
- Flow murmurs across the valves usually mid-diastolic either at mitral or tricuspid valve or an ejection systolic murmur across the semilunar valves.

Q. **What is the site of infective endocarditis in left to right shunt?**

Ans. The infective endocarditis develops where the jet of blood flow strikes the ventricle or the vessel, i.e. right ventricular wall in VSD and wall of pulmonary vessel in PDA. The endocarditis in ASD is rare due to slow flow of blood.

Q. **Which congenital heart diseases can cause atrial fibrillation?**

Ans. The diseases are:
- ASD
- Ebstein anomaly.

CASE 75: SUPERIOR MEDIASTINAL COMPRESSION

A patient (Fig. 1.75) presented with cough, dyspnea, fever, chest discomfort, puffiness of face, hoarseness of voice. The examination showed suffused face, cyanosis, prominent engorged neck veins with absent pulsations and hoarseness of voice. There was enlargement of cervical lymph nodes. Heart was essentially normal.

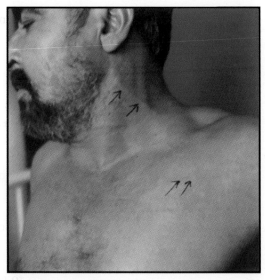

Fig. 1.75: Superior mediastinal compression due to a mass in the mediastinum. Note the prominent neck veins and veins over the upper part of chest above the nipple line

Q. What do the symptoms and signs indicate?

Ans. The symptoms and signs indicate superior mediastinal compression.

Q. What is superior mediastinal compression?

Ans. Superior mediastinum is an area bounded above by thoracic inlet, below by the upper part of heart and vessels, anteriorly by sternum and posteriorly by spines. It contains lymph nodes, thymus, aortic arch, trachea, superior vena cava, esophagus and connective tissue.

Compression in this area due to any cause results in pressure on these structures including superior vena cava leading to clinical picture of superior mediastinal syndrome or superior vena cava syndrome.

Q. What conditions will you keep in mind in such a case?

Ans. All the conditions that produce puffiness of face will come into differential diagnosis.
- Pericardial effusion/constrictive pericarditis
- Cardiomyopathy (restrictive, dilated)
- CHF
- Cor pulmonale
- Valvular heart diseases

Q. What are the causes of superior mediastinal compression?

Ans. They are summarized in Table 1.181.

Table 1.181: Causes of superior mediastinal compression

I.	**Enlarged lymph nodes**
	• Tuberculosis
	• Lymphoma
	• Sarcoidosis
	• Leukemia
II.	**Thymus**
	Thymic hyperplasia or thymoma
III.	**Thyroid**
	Retrosternal goitre
IV.	**Aorta**
	Aortic aneurysm
V.	**Esophageal lesions**
	Carcinoma
VI.	**Tumors**
	• Vascular
	• Teratoma

Q. What are symptoms and signs of superior mediastinal compression or superior vena cava compression (SVC)?

Ans. These are enlisted in Table 1.182.

Q. How the neck veins look like in superior mediastinal compression (SMC)?

Ans.
- The neck veins are engorged, dilated and may be tortuous. JVP is raised.
- Venous pulsations are absent.
- Hepatojugular reflux is positive.
- There is no inspiratory collapse of the veins due to obstruction between veins and right atrium.

Q. How will you investigate such a case?

Ans. The investigations are as follows:
1. *TLC, DLC* for tuberculosis, lymphoma and leukemia
2. *Chest X-ray (PA view)* to identify the anatomical site of tumor and its effects, i.e.
   - Mediastinal widening
   - Collapse or atelectasis
   - Malignancy lung
   - Pleural effusion
   - Raised hemidiaphragm (phrenic nerve palsy)
   - Rarely pericardial effusion
3. *Sputum* for AFB and malignant cells
4. *FNAC or excision biopsy* of palpable lymph node (scalene node, Virchow's gland or any other node)
5. *Pleural fluid* aspiration and pleural biopsy
6. *Barium swallow* for esophageal compression
7. *CT scan of thorax or lung scan or thyroid scan.*

Table 1.182: Clinical features of superior mediastinal compression

Structure compressed	Symptoms and signs
i. **Trachea**	Respiratory distress, stridor, cough
ii. **Esophagus**	Dysphagia (solids and liquids)
iii. **Bronchus**	It is usually not involved except in bronchogenic carcinoma, producing collapse of the lung
iv. **Nerves**	
– Recurrent laryngeal	Hoarseness of voice, bovine cough, stridor
– Phrenic	Breathlessness and hiccough
– Cervical sympathetic	Horner's syndrome
v. **Vessels**	
– Superior vena cava	Suffused and puffy face, visual disturbances, headache, alteration in consciousness, prominent engorged neck veins without pulsations, chemosis
– Azygos vein	Right sided pleural effusion
– Lymphatics	Non-pitting edema of upper thorax, chylothorax

Q. What is inferior vena caval compression (IVC) syndrome?

Ans. Compression or obstruction of inferior vena cava occurs due to ascites, tumors of the abdomen or pelvis, pregnant uterus, thrombosis extending from pelvic veins, membraneous obstruction, oral contraceptives use and myeloproliferative disorders. The clinical picture resulting from IVC obstruction includes:

- Edema (pitting) of legs with dilated veins over the legs
- Collateral veins are seen over the abdomen, flanks and back
- Direction of blood flow in abdominal veins is "below upwards"
- Ascites
- Chronic venous ulcer and staining of ankles in chronic cases
- Signs of portal hypertension (post-hepatic) if venous obstruction is above the joining of hepatic veins.

Q. What is pneumomediastinum?

Ans. Pneumomediastinum means collection of air into the mediastinal space.

The causes are:

1. *Alveolar rupture with dissection of air into the mediastinum*

- Acute severe asthma
- Pneumocystis carinii pneumonia

2. *Perforation of esophagus, trachea or bronchi*

- Aspiration of a foreign body
- Severe straining during coughing or vomiting in children. Weight lifting and glass blowing may also predispose to it.
- Manipulation (iatrogenic)
- Blunt trauma to the chest

3. *Dissection of air from the neck or abdomen into the mediastinum*

- Blunt trauma to neck
- Difficult parturition
- Perforation of a hollow viscus and collection of air into retroperitoneal space and then dissection into mediastinum.

Clinical Signs

- Subcutaneous emphysema in suprasternal notch with pain and dyspnea
- *Hamman's mediastinal sign* – a crunching sound synchronous with heart beat is best heard in left lateral decubitus position on compression of mediastinum with palm of the hand.
- Chest X-ray shows air column parallel to heart and aorta, best seen in lateral film.

The patient presented with chest pain, dyspnea, distension of the abdomen and edema feet. There was past history of fever without cough and hemoptysis. Examination of CVS revealed pericardial rub with enlargement of cardiac area of dullness and feeble heart sounds. The neck veins were engorged and JVP was raised with prominent X-descent. Kussmaul's sign was negative (Fig. 1.76).

Fig. 1.76: Pericarditis with effusion. The diagnostic pericardiocentesis is being done

Q. What is the provisional clinical diagnosis?
Ans. Pericarditis with pericardial effusion.

Q. What are points in favor of your diagnosis?
Ans. 1. Acute febrile onset
2. Symptoms and signs of CHF, e.g. dyspnea, raised JVP, hepatomegaly, ascitis and edema
3. Presence of pericardial rub, prominent X-descent
4. Negative Kussmaul's sign
5. Enlargement of area of cardiac dullness with feeble heart sounds.

Q. What is your alternative diagnosis?
Ans. • Dilated cardiomyopathy
• Myocarditis
• Myocardial infarction with pericarditis.

Q. How do you classify pericarditis?
Ans. Depending on the duration, pericarditis is classifed as:
1. *Acute pericarditis (< 6 weeks)*
• Fibrinous
• Serous or sanguineous
2. *Subacute pericarditis (6 weeks to 6 months)*
• Effusive – constrictive
• Constrictive
3. *Chronic pericarditis (> 6 months)*
• Constrictive
• Effusive (with pericardial effusion)
• Adhesive (non-constrictive).

Q. What are the causes of pericarditis?
Ans. They are tabulated (Table 1.183).

Table 1.183: Causes of pericarditis

A. Idiopathic or nonspecific

B. Infections
• *Viral*, e.g. coxsackie virus A and B, echovirus, mumps, adenovirus, hepatitis, HIV
• *Bacterial*, e.g. tubercular, pyogenic organisms (pneumococci, staphylococci, strepococci and Neisseria)
• *Fungal*, e.g. histoplasmosis, candida, blastomycosis, (coccidioidomycosis)
• *Parasitic*, e.g. echinococcus, amoebiasis and filariasis

C. Non-infectious
i. Postmyocardial infarction
ii. Metabolic, e.g. uremia, hypercholesterolemia
iii. Endocrinal, e.g. myxoedema
iv. Neoplastic, e.g. primary (benign or malignant) and secondary (metastases from lung and breast cancer)
v. Traumatic, e.g. penetrating and non-penetrating injury
vi. Aortic dissection (blood leakage into pericardium)
vii. Post-radiation
viii. Familial mediterranean fever (FMF).

D. Hypersensitivity or autoimmune
• Rheumatic fever
• Collagen vascular disorders, e.g. SLE, rheumatoid arthritis, scleroderma, acute rheumatic fever
• Drug-induced, e.g. procainamide, hydralazine, isoniazide, phenytoin, doxorubicin, methyldopa
• Post-cardiac injury, e.g. postmyocardial infarction (Dressler's syndrome), post-pericardiotomy

Remember five common causes of pericardial effusion
• Tuberculosis
• Viral pericarditis with effusion
• Neoplastic pericarditis
• Myxoedema
• Uremia

Q. What is pericardial rub? What does it indicate? What are its characteristics? How does it differ from pleuropericardial rub?
Ans. It is an adventitious sound produced by rubbing of visceral and parietal pericardium, hence, has a rubbing or scratching quality. It may have presystolic, systolic or early diastolic components which means rub may be heard in a part of systole or throughout systole or in early diastole.

It explains the pain due to pericarditis. The pericardium being painsensitive structure leads to pain during rubbing or scratching of its layers against each other.

Its characteristics are given in the Table 1.184

It does not have any relation to respiration, hence, differs from pleuropericardial rub (Read the Clinical Methods in Medicine by Prof SN Chugh). Its differentiation from continuous murmur are given in Table 1.184.

311

Table 1.184: Differences between a continuous murmur and pericardial rub

Pericardial rub	Continuous murmur
• Rubbing or scratching high pitched sound	Soft musical or machinery sound
• Heard either in a part of systole or diastole	Heard both in systole and diastole
• Best heard in sitting position during expiration with patient sitting up and leaning forward	Heard in all positions
• Associated with pain	Not associated with pain
• Inconsistent and intermittent in character, i.e. may appear and then disappear for few hours	Consistent in character

Q. What are clinical characteristics of acute pericarditis?

Ans. Pain, a pericardial rub and characteristic ECG changes (ST segment elevation with concavity upwards in more than two or three standard leads and V2-V6) are clinical hallmarks (a triad) of acute pericarditis.

Q. What are ECG changes in acute pericarditis?

Ans. Read Practical Electrocardiography by Prof SN Chugh.

Q. When does pericardial rub disappear in pericarditis?

Ans. As pericarditis indicates friction between two layers of the pericardium, the rub persists as long as friction persists in pericarditis, may disappear with appearance of massive pericardial effusion or development of chronic calcific pericarditis. It is possible to hear a pericardial rub in effusive pericarditis (pericarditis with minimal effusion).

Q. What are characteristics of pericardial effusion?

Ans. The pericardial cavity contains about 50 ml or less of pericardial fluid, which may be detected on echocardiography. The pericardial effusion means collection of fluid (exudate, transudate, pus or blood) in the pericardial cavity more than normal but the signs will appear only if it is more than 200 ml.

The symptoms are:
• Pain, central in origin having all characteristics described in pericarditis
• Dyspnea due to compression of lung and bronchi
• Dry hacking cough, hoarseness of voice and dysphagia due to compression of trachea, recurrent laryngeal nerve and esophagus respectively.

The signs of pericardial effusion are given in Table 1.185.

Q. What is cardiac tamponade? What are its salient features?

Ans. It is defined as acute massive collection of fluid leading to an impaired filling of ventricles due to rising intrapericardial pressure. There is decrease in stroke volume due to impaired cardiac contractions.

Note. Tamponade is associated with acute or rapid collection of fluid; whereas large pericardial effusion which has developed slowly may not result in tamponade.

Its salient features are:
• Breathlessness, cyanosis and patient assumes knee-chest position

Table 1.185: Signs of pericardial effusion

General physical signs
• *Pulsus paradoxus*
• Low pulse pressure
• Cyanosis may or may not be present
• Neck veins are distended and Kussmaul's sign is absent
• Pitting edema feet

Systemic examination

Inspection
• Precordium may be bulging including xiphisternum
• Apex is not visible
• No other pulsations are visible

Palpation
• Apex beat is either feeble or not palpable
• A pericardial rub may be palpable
• No other pulsations palpable
• Palpable tender liver (tender hepatomegaly)

Percussion
• Increase in area of cardiac dullness. Shifting cardiac dullness may be present (area of cardiac dullness decreases on sitting)
• There is an area of dullness, on right side of sternum in 5th intercostal space (Rotch's sign)
• An area of dullness in the left interscapular region with bronchial breathing and aegophony (Edward's sign). This is due to compression of base of the lung

Auscultation
• Heart sounds are muffled
• A pericardial rub may be heard

Other signs
• Tender hepatomegaly
• Ascites.

Table 1.186: Distinction between chronic constrictive pericarditis, pericardial effusion and right ventricular failure

Features	Pericardial effusion	Constrictive pericarditis	Right heart failure
A. Clinical			
Pulsus paradoxus	Common	Absent	Absent or rare
Jugular veins, e.g.			
Prominent y descent	Absent	Present	Rare
Prominent x descent	Present	Absent	Rare
Kussmaul's sign	Absent	Present	Absent
Third heart sound (S$_3$)	Absent	Absent	May be present
Pericardial knock (rub)	Absent	Often present	Absent
B. ECG			
Low voltage graph	Present	May be present	Absent
Electrical alternans	Present	Absent	Absent
C. Echocardiography			
Thickened pericardium	Absent	Present	Absent
Pericardial calcification	Absent	Often present	Absent
Pericardial effusion	Present	Absent	Absent
RV size	Usually small	Normal	Enlarged
Right atrial collapse	Present	Absent	Absent
Increasd early filling with increased mitral flow velocity	Absent	Present	May be present
Exaggerated respiratory variation in flow velocity	Present	Present	Absent
D. CT and MRI			
Thickened/calcified pericardium	Absent	Present	Absent
E. Cardiac catheterization			
Equalization of diastolic ventricular pressure pulses-*square root sign*	Present	Present	Absent or present

- Tachycardia
- Pulsus paradoxus, low volume pulse
- Raised JVP. Neck veins full and pulsations present
- Fall in BP with low pulse pressure. There may be hypotension or shock
- Kussmaul's sign (paradoxical rise in JVP during inspiration) is absent
- Muffled heart sounds

Rising venous pressure, fall in arterial pressure and quiet heart constitute a triad of cardiac tamponade

Treatment (Read Medical Emergencies by Prof SN Chugh).

Q. What is chronic constrictive pericarditis?

Ans. The disorder results following healing of acute fibrinous or serofibrinous pericarditis or a chronic pericardial effusion leading to obliteration of the pericardial sac with granulation tissue and ultimately a firm scar encasing the heart is formed. Like pericardial effusion, it also interferes with filling of the ventricles.

The causes of constrictive pericarditis are:

A. *Infectious*
- Tubercular pericarditis (commonest)
- Pyogenic pericarditis
- Acute viral pericarditis
- Fungal (histoplasmosis) pericarditis

B. *Non-infectious*
- Neoplasm
- Post-radiation
- Post-traumatic
- Following cardiac surgery
- Collagen vascular disorder, e.g. SLE, rheumatoid arthritis
- Chronic renal failure treated by hemodialysis.

The clinical features resemble with that of cardiac tamponade, right heart failure (Table 1.186).

A 20 yrs male (patient not shown) presented with palpitations and repeated cough and fever in the winter seasons. The palpitations increased on exertion and produced distress.

Fig. 1.77A: Ventricular septal defect (VSD) line diagram

Figs 1.77B and C: Two-dimensional echocardiogram (long-axis view) showing a ventricular septal defect (arrowed). Color Doppler (C) would provide graphic demonstration of the left to right shunt. RV, right ventricle; IVS, interventricular septum; LV, left ventricle; LA, left atrium

Q. What is your clinical diagnosis.

Ans. The patient has ventricular septal defect (congenital) without pulmonary hypertension, CHF and Bacterial endocarditis.

Q. What is differential diagnosis?

Ans. It has to be differentiated from:
- Mitral regurgitation
- Tricuspid regurgitation
- Papillary muscle dysfunction
- Cardiomyopathy (dilated).

Q. How would you proceed to examine this case?

Ans.

History—Points to be Noted
- H/o dyspnea, fever, cough and reduced exercise tolerance
- History of cyanosis on exertion

General Physical Examination
- Pulse-normal
- BP normal or wide pulse pressure
- Neck for venous and arterial pulsations and JVP show normal pulsations and normal pressure
- Look for anemia, cyanosis, edema, jaundice, etc.

CVS Examination

Inspection
- Apex beat: dynamic or hyperkinetic and laterally displaced
- Precordial pulsations may be present

Palpation
- Apex beat is hyperkinetic, ill sustained
- Left ventricular thrust present
- Left parasternal heave may be palpable
- A systolic thrill palpable across the sternum
- P_2 may be palpable if pulmonary hypertension develops

Percussion
- Area of cardiac dullness widened due to LVH and apex beat corresponds with cardiac dullness
- Pulmonary area may be dull on percussion if pulmonary hypertension develops.

Auscultation
- Both heart sounds are heard
- A pansystolic murmur heard best in 3rd and 4th left intercostal spaces and radiates to the right across the sternum. There is an associated thrill if defect is small.
- A mid-diastolic flow murmur heard at the apex.
- A Graham Steel's murmur heard if pulmonary regurgitation.
- Second heart may be normal or loud due to pulmonary hypertension.

Other System

Respiratory system
- For any evidence of consolidation or chest infection.
- For signs of LVF i.e. end-inspiratory crackles

Abdomen
- For hepatomegaly

Q. What are points in favor of your diagnosis?

Ans.
- Seasonal cough, fever and breathlessness
- A palpable systolic thrill across the sternum
- A pansystolic murmur widely heard across the chest
- No signs of CHF or LHF.

Q. What are the causes of VSD?

Ans.
- Congenital
- Acquired due to rupture of interventricular septum in a patient with myocardial infarction,
- It may be a component of other congenital defect e.g. septum primum, Fallot's tetralogy.

Q. Where does the defect in the septum lies?

Ans.
- Commonly in the membraneous portion of the septum
- Uncommonly in the muscular part of interventricular septum.

Q. Does the defect close spontaneously?

Ans. Yes, it closes in early childhood in 50% cases if the defect is small.

Q. What is the relation of murmur with size of the defect?

Ans.
- Smaller the defect, longer is the murmur
- Larger the defect, shorter is the murmur.

Q. What is maladie de Roger?

Ans. A small membraneous VSD with a loud pansystolic murmur with thrill across the sternum in a patient who is asymptomatic.

Q. When the duration of murmur decreases in VSD?

Ans.
- The duration of murmur decreases if the defect lies in the muscular part of the septum.
- The duration of murmur also decreases with development of pulmonary hypertension.

Q. What are the causes of pansystolic murmur?

Ans. Read the causes in case discussion of MR.

Q. What is Eisenmenger's complex?

Ans. Eisenmenger's complex is VSD with reversal of shunt (R → L).

Q. What will happen to the murmur in VSD if Eisenmenger's syndrome develop?

Ans. The murmur either disappears or becomes short systolic due to reduction in gradient across the defect.

Q. What are the symptoms and signs of Eisenmenger's complex?

Ans. Right to left shunt (reversal of shunt) leads to:
- Cyanosis, clubbing and erythrocytosis
- Sign of pulmonary hypertension (loud P2, narrow splitting of S2, an ejection systolic murmur).
- Decrease in the duration of murmur or no murmur of VSD.
- There may be symptoms and signs of right heart failure (raised JVP, tender hepatomegaly and pedal pitting edema).

Q. What are the complications of VSD?

Ans.
- Pulmonary hypertension with reversal of shunt (Eisenmenger's complex)
- Infective endocarditis
- CHF
- Repeated chest infections
- Aortic regurgitation in high VSD
- Right ventricular outflow tract obstruction (rare in only 5% cases).

Q. How would you investigate such a case?

Ans. *ECG:* It is normal in small VSD. In large defect, there may be LVH, left atrial hypertrophy and conduction defects (bundle branch block)

Chest X-ray: Cardiomegaly with pulmonary plethora (increased lung vascularity if pulmonary hypertension develops then pulmonary conus is prominent with tapering of the peripheral pulmonary arteries and oligemic lung fields)

Doppler echocardiography: Echocardiography will identify the presence and location of the defect while color flow study will identify the magnitude and the direction of shunting.

Q. What is hilar dance?

Ans. It refers to increased pulmonary pulsations seen on fluoroscopy due to increased pulmonary circulation seen in patients with left to right shunts. The increased pulmonary congestion with pulsations is called *pulmonary, plethora.*

Q. What is indication of surgical closure of the defect?

Ans. Large defects should be corrected surgically as early as possible in early life when pulmonary vascular resistance is low, i.e. pulmonary hypertension is still reversible or not yet developed. The ratio of pulmonary to systemic resistance >0.7 is contra-indication for surgery.

Q. Name the conditions where VSD is a part of them?

Ans.
- Fallot's tetralogy
- Double-outlet right ventricle
- Truncus arteriosus
- Septum primum or endocardial cushion defects.

Q. Name the conditions frequently associated with it.

Ans.
- PDA
- ASD
- Tricuspid atresia
- Pulmonary stenosis
- Coarctation of aorta
- Transposition of great vessels.

Q. What is the effect of pregnancy in women with VSD.

Ans.
- Small defects do not cause any problem.
- Patient with moderate or large defect and moderate pulmonary hypertension are at a risk of developing acute right ventricular failure and rapidly progressive worsening dyspnea in pregnancy. They should be managed for heart failure.
- Pregnancy should be avoided in patients of VSD with pulmonary hypertension.

A 45 yrs male (Fig. 1.78) presented with headache, palpitations and breathlessness on exertion. Pulse was normal. BP was 170/110 mm right arm in sitting position.

Fig. 1.78: A patient with hypertension

Q. What is your diagnosis?

Ans. Systemic hypertension without any complication

Q. What important points would you ask on the history?

Ans. *History—Points to be Noted*
- Ask history of syncope, palpitations, dizziness
- Any history of chest pain or dyspnea on exertion
- H/o intermittent claudication
- Any visual disturbance
- In female, ask history of hypertension during pregnancy
- Family history of hypertension
- Drug treatment if any
- H/o renal or endocrinal disease.

Q. How would you proceed to examine this patient?

Ans. *General Physical Examination*
Look for the followings:
- Facial appearance, e.g. cushing face, myxedema, puffiness due to renal disease.
- Neck for carotids pulsations, lymph node and thyroid
- Pulse (rate/volume and radiofemoral delay)
- Blood pressure in both uppear arm, in standing and lying down. BP in the lower limbs
- Fingers for staining (nicotine)
- Fundus examination

Systemic Examination CVS
Inspection
- Look at the apex beat, e.g. normally placed or displaced.

- Look for pulsations in suprasternal notch, precordium and epigastrium

Palpitation
- Palpate the apex beat and note its location (normal or displaced), character and whether forceful or not and whether sustained or not?

Percussion
- Define cardiac dullness (normal or enlarged due to LVH)

Auscultation
- Hear heart sounds in all the areas especially 2nd right intercostal space (Aortic area)
- Hear for any murmurs/rub
- Any 3rd heart sound

Examination of other systems
- Respiratory system for cracklers and rales for LVF

Abdomen
- For polycystic kidneys or for renal artery bruit.

Q. How would you record the BP?

Ans.
- It is measured with sphygmomanometer which should be accurate and calibrated recently.
- Patient should rest for 10–15 minutes before measurement. Make the patient comfortably seated with the arms at the level of the heart. Take the blood pressure cuff of appropriate size of the arm. Cuff should be inflated higher than expected BP and then slowly deflated at 2 mm/sec. and diastolic BP is measured to the nearest 2 mm Hg. Diastolic BP is recorded as disappearance of the sound (sound V) while systolic is measured as appearance of sound. At least 3 consecutive readings at an interval of 10 minutes to be recorded before a patient is declared normal or hypertensive. If the patient is hypertensive, then two readings to be taken at each visit to determine BP threshold.

Q. What is normal and abnormal BP?

Ans. JNC VII classification of normal and abnormal BP is:

Category	SBP (mm Hg)	DBP (mm Hg)
Normal	< 120	< 80
Prehypertension	120-139	80-89
Stage I Hypertension	140-159	90-99
Stage II Hypertension	≥ 160	≥ 100

Q. What are the common identifiable causes of hypertension?

Ans. About 90% cases of hypertension do not have any identifiable cause hence labelled as idiopathic. The identifiable causes (10%) are

Common identifiable causes of Hypertension

Renal
- Chronic Glomerulonephritis
- Chronic pyelonephritis
- Renal artery stenosis
- Diabetic nephropathy

Others
- Coarctation of aorta
- Toxemia of pregnancy
- Collagen vascular disease
- Drug induced, e.g. oral contraceptives and steroids

Endocrinal
- Cushing syndrome
- Excess of corticosteroid
- Hypothyroidism
- Phaeo-chromocytoma

Q. What are conditions that produce discrepancy of BP between the arms or between the arms and legs?

Ans.
- Coarctation of aorta
- PDA (patent ductus arteriosus)
- Supravalvular aortic stenosis
- Thoracic outlet syndrome
- Dissection of aortic aneurysm
- Arterial occlusion of stenosis of subclavian artery (discrepancy between arms)
- Aorto-arteritis
- Thrombotic occlusion of bifurcation of aorta (Lerisch's syndrome)

Q. What are indications of ambulatory BP recording?

Ans.
- Unusual variability in BP recording.
- Hypertension resistant to 3 or more drugs
- To exclude white-coat hypertension
- When symptoms suggest that patient may have hypertension

Q. What is white coat hypertension?

Ans. In some patients, the BP remaining otherwise normal increases to hypertensive range whenever they visit a doctor called white coat hypertension. These are usually labile hypertensives, need ambulatory BP recording before labelling them hypertensive patients.

Q. What is accelerated and what is malignant hypertension? What is the basic difference between the two?

Ans. **Accelerated hypertension** means a significant recent rise over previous hypertension levels associated with vascular damage on fundus examination (hemorrhage and exudate) but without papilledema. The BP may range between 160 and 200 mm Hg systolic and 100 and 120 mm Hg diastolic. It is a hypertensive urgency.

Malignant hypertension is defined as sustained high BP above 200/130 mm Hg associated with vasculopathy and papilledema. It is a hypertensive emergency.

Presence of papilledema in a patient with high BP indicates malignant rather than accelerated hypertension

Q. What is systolic hypertension?

Ans. Isolated rise in systolic BP ≥ 160 mm Hg with diastolic remaining <90 mm Hg is called *systolic hypertension*. Old age, high output states and atherosclerosis are common causes of systolic hypertension.

Q. What is hypertensive urgency and what is hypertensive emergency?

Ans.
- According to JNC VII report, the *hypertensive urgency* is a state of severely elevated BP (>200/120 mmHg) which is not associated with any organ dysfunction wherein BP can be controlled within hours with oral drug therapy given on an outpatient basis.

  Hypertensive emergency means severely elevated BP (>200/130 mm Hg) with symptoms and signs of organ dysfunction (encephalopathy, nephropathy) requiring parenteral drug therapy, close observation in ICU and immediate reduction of BP within hours.

Q. Name few hypertensive emergency and hypertensive urgency conditions?

Ans.

Hypertensive emergency	Hypertensive urgency
• Malignant hypertension or hypertensive encephalopathy	• Accelerated hypertension
• Acute aortic dissection	• Hypertension with coronary artery disease
• Pheochromocytoma crisis	• Uncontrolled hypertension
• MAO inhibitors with tyramine interaction	• Hypertension in patients with kidney transplantation
• Intracranial bleed	• Pre-eclampsia

Q. Name the organs involved in hypertension? What are risks or complications of hypertension?

Ans. Heart, kidney, brain and eyes are the common organs involved. The major risks of hypertension are its devastating complications such as myocardial infarction, aortic dissection, stroke, heart failure and renal failure.

Q. How would you investigate a case with hypertension?

Ans. The investigations done in hypertension are divided into two groups:

I. **Basic (done in all the patients)**
   - Urine for protein, blood and glucose
   - Hematocrit
   - Blood glucose
   - Blood urea, creatinine and electrolytes
   - ECG for LVH and ischemia
   - Chest X-ray for cardiomegaly or heart failure
   - Lipidogram for any hyperlipidemia

II. **Special investigations to screen for the cause**
   - Renal ultrasound or IVP (intravenous pyelogram for kidney disease e.g. polycystic kidneys, if suspected.)
   - Digital substraction angiography for renal artery stenosis, if suspected
   - 24 hour urine catecholamine or VMA at least 3 samples for phaeochromocytoma, if suspected
   - Urinary cortisol and dexamethasone suppression test for Cushing syndrome, if suspected.
   - Plasma renin activity and aldosterone levels for Conn's syndrome if suspected.
   - Angiography/MRI for coaractation of aorta, if suspected.

Q. What is aim of treatment and what should be optimal target BP?

Ans. The aim of treatment of hypertension is to reduce the risk of its complications and to improve life expectancy

The optimal target BP to be achieved is 140/90 mm Hg, and < 130/80 mmHg in patients with diabetes and kidney disease.

Q. What is resistant hypertension? What are its causes?

Ans. According to JNC VII, resistant hypertension is defined as failure to achieve BP control in patients who adhere to full doses of appropriate three drug regimen (including a diuretic). The causes are:
i. Improper BP measurement
ii. Excess sodium intake
iii. Inadequate diuretic therapy (volume overload)
iv. Excess alcohol intake
v. Drug-induced e.g. inadequate doses, non-compliance, over the counter use of drugs (self-medication with NSAIDs)
vi. Unnecessary or concomitant use of other drugs e.g. illicit drugs, sympathomimetics, oral contraceptives
vii. Identifiable causes of hypertension (Read the causes)

Q. What lifestyle modifications would you advise to hypertensive?

Ans. Lifestyle modifications are advised to all prehypertensive and hypertensive patients. They include:
   - **Diet:** Weight reduction in obese patients (BMI < 25 kg/m^2). Low fat diet for hyperlipidemics called DASH eating plan
   - Regular physical exercise predominantly dynamic (brisk walking) rather than isometric (weight lifting)
   - Limit alcohol consumption (<14 units/week for women and < 21 units/week for men).
   - Avoid smoking

Q. What are British hypertensive society guidelines for initiating treatment for hypertension?

Ans. The indications for starting drug treatment are:
   - Sustained SBP over ≥160 mmHg or sustained diastolic BP ≥ 100 mm Hg.
   - Mild hypertension (SBP between 140 and 159 mm Hg and diastolic BP between 90 and 99) in presence of target organ damage, i.e. cardiovascular disease, stroke, diabetes.

Q. What are first line agents for hypertension?

Ans. A diuretic or a beta blocker or a calcium channel brocker.

Note: Regarding questions on drug therapy, i.e. beta blockers, calcium channel blockers, vasodilators, read commonly used drugs in this book.

Rheumatological Diseases

CASE 79: POLYARTHRITIS

A young female presented with history of long duration (few years) of joint pains involving the small joints of both the hands followed by deformities (Fig. 1.79).

Fig. 1.79: Polyarthritis. A young female patient with bilateral symmetrical deforming polyarthritis-rheumatoid arthritis. Note the various deformities

Q. **What is probable diagnosis and why?**
Ans. The probable diagnosis is rheumatoid arthritis. The points in favor of diagnosis are:
1. Small joints involvement (polyarthritis)
2. Bilateral symmetrical distribution
3. Swan-neck deformities with ulnar deviation of hands (deformities).

Q. **What do you understand by rheumatoid hands? How would you proceed to examine them?**
Ans. Hands showing characteristic changes and deformities of rheumatoid arthritis are called *rheumatoid hands*.
Proceed to examine them as follows.
Points to be noted on history
- H/o symmetrical involvement of small joints
- Painful, swollen joints
- Morning stiffness
- Does the patient has difficultty in performing simple tasks, e.g. unbuttoning her clothes or writing

Examination
Examine the hands and comment on the following deformities.
- Swan-neck deformity (Fig.1.79)
- Subluxation at the metacarpophalangeal joint.
- Boutonniere deformity hyperextension at the terminal interphalangeal joints and flexion at the proximal interphalangeal joints)
- Z-deformities of hands
- Dorsal subluxation of ulna at the carpal joint
Look for the Following Signs
- Vasculitic skin lesions and nailfold infarcts
- Palmar erythema
- Wasting of first dorsal interrossei and other small muscles of hands
- Test the median nerve (test for abductor policis brevis and interossei and pin prick sensation over lateral one and half lateral fingers)
- Examine the elbow for rheumatoid nodules
- Examine the other joints.

Q. **What is rheumatoid arthritis (RA)?**
Ans. Rheumatoid arthritis is an immuno-inflammatory system disorder involving the synovial joints and extra-articular tissue leading to bilateral symmetrical polyarthritis with morning stiffness and extra-articular manifestations.

Q. **What are its diagnosis criteria?**
Ans. The American College of Rheumatology (ACR) has laid down criteria for diagnosis and classification (Read Clinical Methods in Medicine by Prof SN Chugh).

Q. **What are the early symptoms and signs in RA?**
Ans. The symptoms and signs for early diagnosis of RA are:
1. Insidious onset of polyarthritis with aches and pains in the joints
2. Prolonged morning stiffness (for 6 weeks or longer)
3. Swelling of multiple involved joints for 6 weeks or longer
4. Slowly progressive signs of inflammation of joints, e.g. pain, tenderness, warmth and erythema for > 6 weeks
5. Symmetric joint involvement.

Q. **What is significance of rheumatoid nodules?**
Ans. The presence of nodules indicate seropositive and more aggressive arthritis.

Q. What are rheumatoid nodules? Where are they found?

Ans. Rheumatoid nodules are firm nontender, subcutaneous nodules present at pressure point or frictions site. Common locations include olecranon bursa, the proximal ulna, the Achilles tendon and occiput.

Q. Which are the joints commonly involved in rheumatoid arthritis?

Ans. The joints commonly involved are:

1. *Small joints of hands*, e.g. proximal interphalangeal (PIP) and metacarpophalangeal (MCP) joints are commonly involved. Distal interphalangeal joints (DIP) are rarely involved
2. Wrist joint(s)
3. Elbow joint(s)
4. Knee joint(s)
5. Arthritis of forefoot, ankle and subtalar joints
6. Axial joints (joints of upper cervical spines)

Q. What are extra-articular manifestations in RA?

Ans. They are given in Table 1.187.

Q. What are skin lesions in rheumatoid arthritis?

Ans. Read the Table 1.187.

Q. What are the causes of anemia in RA?

Ans. The causes are:

1. Anemia of chronic disease
2. Iron deficiency (blood loss, NSAIDs)
3. Bone marrow suppression due to drugs used in the treatment (penicillamine, gold, cytotoxic)
4. Folate and vitamin B_{12} deficiency
5. Hemolysis caused by drugs.
6. Felty's syndrome

   Anemia commonly is due to chronic disease and is normocytic normochromic and correlates well with the disease activity.

Q. What is palindromic rheumatoid arthritis (RA)?

Ans. Palindromic onset is seen in some patients with recurrent episodes of joint stiffness and pain in individual joints lasting only a few hours or days. Hydroxychloroquine prevents such attacks.

Q. What are laboratory findings in RA?

Ans. • Normocytic normochromic anemia
   • Thrombocytosis, eosinophilia
   • Raised ESR
   • Raised C-reactive protein
   • Raised ferritin concentration as an acute phase protein
   • Low serum iron and total iron binding capacity
   • Raised serum globulins
   • Presence of rheumatoid factor (RF)
   • Raised serum alkaline phosphatase activity

Q. What are neurological manifestations of RA

Ans. Read the Table 1.187.

Table 1.187: Extra-articular features in RA

I. Systemic
   • Fever, weight loss, anorexia, fatigue

II. Musculoskeletal
   • Bursitis
   • Tenosynovitis
   • Muscle wasting

III. Skin
   • Rheumatoid nodules
   • Vasculitis
   • Ulcers and gangrene
   • Pyoderma gangrenosa
   • Skin-fold infarcts

IV. Eye
   • Episcleritis, conjunctivitis
   • Sicca syndrome (Sjogren's syndrome)
   • Scleritis (scleromalacia)

V. Cardiac
   • Endocarditis, myocarditis, pericarditis
   • Aortitis, aortic regurgitation (AR)
   • Conduction defects

VI. Respiratory
   • Pleural effusion or pleuritis (seen in 25% cases)
   • Bronchiolitis, fibrosing alveolitis
   • Nodules
   • Caplan's syndrome

VII. Hematological (Reticuloendothelial)
   • Anemia
   • Thrombocytosis, eosinophilia
   • Felty's syndrome
   • Splenomegaly

VIII. Neurological
   • Entrapment neuropathy (carpal tunnel syndrome)
   • Cervical compression (Cervical myelopathy)
   • Peripheral neuropathy (gloves and stocking type)
   • Mononeuritis multiplex

IX. Miscellaneous
   • Amyloidosis
   • Systemic vasculitis

Q. What are pulmonary manifestations of RA?

Ans. Read the Table 1.187.

Q. What are ocular manifestations of RA?

Ans. Read the Table 1.187.

Q. What is rheumatoid factor? What is its significance?

Ans. Rheumatoid factors are autoantibodies reactive with Fc portion of IgG.
   Significance
   • The factor is present in 70% cases of RA
   • The factor is not specific as it is present in 5% of healthy persons

- A large number of conditions are associated with presence of rheumatoid factors such as SLE, chronic active hepatitis, sarcoidosis, interstitial pulmonary fibrosis, infectious mononucleosis, hepatitis B, tuberculosis, leprosy, syphilis, SABE visceral leishmaniasis, schistosomiasis and malaria.

Q. What are the causes of polyarthritis?

Ans. The causes are:
1. Rheumatoid arthritis
2. Viral arthritis
3. Juvenile idiopathic arthritis
4. SLE
5. Psoriatic arthritis
6. Generalized/nodular osteoarthritis
7. Metabolic arthritis (hemochromatosis, acromegaly)
8. Gout
9. Pyrophosphate (crystal-induced)
10. Hyperlipidemia

Note: Causes 1 to 6 produce symmetrical involvement while causes 7 to 10 cause asymmetrical polyarthritis.

Q. What are the causes of arthritis involving the small joints and large joints?

Ans. Depending on the joints involvement, the causes are given in Table 1.188.

Table 1.188: Arthritis of small joints and large joints

Small joint arthritis
- Rheumatoid arthritis
- Reactive arthritis
- Gout
- Enteropathic arthritis
- Nodular osteoarthritis
- Psoriatic arthritis
- SLE
- Metabolic (hemochromatosis)

Large joint arthritis
- Reactive arthritis
- Psoriatic arthritis
- Ankylosing spondylitis
- Inflammatory bowel disease associated arthritis

Note: Reactive arthritis, enteropathic arthritis and psoriatic arthritis involve both small as well as large joints.

Q. What are the causes of proteinuria in Rheumatoid arthritis?

Ans.
- Drug therapy e.g. gold and penicillamine
- Amyloidosis

Q. What are cardiac lesions in RA?

Ans. Read the Table 1.187.

Q. What are valvular lesions in RA?

Ans.
- Aortic incompetence (Aortic valve prolapse)
- Mitral valve prolapse (MVP)

Q. What is Reiter's syndrome? What are its causes?

Ans. It is an inflammatory reactive arthritis associated with rash, urethritis, conjunctivitis, uveitis and oral ulcers. Two types are recognised:
1. Following gastrointestinal infection with *Shigella*, *Salmonella*, *Yersinia* or *Campylobacter* (enteric)
2. Following *nongonococcal* (non-specific) urethritis.

Q. Name the arthritis associated with HLA-B27.

Ans. These are as follows:
1. Ankylosing spondylitis
2. Rheumatoid arthritis
3. Reactive arthritis or Reiter's syndrome
4. Post-dysenteric or enteropathic arthritis
5. Psoriatic arthritis.

Q. What is Felty's syndrome?

Ans. It is characterized by chronic severe RA, splenomegaly, neutropenia and occasionally anemia and thrombo-cytopenia (pancytopenia) due to hypersplenism and leg ulcers. It is associated with positive Rheumatoid factor. Splenectomy ameliorates hypersplenism.

Q. What is Caplan's syndrome?

Ans. It is characterized by seropositive rheumatoid arthritis with pneumoconiosis of the lung (nodular opacities with fibrosis). It is commonly seen in coal-miner's.

Q. How will you treat a case of rheumatoid arthritis?

Ans. The aims of treatment are:
- Relief of pain and reduction of inflammation
- Maintenance of function
- Protection of articular structures from damage
- Control of systemic involvement.

Treatment modalities
1. *Medical therapy*
   i. NSAIDs (Cox-1 and Cox-2 inhibitors)
   ii. Corticosteroids
   iii. *Disease modifying antirheumatic drugs (DMARDs)-* DMARDs are used early in the disease to modify the course of RA, and to retard the development of erosions or facilitate their healing. The agents used include; gold (IM), antimalarial (chloroquine, hydroxychloroquine), penicillamine, sulphasalazine, antimitotics (methotrexate, azathioprine, cyclosporine) and leflunamide
   iv. *Biological agents.* Recently tumor necrosis factors (TNF alpha), blocking monoclonal antibody (etanercept, infliximab) have been used to prevent disease progression

II. *Surgical treatment*
- Decompression for carpal tunnel syndrome and ulnar nerve involvement
- Synovectomy for persistent synovitis
- Excision arthroplasty

- Arthrodesis
- Joint replacement
- Fixation of joint (for atlanto-axial subluxation)

Q. What would you advise if a patient of RA gets gastric upset with NSAIDs?

Ans. Prophylaxis against NSAIDs induced gastric distress can be attempted with current administration of H$_2$ receptor blocker (ranatidine) or proton pump inhibitors (omeprazole) or mesoprostol (prostaglandin analogue) on empty stomach.

Q. What are the causes of seronegative arthritis?

Ans. Absence of rheumatoid factor indicates seronegative arthritis. The causes are:

- Ankylosing spondylitis
- Reiter's syndrome (reactive arthritis)
- Arthritis associated with inflammatory bowel disease
- Psoriatic arthritis
- Undifferentiated spondyloarthropathies
- Juvenile chronic arthritis
- Gout and pseudogout.

Q. What are poor prognostic indicators in RA?

Ans.
- Systemic features (weight loss, extra-articular features)
- Insidious onset
- Presence of rheumatoid factor more than 1:512
- Rheumatiod nodules, persistent disease activity
- Bony erosions
- Raised ESR or C-reactive protein persistently

Q. What is gout and pseudogout? What is gouty arthritis?

Ans. Gout is an inflammatory response to the deposition of monosodium urate monohydrate (MSUM) crystals in the articular and periarticular tissue secondary to hyperuricemia.

Pseudogout: The word pseudogout refers to gout like presentation in calcium pyrophosphate dihydrate (CPPD) crystals induced disease. The crystals evoke an inflammatory response similar to gout. The crystal deposition disease is not a primary disorder but is secondary to osteoarthritis and is a common occurrence.

Gouty arthritis: It may be acute gouty arthritis or chronic erosive, deforming arthritis (tophaceous gout)

Acute gouty arthritis is characterized by acute attack of pain involving the big toe (first metacarpophalangeal joint) with fever and chills occurring at night disturbing the sleep of the patient. Arthritis may uncommonly involve other joints also.

Chronic erosive gouty arthritis occurs after many years of repeated attacks of acute gout, is characterized by deposition of urate crystals (tophi) in and around the joint leading to joint inflammation, erosion and deformity. The common joints involved are big toe, feet and hand joints.

Q. How will you treat gout?

Ans. The treatment is as follows:

I. Treatment of acute attack
- NSAIDs
- Colchicine
- Local and systemic steroids.

II. Recurrent or chronic gout
- Reverse the underlying cause of hyperuricemia, e.g stop diuretics and alcohol
- Treat associated condition if present, i.e. obesity, hyperlipidemia, hypertension
- Correct life-style patterns, e.g. avoid high purine diet, exertion, starvation and dehydration
- Lower plasma urate levels either by allopurinol, probenecid or colchicine
- Continue prophylactic doses of colchicine or NSAIDs for few months even after normalization of hyperuricemia.

Q. What is Sjögren's syndrome (sicca syndrome)?

Ans. It is characterized by keratoconjuctivitis sicca (lack of lacrimal secretion) and, xerostomia (dry mouth due to lack of salivary secretion) in association with a connective tissue disorder usually rheumatoid arthritis. This syndrome may be associated with other autommune disease, i.e. autoimmune thyroiditis.

The *Schirmer filter paper test* for tear production is diagnostic. Filter paper is hooked over the lower eyelid. In normal people at least 15 mm of paper is wet with in 5 minutes; whereas in sicca syndrome it is < 5 mm.

Anti RO (SSA) and *anti SS-B antibodies* are present. Treatment is symptomatic with artificial tears (hypomellose drops or 1% methylcellulose drops), artificial saliva and NSAIDs for arthritis.

Renal Diseases

CASE 80: ADULT POLYCYSTIC KIDNEY DISEASE

A 40-year male patient presented with abdominal pain localized to the flanks with headache hematuria and dysuria. There was history of mass in the right side of abdomen. There was no history of fever. There was history of such a disease in the family. Examination revealed hypertension and bilateral palpable kidneys with soft and cystic feel. The USG (Fig. 1.80) showed the enlarged kidneys with multiple cysts in both the kidneys.

A. Ultrasonography showing multiple (renal cysts in a patient with adult polycystic kidney disease)

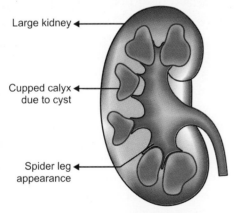

B. Diagrammatic representation of features of adult polycystic kidney disease

Figs 1.80A and B: Adult polycystic kidney disease (ADPKD)

Q. What is probable diagnosis and why?

Ans. The probable diagnosis is adult polycystic kidney disease. The points in favour of the diagnosis are:
1. History of flank pain with dysuria and hematuria
2. Positive family history
3. Presence of hypertension
4. Bilateral palpable kidneys

Q. Describe the mass in the abdomen

Ans. *Inspection*
- There is fullness in both the loins
- Umbilicus is normal.
- Hernial sites are normal
- No scar marks
- Renal angle on the back is full

Palpation
- There are two masses, one each in the lumbar region.
- Each mass is small, nontender having irregular surface, moves slightly with respiration. mass is bimanually palpable and ballotable.
- Fingers can be insinuated between the mass and costal margins
- *Renal angle* on the back is nontender

Percussion
There is resonant note over the mass

Auscultation
There is no bruit, rub or hum.

Q. What is your impression about the masses?

Ans. Bilateral renal masses

Q. What is your differential diagnosis?

Ans.
- Bilateral hydronephrosis
- Bilateral pyonephrosis
- Bilateral masses can be confused with hepatosplenomegaly i.e. liver enlargement with right kidney and enlarged spleen with left kidney. For differentation read clinical methods by Prof SN Chugh.
- Para-aortic and mesenteric lymphadenopathy. These masses are irregular, firm, nontender, nonmobile neither bimanually palpable nor ballotable.

Q. What important points would you like to ask on the history?

Ans.
- Acute pain in loin and hematuria (due to clot colic or hemorrhage into cyst, cyst infection or urinary stone formation)
- Loin discomfort or dragging pain in both lumbar regions due to large kidneys itself.
- Family history of kidney disease
- Symptoms and signs of hypertension, e.g. headache, palpitation, dyspnea.
- Family history of brain hemorhage due to rupture of aneurysm in young age.

323

Q. What is adult polycystic kidneys disease (ADPKD)?

Ans. Adult polycystic kidney disease is a heredofamilial (autosomal dominant and autosomal recessive) disorder in which cysts are present in kidneys making it palpable and enlarged. These cysts cause compression of the intervening renal tissue and progressive loss of excretory function.

Q. How does polycystic kidney present?

Ans. It presents in 3rd and 4 decade with:
- Pain in the lumbar region (s) hematuria, hypertension.
- Urinary tract infection, urinary tract obstruction, symptoms of uremia.
- Subarachnoid hemorrhage due to rupture of associated berry aneurysm.
- Liver cysts may also be associated

Q. What is genetic defect in ADPKD?

Ans. Three forms of autosomal dominant genes have been recognized;
1. *ADPKD1 gene* accounts for 90% of cases and the gene has been localized to short arm of chromosome 16.
2. *ADPKD2 gene* is less common (10%) and is localised to short arm of chromosome 4. These patients develop symptoms and renal failure later than ADPKD1.
3. *ADPKD3 gene* has been documented but has not been mapped to any specific chromosome
   Both ADPKD1 and ADPKD2 encode for the polycystins 1 and 2, the mutation of which leads to the disease.

Q. What are the causes of pain abdomen in ADPKD?

Ans. The causes of acute pain are:
1. Urinary tract obstruction by clot or stone
2. UTI
3. Sudden hemorrhage into a cyst.

Q. What is the cause of hypertension in ADPKD?

Ans. Hypertension is secondary to intrarenal ischemia from distortion of renal vasculature leading to stimulation of renin-angiotensin-aldosterone system.

Q. What are extrarenal manifestations of ADPKD?

Ans. These are as follows:
1. **Cysts in the other organs**, i.e. liver, spleen, pancreas and ovaries. Hepatic cysts are commonest (50-75% cases).
2. **Intracranial aneurysms (berry aneurysms)** can occur in 5-10% cases, may be asymptomatic and may bleed leading to subarachnoid hemorrhage
3. **Diverticulosis** of the colon may occur and patients are more vulnerable to perforation than general population
4. **Mitral valve prolapse** (25% cases).

Q. What are the causes of palpable kidney or kidneys?

Ans. Read the Clinical Methods in Medicine by Prof SN Chugh.

Q. What are the characteristic of renal mass?

Ans. The characteristic of renal mass are:

Inspection of abdomen
- Fullness of renal angle on the side involved

Palpation
- An irregular mass in lumbar region involved.
- Moves slightly with respiration vertically (up and down)
- Soft, cystic or firm in consistency
- Bimanual palpable mass
- Ballottable mass

Percussion
- A band of resonance elicitable over the mass.

Q. What are the causes of mass in lumbar region?

Ans. Read the "Clinical Methods in Medicine" by Prof SN Chugh.

Q. How will you diagnose a case of ADPKD?

Ans. Ultrasound is the preferred technique for diagnosis of symptomatic patients and for screening of asymptomatic family members. It has replaced intravenous pyelography (IVP) used to be done previously for diagnosis.

At least 3-5 cysts in each kidney is standard diagnostic criteria for ADPKD

- *IVP*: It has been superceded by USG. It detects cysts and distortion of pelvicalceal system and gives typical "Spidery–leg appearance"
- *CT scan*: It is more sensitive than USG in detection of small cysts.
- *Genetic linkage analysis:* Genetic probes are available for analysis. The genetic analysis is reserved for cases where radiographic imaging is negative and there is need to confirm the diagnosis, for example, screening of family members for potential kidney donation.

Q. What are indications of dialysis in CRF?

Ans. Dialysis is usually not required in CRF except under following situations:
1. Presence of uremic syndrome.
2. Hyperkalemia unresponsive to conservative management.
3. Fluid overload in end-stage renal disease or CRF
4. Metabolic acidosis refractory to medical therapy.
5. Acute on chronic renal failure.
6. Prior to renal transplantation
7. Creatinine clearance <10 ml/min or oliguria per 1.32 m^2

Q. **What are cause of death in ADPKD?**

Ans. 1. End-stage renal disease and progressive renal failure
   2. Hypertension and its related complications, i.e. CHF, cerebral hemorrhages
   3. Rarely due to unrelated causes

Q. **What are complications of ADPKD?**

Ans. • Recurrent urinary tract infection including infection of the cyst (pyocyst)
   • Urinary tract obstruction
   • Nephrolithiasis (calcium oxalate and uric acid stones) is common
   • End-stage renal disease (ESRD) due to progressive decline of renal function is a late complication
   • Renal failure.

Q. **How will you treat ADPKD?**

Ans. As it is genetically related disorder, hence, there is no definite treatment. The aim of treatment is to retard the progress of the disease and preserve renal function as long as possible by:
   • Control of hypertension by antihypertensives especially ACE inhibitors
   • Treatment of urinary tract infection by appropriate antibiotics
   • Relief of chronic pain by an analgesic. If no relief, cyst may be punctured and sclerosed with ethanol.
   • Dialysis and kidney transplantation when renal failure occurs

Q. **Mention 3 common indications for renal transplantation.**

Ans. • Diabetes mellitus with renal failure
   • Hypertensive renal disease with renal failure
   • Glomerulonephritis with end-stage renal disease and renal failure

Q. **What are the causes of renal cysts on USG?**

Ans. The causes are:
   1. ADPKD (autosomal dominant)
   2. ADPKD (autosomal recessive)
   3. Tuberous sclerosis (Adenoma sebaceum, shagreen patch, benign tumors of CNS, renal angiomyo-lipomas and renal cysts may occur)
   4. *Von Hippel-Lindau disease* (e.g. hemangio-blastoma of retina and CNS; bilateral renal cysts may occur)
   5. Medullary spongy kidney
   6. Medullary cystic disease.

Gastrointestinal Diseases

CASE 81: ABDOMINAL MASS

A patient presented with abdominal pain, dull aching in character associated with slight distention of abdomen and constipation. There was normal passage of flatus. Prior to this, patient gave history of off and on alternate diarrhea and constipation.

Examination revealed dilated loops of gut visible in the central part of abdomen. There was a ill-defined irregular mass palpable in the right iliac fossa (Fig. 1.81A), firm, tender. The abdomen was resonant including the mass on percussion. There were increased bowel sounds on auscultation. The per rectal examination was normal. The barium meals examination of the patient is depicted in Figure 1.81B.

Q. What is your probable diagnosis and why?

Ans. The probable diagnosis is subacute intestinal obstruction due to ileocaecal mass. The points in favor are:
- History (dull abdominal pain, central distention and constipation)
- Visible and palpable dilated loops of gut
- Resonant percussion note
- Increased bowel sound

The mass is ileocecal because:
- The mass is in the right iliac fossa
- It is firm, tender and resonant on percussion
- Associated features of subacute intestinal obstruction present.

Fig. 1.81B: Ileocecal tuberculosis. There is narrowing of terminal ileum and cecum is pulled up on barium meal follow through study

Q. What are causes of a mass in the right iliac fossa? What are causes of ileocecal mass?

Ans. *Causes of mass in right iliac fossa are:*
- An appendicular lump
- An ileocecal mass (read its causes)
- Ileopsoas abscess
- Gallbladder mass
- Undescended kidney or testis
- Uterine or tubo-ovarian mass.
- Transplanted Kidney

Causes of Ileocecal mass
- Hyperplastic ileocecal tuberculosis
- Amoebic typhilitis
- Carcinoma of cecum and colon
- Inflammatory bowel disease
- Fungal granuloma (aspergilloma)
- Lymphoma
- Impaction of round worms
- Carcinoid tumor.

Q. What are characteristics of ileocecal tuberculosis?

Ans. These are as follows:
- An irregular firm tender mass that slips under your fingers on palpation
- Symptoms and signs of intermittent subacute intestinal obstruction, e.g. vomiting, distention, constipation, visible gut loops, increased peristaltic sounds

Ileocecal mass in right iliac fossa

Urinary bladder

Fig. 1.81A: The site of the mass in right iliac fossa

- History of alternate diarrhea and constipation, night sweats and low grade fever
- Weight loss, emaciation
- Supportive evidence of tuberculosis elsewhere, e.g. lung, abdominal or cervical lymph nodes, ascites.

  Barium meal study may show pulled up cecum, ulceration and stricture of ileum, multiple areas of dilatation, narrowing and matting of small bowel loops and a filling defect. The study is not to be performed in the presence of subacute intestinal obstruction where barium enema may be done to visualize the filling defect.

Q. What are the characteristics of carcinoma of colon?

Ans. Read the Clinical Methods in Surgery.

Q. What are characteristic of amoebic typhilitis?

Ans. These are as follows:
- An irregular, firm, tender lump
- Past or present history of amebic dysentery
- History of pain abdomen and tender descending colon
- Stools are positive for *E. histolytica*.

Q. What are the characteristics of Crohn's colitis or disease?

Ans. These are as follows:
- An inflammatory boggy swelling or mass of adherent loops of intestine. It is soft and tender.
- Associated symptoms such as fever, right quadrantic abdominal pain, diarrhea (often without blood), fatigue and weight loss
- Mild anemia, aphthous ulceration of mouth, stomatitis, glossitis, cheilosis due to malabsorption may sometimes be seen.
- There may be associated anorectal complications such as fistulae, fissures and perirectal abscess
- Extracolonic manifestations such as arthritis may also occur
- Sigmoidoscopy and radiological studies are important for diagnosis. Barium meal study may show *cobble–stone appearance* of the mucosa and fistulous tracts. Barium enema may reveal rectal sparing, presence of skip lesions, small ulcerations occurring on small irregular nodules. Fibreoptic colonoscopy and mucosal biopsy will confirm the diagnosis.

Q. What are the characteristics of an appendicular lump?

Ans. These are as follows:
- An irregular, firm, tender lump often fixed but may show slight mobility.
- History of recurrent attacks of periumbilical pain with vomiting, settling down to the right lower quadrant

- Fever and leukocytosis
- Guarding and muscular rigidity on palpation
- Rebound tenderness may be present, indicates peritoneal inflammation around the appendix
- Positive Rovsing's and psoas sign
- Obturator sign may be positive
- USG of abdomen may help in the diagnosis.

Q. What are clinical presentation of abdominal tuberculosis?

Ans. These are:
1. Ascites due to tubercular peritonitis
2. Ileocecal tuberculosis, e.g. hyperplastic and ulcerative
3. Tuberculosis of lymph node (tabes mesenterica)
4. Tuberculous abscess, e.g. liver and spleen.

Q. What are the clinical presentation of intestinal tuberculosis?

Ans. These are as follows:
I. Nonspecific symptoms of pain abdomen, low grade fever with evening rise, night sweats, decreased appetite and weight loss. The abdominal examination may show dilated loops of gut with doughy feel.
II. Patients may present with symptoms and signs of subacute intestinal obstruction. These are due to multiple areas of narrowing.
III. Diarrhea and malabsorption. Diarrhea is common in ulcerative type of tuberculosis. Blood and frank pus in the stool is rare. The malabsorption in intestinal tuberculosis is due to decreased absorptive surface area as a result of;
   - Extensive ulceration
   - Lymphatic obstruction
   - Bacterial overgrowth (Blind loop syndrome)
IV. Acute intestinal obstruction due to stricture formation
V. Perforation and fistula formation is rare in intestinal tuberculosis.

Q. What are the features that suggest the mass to be transplanted kidney?

Ans.
- H/o of chronic renal failure and symptoms of uremia.
- History of hemodialysis
- H/o renal transplantation.
- H/o receiving immunosupppressive drugs
  Following sign on abdominal examination signs suggest transplanted kidney.
1. Lapartomy scar.
2. Arteriovenous fistula in the arm
3. Palpable kidney either in right or left iliac fossa.
4. Signs of hypercortisol state if patient is on steroids as immunosuppressive therapy.

Q. What drugs are used for post-transplant immunosuppression?

Ans. • Steroids, azathioprine and cyclosporine are used independently or combinations.

• Newer drugs include FK 506, rapamycin, sirolimus, mycophenolate mofetil and daclizumab.

Q. What is carcinoid tumor and carcinoid syndrome?

Ans. *Carcinoid tumor* originates from enterochromaffin cells (APUD cells) of the intestine and the common sites being appendix, terminal ileum and rectum. Clinically it is asymptomatic until they metastasise in the liver and produce carcinoid syndrome.

The *carcinoid syndrome* is characterized by:

• Bluish-red flushing on face and trunk due to vasodilatation occurring spontaneously or during an attack of pain abdomen

• Gastrointestinal hurry producing pain and recurrent watery diarrhea

• Cardiac abnormalities, e.g. pulmonary stenosis and tricuspid incompetence

• Bronchial carcinoid produces recurrent attacks of wheezing

• Hepatomegaly due to metastases in symptomatic patients.

Q. What are the causes of flushed face?

Ans. • Carcinoid syndrome.

• Mastocytosis

• Chronic myeloid leukemia with increased histamine release.

• Menopausal syndrome

• As a reaction to alcohol and glutamate.

• Side effects of chlorpromazine, calcium channel blockers and nicotinic acid.

Q. What are various sites of carcinoids?

Ans. Stomach, small intestine, appendix, rectum and bronchus

Q. How would you investigate carcinoid syndrome?

Ans. • Urinary 5- HIAA levels- elevated

• Plasma and platelets serotonin levels-elevated

• Serum chromogranin A levels-elevated.

U N I T

2

Bedside Procedures and Instruments

Bedside Procedures

LUMBAR PUNCTURE (LP)

It is a bedside procedure done to remove cerebrospinal fluid (CSF) from the subarachnoid space by puncturing it at or below L_2-L_3 intervertebral space. The spinal cord ends at the level of L_1 vertebra after which there is a *cul-de-sac* (dilatation of subarachnoid space) from which CSF can be removed. The instrument used for the purpose is called *lumbar puncture (LP) needle* (Fig. 2.1).

Fig. 2.1: Lumbar puncture needle;
Stilet (upper) and needle (lower)

Identification

It can be recognized as a large 16 bore needle having two parts
 i. Needle proper
 ii. A stilet

Indications

I. Diagnostic
CSF is removed for diagnosis of the following conditions:
 i. *CNS infections/inflammation*
 • Encephalitis
 • Meningitis
 • Multiple sclerosis
 • Myelitis
 • Acute post-infective polyneuritis (Guillain-Barre syndrome)
 ii. *Subarachnoid hemorrhage (to be done after fundus examination)*
 iii. *Infiltrative conditions*
 • Carcinomatous meningitis
 • Lymphoma and leukemic infiltration of meninges
 iv. *To confirm raised intracranial pressure when CT scan excludes the danger of brainstem herniation*
 • Benign raised intracranial tension
 • Cerebral venous sinus thrombosis
 v. *Instillation of contrast media or an isotope*
 • Myelography (CT myelography)
 • Cisternography.

II. Therapeutic
Lumbar puncture is done for treatment purpose;
 i. Administration of intrathecal antibiotics or tetanus immunoglobulin
 ii. Administration of antileukemic drugs in ALL
 iii. Spinal anesthesia
 iv. Removal of CSF to lower the pressure in benign intracranial hypertension

III. Other Uses of LP Needle
 i. Used as aspiration needle for tapping fluids from a cavity, e.g. ascites, pleural effusion.
 ii. For cisternal puncture

Contraindications

 i. Thrombocytopenia and coagulation disorders
 ii. Depressed consciousness especially if focal neurological signs present. CT scan to be done initially to rule out raised intracranial pressure or mass lesion. LP should not be performed in presence of raised intracranial pressure or a mass lesion
 iii. Papilledema
 iv. Skin infection at the site of lumbar puncture. It is not a contraindication, LP can be done one space higher
 v. Lumbar meningomyelocele.

Normal CSF and findings in meningitis are given in Table 2.1.

Q. Could we use it as an aspiration needle?
Ans. Yes, without stilet, it can be used as aspiration needle.

Complications

• *Brainstem herniation or cerebellar coning:* To avoid this LP should not be done in presence of gross papilledema. In dire emergency, slow removal of CSF by keeping the stillet inside the needle is advised and signs of brainstem herniation to be looked for (change in size of pupil).

In a patient suspected of ICSOL or SAH, CT scan must be done to rule out raised ICT.

• *Introduction of infection:* To avoid it, aseptic precautions are to be followed.
• *Postspinal headache:* It occurs due to low intracranial tension putting stretch on the meninges. It develops after few hours of either sudden withdraw of a large amount of CSF (>10 ml) or due to continuous leakage of CSF from LP site. Measures to avoid/treat it are:

Table 2.1: Differential diagnosis of CSF findings in meningitis

Finding	Pyogenic meningitis	Tubercular meningitis	Viral meningitis	Fungal meningitis	Carcinomatous meningitis
Gross appearance	Turbid	Clear or straw colored, cob-web seen on standing	Clear	Clear	Clear or hemorrhagic
CSF pressure	Elevated	Elevated	Normal	Elevated	Elevated
Proteins	Elevated (>45 mg/dl)	Elevated	Normal or slightly elevated	Elevated	Elevated
Glucose	Markedly reduced (<30 mg/dl)	Moderately reduced (< 40 mg/dl)	Normal	Reduced	Normal
Cells	>1000 cells/ml mainly polymorphs	>400 cells/ml mainly mono-nuclear	25-500 cells/ml mainly lymphocytes	Mononuclear or lymphocyte pleocytosis	Malignant cells may be seen
Isolation of organism	Gram's stain is positive	Acid fast stained smear positive in 10-40% cases	Not possible	India-ink or fungal wet mounts of CSF positive	—
PCR for detection of DNA sequence	Detection of bacterial DNA is just research test	*M. tuberculosis* DNA positive in 70-80% cases	Viral specific DNA or RNA from CSF positive	Cryptococcal antigen is specific and positive	—
Culture	Positive in >80% cases	Positive <50% cases. It is a gold standard to make diagnosis	Viral culture results disappointing because of cumber-some procedure	Positive for fungi	—

i. Remove the fluid slowly
ii. Put the needle obliquely into subarachnoid space
iii. Put the patient in prone position if headache develops.

Procedure

Site—L$_3$-L$_4$ Interspace

1. The patient is placed on the edge of the bed or a table in the left lateral position with knees drawn upto the abdomen and neck is gently flexed so as to bring them as close as possible.
2. The 3rd and 4th lumbar spines are palpated by rolling the fingers on the spine. The 4th lumbar spine usually lies on a line joining the iliac crests and L$_3$ is just above it. The interspace between L$_3$ and L$_4$ is defined.
3. Under aseptic precaution, local infiltrative anesthesia (xylocaine 2%) is used at the site of puncture (L$_3$-L$_4$).
4. The LP needle is pushed through the skin in the midline, it is pressed steadily forwards and slightly towards the head. When the needle is felt to penetrate the dura mater (a sudden release of resistance), the stilet is withdrawn and a few drops of CSF are allowed to escape.
5. The CSF pressure can be measured by connecting a manometer to the needle. The normal CSF pressure is 60-150 mm H$_2$O. It rises and falls with respiration and heart beat.

7. Specimens are procured in three sterile vials/tubes and sent to laboratory. An additional sample in which sugar level can be measured together with simultaneous blood sugar sample should be taken when relevant (e.g. meningitis).

Note: A three vial test is useful to identify traumatic CSF from SAH.
   i. Traumatic CSF is more red in the first than in the other tubes while non-traumatic CSF is uniformly red.
   ii. The supernatant fluid is clear in traumatic CSF while there is xanthochromia (yellowish brown coloration of CSF) in SAH.
   iii. On standing, the blood will clot in traumatic CSF whereas this does not occur in nontraumatic (SAH) CSF.

8. Now the needle is removed, the site is sealed with a wisp of cotton soaked in tincture. The patient is made to lie flat to avoid a postspinal headache.
   The amount of fluid to be removed is 5-8 ml.

Dry Tap means CSF does not come out through the LP needle, could be due to:

1. Improper positioning of the needle, i.e. needle is not in the subarachnoid space. This is common cause.
2. Subarachnoid space is obliterated by a tumor or adhesive arachnoiditis.

Xanthochromia

Xanthochromia means yellowish brown discoloration of CSF. It indicates either increased proteins or hemolysed blood in CSF. It is seen in meningitis and SAH. CSF may be yellow in a patient with jaundice also.

BONE MARROW ASPIRATION

It is done in adults to aspirate the marrow from sternum or posterior iliac crests because of being superficial and accessible (all flat bones and vertebre contain bone marrow in adults). If aspiration fails then a trephine bone marrow biopsy is done, if necessary. The instrument used in the procedure is bone marrow aspiration needle (Fig. 2.2).

Fig. 2.2: Bone marrow aspiration needle

Identification

It can be recognized easily because:
1. It has a thick metallic body with nail.
2. It has a guard 2 cm from the tip which is adjustable. It prevents through and through penetration of bone.
3. Stilette – A solid metallic rod inside the lumen of needle. It is removed after bone puncture and needle is attached to the body to aspirate the marrow (Fig 2.2).

Indications of Bone Marrow Aspiration

1. **Bone marrow infiltration**
   - Leukemia/lymphoma
   - Secondary carcinoma
   - Myelofibrosis/agnogenic myeloid metaplasia
2. **Cytopenias**
   - Neutropenia
   - Thrombocytopenia
   - Anemias including aplastic
   - Pancytopenia
3. **Myeloproliferative disorders**
4. **Infections,** e.g. bone marrow aspirate is used for culture of typhoid, tuberculosis, where other tests are negative but suspicion is high.

Contraindications

- Severe thrombocytopenia (count <20,000/ml) or a coagulation defect
- Osteomyelitis/infection at the site of puncture.

Complications

- Bone pain
- Hemorrhage
- Infection.

Procedures

Site—Mid-manubrium sterni region in adults and iliac crest in children.
1. The patient is made to lie flat on the bed and skin is shaved over the sternum.
2. The site is cleansed with antiseptic solution many times.
3. The site is infiltrated with local anesthesia under aseptic precaution.
4. The bone marrow needle is introduced at the site vertically and bone marrow is aspirated with the help of syringe attached to the needle.
5. Make the smear of bone marrow on the slide by discarding or shedding off the peripheral blood and send it for examination.
6. Remove the needle, paint the site with a cotton wisp soaked with tincture benzoin.

Dry Tap

No bone marrow aspirated when the needle is in place. It could be due to:
1. Faulty technique.
2. Myelofibrosis, e.g. marrow replaced by fibrosis
3. Marrow packed tightly with infiltrates, hence, is difficult to aspirate.

TISSUE BIOPSY NEEDLE

Biopsy means taking a small amount of tissue percutaneously from the intact organ with the help of a needle called tissue biopsy needle (Figs 2.3A and B). The *Vim-Silverman's needle* (A) is more traumatising than *trucut needle* (B), which is a disposable needle.

Identification

1. *Vim-Silverman's biopsy needle* (Fig 2.3A)
   It has three parts ; (1) inner split needle for bringing the piece of tissue, (2) outer hollow needle to accommodate the inner needle and, (3) stilet which keeps the needle patent during introduction.
2. *Tru-cut needle* (Fig 2.3B). This needle has a sliding knife edge, hence, is less traumatic and best suitable for kidney and liver biopsy.

Uses

It is used to take the biopsy from kidney, liver, pleura in diseased state for diagnosis and differential diagnosis.

Figs 2.3A and B: Tissue biopsy needles:
A. Vim-Silverman B. Trucut (disposable)

Liver Biopsy

Liver biopsy is now performed under ultrasound or CT guidance particularly when specific lesions need to be biopsied.

Laparoscopic guided liver biopsy is done through a small incision in the abdominal wall under local anesthesia.

A transjugular approach is used when liver biopsy is essential but coagulation studies prevent percutaneous approach.

Indications

1. Unexplained hepatomegaly or hepatosplenomegaly
2. Chronic hepatitis and cirrhosis of the liver
3. Persistently abnormal liver function tests
4. Suspected systemic or infiltrative disease, e.g. sarcoidosis, miliary tuberculosis or fever of unknown origin (PUO), Wilson's disease
5. Suspected primary or metastatic liver tumor
6. Screening the relatives of patients with certain diseases, e.g. hemochromatosis
7. Operative biopsy may sometimes be valuable as in the staging of lymphoma.

Contraindications

- Uncooperative patient or patient who refuses to give a written consent.

- Impaired hemostatis (prothrombin time prolonged by 3 sec or more over control or PTT or BT prolonged and platelet count less than $80 \times 10^9/L$).
- Tense ascites.
- Extrahepatic cholestasis.
- When there is possibility of a hydatid cyst.

Complications

- Hemorrhage
- Infection
- Pleurisy, perihepatitis producing shoulder and abdominal pain
- Biliary peritonitis.

Renal Biopsy

Indications

- Asymptomatic proteinuria (>1 g/day) or hematuria (occasional indication).
- Adult nephrotic syndrome. In nephrotic syndrome in children, it can be done only if proteinuria persists after a trial of steroids.
- Unexplained renal failure where kidneys are normal-sized on ultrasound.
- Failure to recover from assumed reversible acute renal failure.
- Systemic disease with renal involvement, e.g. SLE, sarcoidosis, amyloidosis (occasional).

Contraindications

- Uncooperative patient or patient who refuses to give a written consent.
- Single kidney
- Small contracted kidneys (technically difficult, histology is difficult to interpret and prognosis remains unaltered).
- Bleeding diathesis.
- Uncontrolled hypertension.
- Perinephric abscess or pyonephrosis, hydronephrosis or polycystic kidney disease.

Complications

- Macroscopic hematuria (about 20%).
- Pain in the flank, sometimes referred to shoulder tip.
- Perirenal hematoma.
- Transient AV fistula or aneurysm formation.
- Introduction of infection.

Pleural Biopsy

It is done always in the presence of pleural effusion for diagnosis and differential diagnosis.

ASPIRATION (PARACENTESIS)

Paracentesis means aspiration of fluid accumulated in one of the serous cavities. It is done to remove the excess of fluid with the help of a wide bore needle called *aspiration needle* (Fig. 2.4). Excess of fluid can accumulate under pathological conditions in pleural cavity (pleural effusion/empyema) or pericardial cavity (pericardial effusion) and peritoneal cavity (ascites).

Fig. 2.4: Aspiration needle

Identification

This is a long B D needle similar to LP needle but there is no stilet attached to it. It can be attached to a syringe or three – way cannula during aspiration of fluid or pus.

Paracentesis of Pleural Fluid

Indications

A. Diagnostic
- For diagnosis and differential diagnosis of pleural effusion, e.g. transudate or exudate.
- Tubercular pleural effusion when fever and toxemia not subsiding after 4 weeks of anti-tubercular therapy.

B. Therapeutic
- To relieve dyspnea, if there is cardiorespiratory embarassment.
- Empyema thoracis: If fluid removed on first occasion is pus, then intercostal drainage with the help of self-retaining tube/catheter should be attempted.

Complications
- Unilateral pulmonary edema may develop with sudden removal of a large amount of fluid. It is rare.
- *Hydropneumothorax (iatrogenic):* Air may be sucked into pleural cavity during the procedure, hence X-ray chest to be done after aspiration.
- Hemothorax
- Intravascular collapse due to sudden withdrawal of large amounts of fluid.

Paracentesis of Ascites (Ascitic Tap)

Indications
- For diagnosis and differential diagnosis of ascites. About 20-50 ml of fluid is removed.
- Tense ascites producing cardiorespiratory embarrassment; fluid (2-3 L) is removed to relieve dyspnea.

Complications
- Leakage of ascitic fluid (continuous soakage of clothes)
- Introduction of infection
- Repeated frequent tapping may result in anemia, hypoproteinemia.

Paracentesis of Pericardial Fluid

Indications
- For diagnostic purpose to determine the nature of fluid. About 20-50 ml of fluid is removed.
- Cardiac tamponade to relieve dyspnea. Fluid is removed as much as possible.

Complications
- Hemorrhage or bleeding
- Infection
- Injury to liver or diaphragm if subcostal approach is used to remove the fluid.
- Shoulder pain.

Tapping of Liver Abscess

Liver abscess is mostly amebic but could be pyogenic in origin. Tubercular abscess is rare.

Indications

Liver abscess is tapped under following situations:
1. When pyogenic origin of the abscess is suspected. It is tapped to differentiate amebic from pyogenic abscess.
2. A large left lobe abscess (>10 cm).
3. *Impending rupture:* Abscess should be tapped irrespective of its size, if it is superficial and poses a danger to rupture.
4. Abscess not responding to treatment.

TRACHEOSTOMY

Tracheostomy means opening of the trachea to the surface through which a tracheostomy tube (Fig. 2.5) is inserted and cuffed to maintain ventilation and to aspirate the secretions.

Identification

It is a small cuffed tube either metallic (for permanent use) or made of portex. The portex (polyethylene) tube has a cuff which is inflated with air which keeps the tube in position. A plastic plate attached to the tube has ribbons which are used to secure the tube around the neck.

Fig. 2.5: Tracheostomy tube

Fig. 2.6: An endotracheal tube

Indications

1. In unconscious patients with depressed pharyngeal or cough reflexes, e.g. neuromuscular respiratory paralysis.
2. In tetanus to maintain ventilation.
3. In laryngeal/pharyngeal obstruction (nasopharyngeal carcinoma, diphtheria).
4. Systemic anaphylaxis and angiedema when patient becomes cyanosed.

Complications

Early
- Surgical complications, e.g. hemorrhage, pneumothorax.
- Subcutaneous emphysema.

Intermediate
- Erosion of tracheal cartilage.
- Erosion of innominate artery.
- Infection.

Late
- Tracheal stenosis
- Collapse of tracheal rings at the level of stoma.

ENDOTRACHEAL INTUBATION

It refers to putting the endotracheal tube (Fig. 2.6) into the trachea through laryngeal opening via mouth.

Identification

It is usually a curved tube but flexible, made up of polyethylene or rubber, has a 7.5 mm or 8 mm bore inside it. It is called cuffed because it has a small balloon at the upper end. This balloon is inflated with air and it keeps the tube in position. A small side tube is also attached to the main body, is used to inflate the cuff.

Indications

It is done for respiratory support.
1. Cardiorespiratory arrest.
2. Acute respiratory failure.
3. Prophylactic postoperative ventilation in poor risk patients with depressed respiration and profuse secretions.
4. During general anesthesia.
5. Head injuries producing unconsciousness and depressed respiration.
6. Chest injuries/lung contusion.
7. Respiratory depression in poisoning.
8. Systemic anaphylaxis and angiedema when patient is cyanosed.

Contraindications

- Trauma or tumor present in upper respiratory tract.
- Laryngospasm.

Complications

- Tube may slip into one of the bronchus or in esophagus.
- Migration of the tube out of trachea.
- Obstruction of the tube due to kinking or secretions.
- Mucosal edema and ulceration of trachea due to tube.
- Damage to cricoarytenoid cartilage.
- Tracheal stenosis (late complications).

NASOGASTRIC (RYLE'S TUBE) INTUBATION

Ryle's tube (Fig. 2.7), named after the physician who dsigned it, is a fine bore rubber or plastic-silicon tube used for nasogastric intubation. The tube is passed intranasally or through the mouth into the stomach, the position of which is confirmed either by passing the air through the tube into stomach and simultaneous hearing of hussing sound by stethoscope or by aspiration of food material or by X-ray.

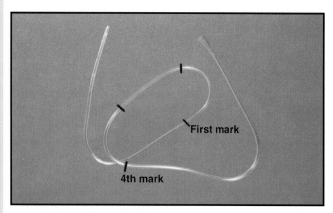

Fig. 2.7: Nasogastric (Ryle's) tube.
(The tube for adult is a long fine bore (30 inches) with distal end blind containing oval bulb and has side-holes. It is passed by this end through nose into stomach. The proximal end is open to which syringe is attached. From proximal to distal end it has four marks indicating end of esophagus, cardia of stomach, pylorus of stomach, and the duodenum)

Identification

A long coiled flexible polyethylene tube, 90 cm in length having a lower bulbous tip containing lead beads (shots) which facilitates its passage through the esophagus by gravity when patient is asked to swallow. The lower end also has a number of side holes for aspiration of gastroduodenal contents. The four markings help in its identification (Read Fig. 2.7).

Indications

1. *Nutritional supplementation:* It is used in hospitalized patients for internal feeding required in those patients who cannot eat, should not eat, will not eat or cannot eat enough, such as:
   • Unconscious patients
   • Neurological dysphagia (dysphagia without esophageal obstruction)
   • Post-traumatic or postoperative or post-radiation weakness
   • In patients with burns.
2. Nutritional support (Ryle's tube feeding) for malnourished children/adults.
3. For gastrointestinal decompression in acute intestinal obstruction, paralytic ileus (perforation), hemorrhage and acute pancreatitis.
4. Gastric lavage in patients with drug overdose or poisoning.
5. To remove fluid for gastric analysis.
6. For drug delivery in unconscious patients.
7. For diagnosis of acute esophageal or gastric bleed.
8. To aspirate gastroduodenal secretion for isolation of AFB in children and even for detection of typhoid carrier and giardiasis.

Complications

Immediate
• Regurgitation and aspiration of gastric contents into lung (pneumonia)
• Blockage of the tube.

Late (prolonged use)
• GI side-effects, the most common being diarrhea
• Metabolic complications after prolonged feeding including hyperglycemia, hyperkalemia as well as low levels of potassium, magnesium, calcium and phosphate
• Ulceration of nasal and esophageal tissues leading to stricture formation.

URINARY CATHETERIZATION

It is a method to remove the urine from the urinary bladder by passing a catheter (Figs 2.8A and B) through the urethera. Catheterization may be done just once or repeatedly by a simple catheter or continuously by putting a self-retaining catheter for few days.

Identification

1. *Simple rubber catheter:* It is a simple single lumened rubber catheter. It is closed at one end and has an eye opening at the same end. Sizes are variable.
2. *Foley's self retaining catheter:* It is double lumen, self retaining disposable catheter made of latex. At proximal end there is an eye opening on the side. The distal end is bifid. The catheter has two lumens one for the passage of urine and other for inflation of balloon with normal saline. The balloon makes the catheter self retaining.

Indications or Uses

Catheterization just once (by simple catheter)
• Retention of urine due to reversible cause
• Before or during delivery
• To differentiate anuria from retention of urine

Figs 2.8A and B: Urinary catheters: (A) Simple rubber catheter (Upper – Large; Lower – Small), (B) Self-retaining catheter (Foley's)

- To obtain urine specimen from an unconscious patient
- To differentiate pelvic swelling from distended bladder
- Before cystoscopy.

Continuous urinary drainage (by self-retaining catheter)
- Unconscious patient
- Peripheral circulatory failure to monitor urinary output
- Paraplegia with bladder involvement (incontinence or retention of urine)
- Neurogenic bladder
- Inoperable prostatic carcinoma.

Other uses
- For cystography
- Simple catheter can be used as a tourniquet, as a stent or as a sling

Contraindications

- Acute urethritis

Complications

- Hemorrhage
- Creation of false passage
- Introduction of infection
- Blockage of urethera leading to retention
- Uretheral ulceration and stricture formation on prolonged use.

Precaution

- Self-retaining catheter should be irrigated with an antiseptic solution daily
- Self-retaining catheter preferably be changed after few days
- Urine culture and sensitivity may be done when patient develops unexplained fever.

Bedside Instruments

OXYGEN DELIVERY DEVICES

Oxygen can be delivered by many devices such as nasal catheter, simple face-mask and venturi-mask (fixed-performance device) to spontaneously breathing patients. Oxygen is initially given either by nasal catheter or via face-masks (Figs 2.9A to C).

In majority of patients, except COPD with CO_2 narcosis, the concentration of O_2 given is not important and O_2 can be given by simple nasal catheter or face mask (Figs 2.9A and B). With these devices, O_2 concentration varies from 35-55% with O_2 flow rates between 6 and 10 L/min. Nasal catheter or simple face mask are often preferred because they are less troublesome and do not interfere with feeding or speaking. Fixed performance mask (venturi mask – Fig. 2.9C) is used in patients with COPD with elevated $PaCO_2$ (type II respiratory failure) where

Fig. 2.9A: Nasal oxygen catheter (holes at the end)

Fig. 2.9B: Nasal oxygen set

Fig. 2.9C: Venturi mask (masks are available to deliver 24%, 28% and 35% O_2)

concentration of O_2 delivered is very important and through this the desired concentration of O_2 can be delivered and controlled.

Indications of Oxygen Therapy

- Type I (hypoxemic) respiratory failure
- Type II (hypercapnoic) respiratory failure (COPD with acute exacerbation)
- Shock
- Asphyxia (e.g. hanging)
- Acute myocardial infarction
- Cardiac tamponade
- Acute severe asthma/status asthmaticus
- Acute pulmonary edema
- Tension pneumothorax
- Carbon monoxide poisoning.

Complications

- Damage to the lung leading to acute pulmonary edema. This is due to liberation of O_2 free radicals due to hyperoxia (high concentration of O_2).

NASOPHARYNGEAL SUCTION CATHETER

It is a small lumen rubber or plastic catheter having holes on the sides for entry of secretion. It is blind at distal end, the proximal end is connected to the suction apparatus (Fig. 2.10).

N.B. *Simple urinary catheter, nasal O_2 catheter and suction catheter resemble one another. For difference, read the legend below the Figure 2.10.*

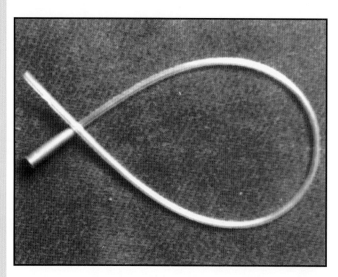

Fig. 2.10: Nasopharyngeal suction catheter

Note: Simple urinary catheter, nasopharyngeal suction catheter and simple nasal catheter can be confused with each other. Note the following:
1. Simple urinary catheter is wide bored rubber tube with a hole on the side at distal end
2. Nasal oxygen catheter is a narrow lumen rubber catheter open on both the ends with many side holes at the distal end
3. Suction catheter is a narrow bored plastic catheter with a hole on one side, and on the tip

Indications for Suction

- Unconscious patient
- Tetanus (through tracheostomy tube)
- Cardiac arrest. It is done during cardiopulmonary resuscitation
- Excessive bronchial secretion during drug overdoses or poisoning (organophosphorus compounds)
- Respiratory failure to maintain clear airways
- Drug anesthesia, surgery and postoperatively.

INTRAVENOUS LINE ACCESS (IV ACCESS)

To procure IV line and its preservation is an important and preliminary step in management of dehydration, shock, cardiac arrest and any unconscious patient. The IV line can be procured and maintained by simple needle, scalp vein set (Fig. 2.11A) and by cannula (Branula Fig. 2.11B).

Identification

Scalp vein needle (set) is recognized easily as it consists of a short stainless steel needle attached to a polyethylene tube which has a stopper at the end for closure (Fig. 2.11A). Between the needle and tube, two flaps in the form of butterfly shape wings are present for fixation of the needle to the skin. These needles are 18-25 G (gauze) and disposable.

Branula (i.v. cannula). It consists of siliconised stainless steel needle with an outer cannula made of polyethylene. The needle fits into outer sheath. It is available as winged cannula (Fig 2.11B). The wings are used for better fixation to the skin with leucoplast.

Figs 2.11A and B: (A) Scalp vein set, (B) Cannula (Branula)

Indications

1. **Emergency:** It should be precured on urgent basis during following conditions:
   - Cardiac arrest
   - Shock
   - Unconscious or comatosed patient
   - Diabetic ketoacidosis or hypoglycemic coma
   - Acute gastroenteritis and pancreatitis
   - Acute dehydration or fluid loss/blood loss.
2. **Immediate**
   - Acute attack of bronchial asthma
   - Respiratory failure
   - Anaphylactic reactions
   - Acute myocardial infarction
   - Thyrotoxic crisis
   - Hypercalcemic crisis
   - Poisoning.
3. **Others**
   - For drug administration
   - For fluid therapy who is not accepting orally, or for nutritional support during therapy for cancer, fistule and severe inflammatory bowel disease
   - Forced diuresis
   - For transfusion of blood and blood products
   - Dialysis.

Complications

Counterpuncture with hematoma
- Thrombophlebitis
- Pain at the site of puncture
- Introduction of infection
- Transmission of hepatitis or AIDS.

INTRAVENOUS INFUSION SET

It is transmission line containing a bulb near the proximal end to see the rate of flow. At one end it has a plastic nozzle for connection to the bottle or bag. At the other end, it is connected to intravenous line (Fig. 2.12).

Fig. 2.12: Intravenous infusion set

Identification

IV set has three parts i.e,
   - i. Proximal part (limb) has a sharp pointed tip made of plastic to be introduced into the infusion bottle or bag.
   - ii. Murphy's chamber. It is a glass chamber to regulate the flow of fluid by adjusting the number of drops/minute.
   - iii. Distal part (limb) consists of a long tubing with a nozzle at the end for connection to venous access (scalp vein or branula). It has a regulator to adjust the rate of flow through chamber.

Indications

- For transfusion of fluids, crystalloid and colloids
- For blood or blood product transfusion.

MOUTH GAG (NASOPHARYNGEAL AIRWAY)

It is a wide noncompressible transparent tube with a wide hole (Fig. 2.13) to maintain patent airway during anes-thesia and in an unconscious patient as tongue may fall back on oropharynx and may obstruct respiratory airway during anesthesia or unconsciousness.

Identification

The nasopharyngeal airway is a plastic or metallic instrument having three parts i.e. flank, bite portion and the body (Fig. 2.13). The flank is circular flat distal end to prevent the slipping of airway into oral cavity. The middle bite portion is flat, fits in between teeth to prevent clenching of teeth and obstruction of airway. The body is curved portion, fits over the tongue and prevents tongue bite.

Fig. 2.13: Mouth gag

Indications

1. To prevent falling of tongue during repeated attacks of epilepsy or status epilepticus. It also protects the tongue from injury during these episodes.
2. To prevent falling of tongue in an unconscious patient.
3. To maintain patent airway prior to endotracheal intubation.
4. Facilitates airway suction.

STOMACH (GASTRIC) LAVAGE TUBE

This is a wide bore rubber tube having a cup at one end for entry and exist of fluid. There is a bulb in the middle. The other end (gastric end) lies in the stomach (Fig. 2.14). The tube is marked with a black ring at 45 cm indicating the distance between teeth and the cardia of stomach.

Indications

• Gastric lavage is attempted in poisoning or drug overdosage.

Contraindications

• Corrosive poisoning

Note: Ryle's tube can be used for gastric lavage also.

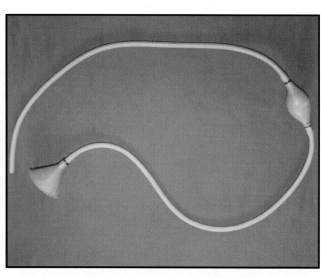

Fig. 2.14: Gastric (stomach) lavage tube

DRUG DELIVERY DEVICES

Insulin Delivery Devices (Fig 2.15A and B)

Identification

This is long narrow syringe of 1 ml resembeling tuberculin syringe, but it can be differentiated by the markings of 5, 10, 15, 20, 25, 30, 40 units. The small needle is No 26, attached to it.

Fig. 2.15A: Insulin syringe and needle (disposable)

Insulin pen

Cartridge

Fig. 2.15B: Insulin pen and its cartridge

Main Use

To deliver insulin subcutaneously, hence, its name.

Other Uses

• It can be used as 1 ml syringe for giving im or sc injections.
• It can be used as a hypodermic syringe similar to tuberculin syringe for testing the drug sensitivity.

Indications of Insulin

• Read insulin under commonly used drugs unit III of this book.
• However indications of insulin are divided into two heads.

I. *Indications in diabetes*
• All type 1 DM
• Type 2 DM with OHA failure
• Type 2 diabetes undergoing surgery, having complications or infections
• Diabetic ketoacidosis or hyperosmolar non-ketotic coma.
• Gestational diabetes.

II. *Non diabetic indications*
• For treatment of hyperkalemia (insulin+glucose)
• Insulin test for GH secretion
• To prevent glucotoxicity postoperatively (glucose neutralization with insulin)

Side Effects e.g. hypoglycemia, lipodystrophy (tumefaction), weight gain, allergic reactions and insulin resistance.

Site of injection: Abdomen is the best site, but it can be given on the thigh and arms also.

Uses of Insulin Pen

- It is useful for self administration of insulin.
- It can be carried easily while travelling and insulin can be given at will even in restaurant, residence or any other place.

Advantages over the Insulin Syringe

- It obviates the need to carry insulin syringe and its vial while touring as it contains an attached cartridge containing insulin.
- It obviates the need to store insulin.

Ordinary Syringes (Fig. 2.16A)

Fig. 2.16A: Ordinary 5 cc syringe

Identification

The ordinary syringe may be made up of glass (nondisposable) or plastic (disposable), has markings on it. They are available in different capacities i.e. 2 ml, 5 ml, 10 ml, 20 ml, and 50 ml. Each syringe has two parts:
1. A cylinder with a nozzle at one end for attaching the needle, scalp vein set or adaptor to it.
2. An air tight piston to push the contents of the cylinder.

Indications for Use

1. 2 ml and 5 ml syringes are used to collect blood samples or to administer drugs subcutaneously (e.g. adrenaline, terbutaline) or intradermally (drug sensitivity testing), intraarterially, intramuscularly and intravenously. They are also used for infiltrating anesthesia before any local invasive procedure i.e aspiration, LP etc.
2. 20 and 50 ml syringe are used for aspiration of large amount of contents i.e.
3. Aspiration of pleural and pericardial fluid, amebic liver abscess.
4. Used for Ryle's tube feeding as well as for gastric aspiration (e.g. pyloric stenosis, intestinal obstruction).
5. For stomach wash or gastric lavage.

Hypodermic (Tuberculin) Syringe (Fig. 2.16B)

Fig. 2.16B: Tuberculin syringe

Identification

This syringe resembles insulin syringe but has blue piston attached to it. It is also 1 ml syringe but has different markings as 0.1, 0.2, 0.3, 0.4, 0.5, 0.6, 0.7, 0.8, 0.9, 1 ml etc. hence, can easily be recognized. It does not have an attached needle. Any hypodermic needle can be attached to it.

Indications for Use

- *Montoux test:* PPD (purified protein derivative) in a dose of 0.1 ml (5 tuberculin units) is injected as a test dose intradermally on the forearm. The result is read after 48-72 hours.
- It can also be used as a hypodermic syringe and needle for drug sensitivity testing.

Inhalers (Fig 2.17A and B)

Metered dose inhaler (Fig 2.17A): It is a device to deliver drug under pressurized aerosol system.

Identification

It consists of a L shaped plastic tube consisting of a mouth piece, and main body which holds the canister of drug to be inhaled. A cap is used to cover the mouth piece.

Advantages of Inhaler over Oral Therapy

- Rapid onset of action
- A smaller dose of drug is required as the lungs provide wider area for absorption
- Lower incidence of side effects
- Easier to carry and cost effective

Disadvantage

The major disadvantage is ignorance about its use and non acceptability of this route of administration. The patient has to rinse the mouth after use otherwise there are chances of superadded candida mouth infection.

Rotahaler (Fig 2.17B)

It is a fixed dose dry powder inhaler.

Fig. 2.17A: Method of use of a multi-dose inhaler. (a) Parts of inhaler. A canister contains multiple dose of bronchodilator. (b) Fixation of lips on the mouth piece. (c) Release of a fixed dose by pressing the inhaler (↓). (d) Removal of the inhaler and holding of breath. (e) Exhalation

Fig. 2.17B: Rota cap inhaler. A fixed dose is pressed into the hole (↓) and is rotated (→) to crush the capsule and release the dose of bronchodilator. Now the inhaler is ready for use

Identification

It has two parts
1. Mouth piece and a side square hole to receive the fixed dose capsule of the drug.
2. The base

Working

- The rotacap capsule is inserted into the hole.
- Rotate the base. On rotation, two halves of the capsule get separated and can be seen through the transparent body.
- The patient puts the mouth piece into his mouth and tighten the lips around it. Patient breaths as deeply as possible to take the drug inside.

Advantages

Easier to use especially in children, older asthmatics etc.

Disadvantages

It requires minimal inspiratory flow rate which is difficult to achieve in dysponeic and handicapped patients.

Uses of Inhaler

1. Acute attack of asthma
2. Chronic asthma
3. COPD
4. Bronchospasm due to any cause

Spacehaler (Fig 2.17C)

It consists of a smooth plastic cylinder. At one end, metered dose inhaler is placed for drug delivery. At the other end, there is mouth piece through which patient inhales the drug (Fig 2.17C). The cylindrical body is the space, holds the drug which is being inhaled.

Fig. 2.17C: Inhalation by a large volume air spacer (a holding chamber). A patient of asthma demonstrating the use of air spacer and inhaler

Advantages

- There are few chances of *Candida* infection.
- Low cost and portable
- Strict coordination of the patient is not required as patient breaths in the cylinder.
- Makes best use of metered dose inhaler

Disadvantages

It is inconvenient to carry such a big device.

Uses

Same as for inhaler

Nebulizer (Fig 2.17D)

It is a device (machine) which delivers higher doses of the drugs, hence, are useful during emergency situations e.g. acute severe asthma or status asthmaticus.

Fig. 2.17D: Nebulizer for nebulization therapy. A patient of asthma being nebulized at bed side

AMBU Bag (Fig 2.18)

The AMBU (Ambulatory Manual, Breathing Unit) bag is compressible self-inflating bag made of rubber. It has following parts:

  i. Outlet. Mask is attached to this end.
 ii. Two valves. There is one way expiratory valve to prevent the expired air to enter the bag and other valve is pressure release valve which is set at 30-45 cm of water.
iii. A compressible rubber bag. The bag refills automatically after compression.
 iv. Two inlets e.g. oxygen inlet and air inlet

Fig. 2.18: AMBU bag

Indications for its Use

- It is used to provide intermittent positive pressure ventilation. It is connected to the face mask (Bag and mask ventilation)

  Through AMBU bag, oxygen can be delivered for ventilation in different concentrations i.e.
- 21% air ventilation when there is no oxygen source.
- With oxygen source but without oxygen reservoir, up to 40% oxygen can be delivered.
- With oxygen source and with oxygen reservoir bag, 100% oxygen can be delivered.

Three Way (Fig. 2.19)

It is a T shaped instrument made of plastic. It has two inlets and one outlet, hence, its name "three way". By the screw either or both inlets can be connected to the outlet. It is disposable, hence, used once.

Fig. 2.19: Three way

Indications for its Use

1. For administration of IV fluids and IV medication simultaneously. It is commonly connected to IV cannula (brannula). Through one intlet, IV fluids can pass and through another inlet medications can be given or this inlet can be used for measuring CVP during fluid administration. The outlet is used during removal of fluids (see below).
2. For paracentesis: It is used during removal of fluid from the body cavity i.e. pleural, pericardial or peritoneal. Its one inlet is connected to the aspiration needle through which fluid is drawn into the syringe and by changing the direction of screw, the fluid from the syringe is pushed through the outlet into the bucket or kidney tray.
3. For exchange transfusion.

CLINICAL THERMOMETER (FIG. 2.20)

Identification

It is recognized by the mercury bulb at one end. The other end is blind. There is marking on it from 94°F to 108°F as well as in °C from 35° to 42°C. It is made up of glass.

Fig. 2.20: Clinical thermometer

TYPES

Maximum Thermometer

It is called maximum thermometer because maximum temperature beyond 108°F once obtained does not return to normal spontaneously.

Rectal Thermometer

This thermometer is graduated upto 28°C to record low temperature. Low temperatures are usually recorded from rectum, hence, called rectal thermometer.

Room Thermometer/Weather Thermometer

They contain ether or alcohol instead of mercury and reflects minimum temperature. They are called minimum thermometer.

Uses

They are used to record the temperature of the body from the external surface (axilla) or from the internal orifices (mouth or rectum).

Normal Temperature

It is 98.6°F or 37°-37.2°C.

Mouth temperature is 0.5 to 1°F higher than the axilla while rectal temperature is 1°F higher than the mouth temperature.

Fever

It is defined as temperature more than normal. It may be low grade or high grade. It may be continuous, intermittent or remittent or hectic. Habitual hyperthermia is low grade fever ranging from 98.6°F to 99.5°F. It is normal temperature in certain anxious patients. All investigations are normal. This does not require treatment.

Hyperthermia

It is defined as temperature more than 41°C occurs in response to certain anesthetics e.g. halothane, methoxyflurane and muscle relaxants (succinylcholine)

Neuroleptic Malignant Syndrome

It is characterized by hyperthermia, altered sensorium, muscular rigidity and autonomic disturbances.

Drugs Used in Cardiology

UNIT

3

Commonly Used Drugs

Drugs Used in Cardiology

Categorization of drugs used in disorders of cardiovascular system is:

CARDIAC STIMULANT

a. Cardiac stimulants, e.g. glycosides, (digoxin, digitoxin, anabine) and amrinone (inamrinone). They are discussed in Table 3.1.
b. Sympathomimetic amines, e.g. noradrenaline, adrenaline, isoproterenol (isoprenaline), dopamine and dobutamine. They have been dealt separately.

ANTIARRHYTHMIC DRUGS (VAUGHAN WILLIAM CLASSIFICATION (TABLE 3.2)

Class I (Block Na Channels)

1A: Drugs that reduce Vmax and prolong action potential duration
- Quinidine
- Procainamide
- Disopyramide

1B: Drugs that do not reduce Vmax but prolong action potential duration
- Mexiletine
- Lidocaine
- Phenytoin
- Tocainide

1C: Drugs that reduce Vmax, primarily slow conduction and can prolong refractoriness
- Flecainide
- Propafenone
- Moricizine

Class II: Beta blockers (block beta-adrenergic receptors)
- Propranolol, metoprolol, alenolol, timolol, oxypre-nolol, sotalol, bisoprolol, nebivolol, carvedilol

Class III: Drugs block potassium channels and block multiple phases of the action potential and prolong repolarization
- Amiodarone, sotalol, bretylium and N-acetylpro-cainamide, ibutilide, dofetilide

Class IV: Calcium channel blockers
- Diltiazem, verapamil and others

Other antiarrhythmic drugs
- Adenosine
- Digitalis

BETA BLOCKERS

Beta receptors can be separated into two categories; (i) that affect the heart ($\beta1$) and (ii) that affect predominantly blood vessels ($\beta2$) or the bronchi. Therefore $\beta1$ receptors produce cardiac stimulation and $\beta2$ receptors produce bronchodilation and vasodilation. Cardioselective $\beta1$ blockers antagonise the $\beta1$-cardiostimulatory effects and have less effect on $\beta2$-responses. Nonselective-beta blockers antagonise the effects of both $\beta1$ and $\beta2$ receptors. At high doses, even selective beta blockers also block $\beta2$ receptors.

Some beta blockers (alprenolol, oxyprenolol, pindolol) possess "intrinsic sympathomimetic activity" i.e. they slightly activate the β-receptors. These drugs are as efficacious as other beta blockers without intrinsic sympathomimetic activity and may cause less slowing of heart rate, less prolongation of AV conduction. They have been shown to produce less depression of LV functions than beta blockers without intrinsic sympathomimetic effect.

Only nonselective beta blockers without intrinsic sympathomimetic activity have been demonstrated to reduce mortality in patients with myocardial infarction.

Classification

Base on cardioselectivity and vasodilatory effect, they are classified into 4 groups (Fig 3.1).

Actions

1. *Antihypertensive*: Both selective and nonselective beta blockers antagonise the sympathetic effects on the heart, thus, lower cardiac output and arterial pressure. Metoprolol and atenolol, both cardioselective beta blockers are preferred as antihypertensives.
2. *Antianginal effect*: Both cardioselective and nonselective beta blockers are used in treatment of angina (stable, unstable and postmyocardial) because they reduce myocardial respsonse to sympathetic stimulation and decrease myocardial O_2 demand.
3. *Antiarrhythmic effect*: All beta blockers are classified class II antiarrhythmics except sotalol (has both class II and III effects). They are used in a variety of cardiac arrhythmias, e.g. sinus tachycardia, anxiety neurosis with tachycardia, atrial flutter, atrial fibrillation, paroxysmal atrial tachycardia and ventricular arrhythmias. The antiarrhythmic effects is achieved by blockade of β_1 receptors in the myocardium rather than quinidine like effect (some beta blockers exert local anesthetic and quinidine like effect). They delay conduction through AV node, hence, reduce heart rate response in atrial fibrillation or PSVT.

Table 3.1: Cardiac stimulants

Drugs	Mechanism of action	Uses	Doses	Side effects	Special remarks
1. *Cardiac stimulants*					
Digoxin	• Positive inotropic effect in normal, nonfailing hypertrophied and failing hearts	• CHF • To slow the ventricular response	Oral: Loading dose 0.25–0.5 mg stat then 0.25 mg every	1. *Early:* Anorexia, nausea, vomiting due to effect of	• Avoid administration within 2 hours of antacid • May be proarrhythmic
	• Negative chronotropic effect (slows conduction through AV node by increasing effective refractory period by an enhanced vagal effect)	in atrial fibrillation and atrial flutter • To terminate PSVT	4 hr × 2 doses Maintenance dose (0.25 mg on alternate days or 5 days in a week) IV Loading dose: 0.25–0.5 mg slow IV bolus, then 0.25 mg IV after 2–4 hours, then followed by oral drug.	drug on medullary centres. • Cardiac e.g. VPCs, bigeminy rhythm, nonparoxysmal SVT with block (Wenckebach) ventricular tachycardia, ventricular fibrillation	• Monitor K⁺ and correct hypovolumia • Its serum level increase with verapamil, quinidine and amiodarone • For digitalis induced arrhythmias use phenytoin, or a betablocker or lidocaine
	• It enhances excitability, automaticity and ectopic impulse formation			• Sinus arrhythmias, (sinus arrest, SA blocks), AV junctional and multi-focal or bidirectional VT 2. Chronic intoxication • Exacerbation of heart failure, weight loss, cachexia, neuralgias, gynecomastia, yellow vision, delirium	• Fab antibodies are used for severe intoxication
Amrinone	• Positive inotropic effect (increases CO), vaso-dilator agent (decreases preload and afterload)	Short-term management of CHF in patients unresponsive to digitalis, diuretics and vasodilators	IV Loading dose: 0.75 mg/kg over 2-3 min, may be repeated after 30 min Maintenance infusion 5–15 mg/kg/min (dose titrated according to response). Do not exceed 10 mg/kg in a day	• GI tract symptoms, e.g. nausea, vomiting, pain abdomen, anorexia • Cardiac symptoms, hypotension, tachycardia arrhythmias • Hepatotoxicity (jaundice) • Hypersensitivity reactions e.g. pericarditis, pleuritus, myositis, vasculitis, ascites • Lungs: nodular pulmonary shadows, hypoxemia, cough, fever, chest pain	• Avoid mixing in dextrose • Incompatible with furosemide • May exacerbate myocardial ischemia or worsen ventricular ectopy

Table 3.2: Antiarrhythmic drugs

Drugs	Mechanism of action	Uses	Doses	Side effects	Remarks
CLASS I					
1A.	**BLOCK NA+ CHANNELS** Reduce V$_{max}$ and prolong action potential duration				
• Quinidine	—do—	VT and SVT; APC/VPC 6-8 hr daily orally PSVT, atrial fibrillation	200-300 mg • Nausea, vomiting, diarrhea 400-600 mg every 2-3 hourly until reverted then 200-300 mg 6-8 hourly	• Hepatitis, cardiac toxicity • Monitor blood, liver, kidney abdominal pain, dizziness sweating, headache • Hemolytic anemia agranulocytosis, thrombocytopenic purpura • Bradycardia, hypotension • Allergy, rash, angioneurotic edema, flushing • Cinchonism, e.g. impaired hearing	• Monitor for GI distress functions • Monitor ECG and serum levels • Contraindications are acute infection, AV block, myocarditis, cardiac insufficiency, thrombocytopenia, prolong Q-T syndrome, myasthenia, digitalis toxicity, pregnancy
• Procainamide	—do—	—do— Cardiac arrhythmias associated with anesthesia, surgery	250-1000 mg every 3-6 hourly IM until oral therapy possible		• Same as above • May induce lupus syndrome
1. B.	**Do not reduce V$_{max}$, shorten action potential duration**				
• Mexiletine	—do—	Ventricular arrhythmias	200-400 mg tid upto upto 1200 mg/day/oral IV 200-250 mg IV infusion at a rate of 1 mg/min	• Nausea, vomiting, constipation • Bradycardia, hypotension • Confusion, convulsions ataxia and CNS disturbance • Hepatitis, blood dyscrasias	• Monitor ECG and BP • Proarrhythmic drug may induce torsades de pointes
• Phenytoin	—do—	• Digital induced ventricular arrhythmias • As an antiepileptic • For neuropathic pains e.g. trigeminal neuralgia, diabetic neuropathy	Oral: 100 mg bid or tid IV: Dilantinisation 500-1000 mg as IV drip followed by 100 mg tid orally or IV	Read side effects in antiepileptic drugs	• Read antiepileptics
• Lidocaine	—do—	Ventricular arrhythmias	Loading dose: 1-1.5 mg/kg IV push, may be repeated as 0.5-1.5 mg/kg IV after 5-15 minutes followed by drip	• Nervousness, dizziness blurred vision, tremors numbness, tinnitis, nausea vomiting • Bradycardia, hypotension cardiovascular collapse	• BP monitoring and ECG control essential • Bradycardia, AV blocks and cardiac decompensation are its contraindications

Contd...

Drugs	Mechanism of action	Uses	Doses	Side effects	Remarks
1. C	**Reduce V$_{max}$ primarily, slow conduction and can prolong refractoriness**				• Monitor ECG • May be proarrhythmic
• Flecainide • Encainide • Propafenone	—do— —do— —do—	Supraventricular and Ventricular arrhythmias e.g. VT	• 50-100 mg 12 hourly orally • 25-50 mg 8 hourly orally • 150 mg tid orally (upto 300 mg tid)		
CLASS II	**BETA BLOCKERS.** Read beta blockers. They are discussed separately				
CLASS III	**DRUGS BLOCK K$^+$ CHANNELS, BLOCK MULTIPLE PHASES OF ACTION POTENTIAL AND PROLONG REPOLARISATION**				
• Amiodarone	—do—	• Potentially life threatening ventricular arrhythmias unresponsive to conventional therapy	*Oral:* Loading dose 800 to 1600 mg/day for 1-3 weeks	• Liver toxicity • GI symptoms • Pulmonary fibrosis • Photosensitivity • Hypothyroidism or hyperthyroidism	• Monitor liver and thyroid function • Half-life is 13-107 days • May be proarrhythmic
		• Supraventricular arrhythmias, e.g. AV nodal, AV reentry, junctional tachycardia, atrial	600-800 mg/day for 4 weeks then 400 mg/day **IV for VT:** 15 mg/min	• Disorders of thyroid function e.g. hyper and hypothyroidism • Cardiac toxicity, e.g.	• Monitor ECG for bradycardia, prolongation of PR, QRS and QT$_C$ intervals
		flutter and fibrillation	as infusion for 10 minutes followed by 1 mg/min for 6 hours for the next several days as necessary	bradycardia, ventricular tachyarrhythmias • Neuropathy	• May increase serum levels of digoxin, class I drugs • High IV dose infusion may cause hypotension
• Bretylium tosylate	—do—	• Life-threatening ventricular arrhythmias unresponsive to conventional drugs • Drug-resistant ventricular tachyarrhythmias	**VF:** 5 mg/kg IV (diluted both 50-100 ml of 5% dextrose) push; if no response, then 10 mg/kg IV push (diluted with 50-100 ml of dextrose) then maintain infusion at 1-2 mg/min (do not exceed 30-35 mg/kg/day)	• Orthostatic hypotension • Nausea, vomiting • Increased salivation and parotid pain	• Rapid IV infusion may cause hypotension • Avoid in digitalis toxicity
• Sotalol	Class II (betablocker) drug but has class III properties also	• Approved only to treat ventricular tachyarrhythmias	Oral: 80 bid to 320 mg/day	• Side effects of beta blockers may occur • Reduce the dose in	• Watch for proarrhythmic effect • Monitor QT interval, renal insufficiency

Contd...

Commonly Used Drugs

Drugs	Mechanism of action	Uses	Doses	Side effects	Remarks
CLASS IV	**CALCIUM CHANNEL BLOCKERS—READ THE TEXT (DISCUSSED SEPARATELY)**				
OTHER ANTIARRHYTHMICS					
• Adenosine	• Slows conduction through AV node, interrupts reentry pathway in AV node • Vasodilator	• Narrow QRS complex paroxysmal supraventricular tachycardia (PSVT) • Used for pharmacological stress testing	IV: 6 mg IV push over 1-3 seconds (follow with 20 ml NS flush), if no response in 1-2 min; then 12 mg rapid IV push	• Flushing; dyspnea, headache, chest pressure • Hypotension • Bradycardia and conduction disturbances	• Can be used to determine origin of wide QRS tachycardia (ineffective in the presence of VT) • Short half-life (<5 sec) • May produce transient bradycardia and ventricular ectopy • Do not use in 2nd and 3 degree AV block or sick sinus syndrome unless pacemaker is *in situ*
• Magnesium	• Hypomagnesemia can precipitate dysarrhythmias and pump failure • Electrolyte plays an important role in initiation and maintenance of cardiac muscle contraction • Membrane stabilising agent and vasodilator	• Refractory life-threatening arrhythmias (VT and VF) not responding to conventional drugs • Torsade de pointes • Post-myocardial infarction arrhythmias • Used for treatment of refractory epilepsy and bronchial asthma	**For refractory VF/VT;** 1-2 g diluted in 100 ml 5% dextrose and infuse over 1-2 min **Post MI:** 1-2 g (8-16 mEq) in 50-100 ml in 5% dextrose and infuse over 5-60 minutes and follow 0.5-1.0 g/hr IV over 24 hr	• Flushing, headache, tachycardia, hypotension	• May cause hypotension or asystole

Fig. 3.1: Clinical classification of beta blockers

4. *Antithyroid*: Nonselective beta blockers without intrinsic sympathomimetic activity are used to block the sympathetic stimulation in thyrotoxicosis, hence, are used for relief of thyrotoxic symptoms. In addition, they depress peripheral conversion of T_4 to T_3 and exert mild antithyroid effect.

Uses of beta blockers: They are used in the treatment of:

- Hypertension
- Angina
- Arrhythmias
- Some patients of CHF (e.g. carvidelol)
- Pheochromocytoma
- Mitral valve prolapse
- Anxiety neurosis
- Thyrotoxicosis
- Migrainous headache
- Essential tremors
- Glaucoma (timolol eyedrops)
- Esmolol is the only beta blocker used in the treatment of narrow QRS tachycardia (PSVT).

Drugs and Dosage

Atenolol	Oral: 25-150 mg daily
Metoprolol	25-450 mg in divided doses/day orally
	IV: Acute MI: 5 mg IV push over 2 min × 3 doses then 50 mg orally every 6 hourly
Propranolol	Oral: 10-80 mg bid or qid upto 320 mg/day
	IV: 0.5-3.0 mg IV push, may be repeated in 2 min then after every 4 hour
Nadolol	Oral: 40-120 mg/day upto 240 mg
Sotalol	Oral: 80 mg bid upto 320 mg/day
Timolol	Oral: 10-20 mg bid to max of 60 mg
Carvidelol	Oral: 3.75 to 12.5 mg/day
Esmolol	IV infusion: Loading dose 500 mg/kg over 1 minute followed by 50 mg/kg/min

infusion over 4 min; may be repeated with increase in maintenance dose at interval of 5 min (do not exceed 200 mg/kg/min)

Adverse Effects

They are due to beta blockade (Box 3.1).

BOX 3.1: ADVERSE EFFECTS OF BETA BLOCKERS	
Cardiovascular	*Noncardiovascular*
• Hypotension, bradycardia, AV blocks, precipitation of CHF, cold extremities, • Raynaud's phenomenon	• Bronchospasm • Hypoglycemia • Allergic manifestations • Dizziness, insomnia, vivid dreams, depression, headache, muscle cramps • Nasal stuffiness, tiredness • Vomiting, diarrhea, constipation

Contraindications

- AV blocks
- Gross CHF refractory to digitalis
- Bronchial asthma or allergic conditions
- Cardiogenic shock
- Anesthesia
- Esophageal stricture and/or obstructive changes in GI tract

Special Precaution to be Observed

- Beta blockers should not be stopped abruptly. They should be withdrawn slowly
- They should not be used in CHF unless patient is fully digitalised. Carvidolol and nebivolol are only used in CHF.
- They should be avoided in combination with calcium channel blockers because of their potentiating effects
- Avoid their use in diabetes mellitus as they may mask features of hypoglycemia, if it develops.

- When used IV, give slowly or with atropine so to avoid severe bradycardia
- Pregnancy safety has not be proved

CALCIUM CHANNEL BLOCKERS

Actions

1. They block slow inward calcium current in all cardiac fibers including SA and AV nodes, thus, reduce the height of action potential, shorten muscle action potential and prolong its duration, hence, are classified as class IV antiarrhythmic.
2. They depress the conduction through AV node. Pacemaker activity of SA node is also depressed.
3. They are vasodilators, hence, reduce the preload, for which they are used in CHF and HT.

Indications (Table 3.3)

Side effects and contraindications/special precaution See the Box 3.2.

Classification

The WHO has classified Ca^{++} antagonists according to their pharmacological and clinical effects.

Class I (Verapamil) agents, *in vivo*, they have most potent negative inotropic effect. Their depressant effect may precipitate CHF. They cannot be used with beta blocker.

Class II (Nifedipine, nicardipine, amlodipine) agents do not depress conduction or contraction, therefore, the risk of precipitation of CHF is reduced. Therefore, they can be used in combination with beta blockers as they even may reverse some of the negative inotropic effects of beta blockers.

BOX 3.2: CALCIUM CHANNEL BLOCKERS

Side effects
- Dizziness, headache, flushes, fatigue, ankle edema
- Nausea, vomiting, constipation
- Reflex tachycardia
- Allergies
- Gynecomastia
- Gingival hyperplasia
- Reversible liver function impairment
- IV administration may lead to decreased HR, (bradycardia), hypotension, depressed myocardial contractility, (CHF) Rarely 2nd and 3rd degree AV block

Contraindications
- Cardiogenic shock
- 2nd and 3rd degree AV block
- Severe bradycardia
- Sick sinus syndrome
- Uncompensated CHF
- Severe LV dysfunction
- Atrial flutter or fibrillation with accessory bypass

Precautions
- Pregnancy, lactation
- Poor cardiac reserve
- First degree AV block, bradycardia, conduction disturbances
- Acute phase of MI
- Concomitant use of beta blockers
- Hepatic and renal impairment

Drug Interactions:
Digoxin, beta blockers, anti-arrhythmics, theophylline, carbamazepine, phenytoin, rifampicin, etc.

Class III agents (e.g. diltiazem). It has a little or negligible negative inotropic effect. It has a selective effect on coronary arteries with little effect on peripheral vessels, hence, does not cause reflex tachycardia.

ANTIHYPERTENSIVES

Drugs used in the treatment of hypertension according to site of action are tabulated (Table 3.4).
a. Diuretics—Read diuretics
b. Antiadrenergic
   i. Central acting, e.g. clonidine, methyldopa
   ii. Autonomic ganglia, e.g. trimethaphan
   iii. Nerve endings, e.g. reserpine, guanethidine

Table 3.3: Calcium channel blockers—indications, drug and dose

Indications	Drug	Route	Dosage
• Antianginal, coronary spasm (Prinzmetal's angina) • Hypertension • Non-Q wave MI (Non-ST elevation MI) • Control of ventricular rate in supraventricular tachycardia, atrial fibrillation and atrial flutter	Diltiazem:	Oral: IV:	30-120 mg tid or qid 0.25 mg/kg I.V push over 2 min; after 15 min 0.35 mg/kg I.V push over 2 minute
• Hypertrophic cardiomyopathy • Vasospastic phenomenon, e.g. Raynaud's phenomenon	Verapamil	Oral: IV	40-120 mg tid or qid 2.5-5 mg I.V push over 2 min after 15-30 min may repeat 5-10 mg I.V push over 2 min to a total of 20 mg
• A combination of Ca^{++} antagonist (nifedipine, amlodipine) with nitrates form an effective combination for treatment of angina with heart failure, sick sinus syndrome or AV conduction disturbance	Nifedipine Sublingual	Oral:	10-40 mg tid or qid upto 160 mg/day 5-10 mg SL to be repeated if necessary
	Amlodipine	Oral:	5-10 mg bid

Note: Nifedipine and amlodipine can only be combined with beta blockers, otherwise combination of diltiazem and verapamil with beta blockers is detrimental

Table 3.4: Antihypertensive drugs

Site of action	Drug	Dosage	Indications	Contraindication/cautions	Common side effects
Diuretics	Have been discussed separately				
Antiadrenergic drugs					
Central	Clonidine	Oral: 0.05-0.6 mg twice daily	• Mild to moderate hypertension • Hypertension with renal disease	—	Postural hypotension, sedation, dry mouth, impotence, constipation, fluid retention, depression, sleep disturbance, rebound hypertension after abrupt withdrawal
	Methyldopa (also acts by blocking sympathetic nerves)	Oral: 250-1000 mg twice daily I.V: 250-1000 mg 4-6 hourly	• Mild to moderate hypertension • Drug of choice for hypertension in pregnancy • Intravenously used for malignant hypertension	• Pheochromocytoma • Hepatic disease • During MAO inhibitor treatment	Postural hypotension, sedation, fatigue, diarrhea, impaired ejaculation, fever, gynecomastia, lactation, positive Coombs' test, chronic hepatitis, ulcerative colitis, SLE like syndrome
Autonomic ganglia blocker	Trimethaphan	IV: 1-6 mg/min	Severe and malignant hypertension	Severe coronary artery disease, severe cerebrovascular insufficiency, diabetes on hypoglycemic therapy, glaucoma, prostatism	Postural hypotension, visual symptoms, dry mouth, constipation, urinary retention, impotence
Nerve endings, e.g. Adrenolytic	Reserpine	Oral: 0.05-0.25 mg daily	• Mild to moderate hypertension in young • Raynaud's phenomenon	Pheochromocytoma, peptic ulcer, depression, MAO inhibitor therapy	Depression, nightmares, nasal congestion, dyspepsia, diarrhea, impotence
	Guanethidine	Oral: 10-15 mg/day	Moderate to severe hypertension	Pheochromocytoma, coronary artery disease, cerebrovascular insufficiency, MAO inhibitor therapy	Postural hypotension, bradycardia, dry mouth, diarrhea, impaired ejaculation, edema, asthma
Alpha receptors blocker	Phentolamine	Oral: 1-5 mg bolus	Suspected or proved pheochromocytoma	Severe coronary artery disease	Tachycardia, weakness, dizziness, flushing
	Phenoxybenzamine	Oral: 10-50 mg once or twice a day	Proved pheochromocytoma	—	Postural hypotension, miosis, tachycardia, dry mouth, nasal congestion
	Prazosin	Oral: 1-10 mg twice a day	• Mild to moderate hypertension • Raynaud's phenomenon	Use with caution in elderly	Sudden syncope, headache, sedation, dizziness, tachycardia, dry mouth, fluid retention
Beta blockers	Read as already discussed				
Alpha and beta receptor blocker	Labetalol	Oral: 100-600 mg twice a day; IV: 2 mg/min	Similar	Similar	Similar to beta blockers with more postural effects

Contd...

Commonly Used Drugs

Contd...

Site of action	Drug	Dosage	Indications	Contraindication/cautions	Common side effects
Vasodilators Vascular smooth muscle	Hydralazine	Oral: 10-75 mg 4 times a day	As an adjuvant to treatment of moderate to severe hypertension	Lupus erythematosus (SLE), severe coronary artery disease	Headache, tachycardia, angina, nausea, anorexia, vomiting, diarrhea, SLE syndrome, rash, edema
	Minoxidil	Oral: 2.5-40 mg twice a day	Severe hypertension	Severe coronary artery disease	Tachycardia, aggravation of angina, fluid retention, hair growth (hypertrichosis), coarsening of facial features, pericardial effusion
	Diazoxide	IV 1-3 mg/kg upto 150 mg rapidly	Severe to malignant hypertension	Diabetes, hyperuricemia, CHF	Hyperglycemia, hyperuricemia, fluid retention
	Nitroprusside	IV: 0.5-8 (mg/kg/min)	Malignant hypertension		apprehension, weakness, nausea, vomiting, diaphoresis, muscle twitching, cyanide toxicity

Calcium Channel Blockers Read as already discussed

Angiotensin Converting Enzyme (ACE) Inhibitors

Site of action	Drug	Dosage	Indications	Contraindication/cautions	Common side effects
The drugs by blocking the ACE, suppress the angiotensin II formation, thus, affect primarily renin-angiotensin aldosterone system	Captopril	Oral: 12.5-75 mg twice a day	• Mild to moderate hypertension • Renal artery stenosis (unilateral) • CHF refractory to digoxin and diuretics • Hypertension with renal failure (S. creatinine < 3.5 mg%) • Nephrotic syndrome to reduce albuminuria	• Renal failure (reduce the dose) • Bilateral renal artery stenosis • Pregnancy	Leukopenia, pancytopenia, hypotension, angiedema, cough, urticarial rash, fever, loss of taste, acute renal failure in bilateral renal artery stenosis, hyperkalemia
	Enalapril Benazepril	Oral: 2.5-40 mg/day Oral: 10-40 mg/day			Same as captopril, but cough and angiedema can be more frequent. All are given once daily dose but side-effects are reduced if given
	Fosinopril Lisnopril	Oral: 10-40 mg/day Oral: 5-40 mg/day			
	Ramipril Perindopril	Oral: 2.5-20 mg/day Oral: 2-4 mg/day		twice a day	

Angiotensin Receptor Blockers (ARBs)

Site of action	Drug	Dosage	Indications	Contraindication/cautions	Common side effects
They block angiotensin receptors	Losartan	Oral: 25-50 mg once or twice/day	• Mild to moderate hypertension • Renal hypertension • Diabetic nephropathy with hypertension	• Pregnancy • Bilateral renal artery stenosis	• Hypotension, acute renal failure in bilateral renal artery stenosis, hyperkalemia
	Irbesartan	Oral: 150-300 mg once or twice/day			

Note: Previously adopted step-ladder pattern of treatment for hypertension is obsolete nowadays. The drug is chosen depending on the situation. Initially, monotherapy is instituted in all grades of hypertension, substituted by polytherapy depending on the severity of hypertension, specific situation and response to treatment. Diuretics and betablockers/calcium channel blockers are preferred for initial therapy.

    iv. Alpha blockers, e.g. phentolamine, phenoxy-benzamine, prazosin

    v. Beta blockers

    vi. Alpha/beta blockers, e.g. labetalol

c. Vasodilators: Vascular smooth muscle relaxants, e.g. hydralazine, minoxidil, diazoxide, nitroprusside

d. Angiotensin converting enzyme inhibitors (ACE inhibitors): They include; captopril, enalapril, benasepril, fosinopril, lisinopril and ramipril

e. Angiotensin receptors blockers: They include losartan, irbesartan, candesartan

f. Calcium channel blockers: They include, nifedipine amlodipine, felodipine, nicardipine, diltiazem, verapamil

Choice of Antihypertensive during Pregnancy

The safety of antihypertensive during pregnancy is depicted in Table 3.5.

Hypertension in Elderly

Antihypertensive therapy reduces the incidence of cardiovascular complications. This benefit is evident upto 85 years of age. The criteria for treatment include diastolic blood pressure ≥100 mm Hg or systolic ≥160 mm Hg over 3 to 6 months observation. A low dose of thiazide is the first drug of choice with addition of a beta blocker when required.

Antihypertensive Drug Choices in Specific Situations (Table 3.6)

ANTIANGINAL DRUGS

Angina can be stable (due to atheromatous plaques in the coronary artery) or unstable (due to plaque rupture) It is important to differentiate between the two. The antianginal drugs include;

Table 3.5: Safety of antihypertensive during pregnancy

Class of drug	Safety	Recommendation
Methyldopa	Safe	Treatment of choice
Beta blockers	Limited experience in first trimester. Use in late pregnancy can cause neonatal hypoglycemia and bradycardia	Avoid in first trimester, if possible
Calcium channel blockers	Limited experience	Second-line treatment
Diuretics	Theoretical risk of compromising uteroplacental blood flow	Avoid
ACE inhibitors	Serious problems in the fetus may occur such as oligohydramnios and renal dysfunction, especially after exposure in 2nd and 3rd trimesters	Contraindicated

Note:
1. In the second and third trimesters, antihypertensive agents are not indicated unless the diastolic pressure exceeds 95 mm of Hg.
2. Hypertensive female becoming pregnant and pregnancy with hypertension (pregnancy-induced hypertension, eclampsia, pre-eclampsia) are different terms but treatment remains same.

Table 3.6: Choice of antihypertensive in specific conditions

Condition	Preferred	Alternative/avoid
Diabetes mellitus	• ACE-inhibitor • ARB (angiotensin receptor blocker) • Calcium antagonist	• Avoid thiazide diuretic • Avoid betablockers
Hyperlipidemia	α_1-antagonist	• ACE inhibitor • Calcium antagonist • Avoid diuretic and beta blockers
Angina	• Beta blockers • Calcium antagonist	
Heart failure	ACE inhibitor	Diuretics and α_1-antagonists
Asthma	—do—	Avoid beta blockers
Peripheral vascular disease	Calcium antagonist	α_1-antagonist, avoid beta blockers
Elderly patients	Low dose thiazide and/or a calcium channel blocker	

1. Nitrates
2. Beta blockers (already discussed)
3. Calcium channel blockers (already discussed)
4. Potassium channel activators

Most patients of angina pectoris are usually treated with beta blockers or calcium channel blockers. However, short-acting nitrates can play an important role both as prophylactic (drug to be taken before exertion) and during acute chest pain occurring at rest or exertion. Nitrates are also used as sole therapy in elderly patients with infrequent attacks.

Nitrates

Actions

1. Their precise mechanism of action is unknown but appears to depend on their conversion to the nitrate ion which is considered to generate oxide. This is possibly the same molecule as "endothelial derived relaxation factor (EDRF), the endogenous nitrate" responsible for vasodilation in hypoxia. Therefore, the predominant effect of nitrates is vasodilation of the venous capacitance vessels (reduction of preload on the heart). This reduction of preload reduces the pressure in the ventricles which, in turn, reduces wall tension, hence, reduces myocardial O_2 demand. They also dilate arteriolar vessels, thus, also reduce afterload on the heart with the result the amount of work of the heart is reduced.
2. In addition, they may increase coronary blood flow (a little effect), but they appear to redistribute blood to ischemic areas particularly the subendocardial regions which are subject to the greatest amount of pressure during systole.

By both these actions, they relieve angina both exertional and vasospastic.

Uses

1. Prophylaxis and treatment of angina. They are used in exertional angina and to relieve coronary spasm in Prinzemetal angina (rest angina).
2. Being smooth muscle relaxant, they find a place in the treatment of gastroesophageal spasms and nutcracker esophagus.
3. Intravenous nitrates can be used in unstable angina, acute myocardial infarction with or without left heart failure, to control blood pressure in preoperative hypertension and treatment of malignant hyperten-sion. They can be used for control of hypertension during surgery.
4. Being, venodilators they reduce portal venous pressure, may, sometimes be useful for treatment of acute variceal bleed due to portal hypertension.
5. Nitrates with calcium channel blockers can be used for treatment of angina with CHF, sick sinus syndrome and conduction disturbance.

Drug Dosage and Route of Administration (Table 3.7)

Potassium Channel Activator (Nicorandil)

Nicorandil belongs to a new class of antianginal agents called *potassium channel activators*. It causes venoarteriolar dilatation. It acts by increasing membrane conductance to K^+ ions which causes hyperpolarization of vascular smooth muscle membrane, thus reducing their excitability and leading to arteriolar dilatation. Unlike, nitrates, tolerance does not develop to nicorandil—an added advantage over nitrates. Being both venous and arteriolar dilator, it increases coronary blood flow and perfusion of poststenotic regions of the myocardium without causing a *"coronary steal-syndrome"* and restores the balance between O_2 supply

Table 3.7: Commonly used nitrates

Drug	Usual dose	Side effects	Contraindications
1. Sublingual nitroglycerine	0.3-0.6 mg	Headache, flushing, dizziness, tachycardia, hypotension	Intolerance or side effects
2. Isosorbide dinitrate (short-acting)	80-120 mg	Flushing, headache dizziness, tachycardia, GI upset and sleep disturbance, methemoglobinemia, cyanosis	As above. There may be worsening of ischemia on withdrawal
3. Transdermal nitroglycerine (skin patch)	0.4-1.2 mg/hr for 12-24 hr	Same as above	Same as above
4. Isosorbide-5 mononitrate (long-acting)	20-30 mg bid or 40 mg od	Same as above	Same as above

and demand of the myocardium and thereby relieving angina. It does not affect HR or BP in patients with angina.

Uses

It is used either as a monotherapy or in combination with other antianginal drugs.

Side-effects

Headache, vasodilation, vomiting, dizziness, asthenia, hypotension, and/or tachycardia at high rates.

ANTIPLATELET AGENTS

These drugs inhibit platelet functions (adhesion and aggregation) and play a role in the management of patients with arterial vascular disease and thrombembolism. Commonly used drugs and their dosage, side effects are given in Table 3.8. These drugs include:

1. Inhibitor of platelet cyclooxygenase activity, e.g. aspirin, dipyridamole
2. Inhibitor of ADP-induced platelet aggregation, e.g. ticlodipine and clopidogrel.

Indications and Contraindications (Box 3.3)

They are used in variety of conditions either alone or in combination with anticoagulants for reduction of frequency of transient ischemic attacks in patients with CVA and progression of unstable angina to myocardial infarction.

ANTICOAGULANTS

These agents retard fibrin deposition on established thrombi and prevent the formation of new thrombi. The drugs include;

1. Heparin—for acute or immediate anticoagulation as well as for long-term administration.
2. Oral anticoagulants—for chronic or long-term anticoagulation.

Indications

1. Acute venous thrombosis and pulmonary embolism.
2. Chronic oral anticoagulation is used to prevent cerebral arterial embolism from cardiac sources such as ventricular mural thrombi, atrial thrombi, or prosthetic

Table 3.8: Commonly used antiplatelet agents

Drugs	Actions	Doses	Side effects
Aspirin	Irreversibly inactivates the enzyme cyclooxygenase and thereby inhibit platelet production of thromboxane A_2	150-300 mg as a single dose in a day	• It may cause allergic or asthmatic reactions, GI intolerance
Tidofidine	Inhibits ADP-induced platelet aggregation	250 mg twice daily with food	• GI symptoms (e.g. nausea, vomiting, abdominal pain, diarrhea) • Skin rashes • Neutropenia, GI hemorrhage • Headache, tinnitus
Clopidogrel	Inhibits ADP-induced platelet aggregation	300 mg as a loading dose followed by 75 mg once daily	• Neutropenia, hemorrhage, agranulocytosis • Skin rash • GI symptoms, e.g. nausea, dyspepsia, gastritis, constipation
A combination of aspirin and clopidogrel	Over all inhibition of platelets aggregation	Aspirin and clopidogrel in usual dosage	• Thrombotic thrombocytopenic purpura

valve thrombi or thrombi from an atherosclerotic, partially occluded or stenosed carotid or vertebral artery.

3. They are used, less successfully, to treat peripheral or mesenteric arterial thrombosis and dural sinus thrombosis.

Acute Anticoagulation with Heparin

Action: Heparin acts as an anticoagulant by inhibiting a number of activated factors (thrombin, XIIa, XIa, Xa, IXa, VIIa) and binds to and activate antithrombin III. It is an extremely potent anticoagulant that can dramatically reduce thrombin generation and fibrin formation in patients with acute venous and arterial thrombosis and embolism. It is given as IV infusion at a rate sufficient to raise the activated partial thromboplastin time (APTT) or INR to 2-2.5 times the patient's preheparin APTT/INR. This requires infusion of approximately 1000 USP units/hour and is continued for 2-3 days while patients are begun on oral anticoagulants simultaneously to achieve appropriate prolongation of prothrombin time during shifting period.

Alternative to continuous IV infusion, heparin can be administered as 5000 units four times a day either subcutaneously or intravenously.

Types of heparin

1. Unfractionated
2. Low-molecular weight heparin
   The low molecular weight heparin has many advantages over unfractionated heparin;

i. The low molecular weight heparin can be administered subcutaneously once or twice daily

ii. Their pharmacokinetics are so predictable that APTT monitoring is not, required.

iii. The low-molecular weight heparin is less immunogenic, hence, less likely to cause thrombocytopenia

iv. Low molecular weight heparin can be given to outpatients

Indication for Anticoagulation with Heparin

Heparin anticoagulation is the treatment of choice for acute venous thrombosis. The indications, dose and route of administration of heparin are given in Table 3.9.

Chronic Oral Anticoagulation

The oral anticoagulants include two groups
1. Coumarins, e.g. warfarin and dicumarol
2. Indandiones, e.g. phenindione

Actions

Both these groups of drugs reduce the activity of vitamin K dependent clotting factors (prothrombin, VII, IX and X) by interfering with their synthesis in the liver. Their effect does not become apparent until the body's existing supplies of vitamin K dependent factors has been exhausted, that is why, they take 2-3 days for the anticoagulant effect to develop fully. Similarly on withdrawal, the anticoagulant activity will not disappear until the liver has once again produced these factors.

Table 3.9: Anticoagulant therapy with heparin

Indications	Dose (USP units)	Route of administration
1. Prophylaxis in general surgery	5000 q 12 hr	Subcutaneous
2. Prophylaxis in medical conditions such as patients with CHF, cardiomyopathy or myocardial infarction	10,000 q 12 h	Subcutaneous
3. Treatment of unstable angina and non-ST elevation myocardial infarction (NSTEMI)	5000 as bolus then 1000 q per hour	Intravenous
4. Acute pulmonary embolism (venous thrombembolism)	5,000 as bolus then 1000 q per hour	Intravenous
5. Venous thrombembolism (prophylaxis in pregnancy, warfarin failure or chronic disseminated intravascular coagulation)	1000 q per hour	Subcutaneous pump
6. Hemodialysis	5000 as bolus then further 5000 if session of dialysis exceeds 4 hr	IV into arterial line of circuit prior to session of dialysis
Low molecular heparin (Flaxaprin, enoxaprin)		
1. *Prophylaxis in general surgery:*	Flaxaprin 3200 U or enoxaprin 2000 U (20 mg) deep subcutaneous 2 hour before surgery then daily for 7-10 days	
2. *Deep vein thrombosis:*	Flaxaprin 6400/day for 5-7 days or Enoxaprin 1-1.5 mg/kg/day until oral anticoagulation is achieved	
3. *Hemodialysis:*	Enoxaprin 1 mg/kg into arterial line of circuit prior to dialysis then 0.5-1 mg/kg may be given again if session exceeds 4 hr of dialysis	

As discussed earlier, patient should remain on heparin until the appropriate dose of oral anticoagulant is achieved.
- Dose and indications of oral anticoagulants (Table 3.10)
- Side effects and contraindications of anticoagulants (Table 3.11).

FIBRINOLYTIC OR THROMBOLYTIC AGENTS

Fibrinolysis is an important part of normal hemostatic process, is initiated by the release of tissue plasminogen activator (tPA) or prourokinase (Pro-UK) from endothelial cells. The fibrinolytic drugs actually accelerate the process of fibrinolysis by preferentially activating plasminogen which, is adsorbed on to fibrin clot, is converted into plasmin (proteolytic enzyme) which lyses the fibrin clot or thrombus to achieve thrombolysis or fibrinolysis.

Drugs

The pharmacologic agents being used to accelerate clot dissolution are either derived from natural products or are chemically modified derivatives. They differ with respect

Table 3.10: Oral anticoagulants

Drugs	Doses	Indications	Effective anticoagulation
Warfarin	5-10 mg/day then titrate the dose to achieve effective anticoagulation	• Treatment, prevention and recurrence of deep vein thrombosis and pulmonary or cerebral embolism	Effective anticoagulation means the prolongation of prothrombin time (PT) of the patient by 1.5 to 2 times than the control. The International Normalised Ratio (INR) or PTI (%) is the well recognised method for effective anticoagulation which is calculated as follows
Dicoumarol	8-12 mg 1st day, 4-8 mg 2nd day, maintenance dose 1-8 mg/day so as to achieve effective anticoagulation	• Prophylaxis for left atrial or ventricular thrombi • Prophylactic therapy for paroxysmal atrial fibrillation or prosthetic valve • Patients with lupus anticoagulants and risk of thrombembolism • Patients with chronic indwelling venous catheter to prevent clot formation at the catheter tip	$INR = \dfrac{(PT \text{ of the patient }) ISI}{Normal\ PT}$ $PTI\ (\%) = \dfrac{PT \text{ of patient}}{Normal\ PT} \times 100$ Note: The intensity of anticoagulation to be achieved depends on the INR or PTI (%) and varies with clinical conditions from 1.5 to 4 times

Table 3.11: Side effects and contraindication of anticoagulants

Drugs	Contraindications	Side effects
Heparin	• Hemorrhagic conditions • Bleeding tendencies • Severe liver or kidney disease • Uncontrolled hypertension	• Hemorrhage is common • Hypersensitivity reactions • Thrombocytopenia • Alopecia • Osteoporosis on prolonged use • Hemorrhage • Dermatitis • Fever • Nausea, diarrhea • A painful purple discoloration of tes and skin necrosis
Oral coumarine derivative	• Pre-existing tendency to hemorrhage e.g. peptic ulcer, cerebrovascular hemorrhage • Severe hepatic or renal disease • Pregnancy *Special precautions* • Antibiotics • Fat malabsorption • Sensitivity to these drugs is increased by aspirin, indomethacin, methyldopa, clofibrate • Sensitivity is decreased by barbiturates, rifampicin, haloperidol, hence, if therapy with these drug is stopped, anticoagulant effect may be increased. Therefore, careful control of dosage with careful and frequent monitoring of PT is essential	

to fibrin specificity and some types of complications. For example, some patients have antistreptococcal antibodies in the blood that may react with streptokinase and reduce its potency and cause immunogenic or fibrile reaction. Similarly streptokinase can only be used once or twice for this purpose because antibodies are formed against it after its first use.

Indications, Dosage, Side Effects

See Table 3.12

Parameters of Fibrinolysis

- Fall in fibrinogen level
- Prolongation of the thrombin time and euglobulin lysis time

Precautions during Streptokinase Therapy

Some patients may develop acute allergic symptoms including urticaria and occasionally serum sickness reactions. The corticosteroids and antihistaminics should be at the bedside for such an event. However, some physicians use concomitant use of corticosteroids and an antihistaminic agent to avoid such reaction. Blood pressure, pulse and ECG should be continuously monitored.

Success of Coronary Thrombolysis in Acute MI

The thrombolysis should be attempted as early as possible within first 6 hr when clot is fibrinous (fresh). Delayed use of streptokinase may make it unsuccessful.

The parameters of successful thrombolysis are:
1. Relief of pain or cardiac symptoms.
2. Return of elevated ST segment to normal or near normal level or reduction in ST elevation by >50%
3. Reperfusion arrhythmias, e.g. nodal ectopics, idionodal rhythm or first degree AV block.

DIURETICS

Definition

These are the drugs which produce natriuresis with obligatory loss of water.

Indications

They are used in following conditions:
1. Congestive heart failure due to any cause
2. Cirrhosis of liver with edema
3. Nephrotic syndrome (nephrotic edema)
4. Hypoproteinemia with edematous state
5. Treatment of hypertension
6. Toxemia of pregnancy
7. Forced diuresis for dialysable poison (salicylates, barbiturate) and hypercalcemia.

All diuretics are effective in eliminating edematous states, but the selection of diuretics is more difficult, and abnormality in serum electrolytes must be taken into account. Overtreatment must be avoided, since, resultant hypovolemia may reduce cardiac output, interfere with renal functions and produce profound weakness and lethargy.

Because of different sites of actions they can be used in combinations. They can be used as an adjunct to

---

Table 3.12: Fibrinolytic agents

Agents	Indications	Doses	Adverse effects
1. Recombinant tissue plasminogen activator (rt PA) *(Source-recombinant)*	Lysis of coronary arterial thrombi in acute MI	• 100 mg IV over 3 hours in hospital only • Current regimen is 15 mg bolus followed by 50 mg IV over 30 min then rest 35 mg over one hour	Localized bleeding, intracerebral hemorrhage, bleeding into GI and urinary tract. Nausea, vomiting, headache, rash, pruritus
2. Urokinase (UK) (source: renal tubular cell cultures)	• Thrombolysis in acute MI, deep vein thrombosis, peripheral arterial occlusion	4400 IU/ kg over 10-30 min IV	• Bleeding (localized or intracerebral or GI tract) nausea and vomiting
3. Streptokinase (source: β-hemolytic streptococci)	• Clot lysis in acute MI • Acute thrombosis of arteries • Pulmonary embolism • Deep vein thrombosis • Veno-occlusive disease of liver	**For acute MI:** 750,000-1.5 million IU over one hour **For deep vein thrombosis** 1.5 million IU over 6 hours	• Hemorrhage, hypotension, arrhythmias, febrile reactions, anaphylaxis (rare) pulmonary edema, nausea, vomiting

Note: Heparin should be started at the same time as an fibrinolytic agent and continued for 7-10 days appropriate therapy directed against the cause of the disease with edema such as these can be combined with digoxin, antihypertensives and so on. They potentiate digitalis toxicity due to hypokalemia.

The hypokalemia is a dangerous side effect of potent loop diuretic, e.g. fursemide, hence, a K⁺ sparing diuretic may be combined, but, this combination becomes again dangerous in hyperkalemia associated with edematous state i.e. renal failure.

Commonly Used Diuretics

Thiazides and Related Diuretics

Actions: They induce diuresis by inhibiting selective renal tubular reabsorption of sodium and chloride chiefly in the early distal tubule (cortical diluting segment). Some also exhibit weak carbonic anhydrase inhibiting activity. All diuretics increase renal excretion of sodium and chloride in approximately equal amounts (Table 3.13).

Loop Diuretics

The loop diuretics are physiologically similar but differ chemically. They are most potent diuretics and remain effective despite the elimination of extracellular fluid volume where other diuretics loose their effectiveness. These drugs are effective orally and intravenously. Due to their effectiveness, they are useful in all emergency edematous states, particularly in refractory heart failure and pulmonary edema. These are even effective in patients with hyponatremia, hypoalbuminemia, hypochloremia, hypokalemia and reductions in GFR and to produce a diuresis in patients in whom thiazide diuretics and aldosterone antagonists, alone or in combination are ineffective. In refractory heart failure, the action of loop diuretics may be potentiated by intravenous administration and the addition of other diuretics.

Actions

They reversibly inhibit the reabsorption of Na⁺, K⁺, Cl⁺ in the thick ascending limb of *Henle's loop*. They may also

Table 3.13: Commonly used thiazide diuretics and similar compounds

Drugs	Doses	Contraindications/cautions	Frequent side effects
Hydrochlorthiazide	Oral: 12.5-25 mg daily or twice daily	Anuria, hepatic coma, concomitant lithium therapy, diabetes mellitus, hyperuricemia, primary hyperaldosteronism and hypersensitivity to thiazides	• **GI symptoms:** Nausea, vomiting, anorexia • **CNS:** headache, dizziness, paresthesias • **Blood:** Blood dyscrasias • **Metabolic:** hyperglycemia, hyperuricemia, hypercalcemia, hypokalemia • **CVS:** Orthostatic hypotension • **Skin:** Photosensitivity, rash
Note: K⁺ supplementation must be made with their use			
Chlorthalidone (not thiazide, but has similar action)	50-100 mg orally on alternate days as single dose	Severe renal failure, pregnancy, lactation, diabetes, gout	• GI symptoms • Cardiac arrhythmias • Hypokalemia, hypomagnesemia • Photosensitivity, rash • Blood dyscrasias • Postural hypotension, fatigue, weakness • Impotence • Rarely jaundice
Metolazone (Quinethazine derivative having similar action to thiazide but is not a thiazide)	5-10 mg/day orally as a single dose	Pregnancy, lactation diabetes, gout,	• Hypokalemia • GI symptoms • Fatigue weakness • Photosensitivity, rash
Note: Metolazone has been reported to be effective in the presence of moderate renal failure			

induce renal cortical vasodilation and can produce rates of urine formation that may be as high as one-fourth of GFR (glomerular filtration rate).

Commonly Used Loop Diuretics (Table 3.14)

This group include bumetanide, fursemide, torsamide and ethacrynic acid

Potassium-sparing Diuretics

This group include:
1. Aldosterone antagonists-spironolactone
2. Triamterene and amiloride.

Actions

Spironolactone competitively inhibits the distal tubular reabsorption of sodium and excretion of potassium by antagonising the action of aldosterone on the distal tubules. Thus, diuresis occurs with excretion of sodium and retention of potassium hence called *potassium-sparing effect*. Its specific indication is to produce diuresis where edematous state is associated with hyperaldosteronism, i.e. cirrhosis of liver, CHF and nephrotic syndrome.

Triamterene and amiloride exert renal effects similar to that of spironolactone (i.e. block Na^+, K^+, H^+ exchange in distal tubules) with a major difference that their action does not depend on the presence of aldosterone, hence, are useful in adrenalectomised state. The dose indications and contraindication and side effects are given in the Table 3.15.

Carbonic Anhydrase Inhibitor (Acetazolamide)

It inhibits renal carbonic anhydrase resulting in increased cation excretion, mainly as sodium and potassium together with bicarbonate. The urine becomes alkaline and the diuresis becomes self-limiting as metabolic acidosis develops.

Inhibition of carbonic anhydrase in the eye results in reduction of intraocular pressure by reducing the formation of aqueous humor.

Uses

- Adjunctive treatment of CHF
- Certain epilepsies, e.g. Petit mal
- Chronic simple glaucoma and postoperatively in acute closed angle glaucoma

Contraindications

Sodium and potassium depletion, marked renal, hepatic and adenocortical insufficiency, hyperchloremic acidosis.

Side Effects

Nausea, vomiting, anorexia, confusion, headache, ataxia, paresthesias, polyuria, rash, blood dyscrasias
Dose: 250-1 g daily orally

Choice of a Diuretic

1. Orally administered thiazides and metolazone are the agents of choice in the treatment of mild to moderate cardiac edema not associated with hyperglycemia, hyperuricemia or hypokalemia.
2. In patients with heart failure or cirrhosis of liver where edema is associated with secondary hyperaldosteronism, a combination of thiazide or loop diuretic with spironolactone is quite effective.

Table 3.14: Commonly used loop diuretics

Drugs	Dosages	Contraindications/cautions	Side effects	Comments
Furosemide	Oral: 20-80 mg as a single dose or divided IV 20-80 mg or IM or slow IV daily or as required Children 1 mg/kg body wt. daily (max 20 mg/day) orally or IV	• Hepatic coma, • Hypovolemia, hypotension • Hyponatremia, hypokalemia • Addison's disease • Caution in patients with diabetes, gout, pregnancy, lactation	• GI upset, malaise • Rash • Deafness • Gout • Blood dyscrasias • Hypokalemia • Hyperglycemia • Hypocalcemia	• It potentiates digitalis toxicity • Potassium must be supplemented when used alone • It can be combined with a potassium sparing diuretic
Torsemide	Oral: 10-40 mg as a single or divided dose I.V 10-20 mg	Same as above	• Electrolyte and metabolic disturbances • Dry mouth, headache • Cramps	• Not recommended for children • GI symptoms • Blood dyscrasias • Hypotension, dizziness

Note: It potentiales digitalis toxicity due to hypokalemia, hence either K^+ is supplemented during its use or a combination of potassium sparing diuretics may be employed

Drugs	Doses	Contraindications/ cautions	Side effects	Comments
Spironolactone	Oral: 25-100 mg three times a day	• Hyperkalemia • Anuria • Renal failure	• GI distress • Mental confusion • Ataxia • Rashes • Gynecomastia • Impotence • Menstrual abnormalities • Hyperkalemia	• Monitor for electrolyte imbalance • Most effective when used with thiazide or loop diuretics • Risk of hypokalemia is reduced by combining it with potassium-losing diuretics
Triamterene	Oral: 100 mg once or twice a day	Same as above	• Nausea, vomiting, diarrhea, headache granulocytopenia, eosinophilia, acidosis, skin rash, orthostatic hypotension, hyperkalemia	Same as above
Amiloride	5 mg once a day (max dose 20 mg)	Same as above	• GI upset, rash, blood dyscrasias, orthostatic hypotension, reduced alertness, acidosis, calcium depletion, hyperkalemia minor psychiatric disturbance (rare)	Same as above

3. Loop diuretics either alone or in combination of spironolactone or triamterene are the agents of choice in patients with severe heart failure refractory to other diuretics.

4. In severe heart failure, the combination of a thiazide, a loop diuretic and a potassium-sparing diuretic is required.

Indications for High Dose Parenteral Furosemide

- Acute renal failure
- Forced diuresis for poisoning and hypercalcemia
- Acute pulmonary edema
- Decongestive therapy in acute cerebral edema
- Hypertensive encephalopathy or related emergencies

SYMPATHOMIMETICS

Sympathomimetic amines activate the adrenergic receptors either directly or release noradrenaline from the sympathetic nerve endings (indirect action). Many drugs have both direct and indirect effects.

1. *Epinephrine (adrenaline) or norepinephrine (noradrenaline):* They stimulate the adrenergic receptors directly. Noradrenaline is employed to support the circulation and elevate the BP in hypotensive states. Vasoconstriction is the major effect, although cardiac stimulation occurs as well. It is used in hypotension and shock.

Adrenaline (epinephrine) is also a pressure agent, has special usefulness in treatment of allergic conditions, especially those associated with anaphylaxis. Adrenaline antagonizes the effects of histamine and other mediators on vascular and visceral smooth muscle and is useful in the treatment of bronchospasm or bronchial asthma in children.

2. *Dopamine:* It is an adrenergic agonist. Its effect is dose-dependant.

At low dose, it exerts a positive inotropic effect by direct action of β_1-cardiac receptors and by indirect release of norepinephrine from sympathetic nerve endings in the heart. At lower doses, it acts as vasodilator of renal and mesenteric vessels and facilitates sodium excretion and diuresis. Because of this action, it is used in oliguric conditions associated with intense vasoconstriction as an adjunct to diuretic therapy.

At higher infusion rates interaction with α-adrenergic receptors result in vasoconstriction, an increase in peripheral vascular resistance and an elevation of BP. Because of this action, it is used in hypotension and shock.

3. **Dobutamine:** A congener of dopamine with relative selectivity for β_1 receptors and with a greater effect on

363

myocardial contractility than on heart rate, is used in treatment of shock and in congestive heart failure in combination with vasodilators. Dobutamine is also in used pharmacological stress testing in conjunction with radionuclide imaging or with echocardiography for the diagnosis of demand-induced myocardial ischemia.

Beta-receptors Agonists

Isoproterenol, a direct acting beta-receptors agonist, stimulates the heart, decreases peripheral resistance and relaxes bronchial smooth muscle. It raises the cardiac output and accelerates AV conduction while increasing the automaticity of ventricular pacemakers. It is used in the treatment of AV block and bronchospasm. Selective β_2-receptors agonists (terbutaline, salbutamol, salmeterol, metaproterenol, etc.) are used as bronchodilators by inhalation (read bronchodilators).

Alpha-adrenergic Agonists

Phenylephrine and methoxamine are direct-acting alpha-agonists (stimulants) that raise the BP by causing peripheral vasoconstriction. They are used in treatment of hypotension and paroxysmal supraventricular tachycardia (PSVT). In the latter case, they decrease the heart rate by increasing cardiac vagal tone through reflex baroreceptor stimulation. Phenylephrine is also used as nasal decongestant for the treatment of allergic rhinitis and upper respiratory infections (URI).

Miscellaneous Sympathomimetics with Mixed Actions

Ephedrine has both direct beta-receptor agonist effect as well as indirect effect by release of norepinephrine on sympathetic nerve endings. It is primarily used as a bronchodilator.

Pseudephedrine a congener of ephedrine is a less potent bronchodilator, hence, is used as a nasal decongestant.

Metariminol (mephentine) has both direct and indirect effects on sympathetic nervous system. It was used in the treatment of hypotensive states but is obsolete nowadays.

Dopaminergic Agonists: The dopamine (D_2) receptors agonist bromocriptine is used to suppress prolactin secretion in prolactinoma and galactorrhea-amenorrhea syndrome.

Apomorphine, another D_2 receptor agoinst is used to induce vomiting.

Dose, Route and Indications

They are tabulated in Table 3.16.

PARASYMPATHOMIMETICS

These include:

Cholinergic Agonists

They stimulate cholinergic receptors. Bethanechol is the only cholinergic agonist in general use, stimulates gastrointestinal and genitourinary smooth muscle with minimal effect on CVS

Uses

1. Treatment of urinary retention without outflow tract obstruction
2. Postvagotomy gastric atony
3. Gastresophageal reflux disease
   Pilocarpine and carbachol are topical cholinergic agonists used in the treatment of glaucoma.

Cholinesterase Inhibitors

Cholinesterase inhibitors diminish the inactivation of acetylcholine, hence, enhance parasympathetic stimulation. Organophosphorous compound are potent cholinesterase inhibitor, used principally as insecticides and are primarily of toxological interest.

The drugs used clinically include:
1. *Physostigmine*—a tertiary amine penetrates the CNS well, hence, acts as central cholinesterase inhibitor. Dose is 1-2 mg IV slowly, when as required.
2. *Neostigmine, pyridostigmine, edrophonium,* etc. are quaternary amines, do not penetrate CNS, act at neuromuscular junction.

Uses

i. For treatment of myasthenia gravis
ii. For termination of neuromuscular blockade following general anesthesia
iii. Reversal of intoxication by agents with a central anticholinergic action
iv. Cholinesterase inhibitors induce vagotonic response in the heart and may be useful in terminating attacks of paroxysmal supraventricular tachycardia. Edrophonium 5 mg IV (after 1 mg as test dose) is used for this purpose

Table 3.16: Some commonly used sympathomimetics

Drugs	Uses	Doses and Routes	Side effects	Comments
Epinephrine (Adrenaline)	• Anaphylaxis • Acute asthma in children • Cardiac arrest (asystole)	300-500 mg SC or IM (0.3-0.5 ml of 1:1000 dilution, infuse 25-50 mg IV slowly every 5-15 minutes, titrate as needed)	• Palpitation, tachycardia and sweating • Hypotension	• Nonselective alpha and beta stimulant, increases BP and HR • Bronchodilation
Norepinephrine (noradrenaline)	• Shock • Hypotension	2-4 mg base/min IV; titrate according to response	—do—	• Alpha and β_1-stimulant • Vasoconstriction predominates • Extravasation causes tissue necrosis; infuse through IV cannula
Isoproterenol	• Cardiogenic shock • Bradyarrhythmias • AV block • Asthma	0.5-5 mg/min; titrate according to response Inhalation	—do—	• Nonselective beta-agonist • Increases HR and contractility • Dilates bronchi and tachycardia can also occur
Dobutamine	• Refractory CHF • Cardiogenic shock • Acute oliguric state • It is not a dopaminergic	2.5-25 µg/kg/min IV infusion	—do—	• Selective β_1-agonist with maximum effect on cardiac contractility than HR
Phenylephrine	Hypotension PSVT	2-5 mg SC or IM 0.1-0.5 mg IV 150-800 mg slow IV push	—do—	Selective α_1 agonist; useful in hypotension due to spinal anesthesia Pressure effect induces vagotonic response
Dopamine	• Shock • Oliguric state	• 2-5 µg/kg/min IV (dopaminergic range, vasodilator effect) • 5-10 µg/kg/min IV (dopaminergic and beta range) • 10-20 µg/kg/min IV (beta range) • 20-50 µg/kg/min IV (alpha range)	—do—	• Pharmacological effects are dose-dependent; renal and mesenteric vasodilation predominates at lower doses; cardiac stimulation and vasoconstriction develop as the dose is increased • It is dopaminergic agonist
Bromocriptine	• Prolactinoma • Amenorrhea-galactor-rhea syndrome • Acromegaly • Parkinsonism	2.5 mg orally bid or tid 5-15 mg orally tid or qid 1.25 to 2.5 mg at bedtime, increased upto 10-40 mg/day in divided doses	Nausea, vomiting, dizziness, fatigue postural hypo-tension, vaso-spasm, CNS	• Selective agonist of D_2 receptor; inhibits prolactin secretion • Useful for parkinsonism sensitive to levodopa • Lowers growth hormone levels in majority of patients with acromegaly

Drug Used in CNS and Psychiatry

ANALGESICS AND ANTIPYRETICS

Analgesics are the drugs that relieve pain while antipyretics bring the temperature down during pyrexia.

Assessment of pain is essential for its correct management because pain is subjective phenomenon based on the individual own interpretation and clinical signs. Pain may be acute or chronic having variable characteristics. The pain may be organic or psychogenic in origin. An attempt should always to made to find out the cause of pain and to treat it appropriately; for example, use of hormone or hormone antagonists in gynecological pain; and consider alternative approaches or adjunct therapy if pain is not controlled.

Analgesic Ladder

The WHO analgesic ladder (Fig. 3.2) ascending from non-opiates through weak opiates to strong opiates according to severity of pain (i. mild, ii. moderate, iii. severe) is widely regarded as best approach to the management of acute pain, chronic non-malignant pain and chronic malignant pain. The goal of treatment in all types of pain irrespective of its cause is to achieve symptom relief and improve the patient's quality of life.

A. NONOPIATE ANALGESICS

1. Salicylates (Aspirin, Salicylamide, Sodium Salicylate)

Actions

All exert analgesic, antipyretic and anti-inflammatory actions which are due to an inhibition of prostaglandin synthesis (cyclo-oxygenase inhibitor). Their analgesic effect is due to their peripheral anti-inflammatory action as well as a central effect on hypothalamus. Aspirin in lower doses also inhibit platelet aggregation (antiplatelet action).

Strong opiate analgesic, e.g. morphine, oxycodone
Weak opiate analgesics, e.g. dextropropoxyphene, codeine, teramadol etc.
Nonopiate analgesic, e.g. aspirin, paracetamol, NSAIDs, etc.

Fig. 3.2: WHO analgesic ladder

Uses

1. They are used as anti-inflammatory agents in the treatment of rheumatoid arthritis, rheumatic fever, osteoarthritis and other rheumatic conditions.
2. Aspirin is used in acute painful conditions such as headache, arthralgia, myalgia and other nonspecific conditions requiring mild analgesia.
3. It is also used as an antipyretic.
4. Aspirin in lower doses (100-300 mg) is used as an antiplatelet agent (Read antiplatelet agents) in the treatment of certain vascular disorders, e.g. transient ischemic attacks, angina. Prophylactically, it is used as an antiplatelet in CVA, postmyocardial angina, atherogenesis in diabetes and hypertension.

Contraindications

- Peptic ulcer and erosive gastritis
- Lactation
- Bleeding disorders
- Previous hypersensitivity
- Concomitant use of probenecid or other uricosuric agents (reduces uricosuric effect)

Caution

- Bronchial asthma
- Low prothrombin time
- Full term pregnancy

Side Effects

- Gastric irritation, pain abdomen and gastric erosion, hematemesis.
- Asthma
- Previous allergy
- Reye's syndrome. The drug controller has recommended that aspirin should not be given to children below 12 years of age because of increased risk of development of Reye's syndrome.

Dose: 600 mg orally to be repeated after 4 hours.

p–Aminophenol Derivatives (Paracetamol)

Actions

These compounds exert analgesic and antipyretic activity but no anti-inflammatory effect. Their mechanism of action is similar to aspirin.

Uses

Relief of pain, fever (pyrexia)

Contraindication

Analgesic nephropathy

Dose

1-2 g orally 3-4 times a day (max 8 g/day)

Side Effects

Nausea, vomiting, dyspepsia, hematological changes; large dose produce hepatotoxicity and analgesic nephropathy.

Nonsteroidal Anti-inflammatory Drugs (NSAIDs)

Besides aspirin, there are several additional nonsteroidal anti-inflammatory drugs (NSAIDs) to treat musculoskeletal and inflammatory disorders.

Actions

All these drugs are cyclo-oxygenase inhibitor (Cox-inhibitor), hence, interfere with prostaglandin synthesis. They have analgesic, anti-inflammatory and antipyretic properties.

Research has further revealed two isoforms of cyclo-oxygenase (Cox). The first isoform (Cox-1) is present in cells and tissues including, stomach, kidneys while Cox-2 is induced in response to inflammation, hence, Cox-1 inhibitor are responsible for most of the side effects such as gastric erosion, renal toxicity while Cox-2 inhibitors (Box 3.4) are presumed to be safe, more potent with fewer side-effects devoid of gastric and renal toxicity. Most of the NSAIDs have property to inhibit both Cox 1 and 2.

BOX 3.4: COX-2 INHIBITORS	
A. *Partially selective cyclo-oxygenase-2 inhibitors*	
Aceclofenac	100-200 mg/day
Meloxicam	7.5-15 mg/day
Nabumetone	500-1500 mg/day
B. *Selective Cox-2 inhibitors*	
Rofecoxib	12.5-25 mg/day
Celecoxib	

Uses

1. They are used as anti-inflammatory analgesic drugs in variety of pain due to musculoskeletal disorders (low back pain, soft tissue rheumatism). Their analgesic property is comparable to paracetamol.
2. They are used as anti-inflammatory drugs for treatment of rheumatoid arthritis, osteoarthritis, ankylosing spondylitis and inflammatory bowel disease.

Safety Profile

Recent evidence on 7 drugs have put some commonly used NSAIDs into three categories (Box 3.5).

BOX. 3.5: SAFETY PROFILE OF NSAIDS		
1. **Low risk**	*Dose*	*Side effects*
Ibuprofen	< 1600 mg/day	Dyspepsia, GI bleeding, rarely thrombocytopenia
2. **Average risk**		
• Diclofenac	75-150 mg/day	• Epigastric pain, nausea, headache, dizziness, rash, edema, peptic ulcer, GI bleed, hepatic and renal toxicity
• Indomethacin	75-150 mg/day	• GI intolerance, dizziness, CNS effects, blood dyscrasias
• Naproxen	500-1000 mg/day	• Rash, GI intolerance, tinnitis, vertigo, blood dyscrasias
• Piroxicam	10-30 mg/day	• GI disturbance, edema, CNS effects, malaise, tinnitis
3. **High risk**		
Azapropazone	1200-1800 mg/day	

Side Effects

- GI tract; nausea, vomiting, abdominal pain and hematemesis due to acute gastric erosion
- Fluid retention
- Nephrotoxicity—interstitial nephritis
- Skin—rash
- Hepatotoxicity
- Rarely asthma and anaphylaxis

Opiates Analgesic

Weak opiates such as dextropropoxyphene, codeine, dihydrocodeine are used along with aspirin and paracetamol for relief of moderate pain.

The side effects of codeine are nausea and constipation. Strong opiates (morphine, oxycodone, fentanyl, hydromorphone, methadone and pentazocine) are strong analgesic but habit-forming and constipating agents.

Indications

- As an antitussive agent, e.g. dihydrocodeine
- As an antidiarrheal agent, e.g. codeine
- Severe continuous pain such as pain of acute myocardial infarction, cancer pain, etc.
- Acute musculoskeletal pain not responding to nonopiate analgesic. They may be added as adjunctive therapy.
- Anesthetic premedication

Doses and Side Effects

See Table 3.17.

Table 3.17: Narcotic analgesic; usual dosage and intervals

Drugs	Parenteral dose (mg)	Oral dose (mg)	Side effects	Comments
Codeine	30-60 q 4 hr	30-60 q 4 hr	Nausea, constipation dependence, CNS depression, hypotension, respiratory depression, decreased urine output	• It is also used as an antitussive agent
Morphine	10 q 4 hr	60 q 4 hr	Constipation, respiratory depression, addiction, diaphoresis, nausea, vagotonic bradycardia	• To be used for short time
Hydromorphine	1-2 q 4 hr	2-4 q 4 hr	Same	• Short acting than morphine
Pethidine	50-100 to be repeated	—	Similar to morphine	—
Methadone	10 q 6-8 hr	20 q 6-8 hr	Similar	• Delayed sedation due to long action
Pentazocin	30-60 mg 4 hrly	15-30 mg 6-8 hrly	• Sedation, dizziness, hallucinations, nausea vomiting, diaphoresis, tachycardia, HT and respiratory depression	
Fentanyl	—	—	—	Transdermal patch used as alternative to morphine

Antidote to opiates is naloxone

Contraindications of Narcotic Analgesics

- Bronchial asthma
- Severe liver disease
- Head injury or raised intracranial tension
- Respiratory depression

Anticonvulsant and Antiarrhythmics as Analgesics

Anticonvulsants and antiarrhythmics increase the threshold for pain, hence, are useful in neuropathic pain such as trigeminal neuralgia, diabetic neuropathy, postherpetic neuralgia.

These include:

Phenytoin	300 mg/day
Carbamazepine	200-300 mg 6 hrly
Clonazepam	1 mg 6 hourly
Mexiletine	150-300 mg at 6-12 hours intervals
Sodium valproate	400-600 mg/day
Gabapentine	

Tricyclic Antidepressants as Analgesics

These agents are extremely useful for the management of patients with chronic pain though they have been developed for the treatment of depression. The mechanism of action is unknown. The analgesic effect of antidepressants has a (i) rapid onset of action and occurs at a lower dose that is required for treatment of depression

(ii) patient who are not depressed also get relief of chronic pain with these drugs (iii) there is evidence that they potentiate the analgesic effects of opiates, hence, are useful adjuncts for treatment of intractable or severe pain of malignant tumors. The painful conditions that respond to antidepressants are given in Box 3.6.

> **BOX 3.6: PAINFUL CONDITIONS THAT RESPOND TO TRICYCLIC ANTIDEPRESSANTS**
>
> - Postherpetic neuralgia
> - Diabetic neuropathy
> - Tension headache
> - Migrain headache
> - Rheumatoid arthritis
> - Chronic low back pain
> - Cancer

Doses

- Amitryptyline 25-300 mg orally in divided doses in a day
- Imipramine 75-400 mg/day in divided doses
- Doxepin 75-400 mg/day in divided doses

Antiepileptics or Anticonvulsants

A seizure is defined as a paroxysmal event due to abnormal excessive hypersynchronous discharges from an aggregate of CNS neurons.

Epilepsy is different from seizure. It is defined as a condition in which a person has recurrent seizures due to a chronic underlying process. This definition implies that a person with a single seizure or recurrent seizures due to correct or removable circumstances does not necessarily have epilepsy. Epilepsy refers to a clinical phenomenon rather than a single disease. The classification of seizures is given in Box 3.7.

BOX 3.7: CLASSIFICATION OF SEIZURES

1. **Partial seizures**
   A. Simple partial seizures (with motor, sensory, autonomic or psychic signs). Consciousness is preserved.
   B. Complex partial seizure where consciousness is lost.
   C. Partial seizures with secondary generalization (tonic-clonic variety).
2. **Primary Generalised Seizure**
   A. Absence (Petit mal). Common in children
   B. Tonic-clonic (grand mal)
   C. Tonic
   D. Myoclonic
3. **Unclassified**
   A. Neonatal seizure
   B. Infantile spasms (seen in < 14 of age)

Jacksonian Epilepsy (Focal Epilepsy)

It implies partial motor seizures with begining of abnormal motor movements in a restricted region such as fingers or toes and gradually progressing over seconds to minutes to include a large portion of the extremity or whole extremity.

Todd's Paralysis

The patients of Jacksonian fits experience a localised paralysis or paresis due to exhaustion of hyperexcitable neurons that occurs minutes to many hours in the involved region following the seizure. Recovery is the rule in this phenomenon.

Epilepsia Partialis Continua

It implies focal or partial seizure that may continue for hours or days. This condition is often refractory to medical therapy.

Complex-partial Seizures

These are characterised by focal seizural activity accompanied by inability to respond to visual and verbal commands during seizure. The patient is unconscious during seizures. It has three stages.
   i. Aura (pre-ictal phase)
   ii. Ictal phase
   iii. Postictal phase, e.g. confusion, automatism or behavioral changes.

Absence Seizures (Petit mal)

These are common in children, characterized by sudden, brief lapses of consciousness accompanied by subtle bilateral motor signs such as rapid blinking of eyelids, chewing movements or clonic movements of the hands. The EEG is characteristic with spike-and-wave discharge.

Grand Mal (Tonic–clonic) Seizures

These are generalised seizures which begin abruptly without warning and have tonic phase (tonic contraction of the muscles throughout the body) and clonic phase (periods of muscle relaxation or tonic muscle contraction leading to muscular flaccidity, excessive salivation and bowel and bladder incontinence). The conscious is lost during seizure and it may be prolonged.

Tonic Seizures

These are variants of grand mal that include pure tonic contractions of the muscles lasting only for a few seconds.

Atonic Seizures

They are characterized by sudden loss of muscle tone lasting for 1 to 2 seconds with impaired consciousness. There is no postictal confusion. A very brief seizure may cause a quick head drop or nodding movement while a longer will cause the patient to collapse and sudden fall.

Myoclonic Seizures

These are characterized by myoclonic jerks, i.e. a sudden and brief muscle contractions that may involve one part of the body or the entire body. These are generalised seizures, hence, consciousness is lost. The EEG is characteristic, i.e. bilateral synchronous spike-and-wave discharges.

Neonatal Seizures

These are characterized by brief episodes of apnea, eye deviation, eye blinking or repetitive movements of arm and legs, hence, are subtle in manifestations. An EEG is critical for diagnosis in such cases.

Infantile Spasms

These are seen in infants (< 1 yr of age) and are characterized by abrupt movements of head, trunk or limbs that often occur in clusters (groups) of 10-20 movements per episode.

The classic spasm is sudden flexion of the neck and abdomen with extension of the limbs (Jack-Knife seizures)

The EEG shows hypoarrhythmia which consists of high-voltage slow multifocal spikes and a variety of other pleomorphic abnormalities.

Febrile Seizures/Convulsions

These are the most common seizures seen in childhood, are associated with fever but without evidence of CNS infection or other defined causes. The patients often have a family history of either febrile convulsions or epilepsy. The typical scenario is a child who develops tonic-clonic seizure during a rising phase of temperature of a febrile episode (i.e. during the first day). These seizures may be simple partial (no loss of consciousness) or complex partial (loss of consciousness). They may be recurrent in one third cases.

Causes

See Table 3.18.

Uses

These drugs are used for:

1. Control of various types of seizures/epilepsy
2. Phenytoin is used for digitalis-induced arrhythmias
3. Phenytoin, carbamazepine and valproate, gabapentine are used for control of pain due to trigeminal neuralgia, diabetic neuropathy and other neuropathies
4. Carbamazepine is used for prophylaxis of manic-depressive illness.

Choice of Drug in Epilepsy

See Table 3.19.

Drugs, Dosage and Side effects

See Table 3.20.

Table 3.18: Causes of seizures

Neonates (< 1 month)	Infants and children (< 12 yrs)	Adolescent	Adults	Old persons
• Perinatal hypoxia and ischemia • Intracranial bleed or trauma • Meningitis • Metabolic-abnormalities (hypoglycemia, hypocalcemia, hypomagnesemia, pyridoxine deficiency • Drug withdrawal (babies born to mothers using neurotoxic drugs) • Developmental disorders • Genetic disorders (metabolic and degenerative)	• Febrile seizures • Genetic disorder (metabolic or degenerative) • Meningitis, encephalitis • Developmental disorders • Head trauma • Idiopathic	• Head trauma • Genetic disorders • Brain tumor • Illicit drug abuse • Idiopathic • Meningitis, encephalitis	• Head trauma • Alcohol withdrawal • Illucit drug abuse • Brain tumor • Idiopathic	• CVA • Brain tumor • Alcohol withdrawal • Metabolic diseases (uremia, hepatic failure, electrolyte disturbances, hypoglycemia • Alzheimer's disease and other degenerative disorder • Idiopathic

Table 3.19: Choice of antiepileptic drugs in various types of epilepsy

Epilepsy	First line drug(s)	Alternatives
1. Grand mal (tonic-clonic)	• Phenytoin • Carbamazepine • Sodium valproate • Primidone	• Phenobarbitone • Clobazam • Clonazepam
2. Focal (partial) seizures	-do-	• Phenobarbitone, primidone, lamotrigene, gabapentine
3. Petit mal	• Sodium valproate	• Ethosuximide
4. Myoclonic	• Sodium valproate • Clonazepam	• Carbamazepine • Phenytoin
5. Status epilepticus	• Clonazepam • Phenytoin	• Diazepam, lorazepam • Paraldehyde

Table 3.20: Commonly used antiepileptic drugs

Drugs	Actions	Uses	Doses and Intervals	Side effects Neurologic	Side effects Systemic	Drug interactions
Phenytoin or dilantin	It increases the seizure threshold in the motor cortex possibly by interfering with movements of ions, e.g. Na^+ and Ca^{++} through cell membranes	• Grand mal seizure • Psychomotor seizures • Focal onset seizure • Cardiac arrhythmias especially digitalis-induced • Trigeminal neuralgia • Seizures following head injury or neurosurgery • Pain due to diabetic or other neuropathy	*Oral: Adults:* Initially 3-4 mg/kg daily or 200-300 mg daily (as a single dose or two divided doses). Usual dose 200-400 (max 600 mg/day) *Children:* Usual dose 4-6 mg/kg (Max. 300 mg) *Injections* 1. *Status epilepticus* • *Adults:* Initially 10-15 mg/kg IV slowly (not exceeding 50 mg/min) then 100 mg IV or orally every 6-8 hours • *Children:* 10-20 mg /kg IV slowly 2. *Neurosurgery prophylaxis* • 250 mg IV slowly 6-12 hourly 3. *Cardiac arrhythmias* • 3-5 mg/kg by slow IV infusion; repeat if necessary	• Alaxia • Confusion • Incoordination • Cerebellar features, e.g. ataxia •	• Gum hyperplasia • Lymph node enlargement/ hyperplasia • Osteomalacia • Excessive hair growth • Coarsening of facial features • Skin rash	• Isoniazid and sulphonamides increase its levels • Phenobarbitone and carbamazepine decrease its levels
Carbamazepine	It increases seizure threshold by inhibiting Na^+-dependent action potentials	• Tonic-clonic seizure • Focal onset seizure • Trigeminal neuralgia • Prophylaxis in manic-depressive illness (mood stabliser/ elevator)	Oral • *Adults,* start 100-200 mg once or twice daily and then increase slowly to 400 mg 2-3 times/day. • *Children* • upto 1 yr: 100-200 mg/d • 1-5 yr: 200-400 mg/d • 6-10 yr: 400-600 mg/d • 11-15 yr: 600-1000 mg/d • Total daily dose is given in divided doses	• Ataxia • Diplopia • Vertigo • Dizziness	• Aplastic anemia • Leukopenia • GI upset • Hepatotoxicity	• Level decreased by phenobarbitone and phenytoin • Level increased by erythromycin and isoniazid
Valproic acid (monotherapy or adjuvant therapy)	It increases brain levels of the inhibitory neurotransmitter GABA	• Tonic-clonic generalised seizures • Focal seizures • Absence seizures • Myoclonic seizures • Prophylaxis in manic-depressive illness (mood elevator /stabiliser)	*Oral* *Adults* 600 mg bid then increase by 200 mg at 3 days interval (max 2.5 g/day) *Children* <20 kg: 200 mg initial dose > 20 kg: Initial dose is 400 mg daily and then increase slowly to achieve control (max 35 mg/day)	• Ataxia • Tremors • Drowsiness or sedation • Skin rash	• Liver toxicity • Thrombocytopenia • GI upset • Weight gain • Alopecia	Levels decreased by phenobarmazepine, carbamazepine and phenytoin

Contd...

Commonly Used Drugs

371

Contd...

Drugs	Actions	Uses	Doses and Intervals	Side effects Neurologic	Systemic	Drug interactions
Primidone (mysoline)	It is converted in the body to phenobarbitone and its antiepileptic properties are due to both phenobarbitone and the parent drug	• Tonic-clonic seizure • Focal onset seizure	*Oral* • Start as 125-250 mg at bed time and double the dose after 3 days, then increase it by 250 mg after every 3 days till control is achieved. Usual dose 750-1000 mg bid or tid.		Same as phenobarbitone	
Phenobarbitone	It exerts anti-epileptic effect by CNS depression	• Tonic-clonic seizure • Focal-onset seizure • As a hypnotic • Used as an anesthetic agent • Status epilepticus • Pre-eclampsia	*Oral:* 30-210 mg daily in divided doses. *IV.* For status: epilepticus 400-800 mg Eclampsia: 300 mg both are given in divided doses 2-4 hourly	• Sedation • Dizziness • Confused state • Depression • Decreased libido	Skin rash	Levels increased by valproic acid and phenytoin
Ethosuximide (Zarontin)	It increases the seizural threshold by CNS depression	• Petit mal	*Oral: Adult:* Start with 500 mg and increase slowly to 1-1.5 g/daily *Children:* Start 250 mg and increase upto 1.0 g/day in divided doses	• Ataxia • Lethargy • Headache	• G I upset • Skin rash • Bone marrow depression	
Gabapentine	Being a structural analog of GABA, increases GABA synthesis and release	• Focal onset seizure • Diabetic neuropathy • Trigeminal neuralgia	*Oral Adult* 1st day-300 mg once/day 2nd day-300 mg twice/day 3rd day-300 mg thrice/day Now increase the dose slowly three times a day to reach max of 800 mg tid. *Children:* Not recommended	• Sedation • Dizziness • Ataxia • Fatigue	• GI upset	
Lamotrigine	It suppresses burst-firing neurons by inhibiting Na$^+$-dependent action potentials	• Focal onset seizure	150-500 mg bid.	• Dizziness • Diplopia • Sedation • Ataxia • Headache	• Skin rash • Stevens-Johnson syndrome	
Clonazepam	CNS depressant	• Absence seizure • Myoclonic seizure	*Oral* *Adult,* Start 0.5 mg bid, then increase 0.5 mg after 3-7 days to reach upto 4-8 mg/day. *Children* 2-5 yr. Initial 0.5 mg in two divided doses then increase it upto 1.5 to 3 mg/day. 6-12 yr 0.75 mg in two divided doses, then increase to reach 3-6 mg/day	• Lethargy • Dizziness • Sedation • Ataxia	Anorexia	

Pregnancy, Lactation and Antiepileptic Drugs

- Most women with epilepsy who become pregnant will have an uncomplicated gestation and deliver a normal baby. During pregnancy, there may be a change in frequency and severity of seizures, hence, monitor the serum level of antiepileptic drugs and see the patient at frequent intervals.
- There is an increased risk of teratogenicity associated with use of antiepileptic drugs; for example, neural tube defects associated with carbamazepine, phenytoin and valproate. Therefore, woman who become pregnant while taking these drugs should be advised antenatal screening (α-fetoprotein measure-ment and USG scan during second trimester).
- To counteract the neural tubal defect, folic acid 5 mg daily should be recommended before and during pregnancy.
- To reduce the risk of neonatal bleeding associated with the use of carbamazepine, phenytoin and pheno-barbitone, prophylactic vit K, is recommended for mothers before delivery and as well as for neonates.
- Breastfeeding is acceptable with all antiepileptic drugs taken in normal doses except barbiturates and etho-suximide.
- Current recommendations are that women who become pregnant on antiepileptic drug should continue it during pregnancy in effective or optimal dose. They are advised to continue folate throughout pregnancy.
- Drugs used in pregnancy include phenytoin, carbamazepine and valproate (Table 3.21).

PSYCHOTROPIC DRUGS

Definition: Drugs used to treat psychiatric illnesses are collectively called as *psychotropic drugs*. They are classified according to there mode of action (Table 3.22).

ANTIPSYCHOTIC (NEUROLEPTIC) DRUGS

Actions: These drugs act by blocking central dopamine receptors (D_1 and D_2), thus reduce the psychomotor excitement and control many of the symptoms of psychotic disorder without causing disinhibition, confusion or sleep. They possess sedative, hypnotic and antipsychotic properties.

Uses

- Acute schizophrenia
- To prevent relapse in chronic schizophrenia
- Mania
- Acute confusional states
- In low doses, they are used to treat anxiety.
- Phenothiazines are useful in the treatment of vomiting (antiemetic), alcoholism, intractable hiccups, over-dosage of hallucinogenic compounds and choreiform movements. Promethazine is used as an antiallergic agent.

Contraindications

- Subcortical brain damage
- Coma
- Circulatory collapse
- Impaired liver function
- Blood dyscrasias

Table 3.21: Safety of common antiepileptics during pregnancy

Drugs	Suspected adverse effects	Comments
Phenytoin	Fetal hydantoin syndrome (Facial dysmorphism, cleft palate and lip, cardiac defects, digital hypoplasia and nail dysplasia)	
Carbamazepine and Sodium valproate	Increased risk of neural tube defects Amniocentesis should be offered if abnormality suggested	• α-fetoprotein should be measured at 16 weeks gestation
Phenobarbitone and primidone	Increased risk of nonspecific defects	• Consider possibility of neonatal withdrawal syndrome
Benzodiazepines	Increased risk of oral clefts syndrome	• Neonatal withdrawal • Taper dose and withdraw before delivery if possible.
Newer drugs, e.g. gabapentin, lomotrigene topiramate, vigabatrin	Risk unknown	• Older agents are preferred during pregnancy at present

Table 3.22: Classification of psychotropic drugs

Actions	Main groups	Uses
Antipsychotics	• Phenothiazines Butyrophenones Thioxanthenes Substituted benzamides Benzisoxazole	Acute and chronic schizophrenia, acute confusion, mania
Antidepressant	• Tricyclic and related drug	• Depressive illness, obsessive compulsive disorder, nocturnal enuresis, neuropathic pain disorders
	• Selective 5 HT (serotonin) inhibitors • Tetracyclic • Mono-oxidase inhibitors	• Depression where sedation is not required • Obsessive-compulsive disorders. Depressive illness Depressive illness, phobic disorders
Mood stabilising	Lithium	Prophylaxis of mania depression, acute mania, mood disorders
Anxiolytics	Carbamazepine Benzodiazepines	Prophylaxis of manic depression • Anxiety and anxiety related disorders • Insomnia • Alcohol withdrawal
	Beta-blockers Buspirone, azapirone	Anxiety (somatic symptoms) Anxiety disorders

Side Effects (Box 3.8)

Dosage: The dosage of various groups of antipsychotic drugs is given in the Box 3.9.

The groups of antipsychotic drugs differ in their indications for use and side effects. Clozapine and resperidone have a much lower incidence of extrapyramidal side effects probably because of their strong blocking effect

BOX 3.8: ADVERSE EFFECTS OF ANTIPSYCHOTIC DRUGS

A. Extrapyramidal
• Acute dystonia
• Parkinsonism
• Tardive dyskinesia
• Akathiasia

B. Autonomic
• Hypotension
• Failure of ejaculation

C. Anticholinergic (atropine-like effects)
• Dry mouth
• Urinary retention
• Constipation
• Blurred vision

D. Metabolic
• Weight gain

E. Rare effects
• Hypersensitivity
• Cholestatic jaundice
• Leukopenia
• Skin reactions

F. Miscellaneous (others)
• Precipitation of glaucoma
• Galactorrhea-amenorrhea
• Cardiac arrhythmias
• Seizures
• Retinal degeneration (with thioridazine in high doses)

BOX 3.9: ANTIPSYCHOTIC DRUG DOSAGES

Group	Drug	Usual dose
Phenothiazines	• Chlorpromazine	100-150 mg/day
	• Thioridazine	50-80 mg/day
	• Trifenperazine	5-30 mg/day
	• Fluphenazine	20-100 mg/day
Butyrophenones	Haloperidol	5-30 mg/day
Thioxanthenes	Flupenthixol	40-200 mg fortnightly
Diphenylbutyl peperidines	Pimozide	4-30 mg/day
Substituted benzamides	• Sulpiride	600-1800 mg/day
	• Remoxipride	150-450 mg/day
Dibenzodiazepine	Clozapine	25-900 mg/day
Benzisoxazole	Resperidone	2-16 mg/day

on serotonin (S_2) receptors and relatively weaker dopamine receptors (D_2) blockade. Neutropenia and agranulocytosis are serious side effect, i.e. the drug has to be monitored by blood count and it must be stopped if neutropenia develops.

Indications of phenothiazines (Parenteral or oral). The parenteral therapy is given during acute conditions.

1. As an antipsychotic drug: They are used in the treatment of acute schizophrenia and to prevent its relapse.
2. Mania and acute confusional states.
3. As an anxiolytic and hypnotics.
4. Antiemetic. Used to prevent nausea and vomiting. They block dopamine receptors in chemoreceptor trigger zone.
5. Alcoholism

6. Premedication in anesthesia
7. Intractable hiccups
8. Overdosages of hallucinogenic compounds, e.g. LSD
9. Promethazine is used as an antiallergic
10. To prevent choreiform movements in rheumatic chorea
11. Induction of hypothermia

Toxicity (Overdosage) of Phenothiazines

Phenothiazines cause less depression of consciousness and respiration than other sedatives. The features of toxicity include:

I. *CVS:* Hypotension, shock, sinus tachycardia and cardiac arrhythmias (particularly with thoridazine)
   Treatment: Arrhythmias may respond to correction of hypoxia and acidosis but antiarrhythmic drugs may also be needed.

II. Dystonic reactions (particularly with prochlorperazine and trifluperazine) and convulsions may occur in severe cases
   Treatment: Dystonic reactions are rapidly abolished by injection of drugs such as benztropine or procyclidine.

Antidepressants and Mood Disorders

Depression: It is a disorder of mood, behavior and affect. It is unipolar primary affective disorder in which patient is gloomy, despodent and sad (depressed mood).

Mood disorders: These disorders are characterized by the disturbance in the regulation of mood behavior and affect. They are divided into:

1. **Primary affective disorders**
   - Unipolar - depression and mania, the recurrences always take either a depressive form (depression) or elation of mood (mania).
   - Bipolar - manic-depression. The recurrences are both manic (elation of mood) and depression (depressive mood).
2. **Secondary affective disorders.** They follow another psychiatric (alcoholism, schizophrenia) or physical illness.

   Treatment of depression requires co-ordination of short-term symptom, remission with long-term continuation and maintenance strategies designed to prevent relapse and recurrence.

ANTIDEPRESSANTS

There is no ideal antidepressant: no current compound has rapid onset of action, moderate half-life, low side effect profile, a meningful relationship between dose and blood level and minimal interaction with other drug. Therefore,

a rational approach to select an anti depressant to use involves knowledge of differences in pharmacokinetic activity and matching of patient preference and medical history with metabolic and side effect profile of the drug considered. About 60 to 70% of all depressed patients respond to any antidepressant drug chosen (Table 3.23) if it is given in a sufficient dose for 6-8 weeks.

Antidepressants should be prescribed in limited quantity at one time as they are dangerous in over dosage. Newer antidepressants (5-HT reuptake inhibitors) are less dangerous as compared to older tricyclics. It takes about a week or more of continuous treatment for suppression of symptoms. Optimal level of therapy should continue for another week before dose reduction is attempted. Premature withdrawal of medication can lead to recurrences of symptoms. Remission generally occurs after 3-12 months or even longer. Some patients respond to maintenance therapy with half of the therapeutic dose for several months to prevent a relapse. In recurrent depression, prophylactic maintenance therapy may be needed for several years.

Prescribing more than one antidepressant at the same time (polytherapy) is not recommended. Not only it may constitute a hazard but there is no evidence that side effects are minimized by the combinations.

Mixed preparations of an antidepressant with an anxiolytic are not recommended because individual doses need to be adjusted separately. Besides, antidepressants are given for long duration while anxiolytics are to be prescribed for brief periods.

Tricyclic Antidepressants

Action: They inhibit the reuptake of amines (noradre-naline and 5-HT) at synaptic clefts and this action has been used to support the hypothesis that affective disorders (e.g. depression) result from a deficiency of these amines which serve as neurotransmitters in the CNS. These are the drug of choice in the treatment of depressive illness. There is a delay of 2 to 3 weeks between the start of treatment and the onset of therapeutic effects.

Uses

1. Primary affective disorders such as depression.
2. Secondary affective disorders, e.g. depression associated with medical illness.
3. Along with anxiolytic, they are used for agitated depression.
4. Nocturnal enuresis or bed-wetting not due to an organic cause. A single dose at bed time for 6 weeks of either imipramine or amitriptyline is prescribed.
5. Neuropathic pains, e.g. trigeminal neuralgia, post-herpetic neuralgia, diabetic neuropathy, etc.

Table 3.23: Some commonly used antidepressants and side effects

Drugs	Usual doses	Adverse effects
A. **Tricyclic** *First generation*		All produce following side effects • Sedation (antihistaminic effect).
Amitriptyline	75-150 mg (<6 yr-10 mg 6>10-20 mg 11-16 yr: 50 mg)	• Anticholinergic effects, e.g. dry mouth, constipation, urinary hesistancy, blurred vision
Imipramine	75-150 mg (<12 yr-25 mg)	• Extrapyrimidal effects, e.g. tremors, dystonia,
Dothiepin	75-150 mg (>12 yr-50 mg)	dyskinesia.
Clomiplamine	75-150 mg	• CVS effects, e.g. hypotension, arrhythmias • Sexual dysfunction, e.g. impotence, impaired ejaculation. • Seizures, insomnia • Other effects, e.g. weight gain, headache, agranulocytosis
Second generation Amoxapine	150-250 (max 300 mg)	More potent, side effects less
Trazadone	150-250 mg	Amoxapine carries the risk of tardive dyskinesia; maprotiline
Maprotiline	150-200 mg	may produce seizure.
B. **Tetracyclic** • *Mianserin*	30-60 mg	Cardiovascular and anticholinergic side effects are less.
C. **Selective 5-HT reuptake inhibitors (SSRIs)**	Fluoxetine Fluroxamine Sertraline Paroxetine	20-80 mg /day 100-200 mg/day Not recommended 50-100 mg/day in children 20-50 mg/day
D. **MAO inhibitors**	Phenelzine Tranylcypromine Moclobemide	60-90 mg/day 20-40 mg/day 300-600 mg/day

Note: Start with the lowest dose and increase it gradually to achieve therapeutic response and then reduce the dose to half as maintenance dose.

Dose and Side Effects (Table 3.23)

Tricyclic antidepressants have anticholinergic and extrapyramidal side effects which are less with second generation tricyclics such as trazadone, amoxapine, bupropion, etc.

Tetracyclic Antidepressants (e.g. Mianserin, Maprotiline)

They differ structurally and in mechanism of action from tricyclic antidepressants. Mianserin is an alpha2-adrenoreceptor antagonist, also inhibits 5-HT uptake (weak effect)

Cardiovascular and anticholinergic effects are markedly reduced. Mianserin has sedatory effect.

Selective Serotonin Reuptake Inhibitors (SSRIs)

They include: Fluoxetine, Fluroxamine, Paroxetine and Sertraline).

Actions: They are selective inhibitors of 5-HT reuptake producing an increase in the amount of this neurotransmitter at central synapses.

Side effects: They have little or no effect on reuptake of other central neurotransmitters and so are virtually free of noradrenergic and cholinergic side effects. The side effects include; headache, nausea, anorexia, sleep impairment, sexual dysfunction, akathisia (an inner sense of restlessness and anxiety). A serious side effect of concern is **serotonin syndrome** thought to result from hyperstimulation of brain-stem 5-HT1A receptors and characterised by myoclonus, agitation, abdominal cramping, hyperpyrexia, hypertension, and potentially death.

Drug Interactions of SSRI

1. MAO inhibitors. They precipitate serotonin syndrome-an absolute contraindication.
2. Serotonin agonists, e.g. tryptophan, fenfluramine
3. Antipsychotics, beta blockers, calcium-channel blockers, codeine, terfenadine, etc.
4. Anticoagulants
5. Quindine

Dose: See the Table 3.23.

Monoamine Oxidase Inhibitors (MAO Inhibitors)

They include: Phenelgine, tranylcypromine.

Actions: They inhibit the metabolism of noradrenaline and 5-hydroxy-tryptamine (serotonin), hence, increase the availability of these neurotransmitters in CNS.

Uses

1. They are less effective than tricyclics for severe depressive illness but are especially effective for milder illness.
2. They are effective particularly when depression is associated with anxiety and phobic symptoms.
3. They are useful in management of primary phobic disorders.

Side effects: The common side effects include orthostatic hypotension, weight gain, insomnia, and sexual dysfunction.

Caution or Drug Interactions

They should not be used with:
  i. Foods rich in tyramine such as cheese, pickled herrings, degraded protein and red wine. There is risk of hypertensive crisis.
  ii. Amphetamines and opiates
  iii. *Dosage:* The dosage of antidepressants are given in the Table 3.23.

Side Effects of Antidepressants and their Management

They are given in the Table 3.24. The side effects are mostly dose-related, hence, to be managed with reduction in the dose and measures to relieve symptoms.

Mood Elevators/Stabilizers

They include:
1. Lithium carbonate: It is used in the treatment of mania and manic-depressive psychoses.
2. Carbamazepine is also effective in mania
3. Sodium valproate is equally effective in acute mania

Dosage and Side Effects: Table 3.25.

ANXIOLYTICS AND HYPNOTICS

These drugs relieve anxiety and its related symptoms and some may induce sleep. Anxiolytics include, benzodiazepine, beta blockers and azapirone (buspirone).

Benzodiazepines

These include: chlordiazepoxide, alprazolam, clonazepam, clobazam, diazepam, flurazepam, lorazepam, nitrazepam and oxazepam.

Actions: They exert sedative, anxiolytic, muscle relaxant and anticonvulsant actions for which they are used in medicine.

Uses

1. Chlordiazepoxide, diazepam, lorazepam and oxazepam, all are used in the treatment of anxiety and tension. Alprazolam is used as a day-time transquilliser. They are also used in phobic disorders, acute stress disorder and post-traumatic stress disorders.
2. Chlordiazepoxide and diazepam are also used in the treatment of muscular spasms e.g. during anesthesia and in tetanus.
3. Nitrazepam and flurazepam are used as hypnotics for insomnia.
4. Parenteral diazepam is used:
   1. As a muscle relaxant to relieve spasms in tetanus and as premedication during anesthesia.
   2. Status epilepticus
   3. Convulsions due to various causes
   4. Acute severe anxiety or medical illness
   5. As a sedative for surgical and other procedures
   6. Alcohol withdrawal.

Table 3.24: Antidepressants side-effects and their management

Symptoms	Management with special comment
Gastrointestinal e.g. nausea, loss of appetite	Usually short lived. Consider temporary dose reduction or administer with food and antacids
Diarrhea	Famotidine 20-40 mg/day
Constipation	Wait for tolerance. Diet change, stool softner and exercise. Avoid laxatives
Sexual dysfunction e.g. impotence, impaired ejaculation	• Consider drug reduction; drug holiday • Bethanechol, 10-20 mg 2 hr before activity or cyproheptadine 4-8 mg 2 hr before activity or amantadine 100 mg bid/tid.
Orthostatic hypotension	Tolerance unlikely, increase fluid and salt-intake. Use calf exercises/calf support; flurocortisone 0.025 mg/day.
Anticholinergic e.g. dry mouth, eyes	Wait for tolerance. Maintain good oral hygiene; Use artificial tears, sugar free gum
Tremors	Antiparkinsonian drugs are ineffective. Use dose reduction/slow increase, lorazepam 0.5 mg bid or propranolol 10-20 mg bid.
Insomnia	Schedule all doses for the morning, trazodone 50-100 mg at night
Sedation	Coffee, tea, schedule all dosing for bed time.
Headache	Evaluate diet, stress, other drugs, try dose reduction, amitriptyline 50 mg/day
Weight gain	Decrease carbohydrate, exercise, consider fluoxetine.

Table 3.25: Commonly used mood stabilizers

Drug	Dose	Side-effects and other effects
Lithium carbonate	Starting dose 300 mg bid/tid Therapeutic blood level 0.8-1.2 mEq/L	• Common side effects — nausea, anorexia, diarrhea, tremors, thirst, polyuria, fatigue, weight gain acne, neutrophilia, hypothyroidism. • Blood levels increased by thiazides, tetracycline, NSAIDs • Blood levels decreased by bronchodilators, verapamil and carbonic anhydrase inhibitors • Rare side-effects-Neurotoxicity, renal toxicity, cardiotoxicity, hypercalcemia.
Carbamazepine	Starting dose; 200 mg/bid Therapeutic blood level: 4-12 mg/ml	Nausea, anorexia, sedation, rash, dizziness, ataxia Rare side effects; hyponatremia, agranulocytosis, Stevens-Johnson syndrome
Valproic acid	Starting dose; 250 mg tid. Therapeutic blood level: 50-125 mg/ml	Nausea, anorexia, weight gain, Sedation, tremors, rash, alopecia Rare side-effects: Pancreatitis, hepatotoxicity, Stevens-Johnson syndrome

Dosage: The dosages of common anxiolytic drug are given in the Box 3.10.

BOX 3.10: COMMON ANXIOLYTIC DRUGS

Group	Drug	Usual dose
Benzodiazepines	Diazepam	2-30 mg/day
	Chlordiazepoxide	5-30 mg/day
	Nitrozepam	5-10 mg/day
	Temazepam	10-20 mg at night
Beta blocker	Propranolol	20-80 mg/day
Azapirone	Buspirone	10-45 mg/day

Note:
1. A short course of benzodiazepine is mostly preferred. Administration should be at the lowest dose possible and perscribed on an as-needed basis as symptoms warrant.
2. Benzodiazepines should not be prescribed for more than 4-6 weeks because of development of tolerance and the risk of abuse and dependence.

Side Effects

1. CNS effects e.g. drowsiness, light headedness, confusion, ataxia, vertigo, drug-dependence.
2. GI symptoms—nausea, gastric upset
3. Hypotension
4. Visual disturbance
5. Skin rashes
6. Urinary retention
7. Change in libido
8. Rare side effects include blood disorders and jaundice

Dependence and Withdrawal Symptoms

The benzodiazepines are known to cause dependence and withdrawal symptoms in many patients who have taken them for 6 weeks or more. Withdrawal symptoms occur especially with short-acting benzodiazepines (alprazolam, oxazepam) and if medication is stopped abruptly, the withdrawal symptoms may appear (listed in the Box 3.11).

BOX 3.11: BENZODIAZEPINE WITHDRAWAL SYMPTOMS

- Anxiety, confusion
- Epileptic seizures
- Heightened sensory perceptions
- Hallucinations
- Ataxia
- Paranoid delusions

Method of Withdrawal

Benzodiazepines withdrawal can be a problem and may be dangerous, hence, they are withdrawn slowly in step-wise fashion i.e one-eight of their daily dose is reduced after every two weeks to prevent withdrawal symptoms. Patients who are taking a benzodiazepine other than diazepam, can be transferred to diazepam in the following manner.

Step 1: Transfer to an equivalent dose of diazepam to be taken at night.

Equivalent doses: Approximately 5 mg of diazepam is equal to:

Chlordiazepoxide	15 mg
Alprozolam	0.5-1 mg
Lorazepam	0.5 mg
Nitrozepam	5 mg
Oxazepam	15 mg
Temazepam	10 mg

Step 2: Reduce the diazepam dose by 2.5 mg every two weeks. If withdrawal symptoms occur, maintain the dose till symptoms improve.

Step 3: Reduce the dose further, if necessary in smaller steps. It is better to reduce too slowly than too quickly.

Step 4: Stop completely. Duration needed to complete withdrawal can take a month or even a year or more.

Beta blockers should only be given, if other measures fail.

Drugs Used in Gastroenterology

Avoid adrenaline in patients with cardiovascular disease.

H₂–Blockers (Anti–hypersecretory Agents)

Action

They block the responses initiated by H₂-receptors stimulation such as gastric acid output.

Preparations

- Cimetidine—Not used nowadays because of side-effects
- Ranitidine
- Famotidine
- Nizatidine

Uses

- Healing of peptic (duodenal) ulcer
- Reflux esophagitis/gastroesophageal reflux disease
- Zollinger-Ellison's syndrome
- Drug-induced acute gastric erosions
- Fulminant hepatic failure to reduce the incidence of gastric erosions
- Poisoning—corrosive, aluminium phosphide
- Cerebrovascular accidents especially subarachnoid hemorrhage to reduce the incidence of stress induced acute gastric erosions
- Nonspecific dyspepsias or nonulcer dyspepsia.

Side Effects

- Dizziness, somnolence, fatigue, confusion and transient rashes
- Liver dysfunction i.e. rise in serum aminotransferases
- Blood—thrombocytopenia and leukopenia
- Hypersensitivity reactions, anaphylaxis

- Breast symptoms such as gynecomastia is seen with cimetidine, rare with ranitidine

Special Precautions

- Famotidine is not recommended for children
- They are not recommended in impaired renal function, pregnancy and lactation

Dose

Oral

Ranitidine—150 mg bid or 300 mg at bedtime
Famotidine—40 mg at bed time daily or 20 mg bid
Nizatidine—300 mg at bed time daily or 150 mg bid

Injections

- Ranitidine 150 mg IV slowly then 150 mg bid I.V infusion 12 hourly depending on the clinical condition
- Famotidine 20 mg I.V slowly over 2 minutes then 20 mg IV infusion 12 hourly depending on the clinical condition

Proton Pump Inhibitors

Hydrogen ions, accompanied by chloride ions are secreted in response to the activity of H^+/K^+ ATPase (proton pump) from the parietal cell membrane of gastric mucosa. The proton pump is the final step in production of gastric acid.

Actions

These are benzimidazole compounds that specifically and irreversibly inhibit proton pump (H^+/K^+ ATPase inhibitors) action and are most powerful inhibitors of gastric acid secretion. The maximum inhibition occurs within 3-6 hours after an oral dose.

Preparations and Doses
see Table 3.26.

Table 3.26: Proton pump inhibitors

Drug	Short-term	Maintenance	Side effects
Omperazole	20-40 mg once daily	20 mg at night	Hypergastrinemia, diarrhea, nausea, headache, skin rashes, dizziness, drowsiness, insomnia, myalgia, arthralgia and drug interactions with warfarin, phenytoin
Lansprazole	30 mg once daily	15 mg at night	Same as above
Pantoprazole	40 mg once daily	Not recommended	Same as above
Esmoprazole	20 mg once daily	do	Side effects are less and it is more potent than others
Rabeprazole	20 mg once daily	do	do

Uses

- NSAIDs and aspirin-induced acute gastric erosions
- Duodenal and gastric ulcers. In *duodenal ulcer*, it is used for eradication of *H. pylori* and to promote healing of the ulcer
- Reflux esophagitis or gastrointestinal reflux disease
- Zollinger-Ellison's syndrome

Contraindications

- Pregnancy and lactation
- Not recommended for children

H. pylori Infections

- The conditions associated with *H. pylori* infection are given in Box 3.12.

BOX 3.12: CLINICAL ASSOCIATION OF *H. PYLORI* INFECTIONS

- Duodenal ulcer—Strong association
- Gastric ulcer—Strong association
- Gastric cancer—Less common association
- Gastric β-cell lymphoma—Less common association

Diagnosis of H. pylori Infection

See Table 3.27.

Eradication of H. pylori

The antibiotic regimen is given in Table 3.28.

Table 3.27: Diagnostic methods of *H. pylori* infection

1. **Noninvasive tests**
   - *Serology:* Kits are available. The test lacks sensitivity and specificity, hence, is good for population studies
   - *Urea breath test.* It has high sensitivity and specificity but is costly
2. **Invasive methods** *(Gastric biopsy)*
   - *Histology.* It is sensitive, specific and cheap but it takes several days to process. False negatives occur
   - *Rapid urease test.* It is cheap, quick and specific but is less sensitive
   - *Microbial culture.* It is gold standard for diagnosis. It is laborious procedure

Anticholinergics (Cholinergic Receptors Blocking Agents)

Definition

Anticholinergics inhibit parasympathomimetic action with the result that:

i. They reduce secretion and motility of the stomach and intestines
ii. They increase heart rate and enhance atrio ventricular conduction
iii. They reverse cholinergic-mediated broncho-constriction and diminish respiratory tract secretions

Preparations

These include: *Dicyclomine, ambutonium, atropine, belladonna alkaloids, glycopyrronium, hyocine, hyoscyamine,*

Table 3.28: Antibiotic regimens for *H. pylori* eradication

1. **Triple Drug Regimens**			
First line		Second line	
OCM/LCM	OAC/LAC	OAM/LAM	BAM
• Omeprazole 40 mg OD or Lansprazole 30 mg 12 hourly plus	• Omeprazole 40 mg OD or Lansprazole 30 mg 12 hourly plus	• Omeprazole 40 mg OD or Lansprazole 30 mg 12 hourly plus	• Bismuth (CBS) 125 mg 6 hourly plus
• Clarithromycin 500 mg 12 hourly plus	• Amoxicillin 500 mg 12 hourly plus	• Amoxicillin 500 mg 12 hourly plus	• Amoxicillin 500 mg 12 hourly plus
• Metronidazole 400 mg 12 hourly	• Clarithromycin 500 mg 12 hourly	• Metronidazole 400 mg 12 hourly	• Metronidazole 400 mg 12 hourly
"Triple Regimen"	*"Triple drug Regimen"*	*"Triple drug Regimen"*	*"Triple drug Regimen"*
Duration 7 days	7 days	7-10 days	14 days
Efficacy 90%	90%	85%	80%
2. **Dual Drug Regimen**			
• Omeprazole 40 mg OD plus	For two weeks. It is less effective but more costly		
• Clarithromycin 500 mg tid			

isopropamide, mepenzolate, pipenzolate, piperidolate, poidine, clidinium and *ipratropium* etc.

Uses

They are used as;

- Antispasmodics to relieve gripping pain by smooth muscle relaxation
- Antidiarrheal agents to reduce motility
- Antipeptic ulcer medication
- Irritable bowel syndrome to relieve spasms
- Atropine is used in complete heart block and OP compounds poisoning (read atropine).

Side-effects

Dry mouth, thirst, dizziness, fatigue, sedation, blurred vision, rash, constipation, loss of appetite, nausea, headache, urinary retention and tachycardia.

Contraindications

- Glaucoma
- Obstructive disease of GI tract and intestinal atony or paralytic ileus
- Obstructive uropathy
- Myasthenia gravis
- Toxic megacolon in ulcerative colitis
- Hiatus hernia associated with reflux esophagitis

Special Precautions

They are to be used carefully in;

i. Pregnancy and lactation
ii. Prostatic enlargement
iii. Pyloric stenosis
iv. Autonomic neuropathy
v. Hyperthyroidism
vi. Children
vii. Where tachycardia is undesirable
viii. Elderly patients

Dosage

Oral

- *Oxyphenonium bromide* 5-10 mg 4 times a day
- *Dicyclomine* (10 mg tab) 10-20 mg 4 times a day
- *Propantheline* (15 mg tab) 15 mg 3 times a day before meals and 30 mg (2 tab) at night
- *Hyoscine* (10 mg tab) 20 mg 4 times a day *children* above 6 years 10 mg three times a day

Parenteral

- *Inj hyoscine* (20 mg/ml) 20-40 mg (IM, SC and IV) 3 or 4 times a day
- *Inj atropine* (0.6 mg/ml) 1-2 mg IV Dose depends on clinical situations (Table 3.29) *Inhalation*
- Ipratropium (Table 3.29)

Atropine and its Congeners/Derivatives

Actions and Uses

1. Atropine blocks muscarinic cholinergic receptors, with little effect on cholinergic transmission at the autonomic ganglia and neuromuscular junctions, hence, CNS effects of atropine or atropine-like drugs are due to blockade of muscarinic synapses. Because of this action, it is used in treatment of organophosphorous poisoning.
2. Atropine increases heart rate and enhances atrioventricular conduction. Because of these actions, it may be useful in combating sinus bradycardia or heart block associated with increase vagal tone (vagolytic effect).
3. Atropine reverses cholinergically mediated bronchoconstriction and diminishes respiratory tract secretions. Because of these actions;
   i. It is used as pre-anesthetic medication.
   ii. Its cogener ipratropium is used in acute severe asthma by inhalation (inhaler)
4. It decreases GI motility and secretion. Because of these actions its various derivatives and congeners such as propantheline, isopropamide and glycopyrrolates are used in patients with peptic ulcer and diarrheal syndromes/diseases.

Table 3.29: Cholinergic receptors blocking agents

Agent	Indication	Dose and route	Comment
1. Atropine	• Bradycardia and hypotension	0.4-1.0 mg I.V 1-2 hours	Competitive inhibition of M_1 and M_2 receptor; blocks hemodynamic changes associated with increased vagal tone
	• Heart block	1-2 mg stat then oral propantheline 15 mg tid	
	• Organophosphorous poisoning	1-2.0 mg every 5-10 min till the signs of atropinsation (dry mouth, mid-dilated pupil and increase in heart rate) appear, then slowly reduce the dose and withdraw it over a period of 5-7 days	• Competitive inhibition of muscarinic receptors
2. Ipratropium	• Asthma • COPD	500 mg by inhalation (nebulizer) tid or qid	Anticholinergic bronchodilator

5. Anticholinergics or atropine like drugs, e.g. benzhexol, benztropine, orphenadrine, procyclidine are used in the treatment of parkinsonism and drug-induced extrapyramidal disorders (read antiparkinsonism drugs).

Anticholinesterase Agents or Acetylcholinesterase Inhibitors

Acetylcholine is a neurotransmitter at the autonomic ganglia, at the postganglionic parasympathetic nerve endings, at the postganglionic sympathetic nerve endings innervating the sweat glands, and at the skeletal muscle end plate (neuromuscular junction).

Anticholinesterase causes hydrolysis of acetylcholine and inactivates the neurotransmitter at cholinergic synapses. This enzyme is present as true cholinesterase within neurons and is distinct from pseudocholinesterase present in plasma and non-neuronal tissue. The pharmacological effects of anticholinesterase agents are due to inhibition of neuronal (true) acetylcholinesterase.

Actions and Uses

Acetylcholinesterase (cholinesterase) inhibitors enhance the effects of parasympathetic stimulation by diminishing the inactivation of acetylcholine (Ach). They are used;
  i. In treatment of myasthenia gravis.
  ii. Termination of neuromuscular blockade following general anesthesia.
  iii. Reversal of intoxication produced by agents having central anticholinergic action e.g. atropine.
  iv. Cholinesterase inhibitors induce a vagotonic response in the heart and may be useful in terminating attacks of paroxysmal supraventricular tachycardia.

Contraindications

• Intestinal and urinary obstruction.

Special Precautions

• Asthma, bradycardia, recent MI, epilepsy, hypoten-sion, Parkinsonism, vagotonia, peptic ulcer, pregnancy and lactation.

Table 3.30: Anticholinesterase agents—doses and indications

Agent	Indication	Dose and route	Comment
Physostigmine	• Treatment of myasthenia gravis	Oral 60 mg 3 to 5 times daily	• Action begins within 15-30 minutes and lasts for 4 hours • At least partial improvement in most myasthenic patients although improvement is complete in few patients
	• Central cholinergic blockade produced by overdose of atropine and tricyclic antidepressants	IV 1-2 mg slowly	• Tertiary amine; penetrates the CNS well and may cause seizure
Edrophonium	Paroxysmal supraventricular tachycardia	5 mg IV (after 1.0 mg of test dose)	• Induces vagotonic response, rapid onset, short duration of action; effects reversed by atropine
Neostigmine	• Myasthenia gravis treatment • Central neuromuscular blockade	Oral: 15-30 mg at suitable intervals through out the day (Total dose 75-300 mg) Children < 6 yr initial dose 7.5 mg > 6 yr initial dose 15 mg *Parenteral (SC or IM)* 1 to 2.5 mg at suitable interval throughout the day (Usual dose 5-20 mg)	• It is quarternary amine, does not penetrate CNS • It is contraindicated in intestinal and urinary obstruction
	• Postoperative intestinal atony • Urinary retention	IM or SC at a dose of of 1 to 2.5 mg IM or SC at a dose of 1 to 2.5 mg	

Side Effects

- Nausea, vomiting, diarrhea, increased salivation and abdominal cramps.

Dosage: See the Table 3.30.

Signs of Overdose

- GI discomfort increased bronchial secretions sweating, involuntary defecation and micturition, miosis, nystagmus, bradycardia, agitation, hypotension, fasciculations and paralysis.

Dopamine Antagonist

Drugs

- Phenothiazines (oral and parenteral)
- Metoclopramide (oral and parenteral)
- Domperidone (oral)

Actions and Uses

1. *Anti-emetic*: Dopamine antagonists suppress proemetic stimuli by blocking D_2 receptors in chemoreceptor trigger zone. They are useful in relieving nausea and vomiting due to variety of conditions including those due to cytotoxic drugs. They are used prophylactically to prevent postoperative vomiting.
2. *Prokinetic effect*: Due to reduction in motility and increasing the tone of lower esophageal sphincter, they are used for treatment of reflux esophagitis or gastro-esophageal reflux disease and gastritis.
3. They are also used for *hyperacidity, nonulcer dyspepsia, hiatus hernia* and *hic-cups*.

Side Effects

- *Extrapyramidal reactions,* e.g. dystonia and tardive dyskinesia, parkinsonism
- *CNS*—depression, restlessness, drowsiness neuroleptic malignant syndrome
- *Raised serum prolactin* levels e.g. galactorrhea in nonlactating mothers.

Contraindications

- Pheochromocytoma and recent GI surgery

Dose

10 mg two or three times daily orally or parenterally.

Prokinetic Agents

Actions

- They facilitate or restore gastrointestinal motility by indirectly enhancing acetylcholine release from myenteric plexus
- They increase the tone of the lower esophageal sphincter
- They reduce gastric acid secretion also

Uses

- Gastro-esophageal reflux disease (GERD)
- Constipation (chronic)
- Gastroparesis associated with diabetes, systemic sclerosis and autonomic neuropathy.

Contraindications

- Not recommended for children
- Personal or family history of prolonged QT or ventricular arrhythmias, irregular heart beats or abnormal ECG and marked bradycardia
- Persistent vomiting or dehydration
- Pregnancy
- GI hemorrhage, obstruction or perforation
- Hypokalemia or hypomagnesemia

Side Effects

- *GI symptoms*—abdominal cramps, borborygmi, diarrhea
- *CNS symptoms*—headache, extrapyramidal effects, convulsions
- *Urinary*—increased urinary frequency
- *Cardiac*-arrhythmias
- *Liver* function abnormalities
- *Hyperprolactinemia.*

Preparation and Dosage

- *Cisapride*—It is a banned drug due to potential arrhythmogenic effect
- *Mosapride*—10 mg 3-4 times a day orally
- *Itopride*—10 mg 2-3 times a day.

Hormones

CALCIUM AND PARATHORMONE

Normal adult plasma calcium level is 2.2 to 2.6 mmol/L (9 to 10.5 mg%) and ionized calcium is 1.1-1.4 mmol/L (4.5-5.6 mg%)

The calcium in plasma is present in three forms i.e. *unbound or free calcium ions* (ionized calcium), *bound calcium* (ions bound to plasma proteins) and *diffusible complexes*. The concentration of ionized calcium influences many cellular functions (neuromuscular) and is subjected to tight hormonal control especially through parathormone (PTH).

Precautions

Never take the blood sample for calcium with the help of tourniquet or by manual compression of arm.

It is ionized calcium which is significant clinically hence, it should be measured by calcium specific electrodes.

If ionized calcium cannot be measured, then protein bound fraction can be calculated as follows

% protein bound Ca = 0.8 × albumin (g/L) + 0.2 × globulin (g/L) + 3

By substracting protein bound calcium from total calcium, one can calculate ionized calcium (approx).

Caution

The serum calcium should not be interpreted in isolation but with concentration of serum proteins which is an important determinant for which correction may be sometimes necessary. The correction is "Add 1 mg/dl to the serum calcium level for every 1 g/dl fall in the serum albumin level below 4 g/dl. For example, if serum calcium is 7.8 mg% but serum albumin is 3 g/dl then stated serum calcium (corrected) will be 7.8 + 1 = 8.8 mg/dl which is within normal range".

Hypocalcemia

Chronic hypocalcemia characterized by neuromuscular irritability and neuropsychiatric manifestations such as paresthesias, numbness (circumoral), cramps, tetany, convulsions, laryngeal stridor and psychosis results from a variety of causes (Box 3.13).

Tetany

Definition

This is a clinical condition characterized by low levels of ionized calcium (<4.8 mg%) leading to increase

---

BOX 3.13: CAUSES OF HYPOCALCEMIA

1. **Increased phosphate levels**
   - Chronic renal failure
   - Phosphate therapy
2. **Drugs**
   - Calcitonin
   - Diphosphonates
3. **Hypoparathyroidism (Congenital or acquired)**
   - Congenital deficiency e.g. DiGeorge's syndrome (intellectual impairment, cataract, calcification of basal ganglia, congenital cardiac and developmental defects, impaired immune response)
   - Idiopathic (autoimmune) hypoparathyroidism
   - Following neck exploration e.g. thyroidectomy, parathyroidectomy
4. **Resistance to paratharmone (PTH)**
   - Pseudohypoparathyroidism
5. **Vitamin D related**
   - Vitamin D deficiency
   - Resistance to vitamin D
6. **Miscellaneous**
   - Acute pancreatitis
   - Citrated blood transfusions

---

neuromuscular excitability. In this condition, total levels of calcium may even remain normal.

Latent tetany: Two clinical signs are helpful in latent tetany.

Trousseau's sign: The inflation of the sphygmomanometer cuff above diastolic blood pressure or 100 mm of Hg for 3 minutes induces tetanic spasms of fingers and wrist.

Chvostek's sign: Tapping over facial nerve near stylomastoid foramen results in twitching of facial muscles. Causes (see the Box 3.14)

For neuromuscular junction, calcium, potassium and magnesium are essential, hence, low levels of these cations lead to tetany. Alkalosis leads to tetany while acidosis prevents it.

BOX 3.14: CAUSES OF TETANY

Hypocalcemic	Alkalotic and hypokalemic
• Malabsorption	• Repeated vomiting
• Osteomalacia	• Excessive intake of alkalies
• Acute pancreatitis	• Hystericol hyperventilation
• CRF	• Primary hyperaldosteronism
• Anticonvulsants e.g. dilantin	• Acute anion load (e.g. citrate, lactate, HCO_3)
Hypomagnesemic	
• Idiopathic	

Indications of Parenteral Calcium Gluconate and Chloride

1. Calcium gluconate
- Tetany due to any cause
- Hyperkalemia
- Hypermagnesemia
- Acute hypoparathyroidism
- Pseudohypoparathyroidism

2. Calcium chloride is used in cardiac arrest and aluminium phosphide intoxications

ANTI–DIABETIC AGENTS

Oral Hypoglycemics (OHA)

Classification: They are classified into two groups;

1. *Insulin secretogogues (they stimulate insulin secretion by β-cells of pancreas)*
   A. Sulfonylureas
      i. *First generation:* Chlorpropamide, tolbutamide, Acetohexamide, Tolazomide
      ii. *Second generation:* Glibenclamide, glipizide, gliclazide, glimepride
   B. Nonsulphonylureas
      i. Meglitinide derivative-Repaglinide, Nateglinide.
2. *Insulin Sensitizers*
   A. Biguanides e.g. metformin, phenformin
   B. Thiazolidinediones derivaties e.g. rosiglitazone, pioglitazone
   C. Anti-obesity drugs
   D. Chromium piconitate
3. Inhibitors of carbohydrate absorption (α-glucosidase inhibitors)
   - Acarbose, miglitol, vouglibose
4. Miscellaneous
   - Glucagon like peptide-I
   - Guargum
   - Vanadium salts

Sulfonylureas

Mechanisms of Action

i. *Pancreatic:* They stimulate β-cells of the pancreas by binding to receptors i.e sulphonylurea receptors.
ii. *Extrapancreatic:* This effect includes an increase in the number of insulin receptors and enhancing the insulin-mediated glucose transport independent of increased insulin binding (pancreatic effect).

Indications of Sulfonylureas

1. Monotherapy: Type 2 diabetes (NIDDM)—Nonobese patients not controlled on diet and excercise are candidates for monotherapy.

2. Combination therapy: They can be used in obese type 2 diabetics not controlled on diet, excercise and maximum dose of metformin (a biguanide)
3. Other uses: Chlorpropamide is useful in the treatment of patients of diabetes insipidous as it sensities the renal tubule to antidiuretic hormone [ADH].
4. Repaglinide or nateglinide has also been used for control of postprandial hyperglycemia.

Dosage (Box 3.15)

Contraindications
- Type I diabetes
- Metabolic decompenzation with acidosis
- Diabetic coma or precoma
- Renal or hepatic insufficiency
- Pregnancy
- Patients exposed to unusual stress
- Hypersensitivity to sulphonamides

Note: The contraindications of OHA are actually indications of insulin.

BOX 3.15: ORAL HYPOGLYCEMIC AGENTS (OHA)			
Agent	Usual daily dose (mg)	Doses per day	Duration of action in hours
First generation drugs			
Acetohexamide	200-500	1-2	12-18
Chlorpropamide	100-500	1	60
Tolbutamide	500-3000	2-3	6-12
Tolazamide	100-1000	1-2	12-14
Second generation drugs			
Glibenclamide	2.5-20	1-2	12-24
Glipizide	2.5-30	2-3	6-12
Gliclazide	40-320	1-2	12-24
Glimepiride	1-6 mg	1	up to 24
Meglitinide			
Repaglinide	1-4	1	up to 24
Nateglinide	30-60	1	up to 24 hr
Biguanides			
Metformin	1500-3000	1-2	up to 24
Thiazolidinediones derivatives			
Rosiglitazone	2-8	1	up to 24
Pioglitazone	15-45	1	up to 24

Nonsulfonylureas (e.g. Repaglinide, Nateglinide)

Action

- They have action similar to sulfonylurea

Uses

- They are used as an alternative to sulfonylurea.
- In addition they are useful as a monotherapy or polytherapy for control of postprandial hyperglycemia.

Side Effects

They include, hypoglycemia, weight gain, nausea, diarrhea, skin reactions, paresthesias, cholestatic jaundice, blood dyscrasias and dilutional hyponatremia.

Insulin Sensitizers

It includes: biguanides and thiazolidinedione derivatives e.g. rosiglitazone, pioglitazone

Actions: Recently, it has been proposed that the insulin resistance—a characteristic feature of type 2 diabetes is due to insulin receptors.

Proliferative Peroxime Activating Receptors gamma (PPAR-γ) are associated with obesity and insulin resistance. Insulin sensitizers (metformin and thiazolidinedione derivatives-rosiglitazone and pioglitazone) act by stimulating these receptors and overcome insulin resistance and hyperglycemia of obese diabetics. By sensitizing the receptors to insulin, they cause peripheral utilization of glucose in peripheral tissues. Both these sensitizers differ slightly in their site of actions i.e. metformin inhibits hepatic ouput of glucose more than peripheral utilization; while thiazolidinedione derivatives are more specific to increase peripheral utilization of glucose than hepatic output. Due to their different site of actions, they can now be combined for obese type 2 diabetes not controlled with either. In addition, they improve the lipid profile of diabetics.

Indications of Biguanides

1. Monotherapy: They are used in obese type 2 diabetics not controlled on diet and exercise
2. Combination therapy: They can be combined with sulfonylurea or thiazolidinedione derivatives if type 2 obese diabetic is not controlled on maximum doses of metformin. It can be used with insulin.
3. Other uses: Metformin is used as antiobesity drug due to its anorectic effect (appetite killer)
4. They are used to lower blood sugar in patients with impaired glucose tolerance (IGT) to prevent diabetes.

Side Effects of Biguanides

Nasuea, vomiting, anorexia, diarrhea, metallic taste, weakness and rashes. Lactic acidosis occurs with metformin but infrequently. Hypoglycemia does not occur with either of them.

Thiazolidinedione Derivatives

Actions. They stimulate PPAR-γ receptors as described above, thus, increase the peripheral utilization of glucose in the tissues. They need the presence of insulin for their action.

Uses

- Monotherapy in type 2 diabetes
- Combination therapy. They can be combined with sulphonylurea or metformin if type 2 diabetes is not controlled with either of them.
- They are used to overcome insulin resistance in polycystic ovarian syndrome
- They can be used in patients with IGT to prevent diabetes.

Side effects of thiazolidinediones: upper respiratory symptoms, headache, light headedness, GI symptoms, weight gain, weakness, edema and occasionally hypoglycemia.

Contraindications

1. Old age >65 years
2. In the presence of renal insufficiency, hepatic insufficiency, cardiovascular disease, pulmonary embolism, tissue hypoxia, pancreatitis, excessive alcohol intake or concomitant use of diuretics.

Insulins

Actions of Insulin (Box 3.16)

BOX 3.16: PHYSIOLOGICAL ACTIONS OF INSULIN

Metabolism	Actions	
	Stimulation	Inhibition
Carbohydrates	• Uptake of glucose by peripheral tissues • Glucogenesis and glycolysis • Phosphorylation of glucose	Gluconeogenesis and glucogenolysis
Lipids	Triglyceride and fatty acid synthesis	• Lipolysis and ketogenesis
Proteins	Protein synthesis and amino acid transport	• Protein degradation
Potassium (K⁺)	Cellular uptake of potassium	——

Insulin Preparations

Insulin preparations contain either bovine, porcine or human insulin. Bovine and porcine insulins are obtained from the pancreas of cattle and pigs respectively, both these insulins are unpurified (contain contaminants >10 parts per million) and antigenic in nature, and may lead to complications. Purification of insulin is done to reduce the level of contaminants to less than 10 parts per million. This purification greatly reduces the antigenicity of the products. In this respect, it must be remembered that bovine insulin which differs from human insulin in their amino acids, is inherently more antigenic than porcine insulin which differ from human by only one amino acid.

Human insulin is obtained by either enzymatically replacing alanine with threonine in the porcine insulin molecule or by recombinant DNA techniques using bacteria *E.coli*. Both processes produce a molecule which is identical to human insulin. These insulins are less immunogenic (antigenic), hence insulin complications such as lipodystrophy, allergic reactions or acquired insulin resistance which were seen with unpurified insulin has virtually been abolished.

Classification of Insulin

The insulins are classified according to there mode of action irrespective of origin of insulin. They are listed in the Table 3.31.

Nowaday human insulins are manufactured by recombinant DNA technology

Table 3.31: Main human (purified) insulins and their duration of action

Insulin	Duration of action (hrs)
I. Unmodified action starts-within half	
A: Rapid/short acting	an hour
(neurtal or acid soluble	Peak- 2-3 hrs
• Actrapid*	Duration-6 hrs
• Nordisulin*	
• Humulin-S**	
II. Modified (Depot)	Action starts 1-4 hrs
(Cloudy solution, contain	Duration-upto 12-36 hrs
protamine in isophane or	
NPH and Zn^{++} in Lente	
prep)	
A. Intermediate Acting	12 hrs (approx)
• Monotard*	
• Insulatard*	
• Humulin-I**	
B. Long Acting	
• Ultratard*	24-36 hrs
• Humilin Zn*	
• Humulin-U**	> 36 hrs
III.Biphasic-Acting	Action starts within half an
(stable premixed preparation	hour, reaches its peak
containing fixed proportions	at 4-6 hr and remains up to
of soluble (rapid acting) and	12 hr
Isophane (intermediate	
acting) insulin such as 10:90,	
20:80, 30:70, 40:60, 50:50.	
• Mixtard 30:70	
• Humulin 30:70	
IV. Insulin analogs	
• Insulin lispro	3-5
• Insulin aspart	3-5
• Insulin galargin	24

In India, insulins are available in 40 units per ml in 10 ml vials; in USA and Britain, they are available as single strength i.e. 100 units/ml.

*Manufactured by Novo-Nordisk
**Manufactured by EI-Lilly

Indications of Insulin

1. Type I diabetes (IDDM)-An absolute indication.
2. Diabetic ketoacidosis or hyperosmolar non-ketotic coma
3. Types 2 diabetes (NIDDM) with primary or secondary sulfonylurea failure in nonobese persons.
4. Type 2 obese diabetics not responding to maximal doses of sulfonylurea, metformin and thiazolidinediones derivatives.
5. Gestational diabetes or diabetes with pregnancy.
   In this case, only purified, soluble human insulin is used for bringing round-the-clock normoglycemia or near normoglycemia.
6. Type 2 diabetics undergoing surgery, having complications, stress or acute infections or not controlled on OHA (Fig. 3.3).
7. *Non-diabetic indications*
   • Insulin with glucose therapy is useful for treatment of hyperkalemia/hypermagnesemia
   • Insulin-induced hypoglycemia is a test for GH secretion.
   • To prevent acute glucotoxicity postoperatively, neutralization of glucose is done by insulin.

Side Effects

1. *Hypoglycemia.* This is main side-effect of all types of insulins; the Somogyi effect and *Dawn phenomenon* may occur (Table 3.32).
2. *Lipodystrophy (tumefaction) at the site of injection.* To prevent this, site of injection of insulin should be changed frequently so that same area is not used more than once a month.

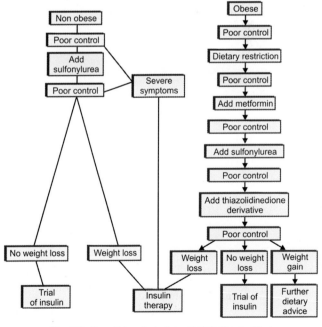

Fig. 3.3: Use of insulin in type 2 diabetes mellitus

Table 3.32: Distinction between Somogyi effect and Dawn phenomenon

Somogyi effect	Dawn phenomenon
• Early hypoglycemia followed by rebound hyperglycemia (Hypoglycemia begets hyperglycemia)	Early hyperglycemia which is not rebound phenomenon
• It is due to excess of night dose of insulin.	It is due to insufficient night dose.
• Early morning symptoms of hypoglycemia	Early morning symptoms of hyperglycemia
• It is due to counter-regulatory hormones mechanism e.g. release of glucagon, epinephrine and norepinephrine, cortisol and GH	It is due to nocturnal release of GH and increased insulin clearance in early morning hours
• It is abolished by reducing night dose of insulin	• It requires an increase in night dose of insulin

3. *Weight gain.*
4. *Insulin resistance.* It is defined as insulin requirement >200 units/day. It is due to anti-insulin antibodies. It is not seen nowadays with purified insulins.
5. *Allergic reactions*

The last two side-effects are not seen usually with purified insulins as they are less immunogenic.

The Somogyi Effect and Dawn Phenomenons

These two phenomena may be seen in patients receiving insulin, more common in children than adults. The differences are given in the Table 3.32.

Warning: Do not jump to increase the night dose of insulin on finding high levels of fasting blood sugar in patients who were previously controlled on the same dose of insulin because it could be due to either of two phenomenons and insulin is useful in one and dangerous in other. To differentiate between the two an early morning sample for blood sugar at 3 AM may be taken. The low value indicates Somogyi phenomenon while high value indicates Dawn phenomenon.

Regimens of Insulin Therapy

1. *Conventional*: single injections with each major meal(s). This is called two-dose or three dose regimen.
2. *Multiple subcutaneous injection of soluble insulin* in gestational diabetes.
3. *Continuous subcutaneous insulin by insulin delivery device such as insulin pump or pen injector.* This is given in educated and motivated patients who do not have visual impairment, can learn and practise the technique. It is easy, convenient, can be used in public places or restaurants or when patient is on tour or travel. This regimen can be used to treat diabetic ketoacidosis with soluble insulin.
   Calcuation of Insulin dose and dosing schedule (Box 3.17).

Assessment of Metabolic Control

• Urine estimation for sugar
• Self-monitoring of blood glucose e.g. fasting and postprandial
• Glycosylated Hb (HbA1 or HbA1c) It is done quarterly in all patients. It is formed by nonenzymatic glycation

---

BOX 3.17: INSULIN DOSE AND DOSING SCHEDULE

Total dose calculation = 0.5-1.0 U/kg/day

1. Two-dose regimen

Type of Insulin	*Dose and Frequency distribution*	
	Pre-breakfast	*Pre-dinner*
Insulin combination such as mixtard (30:70)	2/3 rd of total dose	1/3 rd of total dose

2. Three-dose regimen

Insulin	*Pre-breakfast*	*Pre-lunch*	*Pre-dinner*
Type	Plain	Plain	NPH or Lente
Percentage (%) of total dose	25%	15%	60%

3. Multiple dose

Type of insulin	Lispro	Lispro	Galargine

of amino acids of β-chain of Hb. It gives assessment of control of preceding 3 months. The values of HbA1c is more reliable and 1-1.5% lower than HbA1. Normal value of HbA1c is <6%.

There is close relationship between metabolic control and the incidence of vascular complications. The results of DCCT and UKPDS trials have concluded that diabetic complications are preventable and can be delayed with tight control (near normal glycemia). The targets of assessment defined in various studies is to keep HbA1c < 7% to prevent or delay the complications. The criteria recommended by European NIDDM Policy Group (Box 3.18) are Valid and well accepted.

<table>
<tr><td colspan="4">BOX 3.18: EUROPEAN NIDDM POLICY GROUP TARGET FOR CONTROL OF DM</td></tr>
<tr><td>Parameter</td><td>Good</td><td>Acceptable</td><td>Poor</td></tr>
<tr><td>Blood sugar (mg/dl)
Fasting</td><td>80-120</td><td><140</td><td>>140</td></tr>
<tr><td>Postprandial</td><td>80-160</td><td><180</td><td>>180</td></tr>
<tr><td>HbA1% (HbA1c%)</td><td colspan="3"><8.5(<6.5)8.5-9.5(<7.5) >9.5 (>8.5)</td></tr>
<tr><td>Urine glucose (%)</td><td>0</td><td><0.5</td><td>>0.5</td></tr>
<tr><td>Total cholesterol (mg%)</td><td>200</td><td><250</td><td>>250</td></tr>
<tr><td>HDL cholesterol (mg/dl)</td><td>40</td><td>>35</td><td><35</td></tr>
<tr><td>Triglyceride (mg/dl)</td><td>150</td><td><200</td><td>>200</td></tr>
</table>

Note: Value of HbA1c is lower i.e. <6% is normal, value between 6.0-6.5, 6.5-7.5 and 7.5-8.5% indicate excellent, good and fair control respectively. Values >8.5% indicate poor control.

Antithyroid Drugs

Actions

These drugs block the synthesis of thyroid hormones in the thyroid gland. Propylthiouracil in addition also decreases peripheral conversion of thyroxin (T_4) to tri-iodothyronine (T_3), i.e. a betablock effect.

Drugs

1. *Carbimazole* is a commonly used drug, methimazole is its active metabolite. The period of treatment. dose schedule and side-effects are given in Table 3.33.
2. *Propylthiouracil.* It is used in patients who are sensitive to carbimazole. It is more potent but dosage is 10 times higher than carbimazole. It is drug of choice for patients of thyrotoxicosis with pregnancy.
3. *Potassium Iodide.* It is not routinely used drug. It is indicated in hyperthyroidism to decrease vascularity in patients before undergoing surgery. It is helpful to control thyroid crisis or storm as an adjuvant to other drugs, hence, used in the emergency situation.
4. *Beta blockers.* A nonselective beta blocker (propranolol 120-160 mg/day or metoprolol 50 mg/day) is used for symptomatic relief. They prevent the conversion of T_4 to T_3 in peripheral tissue. They are used;
   i. Along with antithyroid drugs during initial period of 2-3 weeks.
   ii. Following ^{131}I treatment. It is used for short period.
   iii. During preparation of patient for surgery.
   iv. For transient thyrotoxicosis during thyroiditis.

Indications of Antithyroid Drugs

i. Initial treatment of all hyperthyroid patients
ii. Treatment of choice for young patients with hyperthyroidism
iii. Propylthiouracil is used for thyrotoxicosis during pregnancy
iv. Small goiter with thyrotoxicosis.
v. Preparation of patients for thyroidectomy or radioactive iodine therapy

Table 3.33: Two commonly employed antithyroid drugs with their dose and duration in thyrotoxicosis

Period	Drug and dosage	Purpose
1. Initial (0-3 weeks)	High dose • Carbimazole (15-20 mg 8 hourly or 1 mg/kg/day in divided dosage) • Propylthiouracil-150-300 mg every 8 hourly	To overcome the thyroid overactivity
2. Later on (4-8 weeks)	Moderate dose: Carbimazole 10 mg 8 hourly or propylthiouracil 150 mg 8 hourly	To bring euthyroid state
3. Lastly (12-24 months)	Maintenance dose: Carbimazole 5-20 mg/day or propylthiouracil 150 mg/day	To maintain normal T_3, T_4,TSH levels

Contraindications

- Hypersensitivity
- Carbimazole is to be avoided during pregnancy and lactation

Side Effects

- Leukopenia
- Agranulocytosis. Patient on carbimazole should have full blood counts every week
- Allergic rash
- Drug fever
- Arthralgias

Q. What are treatment modalities available for thyrotoxicosis?

Ans.

1. *Antithyroid drugs*—already discussed
2. *Radioactive treatment.* The dose of radioactive iodine ^{131}I is empirical (usually 5-10 mci orally). A second dose may be repeated after 3 months if no improvement.

Indications

- Patients more than 40 yrs of age (after completion of family)
- Recurrence following surgery
- Multinodular toxic goiter (treatment of choice)

Contraindications

- Pregnancy
- Mothers desirous of having a child.
- Older patients who refuse to undergo surgery.

Side Effects

- Hypothyroidism
- Congenital malformations in offsprings
- Susceptibility to carcinogenesis may be increased in the thyroids of children.

3. *Subtotal thyroidectomy*

Indications

- Large goiter or multinodular goiter with thyrotoxicosis
- Frequent relapse on drug treatment
- Young patients with hypersensitivity to drug therapy
- Poor drug compliance

Side effects

- Vocal cord paralysis due to damage to recurrent laryngeal nerve during surgery
- Wound infection
- Hemorrhage
- Hypothyroidism
- Hypoparathyroidism

Thyroxine Replacement Therapy

Preparations

Liothyronine, thyroxine (L-thyroxine), Liotrix (T_4/T_3 4:1) Thyroid extract USP.

Action

They increase the metabolic rate with subsequent increase in catabolism.

Uses

- Hypothyroidism (myxedema, cretinism), subclinical hypothyroidism, postpartum thyroiditis
- Various conditions associated with subnormal metabolism
- To suppress TSH in simple puberty goiter to reduce its size
- Myxedematous coma

Precautions

1. In neonatal, infantile and juvenile hypothyroidism, full replacement therapy or large dose therapy should be instituted as soon as possible, otherwise, the chances of normal intellect development and growth will be poor.
2. In patients of myxedema with heart disease, a small inital dose should be started, otherwise, angina will be precipitated.
3. In some adults, hypothyroidism should be treated rapidly such as myxedema coma or patients prepared for emergency surgery. In these patients, intravenous administration of L-thyroxine, in conjunction with use of hydrocortisone is indicated, but injectable preparation of thyroid hormone is not available, hence, oral therapy is usually employed.
4. In known or strongly suspected cases of pituitary or hypothalamic hypothyroidism, thyroid replacement should not be instituted until treatment with hydrocortisone has been initiated, since acute adrenal insufficiency will get precipitated by increase in metabolic rate induced by thyroxine.
5. Otherwise, in known case of adult hypothyroidism, start with small dose and then increase the dose at interval of 2 weeks till normal metabolic state is achieved.
6. The parameter of metabolic control is return of TSH to normal or near normal level in hypothyroidism due to thyroid origin; while level of T_3 is parameter of control in suprathyroidal hypothyroidism where levels of TSH are erratic and not reliable.

Doses and Side Effects (Box 3.19)

BOX 3.19: DOSAGE AND SIDE EFFECTS OF VARIOUS THYROID PREPARATIONS		
Preparation	*Average daily dose*	*Side effects*
L-thyroxine	100-150 mg/day as single dose (max 300 mg)	Palpitation, tachycardia anginal pain, weight
L-thyronine	50 mg	loss, diarrhea,
Liotrix (T_4/T_3=4:1)	24 units	restlessness, irritability,
Thyroid extract USP	120-180 mg	flushing, headache, sweating

SOMATOSTATIN (INHIBITOR OF GROWTH HORMONE RELEASE)

Actions

It is produced by the pancreas, inhibits the release of GH from pituitary. In addition, it has ability to inhibit secretions of various endocrine and exocrine glands e.g. gastric, pancreatic.

Uses

1. In the management of GI hemorrhage from esophageal varices, gastric or duodenal ulcers or acute erosive or hemorrhagic gastritis.
2. Adjuvant treatment in pancreatic, biliary and intestinal fistule.
3. Prophylaxis and treatment of postoperative complications following pancreatic surgery.
4. Adjuvant treatment in diabetic ketoacidosis.

Dose: 250 mcg by slow IV bolus over 3-5 min, continuous infusion 3 mg administered over 12 hours by infusion in either saline or 5% dextrose.

Contraindication: Pregnancy, immediate postpartum period, lactation

Side-effects: Nausea, vomiting, vertigo, flushing

Precaution: Type I diabetes in whom blood glucose to be monitored every 3-4 hourly.

Somatostatin Analog (Octerotide)

Action

It lowers GH level in acromegaly.

Indications

1. Octreotide is used for short-term treatment of acromegaly prior to pituitary surgery. It lowers GH level to <5 mg/L in 50% cases of acromegaly.
2. Long-term treatment for acromegaly when surgery, dopamine agonists or radiotherapy are ineffective or inappropriate.
3. As an interim measure before radiotherapy becomes effective in acromegaly.
4. It is used in management of GI hemorrhage.

Dose

Adult initially 0.05-0.1 mg 2-3 times daily by SC injection. Optimum dose 0.2-0.3 mg/day and maximum 1.5 mg/day.

Contraindications: Pregnancy, lactation

Side effect: Reaction at injection site, GI upset, gallstones and biliary colic.

Rarely, hyper or hypoglycemia, loss of hair, hepatic dysfunction, acute pancreatitis

SOMATOTROPHIN (GH)

Uses

1. Growth failure in children due to deficiency of endogenous GH.
   Dose: 0.09 IU/kg body weight SC injection daily or 0.02 IU/kg three times a week by SC or IM injection
2. Turner Syndrome (0.09 to 0.1 IU/kg daily by SC injection increasing to 0.11-0.14 IU/kg daily if required)
3. Growth failure in prepubertal children due to chronic renal failure

Dose: 0.15 IU/kg daily by SC injection

Contraindication: Epiphyseal fusion, progressive intracranial lesion

Side effects: Hypothyroidism, edema, pain at injection site and lipoatrophy

ORAL CONTRACEPTIVES

Definition

These are the drugs (pills) used against contraception and contain an estrogen and a progesterone.

Contraindications

1. Thrombophlebitis or thromboembolic disorders or past history of such disorders.
2. Cerebrovascular or coronary artery disease.
3. Known or suspected carcinoma breast and known or suspected estrogen dependent neoplasia.
4. Undiagnosed abnormal vaginal bleeding.
5. Known or suspected carcinoma of genital organs.

6. Known or suspected pregnancy.
7. Hepatic dysfunction, cholestatic jaundice or benign intrahepatic cholestatis, Dubin-Johnson or Rotar syndromes.
8. Sickle cell anemia
9. Abnormal lipid metabolism
10. Depression, migraine, epilepsy, otosclerosis, inappropriate hyperprolactinemia, pills to be used with caution in these disorders.

Adverse Effects/Caution

1. Use of oral contraceptive may be associated with increased risk of thromboembolism, stroke, myocardial infarction, hepatic adenoma, gallbladder disease and hypertension. Should any of these occur or be suspected, treatment should be discontinued. The risk of myocardial infarction is increased in females above the age of 40 years especially in the presence of other coronary risk factors.
2. Optic neuritis and retinal vein thrombosis have been reported. Discontinue drug pending examination if there is unexplained sudden partial or complete visual loss.
3. Ectopic as well as intrauterine pregnancy may occur in contraceptive failure.
4. The first spontaneous ovulation after stopping the oral contraceptive is sometime delayed or there is evidence of temporary impairment of fertility in women who discontinue oral contraceptives, but is not a proven fact.
5. Oral contraceptives may diminish the quantity and quality of the milk of lactating women.
6. Chances of benign breast tumors among the user have been well documented.
7. They impair glucose tolerance and predispose to diabetes. In diabetes, they may increase insulin requirement.
8. Oral contraceptive may cause some degree of fluid retention. Certain disorders such as cardiac or hepatic insufficiency, migraine and asthma may be aggravated.
9. Patient should be warned that vulvovaginal moniliasis may occur or recur, and may require appropriate treatment.
10. Pyridoxine and plasma folate levels may be depressed by oral contraceptives, hence, should be supplemented.

Drug Interactions

1. Antiepileptics (e.g. phenytoin, carbamazepine, ethosuximide), rifampicin, antibiotics (ampicillin, tetracyclines, chloramphenicol), barbiturates, chloral hydrate may reduce the efficacy of oral contraceptives and may lead to contraceptive failure.
2. Oral contraceptives reduce the efficacy of oral anticoagulants.
3. Oral contraceptives reduce the metabolism of antidepressants (imipramine) and lead to increased plasma levels

Missed Pill

Most of oral contraceptive pills are usually taken on 5th day of menstrual cycle and continued daily for 21 days without break for successful contraception. It must be remembered that the critical time for loss of protection is when a pill is omitted either at the begining or at the end of a cycle which lengthens the pill free interval (normal interval is 7 days approx). If a woman forgets to take the pill, she should be advised to take it as soon as possible preferably within 12 hours; and if she takes after that period, it may not work. Even when she restarts taking the pill, she may not be protected for next 7 days, hence, alternative family planning method must be adopted for protection.

Emergency contraception: It is designed to prevent pregnancy after unprotected sex. The precise mode of action is uncertain but the pill probably works by delaying or inhibiting the ovulation.

Preparation: The emergency contraceptive pill consists of 100 mcg of ethinylestradiol and 0.5 mg of levonorgestrel.

Dose: The first dose is to be taken within 72 hours of unprotected sex followed by next dose of same pill 12 hours later. Therefore, 2 tablets will make one course.

Side effects: Nausea, vomiting are common side effects and if they occur within 2 hours of ingestion of either the first or second dose, an extra dose should be taken immediately. An antiemetic drug taken one hour before the dose reduces the risk of nausea and vomiting.

Note: Only preparation of progesterone can also be used in place of a combined pill. The dose is 750 mcg of levonorgestrel. The dose schedule is exactly the same as described above

Follow-up: Abstinence from intercourse or careful use of barrier method should be taken during that cycle. The woman must be seen again after about 3 weeks after treatment to ensure that it has been successful.

Androgens and Antiandrogens

Male Sex Hormone (Androgens-testosterone)

Action: In normal male, they inhibit pituitary gonadotropin secretion and depress spermatogenesis

Uses

1. As replacement therapy in castrated males
2. Male hypergonadotropic hypogonadism (established)

Bedside Medicine

3. Cryptorchidism
4. Delayed puberty (androgen insufficiency)
5. Osteoporosis due to androgen deficiency-androgens act as anabolic hormones
6. Aplastic anemia. Androgens stimulate hematopoiesis.
7. They are used sometimes in cases of advanced breast carcinoma in women

Contraindications: Known or suspected male carcinoma breast or prostatic carcinoma; nephrosis, hypercalcemia, IHD and CHF.

Caution: Used with caution in patients of myocardial infarction, renal insufficiency, hypertension, prepubertal boys, nephrotic syndrome.

Side effects: Priapism, oligospermia and fluid retention, weight gain, increased bone growth, hypercalcemia, virilism in women, premature closure of epiphyses, decreased male fertility.

Dose: Free testosterone or testosterone propionate

- 25-50 mg IM twice a week for 4-6 weeks
  Oral testosterone undecanoate: 120-160 mg/day for 2-3 weeks then 40-120 mg daily according to response.

Danazol

It is a synthetic steroid which suppresses pituitary gonadotropin. It has no estrogenic or progestational activity.

Uses

1. It is used in endometriosis, menorrhagia, benign breast disorders, premenstrual syndrome. Dose is variable.
2. Gynecomastia and precocious puberty 100-400 mg daily for 2-3 months orally. Gynecomastia due to liver disease is a contraindication.

Contraindications: Pregnancy, lactation, porphyria, renal and cardiac edema.

Adverse reaction: Nausea, vomiting, rashes, dizziness, flushing, muscle spasm, anabolic effect (fluid retention, weight gain), headache, emotional lability, jaundice, benign intracranial hypertension.

GONADOTROPINS (FSH AND LH)

Actions

FSH

a. Female: It stimulates maturation of ovarian follicles. It does not cause ovulation.
b. Men: It induces spermatogenesis by acting on seminiferous tubules in the testes.

LH

a. Female: It acts on the matured follicle causing secretion of estrogens, follicle rupture, formation of corpus luteum and secretion of progesterone.
b. Male: It stimulates interstitial cells to form androgens.

Preparations

1. Human chorionic gonadotropin (hCG) from the urine of pregnant women has activity similar to LH.
2. Gonadotropin prepared from the urine of pregnant mares has mixed FSH and LH activity but predominantly FSH activity.

Uses

Combination of FSH and LH are used in:
  i. Anovulatory infertility, threatened habitual abortions
  ii. Hypogonadotropic hypogonadism in males
  iii. Cryptorchidism
  iv. Oligospermia

Side effects: Edema, headache, mood changes, tiredness, hypersensitivity reactions, sexual precocity

Drugs and Impotence

Impotence simply refers to failure to achieve erection, ejaculation or both.

Drug Therapy

1. *Sildenafil:* It is 5-phosphodiesterase inhibitor, prevents breakdown of GMP(cylic) in corpora and prolongs smooth muscle relaxation. It is useful in psychogenic impotence. It is taken orally 50-100 mg one hour before intercourse. Side-effects include, headache, nasal congestion, flushing, visual disturbance. It should be avoided in patients with IHD, CVA, sickle cell disease, hypotension and severe hepatic insufficiency.
2. *Alprostadil (Prostaglandin E-1)* Self injection into corpora covernosa produces erection in men in 90% patients with psychogenic, neurogenic, and mild to moderate vascular impotence. It is also used for neonatal congenital heart defects.
   Contraindications: The diseases which predispose to prolonged erection e.g. anemia, leukemia, multiple myeloma or drugs.
   Dose: 2-5 mcg by direct intracavernosal injection, increasing by 2.5 mcg to obtain desirable effect e.g. erection for not more than 1 hr. Usual dose is 10-20 mcg and maximum is 60 mcg.
   Side effects: Painful erection, prolonged erection, hematoma at site of injection, fibrosis, penile deviations, systemic effects (hypotension, arrhythmias, dizziness, headache, vagal shock and collapse).

3. *Penile prosthesis:* They are alternative to impotent patients refractory to other forms of therapy.

Anabolic Steroids

They include:
- Nandrolone decanoate
- Nandrolone phenylpropionate
- Oxymethalone
- Stanazolol

Actions

Anabolic drugs favor the increased retention of nitrogen, calcium, sodium, potassium, chloride and phosphate (positive balance), lead to an increase in skeletal weight, water retention and increased growth of bone (anabolism), oxymethalone in this group has an erythropoietic effect.

Uses

1. General debility or wasting diseases
2. Uremia
3. Senile and postmenopausal osteoporosis
4. Postsurgical convalescence
5. To promote growth in undernourished children
6. Adjuvant to steroid therapy
7. Oxymethalone and stanazolol may be used to stimulate erythropoiesis in aplastic anemia.

Abuse

They are abused for improving performance by athletes.

Contraindications

- Pregnancy
- Prostatic and male breast carcinoma
- Selected cases of female breast carcinoma

Side Effects

Table 3.34.

RECOMBINANT HUMAN ERYTHROPOIETIN

Action: It stimulates the erythropoiesis by its action on the mesenchymal stem cells in the bone marrow. This action is similar to endogenous erythropoietin secreted by the kidneys.

Indications: Administration of recombinant erythropoietin is the treatment of choice for anemia in patients with chronic renal failure both before and after dialysis. Treatment is instituted if the hematocrit is less than 30%.

Dose: The starting dose is approximately 25-50 units /kg/ three times a week either subcutaneously (SC) or intravenously (IV). Increase in dosage may be needed after 8-12 weeks with monitoring of hematocrit after every 2-4 weeks.

Causes of Erythropoietin Resistance

- Iron deficiency
- Aluminium toxicity
- Marrow fibrosis from hyperparathyroidism
- Chronic inflammatory states
- Primary hematological disease.

Special precaution: About 30% patients on chronic erythropoietin therapy may have increase in severity of hypertension which should be treated appropriately by antihypertensive therapy.

Causes of anemia in CRF: The anemia is normocytic normochronic. It is due to;
- Iron or folate or both deficiency
- Hemolysis (extracorpuscular destruction)
- Bone marrow suppression by uremic toxins

Table 3.34: Common anabolic steroid

Drug	Dosage	Side effects	Comment
• Nandrolone phenylpropionate	*Adult* 25-50 mg I.M/week *Children* 5-10 mg I.M/week	• Edema, virilization in women, hypercalcemia	• Short-acting preparation
• Nandrolone decanoate	*Adult:* 25-50 I.M every 3 weeks *Children:* 5-15 mg I.M after every 3 week *Oral: Adult.* 2 mg tid *Children.* 2 mg bid	- same -	• Long-acting preparation
• Stanazolol	*Oral:* 2-4 mg tid with meals	• Hepatotoxicity, virilisation in women and pre-pubertal children, rashes, dyspepsia, cramps, headache.	• Can be used in aplastic anemia
• Oxymethalone	*Oral:* 2 mg/kg/day in divided doses	• Hepatotoxicity, jaundice, edema, virilization, hypercalcemia, hyperlipidemia	• For aplastic anemia, therapy is used for 2-6 months

- Impaired erythropoietin synthesis
- Bleeding from GI tract (chronic blood loss)
- Blood loss is exaggerated in patients on hemodialysis because of use of heparin during dialysis and the retention of blood in the dialyzer and associated tubing.

CORTICOSTEROIDS

The adrenal cortex secrets glucocorticoid (hydrocortisone or cortisol) which has major effect on intermediary metabolism, and mineralocorticoid (aldosterone) which has major effect on minerals (sodium and potassium) metabolism.

Normal glucocorticoid secretion is 15-30 mg with pronounced circadian rhythm; increases up to 300 mg during acute stress.

Normal mineralocorticoid secretion is 50-250 mg. Corticosteroids secretion is controlled by ACTH by feedback mechanism.

Actions

1. *Metabolic functions*: Physiological effects of glucocorticoids include the regulation of carbohydrate, protein, nucleic acid and lipid metabolism.
   - *Carbohydrate metabolism*: Glucocorticoids raise blood sugar levels by promoting hepatic glucose synthesis (gluconeogenesis) and inhibit peripheral utilization of glucose by inhibiting insulin action (anti-insulin effect)
   - *Protein metabolism*: Glucocorticoids result in protein catabolism with the result that there is increased protein breakdown and nitrogen excretion. This action results in mobilization of proteins from peripheral tissues such as bone, muscle, skin and connective tissue for catabolism
   - *Nucleic acid*: They inhibit the synthesis of nucleic acid in most body tissues
   - *Fat metabolism*: They regulate fatty acid mobilization by enhancing the activation of cellular lipase by lipid-mobilizing hormones (e.g. catecholamines and pituitary peptides). This results in redistribution of fat
2. *Anti-inflammatory*: They have anti-inflammatory properties probably related to suppression of inflammatory cytokines (inhibit the production and action of the mediators of inflammation e.g lymphokines and prostaglandins).
3. *Antiallergic*: They inhibit the release of allergic substances from the eosinophils.
4. *Immunosuppressive*: At higher doses (1 mg/kg), the antibody production is reduced and lysosomal membranes are stabilized. Due to this effect, corticosteroids are used as immunosuppressive drugs.
5. *Water and electrolyte metabolism*: Cortisol at high doses promotes renal tubular sodium reabsorption and its subsequent retention and in exchange causes loss of potassium in the urine. There is passive movement of water along with sodium. This results in hypokalemia with fluid and Na^+ retention resulting in hypertension and edema.

   It also regulates the extracellular fluid volume by retarding the migration of water into the cells. This fluid overload is overcome by solute free water clearance by inhibition of vasopressin secretion by corticosteroids. This action prevents water intoxication.
6. *Suppression of pituitary peptides (ACTH, β-endorphin and β-lipoproteins)*: Cortisol suppresses the secretion of pituitary peptides and the secretion of hypothalamic CRH and vasopressin. The suppression of ACTH and CRH is via pituitary adrenal axis. Due to this action, it is used as a diagnostic tool (dexamethasone suppression test) for diagnosis and differential diagnosis of Cushing's syndrome.

Uses

Because of above mentioned actions, they are systemically used in variety of disorders. Before using them, one must consider that "*they are like a glass to be handled with care*". Therefore, corticosteroids should not be used unless the benefits clearly overweigh the hazards. In any event the lowest dose which will produce desired response should be employed. In certain diseases such as exfoliative dermatitis, pemphigus, acute leukemia, higher doses may be required justifiably because complications of treatment are likely to be less serious than the effects of the disease itself. The initial dose of the drug should be tapered slowly so as to avoid "Addisonian crisis". Their prolonged use may result in "steroid-dependence". The common uses are given in the Table 3.35.

Side Effects

The clinical picture of Cushing's syndrome is due to excessive secretion of endogenous glucocorticoids. If corticosteroids are given from outside for prolonged period, will also result in features simultating Cushing's syndrome (cushingoid features), conveniently called *iatrogenic Cushing's syndrome*. The side effects are summarized in the Table 3.36.

1. **GI tract disorders**
   - Celiac disease (gluten-induced enteropathy)
   - Inflammatory bowel disease
2. **Liver disease**
   - Autoimmune hepatitis
   - Alcoholic liver disease (severe)
   - Primary biliary cirrhosis
3a. **Lymphoreticular disorders**
   - Hodgkin's disease (MOPP regimen)
   - Non-Hodgkin lymphoma (CHOP regimen)
3b. **Skin disorders**
   - Exfoliative dermatitis
   - Skin allergies
   - Pemphigus
   - Anaphylaxis (systemic) and urticaria
4. **Blood disorders**
   - Autoimmune hemolytic anemia
   - Acute leukemias
   - Multiple myeloma (melphalan plus prednisolone)
   - Idiopathic thrombocytopenic purpura
   - Blood transfusion reactions
5. **Joint and connective tissue disorders**
   - Rheumatoid arthritis
   - Collagen vascular disorders such as SLE, dermato-myositis, Sjögren's syndrome
   - Eosinophilic fasciitis
   - Relapsing polychondritis
   - Systemic vasculitis
6. **Neurological disorders**
   - Cerebral edema
   - Demyelinating disorders
   - Bell's palsy
   - Myasthenia gravis
7. **Respiratory disorders**
   - Bronchial asthma
   - Hypersensitivity pneumonitis (severe)
   - Idiopathic pulmonary fibrosis (interstitial lung disease)
   - ARDS (early stage)
8. **Renal disorders**
   - Immune-complex glomerulonephritis and nephrotic syndrome
   - Nephropathy associated with collagen vascular disorders
   - Hypersensitivity nephropathy
9. **Cardiovascular disorders**
   - Acute rheumatic carditis in children
   - Some cases of myocarditis associated with conduction blocks
10. **Endocrinal disorders**
    - Adrenocortical insufficiency (Addison's disease) or following bilateral adrenalectomy
    - Panhypopituitarism
    - Thyrotoxic crisis
    - Grave's ophthalmopathy (severe)
    - Subacute thyroiditis

Table 3.36: Side effects of systemic corticosteroids

Endocrine
- Moon-like face
- Truncal obesity, camel hump
- Excessive hair growth (hirsutism)
- Impotence

- Menstrual irregularity
- Growth suppression
- Suppression of hypo-thalamo-pituitary-adrenal axis

Metabolic
- Fluid and sodium retention leading to edema
- Negative Ca^{++}, K^+ and nitrogen balance
- Hyperglycemia
- Hyperlipoproteinemia
- Hypokalemic alkalosis

Skin
- Acne, strie (pink)
- Bruising
- Skin atrophy
- Impaired wound healing

Immunological
- Reactivation of tuberculosis
- Suppression of delayed hypersensitivity (tuberculin test will be negative in a person on steroids)
- Susceptibility to infections

Musculoskeletal
- Myopathy and weakness
- Osteoporosis, spontaneous fractures
- Avascular necrosis
- Suppression of bone growth in children

GI tract
- Peptic ulcer
- Pancreatitis

Cardiovascular
- Hypertension
- CHF

Ocular
- Glaucoma
- Cataract

CNS
- Change in mood and personality
- Steroid psychosis
- Benign intracranial hypertension

Q. What are life-saving indications of steroids?
Ans.

1. *Adrenal crisis*: It is acute adrenal insufficiency precipitated by sepsis, trauma, anticoagulant therapy or sudden withdrawal of steroids from a patient with presumed adrenal atrophy owing to chronic steroid administration.
2. *Acute systemic anaphylaxis.*
3. *Acute severe asthma* with hypoxia (status asthmaticus).
4. *Acute cerebral edema.*
5. *Waterhouse-Friderichsen syndrome*: It is acute adrenal insufficiency associated with septicemia due to Pseudomonas or meningococcemia in children without an evidence of prior adrenal insufficiency (healthy children).
6. *Acute attack of multiple sclerosis or acute disseminated encephalomyelitis.*
7. *Unexplained shock.*

Contraindications

The patients must be screened for following disorders before use either by history or by investigations.

1. *Chronic infection* such as tuberculosis. Steroids may reactivate the tuberculosis. It should not be used in presence of viral and fungal infections. In addition, person on steroids should not undergo immunization.
2. *Diabetes mellitus.* Steroids may unmask or aggravate diabetes mellitus. Patient of glucose intolerance may develop frank diabetes called *chemical diabetes.*
3. *Osteoporosis* due to any cause.
4. *Peptic ulcer, gastric hypersecretion* or *esophagitis.* There will be exacerbation of symptoms and increased risk of peptic ulcer perforation.
5. Hypertension, CHF, thrombembolic tendencies.
6. Psychological diseases—psychosis
7. Renal failure.

Preparations

The various preparations with their duration of action and glucocorticoid and mineralocorticoid activity are summarized in the Table 3.37.

Precautions Before Use

- Use them when absolutely necessary. Balance the risks vs benefits of steroids
- Use the smallest effective dose. The dosage of steroids is less when used as anti-inflammatory agents than for immunosuppression
- Withdrawal of glucocorticoids following long-term use: Reduce the dose of steroid gradually by 5 mg every 3-5 days and eventually to discontinue a daily steroid dose under most circumstances. Withdrawal of steroids should be initiated by first shifting the patient on alternate day schedule on the same dose. Patients who have been on alternate day program for a month or more experience less difficulty during termination regimen. The dose is gradually reduced and finally discontinued after a replacement dose has been reached (e.g. 5 to 10 mg prednisolone)

  In patients on high dose daily steroid therapy, it is advised to reduce the dose slowly to 20 mg prednisolone daily as a single dose before shifting to alternate-day therapy. If a patient cannot tolerate an alternate-day regimen, consideration should be given to the possibility that the patient has developed primary adrenal insufficiency.
- When used as replacement therapy for Addison's disease, two-third dose should be given in the morning and one-third dose in the evening to maintain circadian rhythm.
- For long-term use of steroids, initial steroid program often requires daily or more frequent doses of intermediate acting steroid (prednisolone) to achieve the desired effect. Once desired effect is achieved, attempt should be made to switch on alternate-day-morning program before withdrawal.

Route of Administration

The routes are oral, parenteral, intra-ocular, intradermal, topical, intrarectal (retention enema), intrapleural and intrarticular.

Table 3.37: Commonly used glucocorticoid preparations

Name	Biological half life (hrs)	Dose	Comment
Short acting Hydrocortisone Cortisone	< 12 hours	IV 100-200 mg after 6 hrs	• They have equal glucocorticoid and mineralocorticoid activity
Intermediate acting Prednisone	12-36 hrs		• They are 4-5 times more potent than short acting drugs
Prednisolone		Oral 10-20 mg/day as single dose 60 mg/day (severe case)	• They have potent glucocorticoid activity with less mineralocorticoid effect
Methyl prednisolone		IV or IM 1gm/day	• Methyl prednisolone has least mineralocorticoid effect
Triamcinolone			
Long-acting • Betamethasone	> 48 hrs	Oral 0.5-5 mg/day I.V or I.M 4-20 mg three or 4 times a day if required	• They are 5 times more potent than intermediate acting and 20-25 times than short acting drugs
• Dexamethasone		Oral 0.5-10 mg IV or IM 0.5-20 mg repeated as required	• They have excellent glucocorticoid activity with least mineralocorticoid effect

397

ACTH

- It is a naturally synthesized hormone by pituitary gland

Uses

- It is used in pituitary adrenal insufficiency
- It is used as a diagnostic test for differential diagnosis of Cushing's syndrome to determine its cause
- It can be used in all other conditions where steroids are indicated except as replacement therapy where steroids only are given.

Q. What are indications for high-dose corticosteroid therapy?

Ans.
- Status asthmaticus (acute severe asthma)
- Cerebral edema
- For immunosuppression
- Unexplained shock
- Enteric encephalopathy: It is used as an adjunct to antimicrobial therapy.

Infections, Infestations and Vaccination

ANTIMICROBIAL DRUGS/AGENTS

- These are drugs/agents used against microbes
- Infection means presence of bacteria in the host
- Disease means reaction to the infection

Stages of Bacterial Infection and Disease

I. Bacterial entry and colonization of the host
II. Invasion by bacteria and growth in host tissue and liberation of toxic substances (toxins)
III. The host response.

The organisms causing infection are given in the Box 3.20.

BOX 3.20: GRAM-POSITIVE AND NEGATIVE ORGANISMS

Gram-positive organisms
- *Cocci* e.g. staphylococci, streptococci
- *Bacilli* e.g. *C. diphtheria, Listeria, Clostridium, B. anthrax*

Gram-negative organisms
- *Cocci* e.g. meningococci, gonococci
- *Bacilli* e.g. *Brucella, Bordetella (Pertussis, Hemophilus, V. cholerae*, enterobacteriacea (e.g. *E. coli, Salmonella, Shigella), Compylobacter, Helicobacter, Yersinia, tularemia, Pseudomonas, Klebsiella, Legionella* etc.

Mechanisms of Action

1. *Inhibition of cell wall synthesis*
   - β-lactams (penicillins and cephalosporins)
   - Vancomycin
   - Bacitracin
2. *Inhibition of protein synthesis*
   - Macrolides
   - Lincosamides
   - Chloramphenicol
   - Tetracyclines
   - Aminoglycosides
   - Mupirocin
3. *Inhibition of bacterial metabolism*
   - Sulphonamides and trimethoprim
4. *Inhibition of nucleic acid synthesis or activity*
   - Rifampicin
   - Nitrofurantoin
   - Novobiocin
   - Metronidazole
   - Quinolones
5. *Alteration of cell membrane permeability*
   - Gramicidin
   - Polymyxins

Q. What is spectrum and uses of penicillin G?

Ans. The organisms sensitive to penicillin and diseases caused by them are as follows:

Organisms	Diseases
• *Spirochetes*	Syphilis, yaws, leptospirosis
• Streptococci (group A and B viridan and *Streptococcus pneumoniae*)	Group A and B streptococcal infections i.e. upper and lower respiratory tract infections, urinary tract infection, cellulitis, endocarditis, peridental infection, brain abscess, meningitis, puerperal sepsis, empyema
• Meningococcal infection	Meningococcemia and meningococcal meningitis
• *Neisseria*	Gonococcal infections i.e. uretheritis
• Clostridia except myonecrosis	Tetanus and clostridial infection, e.g. clostridia perfringens (gas gangrene). Penicillin is not effective against C. difficile infection i.e. pseudomembranous colitis
• *Actinomyces*	Actinomycosis
• *Bacteroides*	Peri-dental infections
• *Anthrax*	Anthrax infection

Indications of Ampicillin/Amoxicillin

i. In addition to above mentioned diseases where ampicillin can be used, the other indications are infections caused by;
   - *E. coli* producing urinary tract infection
   - *Salmonella* causing enteric fever and *Salmonella* enteric infections
   - Shigella causing bacillary dysentery
   - *H. influenze* causing meningitis
ii. Ampicillin/amoxicillin is used in regimen for *H. pylori* eradication.

Name the β-lactamase inhibitors and what are their Uses?

β-lactamase inhibitors are:
- Clavulanic acid
- Sulbactam
- Tazobactam

Uses

They are added to ampicillin, amoxicillin, ticarcillin or piperacillin to extend the spectrum of these agents to cover many other organisms such as *E. coli, Klebsiella*, B-proteus, *H. influenze* and β-lactamase producing staphylococci.

Q. Name the antipseudomonal penicillins
Ans. • Read the classification (Table 3.38).

Table 3.38: Classification and parenteral preparations of β-lactam antibiotics

Class	Parenteral preparations
1. *Penicillins*	
A. *β-lactam susceptible*	
• Narrow spectrum	Penicillin G, procaine penicillin, benzathine penicillin
• Enteric active	Ampicillin, amoxicillin
• Enteric-active and	Carbenicillin, ticarcillin
anti-pseudomonal	mezlocillin, azlocillin, piperacillin
B. *β-lactam-resistant*	
• Antistaphylococcal	Methicillin, oxacillin, nafcillin
• Combination with	Ticarcillin plus clavulanic acid
β-lactamase inhibitors	Ampicillin plus sulbactam
	Piperacillin plus tazobactam
2. *Cephalosporins*	
A. *First generation*	cefazolin, cephalothin, cephradine, cephalexin, cefadroxil
B. *Second generation*	
• Hemophilus active	cefamandole, cefuroxime, cefonicid, ceforanide
• Bacteroides active	cefoxitin, cefotetan, cefmetazole
C. *Third generation*	
• Extended spectrum	ceftriaxone, cefotaxime, ceftizoxime
• Extended spectrum	ceftazidime, cefoperazone
and antipseudomonal	
D. *Fourth generation*	cefepime, cefpicome
3. *Carbapenems*	Imipenem cilastatin
4. *Monobactams*	Aztreonam

Q. Name the long-acting penicillins. What are its indications?

Ans. Benzathine penicillin—(commercial vials contain, 6 millions and 12 millions units for IM use)

Oral Penicillins

• Becampicillin hydrochloride
• Phenoxymethyl penicillin (penicillin V)
• Penicillin potassium

Uses

• Prophylaxis against SABE
• Used for treatment of recurrent streptococcal infections where therapy for prolonged period with penicillin is desired such as syphilis, pyoderma, post-traumatic tetanus

Side Effects

It includes
• Skin rashes
• Pruritus
• Urticaria
• Herxheimer's reaction e.g. *Jerisch Herxheimer reactions*
• GI tract symptoms—nausea, vomiting, pseudomembranous colitis
• Blood—thrombocytopenia, leukopenia, eosinophilia
• Rise in transaminases

• Irritation at the injection site. IV therapy may cause vein irritation and phlebitis
• High parenteral therapy may produce CNS toxicity including convulsions
• Prolonged therapy will result in opportunistic infection by resistant organisms

Precautions

Serious and sometimes fatal hypersensitivity reactions (anaphylactoid) may occur, hence, care should be taken in patients with known allergies such as hay fever, asthma, urticaria, nasal allergy, etc. It should be used with caution in patients with infectious mononucleosis, or lymphatic leukemia since they are susceptible to penicillin induced rashes. During prolonged therapy, blood counts, hepatic and renal functions are to be monitored.

Dosage Schedule

See Table 3.39.

Injectable Penicillin Combinations

The common combinations used are;
• Ampicillin plus cloxacillin
• Ampicillin plus salbactum
• Amoxicillin plus cloxacillin
• Amoxicillin plus clavulanic acid
• Ticarcillin plus clavulanic acid

Meningitis		
1. Pneumococcal	Benzyl penicillin or cefotaxime	24 million units of penicillin/24 hr given in divided doses at 4 hours interval or cefotaxime 2 g every 6 hr. Duration of therapy is 10-14 days.
2. Meningococcal	Penicillin as above	In addition give rifampicin for 2 days before hospital discharge
3. *H. influenze*	Chloramphenicol or cefotaxim	Chloramphenicol (1 g I.V every 6 hrly) or cefotaxime IV 2 g after every 6 hr.
Endocarditis		
	1. Penicillin sensitive streptococci	

Penicillins injectable preparations sharing pharmacological class
Generic name and their combinations

Ampicillin (injections and oral) Combinations	*Amoxicillin (available as oral and parenteral prep)* Combinations
• Ampicillin + cloxacillin	Amoxicillin + cloxacillin
• Ampicillin + cloxacillin	Amoxicillin + clavulanic acid
• Ampicillin + sulbactam	
• Tircacillin + clavulanic acid	Piperacillin Tazobactam

Monotherapy vs Combination Therapy

The common rule for antibacterial therapy is that if the infecting organism is identified, the most specific agent according to culture and sensitivity may be used. The advantage of monotherapy are:

i. It does not alter the normal flora and thus limits the overgrowth of resistant nosocomial organisms e.g. *Candida albicans*, enterococci, *Clostridium* difficile or methicillin resistant staphylococci.

ii. It is devoid of potential toxicity of multi-drug regimens.

iii. Less costly.

Advantage of Combination Therapy

In certain circumstances, there is need for the use of more than one antimicrobial agent such as:

• Prevention of emergence of resistant mutants

• Synergistic or additive activity. The combination therapy may be more effective if it contains drugs having synergistic action. The best example is combination of trimethoprim plus sulphamethoxazole (cotrimoxazole)

• Infections caused by multiple potential pathogens e.g. intra-abdominal or pelvic abscess, brain abscess, infection of a limb in diabetics, fever in neutropenic patients, aspiration pneumonia in hospitalized patients, septic shock or sepsis syndrome.

Action of Penicillins

All penicillins exert a bactericidal action against susceptible bacteria by inhibiting cell wall synthesis.

Spectrum of Penicillins

1. **Narrow spectrum penicillins:** *Benzathine penicillin, benzyl penicillin, phenoxymethyl penicillin and procaine penicillin* have narrow spectrum of activity and are mainly active against gram-positive bacilli, both gram-positive and gram-negative cocci and spirochetes.

   Cloxacillin and flucloxacillin have a similar spectrum of activity to benzylpenicillin but are also active against penicillinase (α lactamase) producing organism such as *S. aureus*.

2. **Broad spectrum penicillins:** Amoxicillin, ampicillin, carbenicillin have a broader spectrum of activity than benzylpenicillin because of being active against a much larger number of gram-negative organisms including *E. coli, Salmonella* and *H. influenze*. Carbenicillin is also active against *Pseudomonas eruginosa*.

Cephalosporins

Action

The cephalosporins are broad-spectrum bactericidal agents which inhibit bacterial cell wall synthesis.

Spectrum

Susceptible organisms include a wide variety of gram-positive and gram-negative organisms. These include *a hemolytic streptococci, Strept. pneumonie, Staph. aureus* (both penicillin sensitive and resistant), *Neisseria gonorrhea, N. meningitides, P. mirabilis* and some strains of *E. coli, Klebsiella sp.* and *H. influenze.*

Second and third generations cephalosporins show improved activity against a range of organisms including *E. coli, indole-positive Proteus sp., Enterobacter* and *Hemophilus sp.* Third generation cephalosporins also show activity against *Pseudomonas eruginosa.*

Uses

Based on their antibacterial spectrum, they are used in treatment of;
  i. Respiratory tract infections
 ii. Genitourinary infections
 iii. Soft tissue infections
 iv. Bone and joint infections
  v. Septicemia
 vi. Intra-abdominal infections

Preparations

Both oral and parenteral preparations are available (Box 3.21).

BOX 3.21: PREPARATIONS OF CEPHALOSPORINS

	Oral	Parenteral
First generation	Cephalexin	—
Second generation	Cefaclor cefadroxil	—
Third generation	—	cefotaxime, cefoperazone, ceftriaxone ceftazidime
Fourth generation	—	Cefepime

Side Effects

• False positive reactions in the urine for glucose
• Blood e.g. positive direct Coomb's test, leukopenia, eosinophilia, granulocytopenia
• Liver e.g. transient rise in transaminases (SGOT/SGPT), and alkaline phosphatase
• Kidney e.g. elevation in serum creatinine and blood urea especially with first generation
• GI tract e.g. nausea, abdominal pain, diarrhea, vomiting, phlebitis at injection sites
• Hypersensitivity reactions e.g. fever, rash (maculo-papular), urticaria.

Precautions

• Impaired renal function. The third generation are safe. Dose may be adjusted

• Overgrowth of opportunistic infections after prolonged use.
• Use first generation cephalosporin with caution in patients receiving aminoglycoside antibiotic as combination may potentiate nephrotoxicity.

Macrolides

Drugs/Preparations

Erythromycin, roxithromycin, azithromycin, clarithromycin, all are *oral* preparations. No parenteral preparation is available.

Actions

They inhibit bacterial protein synthesis.

Bacterial Spectrum

Erythromycin	Azithromycin	Clarithromycin
Streptococci, pneumococci staphylococci, mycoplasma *H. influenze*, Legionella, *N. gonococci*, *T. pallidum* and *Chlamydia*	Same as erythromycin but more effective against *Chlamydia* infection	Same as erythromycin. It is used in combination with proton pump inhibitor for gastric infections due to *H. pylori*

Indications

• Skin infections
• Ear infections
• Respiratory infections. Drug of choice for mycoplasma pneumonie
• Gonococcal infections
• Used as an alternative to penicillin in patients with penicillin hypersensitivity such as prophylaxis against bacterial endocarditis
• Clarithromycin is used in combination with proton pump inhibitor for gastric infection caused by *H. pylori.*

Side Effects

• GI symptoms—nausea, vomiting, abdominal pain
• Skin—rashes, urticaria, allergic reactions such as anaphylaxis
• Cholestatic jaundice

Aminoglycosides

Actions

The aminoglycosides are bactericidal agents *in vitro* at low concentrations with activity limited to facultative gram-negative bacteria and staphylococci.

Bacterial Spectrum

- Gram-negative bacilli e.g. *E. coli*, *Kleb. pneumonie*, *Pseudomonas*, *B. proteus*, *Enterobacter*, *Serratia* species.
- *Staphylococci* including penicillin-resistant strains

Preparations

Oral—Neomycin
Parenteral—gentamicin, amikacin, tobramycin, kanamycin, streptomycin, spectinomycin

Indications

1. They are among the drug of choice for any suspected gram-negative bacterial infection particularly in neutropenic patients and in patients with hematological malignancies.
2. They are synergistically bactericidal in combination with a penicillin, hence, the combination is used for the treatment of staphylococcal, enterococcal or streptococcal viridans endocarditis.
3. They are usually combined with a β-lactam antibiotic for treatment of gram-negative septicemia.
4. They are used for severe respiratory tract infections.
5. Streptomycin is still one of the drugs of choice in initial therapy for tularemia, plague, glanders and brucellosis. It is first-line agent for the treatment of tuberculosis. Amikacin, kanamycin, capreomycin all injectable preparations are used as second line antitubercular drugs.
6. Neomycin is also used topically for skin infections due to susceptible organisms and orally for sterilization of gut in hepatic encephalopathy.

Side Effects

- Reversible ototoxicity, nephrotoxicity, headache, rashes, thrombocytopenia and joint pain.
- Streptomycin in addition to above produces perioral paresthesias, hepatotoxicity and superinfections.

Special Precautions

Being nephrotoxic, renal function should be manitored and dose of the drug (e.g. gentamicin a commonly used aminoglycoside) should be adjusted according to serum creatinine level.

Contraindications

- Severe renal failure
- Pregnancy. It crosses the placenta and can cause eighth nerve damage in the fetus
- Neonates (except in life-threatening situations)

- Streptomycin is contraindicated in patients receiving neuromuscular blockers
- Hypersensitivity

Lincosamides

Action

They inhibit bacterial protein synthesis. Bacterial spectrum includes gram-positive cocci similar to erythromycin. It is effective against anerobes.

Preparations

It includes
- Clindamycin (parenteral)
- Lincomycin (oral and parenteral)

Uses

- Staphylococcal bone and joint infections
- Peritonitis
- Endocarditis prophylaxis
- Anerobic infections

Contraindications

- Diarrheal states
- Neuromuscular blocking agents use

Special Precautions

- Hepatic and renal impairment
- Discontinue its use if persistent diarrhea or colitis develops
- Monitor liver function and blood counts on prolonged therapy
- Avoid it during pregnancy and breastfeeding

Side Effects

GI tract—diarrhea, pseudomembranous colitis
Liver—jaundice, altered liver functions
Skin—rash, pain, induration and abscess after IM inj
Blood—agranulocytosis and thrombocytopenia.

Chloramphenicol

Action

It inhibits bacterial protein synthesis (bacteriostatic).

Microbial Spectrum

- All species of rickettsia
- Large viruses of psittacosis, lymphogranuloma group

- Gram-negative bacterial infections e.g. *Salmonella typhi*, *Hemophilus influenze*, *B. pertussis*, *E. coli* and *Shigella*, *Brucella*, *Klebsiella* and *Proteus sp.* and *Treponema pallidum*
- Its activity against gram-positive bacteria is much less than penicillin

Uses

1. This antibiotic is rarely used in adults because of the rare idiosyncratic side effect of irreversible bone-marrow aplasia. It is used only when it is the only suitable drug in the treatment of life-threatening infections.
2. It remains one of the drug of choice for treatment of *typhoid* and *paratyphoid* fevers, *plague*, *H. influenze* and other severe Salmonella infections.
3. It is still useful for treatment of *brucellosis* and *Pneumococcal meningitis.*

Contraindications

- Hypersensitivity
- Porphyria
- Pregnancy and lactation
- Concomitant use of penicillin

Precautions

- Avoid repeated use and prolonged treatment
- Monitor regular blood counts before and after therapy
- Reduce the dose during hepatic and renal impairment
- There is possibility of superinfections

Drug Interactions

- Rifampicin
- Phenobarbitone and phenytoin
- Anticoagulants (warfarin) and sulphonamides action is enhanced

Side Effects

- *Blood dyscrasias* e.g. aplastic anemia (both idiosyncracy and dose related) and bone marrow suppression
- *Grey syndrome* in newborn and premature infants (Grey-baby)
- *GI symptoms*—nausea, vomiting, diarrhea, dry mouth
- *CNS*—optic and peripheral neuropathy
- *Skin*—allergic skin reactions
- *Nocturnal hemoglobinuria reported.*

Preparation

Both oral and injectable (vial)

Tetracyclines

Actions

They have broad spectrum bacteriostatic (inhibit protein synthesis) activity. Their value has considerably decreased owing to increased bacterial resistance.

Microbial Spectrum

Susceptible organisms include

- Chlamydia infection (trachoma, psittacosis, salpingitis, uretheritis and lymphogranuloma venereum). Doxycycline is drug of choice
- Rickettsia (Q fever)
- Mycoplasma (respiratory and genital infections)
- Brucella (doxycycline with rifampicin)
- Spirochete (Lyme disease and relapsing fever leptospirosis, syphilis) infection
- Actinomycosis (used when there is penicillin hypersensitivity because penicillin is the drug of choice)
- Gram-positive cocci
- Vibrio infection (cholera)

Preparations

Tetracycline—only oral
Oxytetracycline (both oral and injectable—terramycine)
Chlortetracycline (oral)
Dimethylchlortetracycline (oral)
Doxycycline (oral)
Minocycline (oral)

Uses

- Acute exacerbation of chronic bronchitis
- Acne vulgaris
- Cholera
- Brucellosis, chlamydia, mycoplasma and rickettsial infections
- Pleural effusions due to malignancy or cirrhosis. It is instilled into pleural effusion for pleurodhesis
- Pelvic inflammatory disease in combination with metronidazole

Side Effects

- *GI symptoms*—gastric upsets, glossitis, stomatitis, proctitis
- *Skin*—rashes, photosensitivity
- *Superinfection* e.g. by fungi
- *Teeth discoloration* (yellow-grey brown), enamel hypoplasia, reduces fibula growth in children
- *Allergic reactions*, pain and local irritation on IM injection
- *Hepatotoxicity*

Contraindications

- Pregnancy
- SLE
- Lactation
- Severe renal insufficiency

Special Precaution

- Avoid its use with milk, food, antacid, iron supplement, oral contraceptive, penicillin and anticoagulants
- Avoid its use in children below 8 years
- Reduce the dose in renal failure
- Use carefully in hepatic insufficiency.

Fluoroquinolones

The fluoroquinolones have excellent activity against most facultative gram-negative rods, fair activity against staphylococci, variable to poor activity against streptococci and no activity against anerobes.

Actions

They are bactericidal drugs and act by inhibiting the enzyme responsible for maintaining the structure of DNA.

Preparations

Both oral and parenteral preparations are available. The oral absorption of these drugs is good to excellent and there is greatest activity against *P. eruginosa* especially of ciprofloxacin.

Formulations

Parenteral
- Ciprofloxacin
- Ofloxacin
- Pefloxacin

Oral
- Norfloxacin
- Ciprofloxacin
- Ofloxacin
- Lomefloxacin
- Levofloxacin
- Pefloxacin
- Sparfloxacin
- Gatifloxacin

Indications

1. Oral norfloxacin can be used for urinary tract infections and has been recommended for infectious diarrhea.
2. However, quinolones other than norfloxacin should be used for gram-negative infections. The injectable ciprofloxacin and ofloxacin are best for this purpose.

3. The quinolones are among the drug of choice for complicated urinary tract infections, bacterial gastrenteritis and typhoid fever and may be useful in therapy for chronic infections caused by gram-negative organisms such as osteomyelitis and chronic otitis external.
4. They are useful in respiratory and soft tissue infections and gonococcal infections.
5. They are used in prophylaxis in surgery and endoscopy.
6. Ofloxacin and ciprofloxacin are used as second-line antitubercular drugs.

Cautions

Fluoroquinolones should be used with caution in patients with epilepsy or a history of epilepsy, in hepatic and renal impairment, in pregnancy, during breastfeeding, and in children and adolescents (arthropathy has developed in weight-bearing joints in young animals but human evidence lacking).

Side Effects

Common
- **GI tract**—nausea, vomiting, abdominal pain, diarrhea (rarely pseudomembranous colitis)
- **CNS**—headache, dizziness, sleep disorders
- **Allergic**—fever, rash, anaphylaxis, photosensitivity and pruritus
- **Kidneys**—rise in blood urea and S. creatinine
- **Liver**—rise in serum transaminases and bilirubin
- **Blood**—eosinophilia, leukopenia, thrombocytopenia and altered prothrombin concentration

Less Common
- Loss of appetite
- Disturbance of vision, taste and smell
- Hypoglycemia, renal and hepatic impairment
- Restlessness, depression, hallucinations and confusion
- Raised intracranial tension

Note: The drug should be discontinued if mental, neurological or hypersensitivity reactions occur.

Nitroimidazoles

Action

They have bactericidal activity against anerobic bacteria and are amebicidal drugs.

Preparations

- Metronidazole (oral and injectable)
- Tinidazol (oral)
- Secnidazol (oral)

- Satronidazole (oral)
- Ornidazole (oral).

Uses

1. They are principally used for infections caused by anerobic bacteria such as Vincent's angina (purulent gingivitis) and pelvic inflammatory disease, lung infection, e.g. bronchiectasis.
2. Nonspecific vaginitis or trichomoniasis.
3. They are useful for intestinal and extra-intestinal amebic infection, specifically used for amebic liver abscess.
4. They are useful against giardiasis.
5. They are used for intra-abdominal infection, peritonitis, genital or puerperal sepsis.

Contraindications

- Ist trimester of pregnancy, blood dyscrasias, lactation, hypersensitivity and neurological disorders

Drug Interactions

- Alcohol (antabuse effect or disulfiram-like reactions)
- Anticoagulants, phenobarbitone, phenytoin, disulfiram

Side Effects

- Abdominal distress, furred tongue, pseudomembranous colitis (rare) stomatitis, glossitis (occasional), unpleasant metallic taste, neutropenia, urticaria, angiedema, CNS disturbances, dark urine, neuropathy and epileptiform seizures on long-term use.

Indications of Metronidazole Infusion (500 mg/100 ml bottle)

- *Anerobic infection* i.e. gut perforation, peritonitis post-puerperal sepsis
- *Amebic liver abscess* if patient is not taking orally
- *Antibiotic prophylaxis for surgery*
  Dose: 100 ml (500 mg) 8 hourly in adults and children above 12 yrs.
  Below 12 years—7.5 mg/kg 8 hourly
- For *prophylaxis*, for vascular, urological, biliary tract surgery
  500 mg IV infusion on induction only
  For appendicectomy and colorectal surgery
  500 mg IV on induction plus 8 and 16 hours postoperatively.

Antitubercular Drugs

First Line (Table 3.40)

- Isoniazid
- Rifampicin

- Pyrazinamide
- Ethambutol
- Streptomycin (injectable)

Second Line

- PAS (paraminosalicylic acid)
- Ethionamide
- Cycloserine
- Kanamycin, amikacin, capreomycin
- Thiacetazone
- Rifabutin
- Quinolones (ciprofloxacin, ofloxacin and sparfloxacin)

First line drugs being most effective are a necessary component of any short-course therapeutic regimen, while second line drugs are less effective than first line and much more frequently elicit severe reactions. They are used only for treatment of patients with tuberculosis resistant to first-line drugs.

Treatment Regimen

1. Pleuropulmonary tuberculosis
   A short course regimen
   a. Initial phase (2 months)—4 drugs
      — Rifampicin (450 mg)
      — Isoniazid (300 mg)
      — Pyrazinamide (1.5 g)
      — Ethambutol (800 mg)
      Note: Initial phase (intensive phase) is designed to reduce the population of viable bacteria as rapidly as possible and to prevent emergence of drug resistant bacteria.
   b. Continuous phase (4 months). Two drugs used are"
      - Rifampicin (450 mg)
      - Isoniazid (300 mg)
2. Extrapulmonary tuberculosis (bone and joint, meningitis, pericardial disease)
   The continuous phase in these type of tuberculosis is extended up to 1 year or more while initial phase is same.

Treatment During Special Circumstances

Although clinical trials of extrapulmonary tuberculosis are limited, therefore, the available data indicate that all forms of tuberculosis can be treated with short course 6 month regimen used for pulmonary tuberculosis. However, the American Academy of Pediatrics recommends that children with bone and joint tuberculosis, tubercular meningitis, or miliary tuberculosis receive a minimum of 12 months of treatment. Nowadays it is applicable to adults also.

Table 3.40: Common antitubercular drugs

Drug	Mechanism of action	Side effects	Dose	Management in case of toxicity
1. Isoniazid (both oral and injectable)	It is both bacteriostatic and bactericidal drug. It is bacteriostatic against resting bacilli and bactericidal against rapidly multiplying organisms both extra-cellularly and intracellularly	• Hepatotoxicity • Peripheral neuropathy • Rash and fever • Acne • Anemia • Arthritic symptoms • SLE like syndrome • Optic neuropathy, seizures and psychiatric symptoms	1. Usual dose 300 mg (5 mg/kg) in adults. In children: 10-15 mg/kg with maximum of 300 mg 2. For intermittent therapy, a maximum dose of 900 mg twice or thrice a week is used with vitamin B_6	• Limit alcohol consumption • Monitor SGPT and hepatitis symptoms • Stop the drug at first symptom of hepatitis (nausea, vomiting, anorexia and flu-like symptoms) • Concomitant administration of vitamin B_6 reduces the incidence of peripheral neuritis, optic neuritis and seizures • Now a days all oral packs of of anti-tubercular drugs incorporate vitamin B_6
2. Rifampicin (oral)	i. It has both intracellular and extracellular bactericidal activity i.e. blocks RNA synthesis by inhibiting DNA dependent RNA polymerase ii. It is also effective against a wide spectrum of gram-positive and gram-negative organisms	• Hepatotoxicity • Rash • Flu-like syndrome • Red-orange colored urine • Drug interaction	Adult: 450-600 mg (10 mg/kg) daily or twice a week children. 10-20 mg/kg	• Limit alcohol consumption • Monitor SGPT and hepatitis symptoms • Reassure the patient that dark urine is due to drug itself • Stop the drug if symptoms of hepatitis or jaundice develops.
3. Pyrazinamide (oral)	• Bactericidal drug, used in short-course therapy for tuberculosis. It has excellent CSF penetration, hence, a preferred drug in tubercular meningitis	• Hepatotoxicity • Hyperuricemia • Polyarthralgias	Adults: 1.5 g to 2 g daily (15 to 30 mg/kg)	• Monitor SGPT and hepatitis symptoms • Limit the dose to 15-30 mg/kg • Monitor uric acid levels in patients of gout or renal failure
4. Ethambutol (oral)	Bacteriostatic against rapidly growing *Mycobacterium*	• Retrobulbar optic neuritis (dose related) • Hyperuricemia (rare)	Adults: 15 mg/kg as a single dose daily. For retreatment 25 mg/kg daily for 2 months then 15 mg/kg daily. For intermittent therapy 50 mg/kg twice a week	• Avoid in children due to its visual toxicity • Use the lowest dose 15 mg/kg/day • Monitor visual acuity (eye chart) and red-green colour vision (ishihara color chart/book) monthly, stop the drug at first change in vision
5. Streptomycin, amikacin, capreomycin	These drugs inhibits bacterial protein synthesis (bactericidal) for rapidly dividing extracellular mycobacteria. These drugs poorly diffuse into CSF	• Ototoxicity • Renal toxicity • Less common are i.e. peri-oral paresthesias, eosinophilia, rash and drug fever	Adults: 0.5 to 1.0 g (10-15 mg/kg) daily or five times a week. Children: 20-40 mg/kg with a maximum of 1.0 g/day	• Limit the dose and duration of therapy as far as possible • Avoid daily therapy in old persons (> 60 yrs) • Monitor blood urea and serum creatinine levels • Ask daily for symptoms of ototoxicity i.e. tinnitis, vertigo, dizziness and decreased hearing • Perform audiometry if possible before and during course of therapy if needed • Stop the drug at first development of adverse effect

Commonly Used Drugs

1. *Renal failure*: As a rule patient with renal failure should not receive aminoglycosides as they are nephrotoxic. Ethambutol in renal failure should be used only if serum levels can be monitored. Isoniazid, rifampicin and pyrazinamide may be given in the usual dosage in cases with mild to moderate renal failure but dosage of isoniazid and pyrazinamide should be reduced for all patients with severe renal failure except those undergoing hemodialysis.

2. *Hepatic disease*: The majority of first line antitubercular drugs i.e. isoniazid, rifampicin and pyrazinamide being hepatotoxic should be avoided in hepatic disease. Patients with severe hepatic disease may be treated with streptomycin and ethambutol and, if required, with isoniazid and rifampicin under close supervision. The use of pyrazinamide by patients with liver cell failure should be avoided.

3. *HIV or AIDS*: Patients with HIV or AIDS appear to respond well to standard 6 months therapy, although treatment may need to be prolonged if the response is suboptimal.

4. *Pregnancy*: The regimen of choice for pregnant women is 9 months of treatment (HRE for 2 months and HR for 7 months). Streptomycin is contraindicated during pregnancy as it causes 8th nerve damage in fetus. Pyrazinamide should be avoided during pregnancy.

5. *Lactation and breast feeding*: Treatment of tuberculosis is not a contraindication to breastfeeding; most of the drugs administered will be present in small quantities in breast milk, but their concentration will be too low to provide any benefit or damage.

Preventive of Tuberculosis

It includes:

i. Treatment of infectious cases with appropriate therapy until cure.
ii. BCG vaccination
iii. Preventive chemotherapy

BCG Vaccination

BCG vaccine was derived from a attenuated strain of *M. Bovis* and was first administered in human in 1921. Many BCG vaccines are available worldwide but vaccine efficacy varies from 80% to nil. A Cohort study conducted in areas where infants are vaccinated at birth has found higher rates of efficacy in the protection of infants and young children from serious forms of tuberculosis i.e. tubercular meningitis and miliary tuberculosis.

BCG vaccine is recommended routinely at birth in countries with high tuberculosis prevalence. In countries such as USA where it is not recommended for routine use, the vaccination is indicated only for PPD negative infants and children who are at high risk of intimate or prolonged exposure to patients with tuberculosis and who cannot take prophylactic isoniazid.

BCG vaccination is safe. The local tissue response begins 2-3 weeks after vaccination with scar formation and healing occurs within 3 months. Side effects include; ulceration at vaccination site and regional lymphadenitis, osteomyelitis (rare), disseminated BCG infection in HIV patients.

Preventive Chemotherapy

It is a major component of tuberculosis control in USA, involves the administration of isoniazid to persons with latent tuberculosis and a high risk of active disease. It is recommended that 6-12 months course of isoniazid reduces risk of active tuberculosis in infected people by 90% or more. In the absence of reinfection, the protection is life-long. It has now been shown that isoniazid prophylaxis reduces rates of tuberculosis among person with HIV infection.

For prophylaxis, candidates are identified by PPD skin testing (Mantoux test 5 units of PPD intradermal). The positive reactions for close contacts of infectious cases, person with HIV infection, and previously untreated persons whose X-ray is consistent with healed tuberculosis are considered for prophylaxis if an area of induration is 5 mm in diameter at 48 to 72 hours (Table 3.42). A 10 mm cut off is used to define positive reactions in most other persons at-risk. For persons with low risk of developing tuberculosis, if infected, a cutoff of 15 mm is used.

Contraindications for Prophylaxis

- Presence of active liver disease
- Older patients
- Alcoholics

Drug Resistant Tuberculosis

Resistance to individual drug arises by spontaneous point mutation in the mycobacterial genome which occurs at low rate. There is no cross resistance among the commonly used anti-tubercular drugs. The development of drug resistance is invariably the result of monotherapy i.e. patient is not taking the two initial drug or poor compliance of the patient to properly prescribed therapy either due to poverty or ignorance. Drug resistance may be primary (a patient who has not been previously treated) or acquired (during the course of treatment with inappropriate regimen). Multidrug resistant tuberculosis or isoniazid/rifampicin resistant tuberculosis is emerging fast but can be prevented by adherence to the principles of sound therapy; the inclusion of at least two bactericidal drugs to

Table 3.41: Recommended regimens for the treatment of tuberculosis

Indication	Initial phase (Bactericidal phase)		Continuation phase (sterilization phase)	
	Duration (months)	Drugs	Duration (months)	Drugs
New smear or culture positive case	2	HRZE	4	HR*
New culture negative case	2	HRZE	2	HR*
Intolerance to H	2	RZE	7	RE
Intolerance to R	2	HES (± 2)	16	HE
Intolerance to Z	2	HRE	7	HR
Pregnancy	2	HRE	7	HR
Failure and relapse †	—	—	—	—
Standard retreatment (susceptibility testing not available)	3	HRZES ‡	5	HRE
Resistance to H+R	Throughout (12-18)	ZE + 0 + S (or another injectable drug)	—	—
Resistance to all first line drugs	Throughout (24)	Injectable agent x + 3 of these 4: ethionamide, cycloserine, PAS, 0	—	—

All drugs can be given daily or intermittently three times a week throughout or twice a week after initial phase of daily therapy. Regimen is tailred according to the results of drug susceptibility test.
‡ Streptomycin treatment should be discontinued after 2 months
x Amikacin, kanamycin or capreomycin (all injectable aminoglucosides). Treatment with all of these agents should be discontinued after 2 to 6 months depending on the response and patient's tolerance.
Abbreviation
H = Isoniazid, R = Rifampicin, Z = Pyrazinamide, E = Ethambutol, S = Streptomycin, O = Ofloxacin, PAS = Para-aminosalicylic acid

Table 3.42: Recommendations for isoniazid prophylaxis (American Thoracic Society and the Centre for Disease Control and Prevention 1994)

Risk group	Mantoux test (mm at 48-72 hr)	Duration of treatment (months)
• HIV infected persons	≥ 5*	12
• Close contacts of tuberculosis patients	≥ 5 †	6 (9 for children)
• Persons with healed fibrotic lesion at chest X-ray	≥ 5	12
• Recently infected persons	≥ 10	6
• Persons with high-risk medical conditions (DM, prolonged steroids therapy, other immunosuppressive therapy, hematological or RES disease, drug abuser, end stage renal disease, etc.)	≥ 10	6-12
• High-risk group < 35 yrs of age ‡	≥ 10	6
• Low-risk group (< 35 yrs)	≥ 15	6

* Anergic HIV infected persons with an estimated risk of tuberculosis of 10% may also be considered candidates
† Tuberculin negative contacts especially children should receive prophylaxis for 2 or 3 months after contact ends and should be retested (Mantoux test). Those whose results remain negative should discontinue prophylaxis.
‡ It includes persons born in high-prevalence countries, members of medically underserved low-income populations and residents of long-term—care facilities.
Isoniazid is administered in a dose of 5 mg/kg/day (up to 300 mg) or 15 mg/kg (up to 900 mg) twice a week for 6 to 12 months; the longer course is recommended for persons with HIV infection and for those with abnormal chest X-ray.

which the organism is susceptible. In clinical practice, five drugs are commonly used in the initial phase.

The treatment of individual drug resistant tuberculosis is given in the Table 3.41. For strains resistant to isoniazid and rifampicin, combination of ethambutol, pyrazinamide and streptomycin is used and if there is resistance to streptomycin also then amikacin is used. The treatment is continued for prolonged period of 12-18 months and for at least 9 months after sputum culture conversion. Many authorities add ofloxacin to this regimen.

If there is resistant to all first-line drugs, cure may be obtained with a combination of three drugs chosen from ethionamide, cycloserine, PAS and ofloxacin plus one drug chosen from amikacin, kanamycin and capreomycin (Table 3.41). The optimal duration of therapy for MDR tuberculosis in 24 months.

ANTI-AMEBIC DRUGS (AMEBICIDAL DRUGS)

The drugs used to treat amebiasis can be classified into two groups depending on the site of action.

i. **Luminal amebicides:** They are poorly absorbed and reach higher concentrations in the intestines. Their activity is limited to cysts and trophozoites close to mucosa. The drugs are:
    - Iodoquinol
    - Paromomycin
    - Diloxanide furoate

    Indications (Table 3.43)
    - Eradication of cysts in patients with amebic colitis or a liver abscess
    - Treatment of asymptomatic carriers
      Nowadays probes are available for differentiation of nonpathogenic from pathogenic cysts, however, it is prudent to treat asymptomatic individuals who pass cysts.

ii. **Tissue amebicides:** They reach higher concentration in blood and tissues after oral or parenteral administration. The drugs are nitroimidazole compounds:
    - Metronidazole (oral and IV)
    - Tinidazole
    - Secnidazole
    - Satronidazole
    - Ornidazole

    Indications (Table 3.43)
    - Patient with amebic colitis should be treated with IV or oral metronidazole (400-800 mg tid for 5-10 days orally) or tinidazole (600 mg bid for 5 days orally) or ornidazole (400 mg bid for 5 days)
    - For giardiasis, oral metronidazole 200-400 mg tid for 5-10 days

- Amebic liver abscess. Metronidazole (oral or IV) is the drug of choice. The usefulness of nitroimidazole in single-dose or abbreviated regimens is important in endemic areas where access to hospitalization is limited.

Table 3.43: Drug therapy for amebiasis

1. **Asymptomatic carrier (luminicidal agents)**
   - Iodoquinol (650 mg tab): 650 mg bid for 20 days
   - Iodochlorohydroxyquine (250 mg tab): 500 mg tid for 10 days
   - Diloxanide furoate (500 mg tab): 500 mg tid for 10 days
   - Paromomycin (250 mg tab): 500 mg tid for 10 days
2. **Acute amebic colitis (amebic dysentery)**
   - Metronidazole (200 or 400 mg tab or 200 mg bottle for infusion): 400-800 mg orally or 200 mg IV infusion tid for 5-10 days
     or
   - Tinidazole (300 or 600 mg tab): 600 mg bid orally for 10 days
     plus
     Luminal agent as given above. Nowaday combinations of oral metronidazole or tinidazole with diloxanide furoate are available
3. **Amebic liver abscess**
   - Metronidazole: 800 mg oral or 200 mg IV tid for 5 to 10 days
     or
   - Tinidazole: 600 mg bid orally for 10 days or 2.0 g oral as single dose
     or
   - Secnidazole: 2.0 g oral as single dose
     plus
     Luminal agent (diloxanide furoate 500 mg tid × 10 day)

Infection by Free Living Amebas

Genera include:
1. Acanthameba
2. Negleria

Naegleria Infection

Source of infection: Lakes, taps, hotsprings, swimming pools, heating and air-conditioning units and even from the nasal passages of healthy children.

Portal of entry: Nasal route

Infecting agent: Infection follows the aspiration of water contaminated with trophozoites or cysts or the inhalation of contaminated dust.

Disease: Amebic meningencephalitis

Diagnosis

- CSF shows elevated proteins and low sugar. The CSF pressure is elevated with high WBC count (upto 20,000 cells/ml)

- Detection of mobile trophozoites in wet mounts of fresh CSF

Treatment: High doses of amphotericin B and rifampicin may be used but prognosis is poor.

Acanthameba Infection

Source of Infection

The primary focus lies in the sinuses, skin or lungs.

Mode of spread: Hematogenous

Clinical Manifestations

1. Granulomatous amebic encephalitis
2. Keratitis

Predisposing factors: It occurs typically in chronically ill or debilitated patients. Risk factors include lymphoreticular disorders, chemotherapy, steroids therapy, SLE and AIDS.

Diagnosis

- The syndrome mimics a space occupying lesion
- CT scan reveals cortical and subcortical lesions of decreased density consistent with embolic infarct
- CSF is having elevated pressure, hence, its examination may not be indicated in all patient; wherever it is done, trophozoites may be isolated on fresh mount of CSF.

ANTIMALARIAL DRUGS

The properties of antimalarial drugs are summarized in the Table 3.45.

Treatment Goals

1. To suppress acute proxysm of uncomplicated malaria.
2. Radical cure to prevent relapse except in falciparum infection. Primaquine is the only drug used for this purpose.

Indications of Antimalarials

- Treatment of uncomplicated and complicated malaria
- Eradication of malarial parasite (radical cure)
- Prevention and prophylaxis of malaria. Drug used for prophylaxis are given in the Table 3.44
- Antimalarial chloroquine is also used in treatment of amebic liver abscess, as a disease modifying agent in rheumatoid arthritis (DMARD) and in skin lesions of systemic lupus erythrematosus

Treatment of Malaria

1. *Uncomplicated malaria (acute attack)*
   - Relief of fever by using antipyretic (paracetamol) and tepid sponging
   - Infection due to *P. vivax, P. ovale* and *P. malarie* and known strains of *P. falciparum* should be treated with oral chloroquine (Box 3.22)
2. For severe malaria or when patient is not able to take medicine orally then injectable dose of chloroquine (Box 3.23) may be given initially followed by oral treatment as soon as patient improves and start taking orally.

> **BOX 3.22: TREATMENT OF UNCOMPLICATED MALARIA**
>
> Oral chloroquine 600 mg base (10 mg/kg) followed by 300 mg (5 mg/kg) after 6 hr and then 150 mg twice a day for 2-3 days *plus* Primaquine 15 mg daily for 14 days is added for radical cure for patients with *P. ovale* or *P. vivax* infection after laboratory tests for G6PD deficiency have been proved negative.

> **BOX 3.23: TREATMENT OF SEVERE MALARIA**
>
> For severe malaria or patient is unable to take oral drug, chloroquine 300 mg base (5 mg/kg) by constant rate infusion over 4-8 hrs followed by three 8 hours infusions of 5 mg/kg (300 mg base) each

Treatment of Chloroquine Resistant Malaria (Table 3.44). In areas of chloroquine resistant strains, a

Table 3.44: Recommended dosage of antimalarial drugs used in chloroquine resistant cases

Drug	Uncomplicated malaria (oral)	Complicated malaria (parenteral)
Tablet of *sulphadoxine* (500 mg) plus *pyrimethamine* (25 mg) (combination)	2 tablets as single oral dose	—
Mefloquine	• For semimmune: 15 mg/kg base as a single dose • For resistant or nonimmune case; 15 mg/kg followed by second dose of 10 mg/kg after 8-12 hours	—
Quinine	• 600 mg (10 mg/kg) at 8 hours intervals daily for 7 days combined with tetracycline 250 mg qid or doxycycline 3 mg/kg (200 mg) once daily	• 20 mg/kg IV infusion over 4 hours than 10 mg/kg after every 8 hours till patient starts taking orally.
Artesunate or *Artemether*	• Two doses of 100 mg (3 mg/kg) on the Ist day followed by 50 mg (1 mg/kg) twice daily on the following 4-6 days. Total dose is 10 mg/kg or 600 mg	• 120 mg (2.4 mg/kg) IV or IM stat followed by 60 mg (1.2 mg/kg) daily for next 4 days

411

combination of sulfadoxine and pyrimethamine may be used. When there is resistance to this combination as well, either quinine *plus* tetracycline/or doxycycline or mefloquine or artesunate/artemether should be used. Tetracycline and doxycycline cannot be given to pregnant women or to children below 8 years of age. Recommended dosage of drugs used in chloroquine resistant malaria and severe malaria are given in the Table 3.44.

Chemoprophylaxis for Malaria

Antimalarial prophylaxis is still a matter of controversy. Chemoprophylaxis is never entirely reliable and malaria remains in differential diagnosis of fever in patients who travelled to endemic areas, even if they are taking prophylactic antimalarial drugs.

Recommendations for prophylaxis depend on:
  i. A knowledge of local patterns of plasmodium sensitivity to drugs.
  ii. Chances of acquiring malarial infection.

Indications

1. All pregnant women at risk should receive prophylaxis.
2. Antimalarial prophylaxis should be considered for children between the ages of 3 months and 4 years in areas where malaria causes high mortality in childhood.
3. Children born to nonimmune mothers in endemic areas should receive prophylaxis from birth.

4. Travellers visiting the endemic areas of malaria. They should start taking antimalarial drugs at least 1 week before departure to endemic areas and continue for 4 weeks after the traveller has left the endemic area.

Drugs (Table 3.45)

1. Chloroquine remains the drug of choice for prevention of infection with drug sensitive *P. falciparum* and with the other human malarial species. It is well tolerated, cheap and safe during pregnancy. The side effects of the drug are depicted in Table 3.45.
2. Mefloquine has become the antimalarial prophylactic agent of choice for much of the tropics because it is effective against chloroquine and multidrug resistant falciparum malaria. It is also well-tolerated drug but is costly.
3. Doxycycline is an effective alternative to mefloquine.
4. In the past, pyrimethamine and proguanil have been administered widely, but resistant strains of both *P. falciparum* and *P. vivax* have limited their use. Proguanil is considered the safest drug during pregnancy. The prophylactic use of pyrimethamine and sulfadoxine is not recommended because of severe side effects.
5. Recently daily primaquine (8-aminoquinoline used for radical cure) has been found effective for prophylaxis of *P. falciparum* and *P. vivax* malaria, further studies are needed for confirmation.

The drugs used and their dosages for chemoprophylaxis of malaria are summarized in Table 3.46.

Table 3.45: Properties of antimalarial drugs

Drug(s)	Pharmacokinetics	Action	Minor side effects	Major side effects
Quinine, quinidine	Good oral and IM absorption	Acts mainly on trophozoite stage of all malarial species in blood, kills the gametocytes of *P. vivax*, *P. ovale* and *P. malarie*. No action in liver stages	• Bitter taste, • Cinchonism, • Tinnitis • Heating loss • Nausea, vomiting • Postural hypotension • QT prolongation on ECG Rare Diarrhea, rash and visual disturbance	Common Hypoglycemia Rare Hypotension, blindness, deafness, cardiac arrhythmias hemolytic anemia, thrombocytopenia cholestatic jaundice, neuromuscular paralysis
Chloroquine	Good oral absorption, very rapid IM and SC absorption	Similar to quinine but more rapid	Bitter taste, nausea, dysphoria, pruritus postural hypotension *Rare* Accommodation difficulties, rash	Acute • Hypotension or shock (IM) • Cardiac arrhythmias • Neuropsychiatric reactions Chronic • Retinopathy • Skeletal and cardiac myopathy
Mefloquine	Adequate oral absorption. No parenteral prep.	As for quinine	Nausea, giddiness, dysphoria, confusion Sleeplessness, nightmares	• Neuropsychiatric reactions, convulsions

Contd...

Drug(s)	Pharmacokinetics	Action	Minor side effects	Major side effects
Tetracyclines	Excellent absorption	Weak antimalarial, should not be used alone for treatment	GI intolerance, discoloration of teeth, deposition in growing bones, photosensitivity, moniliasis, benign raised intracranial hypertension	• Renal failure in patients with impaired renal functions
Halofantrine	Variable absorption	As for quinine, but more rapid	Diarrhea	Prolonged QT on ECG, AV conduction delay, cardiac arrhythmias
Artemisinin derivatives, artemether, artesunate	Good oral absorption variable in IM absorption	Broader range, specificity and more rapid action than other drugs	Fever and reduction in reticulocyte count	Neurotoxicity reported in animals but not in humans
Trimethoprim	Good oral absorption variable IM absorption	• Acts on the mature forms at blood stages • Casual prophylactic	Well tolerated	Megaloblastic anemia, pancytopenia, pulmonary infiltrates
Proguanil (chloroquanil)	Good oral absorption	• Casual prophylactic drug, not used for treatment	Mouth ulcers and alopecia (rare)	Megaloblastic anemia
Primaquine	Complete oral absorption	• Radical cure • Some activity against blood stage infection, used to eradicate exoerythrocytic (hepatic) forms of *P. vivax* and *P. ovale* and to prevent relapses • Kills gametocytes of *P. falciparum*	Nausea, vomiting diarrhea, abdominal pain, hemolysis, methemoglobinemia	Massive hemolysis in patients with G6 PD deficiency

Note
- Tetracycline and doxycycline should not be used in pregnancy and in children below 8 years
- Halofantrine should not be used by patients with long QT intervals or known conduction disturbances or in those taking a drug that affect ventricular repolarization, i.e. quinine/quinidine, mefloquine, chloroquine, neuroleptics, tricyclic antidepressants, terfenadine or astemizole

Table 3.46: Chemoprophylaxis of malaria

Drug	Indication	Dose	
		Adult	**Children**
Chloroquine	Used in areas where malaria is chloroquine sensitive	300 mg base/week orally	5 mg/kg orally once a week
Mefloquine	Used in areas where there is chloroquine resistant malaria	250 mg salt/week orally	• < 15 kg (5 mg/kg) • 15-19 kg (1/4 tab/week) • 20-30 kg (1/2 tab/week) • 31-45 kg (3/4 tab/week) • > 45 kg (1 tab/week)
Doxycycline	An alternative to mefloquine	100 mg/day orally	• > 8 yr of age (2 mg/kg/day with maximum of 100 mg daily orally)
Proguanil	Used simultaneously with chloroquine as an alternative to mefloquine or doxycycline	200 mg orally once a day in combination with oral weekly chloroquine	< 2 yr (50 mg/day) 2-6 yr (100 mg/day) 7-10 yr (150 mg/day) >10 yr (200 mg/day)
Primaquine	Used for travellers only after testing for G6PD deficiency, postexposure prevention for relapsing malaria	15 mg base orally once a day for 14 days	0.3 mg of base/kg orally once a day for 14 days

Multidrug Resistant Malaria

Drug used are:
1. Mefloquine
2. Artemisinin and derivatives (artemether and artesunate).

Complications of Malaria

These are commonly observed with falciparum infection.
1. Cerebral malaria
2. Black-water fever. This is common due to drugs used in malaria rather than malaria itself.
3. Acute renal failure (ARF)
4. Granulomatous hepatitis
5. Hypoglycemia (may be quinine induced)
6. Hematological abnormalities—anemia, thrombocytopenia, pancytopenia, DIC
7. Aspiration pneumonia
8. Lactic acidosis
9. Noncardiogenic pulmonary edema

Q. What are the features of severe falciparum infection (>20% RBCs are parasitised)?

Ans. The features are;
- **CNS**—Cerebral malaria (coma, convulsions)
- **Renal**—Blackwater fever (hemoglobinuria) and acute tubular necrosis
- **Blood**—Anemia, thrombocytopenia, pancytopenia and DIC
- **Respiratory**—ARDS
- **Metabolic**—Hypoglycemia (children), metabolic acidosis
- **Liver**—Jaundice (hemolytic, hepatocellular)
- **GI tract**—Diarrhea
- **Miscellaneous**—Shock, hyperpyrexia.

Q. What are chronic complications of malaria in endemic areas (endemic malarial infections)?

Ans.
- *Tropical splenomegaly* (hyper-reactive malarial splenomegaly—an abnormal immune response to repeated malarial infections)
- *Quartan malarial nephropathy* (malarial induced nephrotic syndrome due to soluble immune complex glomerular injury due to repeated malarial infections)
- *Burkitt's lymphoma and Epstein-Barr virus infection* due to immunosuppression induced by repeated malarial infections

Other uses of Chloroquine:
1. As DMARD in rheumatoid arthritis.
2. For treatment of amebic liver abscess
3. For SLE
4. For treatment of cutaneous porphyrias

Acyclovir and Valacyclovir (available both oral and IV preprations)

Mechanism of Action

They act by interfering with DNA synthesis. To become effective, it must first be phosphorylated by a virus-specific enzyme thymidine kinase in the virus infected cells; this process does not occur in non-infected cells. Therefore, the drug causes selective inhibition of DNA synthesis in virus-infected cells only.

Indications

1. Herpes simplex virus (HSV) type I and II infections such as genital infections, encephalitis, etc.
2. Varicella zoster (chickenpox, shingles) infections
3. Epstein-Barr virus (EBV) infections
4. On emperical basis in Bell's palsy

Note: It does not eradicate viruses and is effective only if started at the onset of infection. It can save lives in herpes simplex and varicella-zoster infections in the immuno-compromised host. It can also be given to immuno-compromised patients for prevention of recurrence and prophylaxis of herpes simplex infection. It causes chromosomal breakage at high doses, hence, should be avoided during pregnancy.

Indications, route or *administration* and *dosage* are tabulated (Table 3.47).

Valacyclovir

Valacyclovir exhibits 3-5 times more greater viability than acyclovir.

Uses (Read the uses of acyclovir)

Dose

- Oral: 1 g tid for 7 days
- I.V: 5 mg/kg every 8 hours.

Side Effects

These are well-tolerated drug with fewer side effects.
1. Renal dysfunction
2. CNS changes—lethargy and tremors

Caution in Pregnancy

Both the drugs should be avoided during pregnancy.

Gancyclovir

It is an analogue of acyclovir, is active against HSV and VZV and is more active than acyclovir against CMV. The mechanism of action is similar.

Infection	Route	Dosage	Comment
1. Varicella			
• Immunocompetent host	Oral	20 mg/kg (max 800 mg) 4 or 5 times a day	Treatment benefits reported if started within 24 hours of rash
• Immunocompromised host	IV	500 mg/m² q 8 h for 10 days	Same
2. Herpes-simplex encephalitis	IV	10 mg/kg q 8 h for 10 days	It is a drug of choice
3. Neonatal herpes simplex	IV	30 mg/kg per day as continuous infusion over 12 hr for 14-21 days	Serious morbidity is frequent despite therapy
4. Genital herpes simplex			
• Primary (Treatment)	IV	5 mg/kg q 8 hour for 5-10 days	The IV route is preferred for severe
	Oral	200 mg 5 times a day for 10 days	infections or with neurological
• Recurrent (Treatment)	Oral	200 mg 5 times a day for 10 days	complications
5. Mucocutaneous herpes simplex in immunocompromised host			
Treatment	IV	250 mg/m² q 8 h for 7 days	Choice of route of administration
	Oral	400 mg 5 times a day for 10 days	depend on severity of infections
Prevention of recurrences	Oral	200 mg qid	It is administered during period of
during intense immuno-suppression	IV	5 mg/kg q 12 h	immunosuppression, e.g. antimitotic drugs or after transplantation
6. Herpes zoster infections			
Immunocompromised host	IV	500 mg/m² q 8 h for 7 day	It is effective in localized zoster, particularly when given early
Immunocompetent host	Oral	800 mg 5 times daily for 7-10 days	It causes faster resolution of skin lesion

Indications

It is approved for the treatment of CMV retinitis in immunocompromised host and for prevention of CMV disease in transplanted recipients.

Dose

Oral 1.0 g three times a day for the period of immuno-suppression

Parenteral initial therapy 5 mg/kg I.V every 12 hours for 14-21 days then 5 mg/kg per day or 5 times a week as a maintenance dose for the period of immunosuppression.

Side effects: Neutropenia and bone marrow suppression.

Vidarabine (Available as IV Prep)

Mechanism of Action

It inhibits DNA synthesis. It is effective similar to acyclovir against HSV-1 and HSV-2, VZV and EBV.

Indications

Similar to acyclovir

Dose

10-15 mg/kg/day as constant infusion over 12 hours

Side Effects

• **Hematological**—anemia, leukopenia, thrombocytopenia
• **Neurotoxicity**—neuropathy

Ribavirin (Aerosolized, Oral and IV Prep)

It inhibits wide range of DNA and RNA viruses.

Indications

1. It has been used to treat respiratory syncytial virus (RSV) infections in infants and less extensively to treat parainfluenza virus infections in children and influenza virus A and B infections in adults. Aerosolized ribavirin has been licensed for treatment of bronchiolitis in infants.
2. Acute hepatitis
3. Herpes virus infections

Dose: Oral 200 mg 4 times daily for 3-5 days in adults and 10 mg/kg/day in children.

Side effects: Hypotension, cardiac arrest and respiratory effects.

Contraindications: Pregnancy, severe hepatic and renal impairment.

Amantadine and Rimatadine (Oral Prep. only)

Mechanism of Action

They inhibit viral replication probably by preventing uncoding of the infecting virus particles.

Indications

- They are used for the prophylaxis and treatment of influenza A virus.
- Amantadine is used for treatment of parkinsonism.

Dose Adult: 200 mg/day orally for period at risk (2-3 weeks) if used for prevention and for 5 to 7 days if used for treatment

Children: 9 yr (5 mg/kg/day max. upto 150 mg/day)

Side effects: Livedo reticularis, peripheral edema, rash and CNS disturbances.

Contraindications: Pregnancy, lactation, severe renal disease, H/O convulsions or peptic ulceration.

Interferons (Parenteral preparation only)

Interferons (α, β and γ) are cytokines that exhibit antiviral, immunomodulating and antiproliferative properties.

Indications

1. They show beneficial effects on genital warts when administered intralesionally or systemically.
2. Chronic hepatitis B
3. Chronic hepatitis C or non-A, non B

Dosage: See the Table 3.48.

ANTIRETROVIRAL DRUGS (ANTI–HIV DRUGS)

The drugs used in HIV infection include:
- Zidovudine
- Stavudine
- Didanosine
- Zalcitabine
- Squinavir
- Lamivudine

Mechanism of Action

They inhibit the replication of HIV-1 and HIV-2 through competitive inhibition of reverse transcriptase and through chain termination of viral DNA synthesis.
Dosage: The drugs are discussed in brief in the Table 3.49.

Side Effects of Nucleoside Analogues

- **Hemopoietic**—anemia, neutropenia, leukopenia
- **GI tract**—abdominal upset, anorexia, nausea, malaise
- **Hypersensitivity**—anaphylaxis, fever, rash
- **Neurological**—fatigue, asthenia, headache, convulsions, neuropathy, paresthesias
- **Liver**—jaundice, hepatomegaly
- **Lactic acidosis**
- **Rare**—pancreatitis.

VACCINES AND ANTITOXINS

Immunoglobulins

They are used for passive immunisation. The protection offered is immediate but shortlasting.

Classes

1. *Normal immunoglobulin*
   i. It is prepared from pooled human plasma and are used for protection against hepatitis A and measles.
   ii. It has also been used to protect against rubella in susceptible pregnant women.
   iii. Used as long-term replacement therapy for congenital agammaglobulinemia.
   iv. Used for the management of idiopathic thrombocytopenic purpura not responding to conventional therapy.
   v. Used for the management of Guillain-Barre syndrome either alone or with plasmapheresis
      Preparations
      Both IM and IV preparations are available.
2. *Specific immunoglobulins*: They are prepared from immunized donors or convalescent patients. They are used for protection against.

Table 3.48: Interferones

	Disease	Drug	Route	Dose	Comment
1.	Chronic hepatitis B	Interferon a2B	SC or IM	5 million units daily for 16 weeks	Hepatitis B antigen (HBAg) and DNA are eliminated in 33-37% cases. Histological improvement occurs
2.	Chronic hepatitis C or non-A, non B	Interferon a2B	SC or IM	3 million units thrice weekly for 24 weeks	Serum alanine transferase values return to normal in 40-50% cases but relapse occurs in half after stoppage of treatment

Table 3.49: Anti-HIV drugs

Name	Route	Dosage	Comment
1. **Nucleoside analogs**			
Zidovudine (ZDV)	Oral IV	200 mg q 8h 1-2 mg/kg q 4h	ZDV is recommended for treatment of patient with HIV infection and CD4 count of < 500/ml. Administration during pregnancy, during delivery and to newborn infants reduces the rate of potential HIV transmission
Didanosine (ddI)	Oral	150-200 mg tablet bid	ddI is licensed for treatment of HIV patients who either do not tolerate or do not respond to ZDV
Zalcitabine (ddc)	Oral	0.75 mg q 8h	ddc is used in combination with ZDV in patients with advanced HIV infection who are not responding to ZDV as monotherapy otherwise also, combination of ZDV and ddc is superior to ZDV alone in patients with less advanced disease
Stavudine (d4T)	Oral	30-40 mg bid	Used for advanced HIV infection who are intolerant to or fail to respond to approved therapy
Lamivudine (3TC)	Oral	150 mg bid	It is used in combination with ZDV or stavudine in patients with HIV infection and clinical or immunological disease progression. It is also used for hepatitis B infection.
2. **Protease inhibitor**			
Squinavir	Oral	600 mg bid	This is protease inhibitor and is approved for combination therapy with nucleoside analogues in advanced HIV infection

- Hepatitis B
- Tetanus
- Varicella-zoster
- Rabies

Vaccines

They are used for induction of active immunity.

Types

1. *Live vaccines*: These contain an attenuated strains of micro-organism intended to cause a subclinical infection. Some vaccines notably measles vaccine may cause a mild febrile illness. Viral vaccines both attenuated and inactivated virus are prepared in tissue culture (which may contain antibiotics) or in chick embryos. They are contraindicated in patients allergic to egg protein. Examples include: oral polio (sabin), MMR vaccine, BCG vaccine and typhoid vaccine (TY 21 a).

2. *Killed micro-organisms*: These vaccines contain either the intact killed organism (e.g. typhoid, pertussis or rabies) or specific antigens as in the case of influenza and hepatitis B (virus surface antigens). Examples include vaccines for Hepatitis A, pertussis, typhoid (whole cell or Vi antigen), polio (salk), meningococcal (gray A and C) pneumococcal and *H influenze*.

3. *Bacterial toxins (toxoid vaccines)*: The inactivated bacterial toxins are used in vaccine preparations. Tetanus and diphtheria are two examples.

Contraindications for Vaccination

1. In general, vaccination should be postponed if the subject is suffering from acute illness. Minor infection without fever or systemic upset are not contraindications.

2. Live vaccines should not be routinely used for pregnant women because of possible harm to fetus. They should also not be given to immunocompromised host, i.e. HIV patients or patients receiving corticosteroids or radiotherapy or immunosuppressive drugs.

3. They should not be given to patients of malignant disease or tumors of reticulendothelial system.

Vaccination and immunization are interchangeably used terms but vaccination refers to administration of vaccine or toxoid; whereas the immunization describes the process of inducing or providing immunity by any means whether active or passive. Thus vaccination does not guarantee immunization. Active immunization refers to induction of immunity by administration of appropriate antigens; whereas passive immunization refers to providing temporary protection by administering exogenously produced immune substances. The examples of available active and passive immunization are given in the Box 3.24. The immunization schedule recommended by WHO for developing countries is depicted in Table 3.50 and prevalent in UK in Table 3.51.

Vaccination for Dogbite and Snakebite

Dogbite: Rabies or hydrophobia is caused by rabies virus usually acquired by man from stray or domestic dogbite (unvaccinated dog). Infection can also be transmitted by some other animals such as cats, vampire bats, fox, wolf, monkeys. The disease has a long incubation period (1 month to 1 year). The disease once develops ends fatally.

Prevention

- Local treatment of the wound is of great value and should be carried out as quickly as possible. The wound should be cleansed with soap or a detergent. Alcohol or antiseptic solution be applied to the wound

- Animal saliva must be wiped off from the surrounding skin
- Bleeding should be encouraged by application of a ligature
- Do not suture the wound
- An injection of tetanus toxoid should be given immediately.

Vaccination with antirabies vaccine: It should begin on the day of the bite and continued as recommended.

i. **For postexposure case (adults and children):** Six doses of 1 ml IM each on day 0, 3, 7, 14, 30 and 90

ii. **For prophylaxis** (adults and children): Three dose of 1 ml each on days 0, 28, 56 (or day 0, 7, and 21 in urgent cases)

Reinforcing vaccinations after 1 year and between 2 and 5 years.

Table 3.50: Immunization schedule recommended by WHO for developing countries

Age	Vaccine	Route	Efficacy (%)	Adverse events
Birth or first contact	BCG (Bacillie-Calmette-Guerin)	Intradermal	75-86	Regional adenitis, disseminated BCG infection, osteomyelitis
6, 10, 14 weeks	DPT and OPV	I.M	90-95	Local reactions, hypersensitivity reactions to toxoid
		Oral	95	No significant reaction. Rarely vaccine-associated polio
9 months	Measles, Mumps Rubella (MMR)	S.C	90-95	Acute encephalopathy (measles) Rare parotitis or orchitis (mumps)
12 months	Yellow fever in endemic area	S.C	High	Encephalitis, encephalopathy
18-12 months (second dose)	DPT and OPV			
5 yrs (Booster dose)	DPT and OPV			

MMR: Measles, mumps, rubella; DPT: Diphtheria, pertussis, tetanus (triple vaccine); IM: Intramuscular; SC: Subcutaneous OPV: Oral polio vaccine

Table 3.51: Immunization schedule in UK

Age	Visits	Vaccine	Intervals
3-12 months	3	Three simultaneous administration of DPT + OPV and *Hemophilus influenzae* type B	4 weeks (ideal start at 3 months of age) or at 3, 4 and 6th months)
12-24 months	1	MMR	
Ist year at school	1	Booster DT + OPV	
10-13 years	1	BCG for tuberculin-negative	
Girls 11-13 yrs	1	Rubella vaccine	
15-19 years or	1	Rubella vaccine	
15-19 years or on school leaving	1	Td + OPV	

Abbreviation
DPT: Diphtheria, pertussis, tetanus (triple vaccine)
OPV: Oral polio vaccine
DT: Diphtheria, tetanus
Td: Tetanus, low dose diphtheria toxoid
MMR: Measles, mumps and rubella

BOX 3.24: IMMUNIZATION

1. **Available active immunization**

   Live Vaccine
   - Oral polio (sabin)
   - Measles
   - Mumps
   - BCG
   - Typhoid (TY 21a)
   - Toxoids
   - Diphtheria
   - Tetanus
   - *H. influenze*

   Recombinant vaccines
   - Hepatitis B

   Dead Organism
   - Hepatitis A
   - Pertussis
   - Typhoid (whole cell and Vi antigen)
   - Polio (salk)
   - Influenza
   - Cholera
   - *Meningococcus*
   - Rabies
   - *Pneumococcus*

2. **Available passive immunization**
   (Prepared antibody)
   - DT (Diphtheria, tetanus).
   - Botulism

   Viral
   - Hepatitis A and B
   - Measles
   - Rubella
   - Rabies
   - Varicella zoster

- *Passive immunization with antirabies antisera of either equine or human origin*: In some cases where the bite is extensive or from a suspected rabid animal, passive immunization with human rabies immunoglobulin (HRIG) or equine rabies antisera should be done. Since equine antiserum can cause serum sickness, it is better to use human rabies immunoglobulin.

  Dose: Half of the total dose, e.g. 20 units/kg of HRIG (or 40 units/kg of equine antisera) is given by local infiltration of the wound and the rest by IM route into the gluteal region.

- Pregnancy is not a contraindication to postexposure prophylaxis. If there is substantial risk of exposure to rabies, pre-exposure prophylaxis may be indicated during pregnancy, but in such a situation, human diploid cell vaccine should be used.

- *Medical staff*: The medical staff attending a patient of rabies or suspected to be suffering from rabies must be immunized. Four intradermal doses of rabies vaccine should be given on the same day at different sites.

  The commonly employed vaccines and other side effects are depicted in Table 3.52.

Table 3.52: Special use vaccines

Vaccine	Type of vaccine	Route	Indications	Efficacy (%)	Side effects
Anthrax	Inactivated avirulent bacteria	SC	High risk exposure (i.e. person in contact or involved in manufacture of animal tides, fur, bone meal wool, goat hair, etc.	90	No serious side effects
Tuberculosis (BCG)	Living bacteria (attenuated *M. bovis*)	ID	PPD negative persons in prolonged contact with active TB patient	75-86	Lymphadenopathy disseminated BCG infection, osteomyelitis
Hepatitis A	Killed virus antigen	IM	Traveller's or person living in high-risk areas	94	Local reaction
Cholera	Inactivated bacteria	SC or IM	Not recommended for public health use	50% (short lived)	Fever, pain and local swelling
Meningococcus A	Bacterial polysaccharide of 4 serotypes	SC	Military personnel, traveller's to epidemic areas	90%	Rare
Plague	Inactivated bacteria	IM	Laboratory workers, foresters in endemic area, travellers	90%	Local reaction, hypersensitivity
Rabies (Human diploid)	Inactivated virus	IM or ID	Travellers, laboratory workers, veterinarians	100%	Local reaction, arthropathy, arthritis, angiedema
Japanese encephalitis	Inactivated virus	SC	Travellers	80-90	Anaphylactic/severe delayed allergic reactions common, recipient to be observed for 10 days
Typhoid	Killed whole bacteria	IM	Used for travellers, contacts of carriers	50-70	Fever, local swelling and pain

Abbreviations

SC: Subcutaneous; BCG: Bacille-Calmete-Guerin; ID: Intradermal; IM: Intramuscular

* Recommendations of the Committee on Immunization practices, the American Academy of Pediatrics and the American College of Physicians

Nutrition

MINERALS AND VITAMINS

Iron

It is important mineral for synthesis of heme fraction of hemoglobin. It is also present in myoglobin and cytochrome system.

Normal serum iron (ferritin) level:
- Male 50-150 µg/L
- Female 15-50 µg/L

Transferrin iron binding capacity (TIBC):
- 300-360 µg/dl

Serum iron and iron binding capacity in different condition are given in the Box 3.25.

Iron saturation (%) = It is calculated by serum iron divided by iron binding capacity × 100. The normal value is 30-50%. Iron deficiency states are associated with saturation < 20%, while iron overload occurs if saturation exceeds 50 to 60%.

BOX 3.25: SERUM IRON AND IRON BINDING CAPACITY IN DIFFERENT CONDITIONS		
Microcytic hypochromic anemia	Serum iron	Total iron binding capacity
1. Iron deficiency anemia	Decreased	Increased
2. Inflammatory diseases associated with anemia	Decreased	Decreased
3. Sideroblastic anemia	Increased	Normal
4. Thalassemia	Normal	Normal

Iron Deficiency Anemia

It is microcytic hypochromic anemia.

Other causes of microcytic hypochromic anemia are:
- Sideroblastic anemia
- Thalassemia

Iron Preparations

Oral preparation (Table 3.53).

Parenteral Preprations

1. Iron dextran injection (100 mg elemental iron)
2. Iron sorbitol citric acid complex (75 mg elemental iron)

Indications of Iron Therapy

1. Increased physiological demands, e.g. pregnancy, lactation, infants, children.
2. Iron deficiency anemia due to
   - Poor intake (nutritional)
   - Malabsorption
   - Parasitic infestation, e.g. hookworm disease
   - Blood loss, e.g. menstrual, hematemesis, piles or hemorrhoids
3. Parenteral preparations are used (i) in patients who are unable to tolerate oral iron or who suffer from malabsorption syndrome and (ii) in patients receiving recombinant erythropoietin therapy to guarantee adequate iron delivery to support erythropoiesis.

Dose. The amount of iron needed can be calculated as follows:

Total dose (mg) = Body wt (kg) × 2.3 × (15 minus patient's Hb in g%) + 500 to 1000 mg (to replenish iron store).

Precautions

1. Iron dextran complex should be administered after a test dose of 0.5 ml and patient observed for complaints of itching, chest or back pain and breathlessness. The BP should be monitored throughout the period of administration.
2. To be given as deep intramuscular injection. Phenol free preparation of iron-dextran can be given by IV route also.
3. Side effects of parenteral therapy include anaphylactic reactions or serum sickness (fever, arthralgia, rash, malaise and lymphadenopathy).

Table 3.53: Oral iron preparations

Generic name	Dose		
	Tablet (iron content) mg		Elixir (iron content) mg
Ferrous sulphate	325 (65)	300 (60)	200-250 mg of
	195 (39)	90 (18)	elemental iron/
Slow release	525 (105)	—	day
Ferrous fumarate	325 (107)	—	
	195 (64)	100 (33)	
Ferrous gluconate	325 (39)	300 (35)	

Precautions

1. To be given after meals to avoid GI tract symptoms.
2. Patient should not be on antacid or tetracycline therapy as they interfere its absorption.

Side effects: Oral preparations are safe and produce GI upset which can be minimized if iron is taken after meals.

Vitamins

These are organic compounds not synthesized within the body and are taken in diet. Only a small amount of vitamins is required in the diet because they are not energy yielding substances but act as catalytic co-factors for biological reactions.

Causes of Vitamin(s) Deficiency

1. General malnutrition-poor intake
2. Increased demands during growth, pregnancy and lactation
3. Food-faddism: consumption of staple diet
4. Malabsorption; diarrhea, parasitic infestations, etc.
5. Hemodialysis
6. Parenteral nutrition
7. An inborn error of metabolism
8. High processing, boiling or other sophisticated measures may destroy vitamins.

Diagnosis

Biochemical means of proving vitamin deficiency, once suspected are limited and the role of vitamin deficiency in disease state is not recognized because nonspecific vitamin therapy is a common part of standard supportive care, i.e. prescribed without proven deficiency. As a consequence, knowledge of manifestations of vitamin deficiency and a high degree of suspicion in appropriate setting are essential for considering the diagnosis and demonstration of a response to replacement therapy may be the most accurate way to confirm the diagnosis.

Hypervitaminosis

Excess of vitamins can be consumed either as a result of indirect consequence of dietary practice or by deliberate ingestion. Excess of vitamins A and D consumption and subsequent syndromes development are well recognized; while toxicity syndromes resulting from excessive consumption of water soluble vitamins are inconsistent and less well understood.

Normal requirement of fat soluble vitamins A, D, E, and K are given in the Table 3.54.

Vitamin A

Sources (Box 3.26).

BOX 3.26: SOURCES OF VITAMIN A

1. Animal source (vit A or retinols)
  • Milk, butter, cheese, eggs yolk, fish, liver oils, etc.
2. β-carotene (Plant sources)
  • Carrots, dark green leafy vegetables, yellow fruits, red-palm oil, etc.

Clinical Significance

1. It is an anti-oxidant vitamin along with vitamin C and E, is used to prevent acceleration of atherosclerosis, e.g. diabetes, CVA, IHD, etc.
2. It is used as a part of protection against epithelial cancer
3. Vitamin A deficiency predisposes to infection.
4. Its requirement increases during pregnancy, lactation and growth.
5. It is used for acne and other dermatological conditions
6. It must be supplemented in deficiency states.

Deficiency Signs/Symptoms

- Night blindness
- Xerophthalmia
- Keratomalacia
- Xerosis
- Hyperkeratosis of skin
- Bitot's spot

Prevention

1. Pregnant women, lactating mother, growing children should be advised to take adequate amounts of dark green leafy vegetables and green or yellow fruits.
2. Controlled trials in Indonesia, Nepal, Ghana, India have shown that in communities where xerophthalmia is prevalent, a single dose of 60 mg retinol (200,000 IU of vitamin A as palmitate) to preschool children significantly reduced mortality from gastrenteritis and respiratory infections by 33%.

Table 3.54: Requirements of fat soluble vitamins

	Vitamin A(mgRE)	Vitamin D (mg)	Vitamin E (mgα–TE)	Vitamin K (mg)
Infant	375	7.5-10	3-4	5-10
Children (1-10 years)	400-700	10	6-7	15-30
Adult Male	1000	2.5	10	50-80
female	800	2.5	8	50-65
Lactating or pregnant women	1000-1200	10	11	65

Treatment

1. Night blindness-30,000 IU of vit. A daily for 7 days
2. Corneal damage-20,000 IUkg/day × 5 days
3. Children who are at risk for vitamin A deficiency and who develop measles should be given 200,000 IU orally each day for 2 days
4. Associated malnutrition must be treated and superadded bacterial infection should be treated with antibiotics
5. Referral to ophthalmologist is necessary for severe cases.

Hypervitaminosis A (Vitamin A toxicity)

Hypervitaminosis A can result from accidental ingestion of polar bear, liver by hunters or explorers, food faddism or as a side effect of inappropriate therapy.

Acute toxicity results from ingestion of a large dose and is characterized by abdominal pain, nausea, vomiting, headache, dizziness and in infants a bulging fontanelle followed by desquamation of skin. Recovery occurs within few days.

Chronic toxicity occurs following ingestion of large doses for prolonged periods; for example, when taken for acne or other dermatological conditions. The features include; bone and joint pain, hyperostosis, hair loss, dryness of lips, weight loss, benign intracranial hypertension and hepatosplenomegaly. Relief is prompt on withdrawal of vitamin.

Vitamin D

Synthesis: Natural form of vitamin D (cholecalciferol, vitamin D_3) is synthesized in the skin by the action of UV light on 7-dehydrocholecalciferol. Cholecalciferol is inactive in the present form, becomes active after hydroxylation twice, first in liver and then in kidneys. The active end-metabolite formed in the kidneys is 1-25 dihydroxy-cholecalciferol. Therefore, patients with renal disease requiring vitamin D should have hydroxylated derivatives (alfacalcidol or dihydrochole-calciferol).

Sources of Vitamin D

1. Natural from skin.
2. Dietary-main sources include; fish liver oil (cod liver oil), fatty fish and infant milk formula fortified with vitamin D.

Functions

It stimulates the absorption of calcium from the small intestine and inhibits mobilization of calcium from bone resorption.

Deficiency Syndromes

1. Rickets in children
2. Osteomalacia in adults

Causes of Vitamin D deficiency (Box 3.27)

BOX 3.27: CAUSES OF VITAMIN D DEFICIENCY
1. Poor dietary intake or less synthesis through skin (common in muslim ladies using purdah).
2. Defective absorption, e.g. celiac disease in children, pancreatic or biliary duct obstruction or GI surgery.
3. Defective metabolism, e.g. interference by drugs (dilantin rifampicin) and chronic renal failure.

Rickets may be due to:
  i. Hypocalcemia due to vitamin D deficiency
 ii. Hypophosphatemia, e.g. familial, inherited or acquired renal tubular defects (Fanconi's syndrome calcinosis, multiple myeloma, cadmium poisoning, outdated tetracyclines)

Uses of Vitamin D (Box 3.28)

BOX 3.28: USES OF VITAMIN D	
Deficiency state	Dose
1. Ricket	• 25-125 mg (1000-5000 IU) daily for 6-12 weeks then 200-400 IU daily orally
2. Osteomalacia	• Same dose
3. Osteomalacia due to malabsorption	• 5,000-10,000 IU orally daily and large doses of calcium OR 10,000 IU daily IM depending on calcium and vitamin D levels
4. Anticonvulsant therapy	• Add 1000 IU/day to drug therapy
5. Renal disease	• Initially alphacalcidol 0.5 µg/d or calcitriol 0.25 µg/d and increase the dose as per response (usual dose is 1µg/day for α-calcidiol and 0.25-0.5 µg for calcitriol) and continue for 2-4 weeks. serum calcium levels are to be monitored
6. Refractory osteodystrophy	• 1.0-2.5 µg three times/week intravenously and in patient on dialysis titrate the response to calcium and PTH levels
7. Hyperthyroidism	• Small dose of vitamin D_3 and calcium supplementation

Hypervitaminosis D (Vitamin D Intoxication)

The symptoms include nausea, vomiting, constipation, drowsiness, dizziness and metastatic calcification; and are mainly due to hypercalcemia. Renal damage may occur breast milk from women taking vitamin D may cause hypercalcemia in breastfed infants.

Vitamin E (Tocopherols)

Eight naturally occurring tocopherols possess vitamin E activity and α tocopherol is widely distributed and most active of all tocopheroles.

Requirement: Adult 10-30 mg/day

Action: It is an antioxidant vitamin and prevents formation of toxic oxidation products.

Clinical Deficiency

Isolated deficiency is rare and occur with selective malabsorption of the vitamin or when an autosomal recessive mutation causes vitamin E deficiency and ataxia. The manifestations of deficiency include areflexia, gait disturbance, decreased proprioceptive and vibration sense and paresis of gaze associated with posterior column degeneration.

Uses

1. Vitamin E deficiency due to malabsorption, cholestatic jaundice
2. Abetalipoproteinemia
3. As an antioxidant vitamin along with vitamin A or C
4. Fibrocystic breast disease
5. Empirically used for muscle cramps

Dose: 50-100 IU/day

Vitamin K

It is present in two forms, i.e. vitamin K_1 (Phytonadione) in green leafy vegetables and K_2 (menaquinone) synthesized by intestinal bacteria. It is coagulant vitamin required for the synthesis of four clotting factors, i.e. II, VII, IX, X-called vitamin K dependent clotting factors.

Daily requirement: 80 mg/day.

Causes of deficiency: Deficiency of vitamin K causes hemorrhagic disease in newborn and clotting disorders in adults.
1. Primary deficiency in newborn occurs due to inefficient transfer of vitamin K from the mother to fetus leading to hemorrhagic disease.
2. Obstructive (cholestatic) jaundice or hepatocellular failure causes decreased synthesis of vitamin K dependent factors leading to coagulation disorder
3. Anticoagulants, i.e. warfarin and related anti-coagulants antagonise vitamin K
4. Antimicrobial therapy (prolonged) eliminates the bacteria required for its synthesis.

Dose: Patients with PTI <70% should receive parenteral vitamin K 10 mg/day for 3-5 days till PTI becomes normal or tolerable (>70%).

Water Soluble Vitamins

It includes: Vitamins C and B-complex group.

Vitamin C (Ascorbic Acid)

Functions

1. It helps in collagen formation of connective tissue by hydroxylation of proline to hydroxyproline—the characteristic amino acid of the collagen. By this action, it helps in healing of the wound.
2. It is most effective reducing agent in aqueous phase of living tissue
3. Vitamins A, C and E are antioxidant vitamins.
4. It is anti-scurvy vitamin.

Daily requirement: 30-70 mg/day. Requirement increases during pregnancy and lactation.

Dietary Sources

Vegetable sources, e.g. guava, potates, cabbage, cauliflower (row) and citrus fruits.
  Animal sources, e.g. meat (liver, kidneys, fish)
  Deficiency disease - Scurvy

Uses

1. Prevention and treatment of scurvy
2. As an antioxidant vitamin
3. Pregnancy and lactation
4. During trauma, surgery, burns, infections, smoking
5. Higher doses have been used in URI without much success.

Dose

In adult scurvy: 500-1000 mg two or three times a day.

In infection: 1.0 g 2-3 times a day.

Children < 4 years: 1/4 of adult dose
         5-12 years: 1/3 of adult dose
         13-14 years: 1/2 of adult dose

Hypervitaminosis C (vitamin C Toxicity)

1. Large amount of iron may be absorbed and may precipitate hemochromatosis
2. Precipitate oxalate stone formation by producing oxaluria
3. Long-term use may interfere with absorption of vitamin B_{12}.

Vitamine B Complex

It includes:
B_1 = Thiamine B_2 = Riboflavin
B_3 = Nicotinic acid (nicotinamide) B_5 = Pentothenic acid
B_6 = Pyriodxine
B_{12} = Cyanocobalamine, hydroxocobalamin.

The vitamin B complex, their source, daily requirements, deficiency states and their uses are tabulated (Table 3.55).

Table 3.55: Vitamin B complex—dietary source, daily requirement, deficiency states and indications for their use

Name	Dietary source	Daily requirement	Deficiency syndrome	Use
Thiamine (B_1) It acts as an coenzyme in • Decarboxylation of pyruvate to acetyl coenzyme in (Krebs' cycle) • For transketolase in hexose-monophosphate shunt • Decarboxylation of ketoglutarate to succinate in Krebs' cycle	• Wheat flour (bran), bread • Yeast, legumes, nuts • Oat meal or fortified cereals • Meat	1.5 mg/day	• Beri-beri, e.g. dry, wet, infantile • Wernicke's encephalopathy (cerebral Beri-beri) • Korsakoff psychosis *Causes of deficiency* Alcoholism, malnutrition malabosrption, antidiabetic therapy, dialysis, folate deficiency intake of machine-milled rice or cereals	1. For *beri-beri:* Initially, 50 mg IM is given for several days after which it is given orally 2.5-5 mg 2. For therapeutic test for beri-beri; A single injection 100 mg produce a prompt relief of symptoms when beri-beri is in doubt 3. As a neurotropic vitamin in association with Vitamin B_6 and B_{12} used in various types of peripheral neuropathies
Riboflavin (B_2) • As a coenzyme in oxidation-reduction reactions	— 1.2-1.6 mg/day	•	• Sore throat, (hyperemia, edema of oral mucous membrane, cheilosis, angular stomatitis, glossitis, seborrheic dermatitis and normocytic normochronic anemia due to bone marrow hypoplasia	• *In deficiency state* 2.5-5 mg daily orally for few days
Nicotinamide (Niacin) • As coenzyme in; oxidation-reduction reactions as NAD and NADP	Cereals	14–18 mg	• *Pellagra* (diarrhea, dermatitis dementia) *Cause:* Consumption of staple diet such as maize, jowar sorghum containing high leucine content for long period	• Oral niacin 10 mg/day to treat endemic pellagra
Pyridoxin (Vit B_6) • Pyridoxal phosphate acts as coenzyme in many amino acid metabolism, e.g. transaminases, synthetases, hydroxylases • Required for synthesis of heme precursors • Plays a role in neuronal excitation	Widely distributed in all foods, e.g. meat, liver, vegetables, cereals	2 mg/day	• There is no isolated deficiency syndrome described but certain disorders depend on pyridoxine. • Infantile convulsions • Homocysteinuria • Sideroblastic anemia	• In deficiency due to pregnancy, oral contraceptives or isoniazid induced; 30 mg/day oral is sufficient • For patients taking penicillamine, 100 mg/day • For peripheral neuropathies in conjunction with Vitamin B_1 and B_{12}
Vitamin B_{12} (Cyanocobalamin) Two metabolic active i. Methyl-cobalamine: It is a co-factor for conversion of homocysteine to methionine, hence, its deficiency results in	• Fortified cereals, spinach, peas, dried beans, cauliflower, whole meal bread, vegetables	Adult requirement is 2 mg/day Children: 1.4 mg/day Pregnant and lactating mothers:	• Pernicious anemia • Homocysteinemia and thrombosis of vessels • Subacute combined degeneration of spinal cord • Peripheral neuropathies of	Therapeutic preparations used are: cyanocobalamin and hydroxocobalamin • *For pernicious anemia* Hydroxocobalamin parenterally as 1000 mg twice a week for 2 weeks, then 1000 mg/week for 6 weeks.

Contd...

Name	Dietary source	Daily requirement	Deficiency syndrome	Use
dearranged folate metabolism and megalobastic anemia, elevation of plasma homocysteine levels that predispose to thrombosis and to some extent neurological complications ii. Adenosylcobalamin: It converts methylmalonyl coenzyme A (CoA). Lack of this factor leads to accumulation of methylmalonyl CoA and its precursors which may contribute to neurological complication		2.6 mg/day	metabolic, drug induced or idiopathic: *Causes of vitamin B_{12} deficiency are:* • Inadequate dietary intake • Gastrectomy (loss of intrinsic factor) • Disease of terminal ileum (loss of absorption site) • Blind loop (bacterial colonization of small intestine with consumption of vitamin B_{12})	Monitor the response The maintenance dose is 1000 mg IM after every 3 months throughout life • For malabsorption it is given along with an antibiotic course for short-term • For neuropathies, it is given along with $B_1=100$ mg $B_6=50$ mg $B_{12}=1000$ mg daily for 10 days *Note:* Folic acid should not be given in Vitamin B_{12} deficiency with neurological features
Folic acid • It an essential hemopoietic vitamin. The activity of folic acid and vitamin B_{12} is essential for normal erythropoiesis	Fortified cereals spinach, peas, beans, cauliflower, vegetables, whole bread	Adults: 100 mg/day Children: 50 mg/day Pregnant women: 400 mg/day Lactating mothers: 260 mg/day	• Megaloblastic anemia • Tropical nutritional paraplegia • Homocysteinemia and subsequent vascular thrombosis • Congenital neural tube defects if deficiency persists during pregnancy *Causes* • Inadequate dietary intake or alcoholism • Malabsorption • Infection • Pregnancy • Drug induced, e.g. phenytoin, methotrexate, oral contraceptives, • Di Guglielmo's syndrome	*Uses and dosage* • For megaloblastic anemia 5 mg/day for few days then 5 mg/week. Folate will aggravate the neurological complication of vitamin B_{12} deficiency if given alone in combined deficiency. Hence, it is customary to use both simultaneously in megaloblastic anemia • Dimorphic anemia: It is used as an adjuvant to iron therapy • Pregnancy: Folate supplements 350 mg/day • For prevention of stroke and coronary occlusion in cases with high levels of homocysteine • Used as an adjuvant to antifolate drugs

Drugs Used in Respiratory Diseases

Antihistamines (H1 Blockers)

Actions

The antihistamines block those responses to histamine that are mediated by H_1 receptors (bronchoconstriction, contraction of GI tract smooth muscles, vasodilation and pruritus), hence, are also called *H_1 blockers*. These compounds exert their actions by competitively inhibiting H_1 receptors. They do not prevent the release of histamine. In addition, these drugs also exert anticholinergic and antiserotonergic activity.

Preparations

These include *chlorpheniramine, brompheniramine, clemastine, cyclizine, cyproheptadine, dexchlorpheniramine, diphenhydramine, hydroxyzine, meclozine, methdiazine-pheniramine, promethazine*, etc.

Acrivastine, cetrizine, loratadine, fexofenadine are new antihistaminics.

Uses

1. Allergic conditions such as hay fever, allergic rhinitis, urticaria, contact dermatitis, pruritus.
2. Insect bites, stings and drug rashes/allergies.
3. Some, e.g. cyclizine, diphenhydramine and meclozine are also used in Meniere's disease, motion sickness and other forms of vertigo, nausea and vomiting.
4. Some, e.g. cyproheptadine has also been used in the treatment of migraine.
5. Injections of chlopheniramine or promethazine are used as an adjuvant to adrenaline in the emergency treatment of angiedema, urticaria and systemic anaphylaxis (type 1 hypersensitivity reactions).
6. Systemic mastocytosis.

Contraindications

- Previous hypersensitivity
- Nursing mothers and premature or newborn infant
- Narrow angle glaucoma
- Epilepsy
- Concomitant therapy with MAO inhibitors
- Treatment of lower respiratory tract infections or acute asthmatic attacks
- Urinary retention and prostatic hypertrophy.

Side Effects

1. *CNS:* Mainly sedation but CNS stimulation accompanied by hallucinations and convulsions, headache, dizziness. Fever may occur after large dose in children.
2. **GI tract**, e.g. abdominal upset and distension.
3. *Blood dyscrasias*
4. *Anticholinergic effects*—dry mouth, blurring of vision
5. *Arrhythmias:* Astemizole and terfenadine prolong QT interval and are arrhythmogenic, hence, not to be used with drugs that prolong QT interval.

Anaphylaxis and Angiedema (Type 1 Hypersensitivity Reactions)

Definition

The life-threatening anaphylaxis (anaphylactic shock) occurs in a sensitized human within minutes after administration of specific antigen and is manifested by laryngeal edema, bronchospasm and hypotension or shock or vascular collapse. Cutaneous manifestations such as pruritus, urticaria, angiedema are characteristics of systemic anaphylaxis. GI tract manifestations include nausea, vomiting, crampy abdominal pain and diarrhea.

Causes

1. Heterologous proteins such as hormones, enzymes, pollen extracts, food, antiserum or vaccines, etc.
2. Insect bites/stings
3. Drugs
   - Antibiotics (penicillins, cephalosporins, amphotericin B)
   - Local anesthetics (procaine, lidocaine)
   - Iron injections
   - Vitamin injections
   - Heparin
   - Neuromuscular blocking agents.

Treatment

1. Make the patient to lie flat with foot end raised.
2. IV adrenaline (1:1000 sol) 0.5 to 1 ml every 10 minutes till patient improves.
3. Repeated slow IV injection of chlopheniramine after adrenaline may be helpful and should be continued for 24 hours.
4. In the absence of adequate improvement, administer IV fluids, IV aminophylline, O_2 and assisted ventilation; if required, tracheostomy may be done on emergency basis especially in angiedema.
5. IV corticosteroids are of secondary help because their onset of action is delayed for few hours. They should be used simultaneously in severe reaction and shock.

Bronchodilators (Oral, Parenteral and Inhaled)

These drugs relax the bronchial mucosa and produce dilatation of bronchial system hence called *bronchodilators*. These include:

Sympathomimetics (adrenergic stimulants): They produce bronchodilation by stimulating β_2 adrenergic receptors in bronchial smooth muscles. The drugs in this category include; *catecholamines* (adrenaline or epinephrine, ephedrine, isoprenaline, etc.), *resorcinols* (metaproterenol, terbutaline and fenoterol) and *saligenin* (albuterol or salbutamol).

The catecholamines are short-acting (30 to 90 min) and are effective only when administered by inhalational or parenteral routes. These are not β_2 selective agent and have considerable chronotropic and inotropic effects. These are used in emergency situation of asthma and type I hypersensitivity (anaphylactic) reaction (e.g. subcutaneous or IV adrenaline 0.5 ml of 1:1000 sol or isoproterenol is used 1:200 solution by inhalation).

Side effects include; tachycardia, palpitation, cardiac arrhythmias, precipitation of angina, CNS stimulation, dry mouth, sweating, headache, dizziness, nausea, vomiting, nervousness, anxiety and tremors.

The commonly used resorcinol (terbutaline) and saligenin (salbutamol) are highly selective β_2 stimulants for respiratory tracts and are virtually devoid of significant cardiac effects except at high doses. They are active by all routes and their effects are long-lasting 4-6 hours.

Uses

1. Bronchospasm due to any cause, e.g. allergies
2. Bronchial asthma
3. Chronic bronchitis or COPD

The doses and side effects are given in the Table 3.56.

Xanthine Derivatives

Actions

They produce bronchodilation by inhibiting the enzyme phosphodiesterase leading to increase in intracellular levels of cyclic AMP. In addition:

1. They are cardiac stimulants.
2. They produce diuresis
3. CNS and respiratory stimulants.

Uses and dosage: See the Table 3.57.

Table 3.56: Commonly used selective β_2 stimulants

Drug	Uses	Dose	Side effects
1. Terbutaline	• Bronchial asthma • Bronchitis • Mucoviscidosis	• Oral: 2.5-5 mg tid in adults Inj: 0.5-1 ml SC or IM up to 4 times a days • Inhalation: 0.25 mg per metered dose 1-2 puffs during acute attack and then as required max 8 puffs in 24 hrs • Nebulizer: 5-10 mg diluted and nebulized 2-4 times daily	• Fine tremors • Peripheral vasodilatation • Hypotension • Headache • Palpitation • GI upset • Muscle clamps • Sleep disturbance • Hypokalemia
2. Salbutamol	• Bronchial asthma • Chronic bronchitis or acute exacerbation of COPD • Bronchospasms due to any other cause • For prophylaxis of asthma	• Oral: Adults 2-4 mg 3-4 times a day • Inhalor: Adult 200-400 mcg as a single dose Children 200 mcg (single dose) For prophylaxis 400 mcg 3-4 times a day in adult and half the dose in children	• GI symptoms, e.g. nausea, vomiting diarrhea • Fine tremors • Insomnia, hyperactivity, nervousness, headache • Palpitation, sweating • Peripheral vasodilatation
3. Salmeterol	• Regular treatment of asthma. Not to be used in acute attack	• Inhalor: Two puffs (40 mcg) twice a day (25 mcg per metered. In severe cases 4 puffs bid dose) Not to be used in children	• Muscle cramps (rare) • Hypokalemia (rare)
4. Formoterol	• Regular treatment of bronchial asthma	• Inhalor: *Adults.* 6 mcg/per metered dose. 1-4 puffs twice a day, titrated to the lowest effective dose *Children:* Under 6 years not recommended over 6 years, half the adult dose	Same as above

Note: Special precautions in cardiac disease, diabetes, hyperthyroidism, gastric ulcer, pregnancy, lactation, hypertension, arrhythmias, hepatic and renal impairment.

Drug	Uses	Dose	Side effects
Aminophylline	• Anaphylaxis • Acute asthma • COPD • Cor pulmonale • CHF • Dobutamine induced coronary steal causing ischemia during dobutamine stress testing	Adults: IV aminophylline/theophylline 250 mg (or 6 mg/kg) as a bolus followed by 1 mg/kg/hr (250 mg over 4 hr) as slow IV infusion for 12 hours then 250 mg as an infusion over 6 hrs for 24 hrs or as long as required	• *GI tract:* Nausea, vomiting, anorexia, epigastric pain, diarrhea, hematemesis • *CNS:* headache, convulsions, insomnia • *CVS:* Tachycardia, flushing, hypotension extrasystoles and life threatening arrhythmias • *Renal:* Albuminuria • *Miscellaneous,* e.g. hyperglycemia tachypnea *Special precautions* Pregnancy, lactation, hyperthyroidism, gastric ulcer, myocardial insufficiency, diabetes
Theophylline	– do –	Adults: IV dose as discussed above Oral: 300 mg 2-3 times a day	Same as above

Note: These can be used in combination with β_2 adenergic stimulants.

Anticholinergics (Ipratropium Bromide Oxitropium Bromide Inhalation)

Anticholinergic drugs produce bronchodilation by smooth muscle relaxation and are useful as bronchodilators in bronchial asthma and chronic bronchitis. They may be of particular benefit for patients with coexistent heart disease in whom use of xanthine derivatives and β_2 adrenergic stimulants may be dangerous. There is some evidence that addition of anticholinergics may enhance the bronchodilation achieved by sympathomimetic. They are slow to act (60-90 min for peak action) and are only of modest efficacy.

Drug and Dose

Drug: Ipratropium bromide inhaler 20 mcg/per metered dose.

Dose: Adult 1-2 inhalations 3-4 times a day.

Side effects: Dry mouth, urinary retention, constipation, headache, nausea, throat irritation and cough.

Corticosteroids (Oral or Inhaled)

They are not bronchodilators but are potent anti-inflammatory agents. They prevent attacks by reducing airway hyper-responsiveness, mucosal edema and bronchial secretions.

Uses

• Acute severe branchospasm not responding to other bronchodilators
• Acute severe asthma

Doses and drugs: See Table 3.58.

Side effects: Read corticosteroids.

Mast Cell Stabilizers (Sodium Cromoglycate, Nedocromil)

Action

They inhibit the degranulation of mast cells, thereby preventing the release of the chemical mediators of anaphylaxis.

Uses

• They are most effective in atopic patients who have either seasonal or perennial airway obstruction
• Prophylactic use: When given prophylactically, they will block the acute obstructive effects of exposure (acute bronchial asthma) to antigen, industrial chemicals, exercise or cold air. They should be used intermittently before provocation of acute episode of asthma, i.e. the drug to be taken 15-20 minutes before contact with precipitant.

Doses: See Table 3.59.

Antihistaminic (Ketotifen)

It acts like sodium chromoglycate but has antihistaminic properties which limits its use as an antiasthmatic.

Uses

• Prophylaxis of bronchial asthma similar to sodium chromoglycate.

Doses: See Table 3.60.

Table 3.58: Drugs and their dosages

Drugs	Dose	Comment
• Hydrocortisone	Adult: In acute asthma or status asthmaticus IV hydrocortisone 200 mg after every 6 hours followed by oral prednisolone 40-60 mg daily for 2 weeks in tapering dose	• It is used in conjunction with other therapy to acute severe asthma
• Prednisolone	Oral 30-40 mg given once daily in acute asthma, then it is tapered slowly by 5-10 mg every 5-7 days. Sudden withdrawal or rapid tapering of steroids result in frequent recurrence	• Its effect is not immediate, hence, it must be used with bronchodilators to achieve rapid and vigorous bronchodilation
• Beclamethasone	Inhaler 400 mcg in 2-4 divided doses daily Severe cases 600-800 mcg initially and then reduce the dose according to response Children 6-12 years: 50-100 mcg 3-4 times a day Rotahaler 200 mcg inhaled in rotahalor 3-4 times a day Children: 100 mcg 2-4 times a day	• Only for patients who require chronic treatment with corticosteroids for control of symptoms of bronchial asthma
• Budesonide	Inhalation: Adults—100 mcg/per metered dose; 1-2 puffs twice a day Children—1 puff bid	• Useful adjunct for control of asthma alone or with β₂-stimulant
• Fluticasone	Inhalation 25-125 mcg/per metered dose Adults—100-1000 mcg twice daily Children—between 4 and 12 years: half the dose < 4 years not recommended	• Useful for control of acute asthma

Table 3.59: Mast cell stabilizers—sodium chromoglycate

Drug	Dosage	Comment
Sodium chromoglycate (5 mg/metered dose)	Inhalor: Adult and children 2 puffs 3-4 times a day	• Avoid sudden discontinuation of therapy if used with steroids concurrently • Side effect—cough and throat irritation

Table 3.60: Ketotifen

Drug	Dose	Comments
Ketotifen	Adults 1-2 mg twice a day orally with food Children over 2 years as 1 mg twice a day with food Not recommended for children below 2 yrs	• Avoid its use during pregnancy and lactation • Slow withdrawal over a period of 2-4 weeks • Side effects—Drowsiness, dizziness, dry mouth impaired reactions (not to drive vehicle while on drug), occasionally CNS stimulation, weight gain

Leukotriene Receptor Antagonists (Montelukast and Zafirlukast)

They are selective CysLT1 receptors antagonists that bind with high affinity to the receptors sites, prevent the inflammtory mediators (leukotrienes) to exert their effect. By this mechanism, they reduce the early and late phase of the asthma. They are useful in mild to moderate asthma not controlled by steroids and β-agonists.

Montelukast is used orally as 10 mg at bed time. In children (4-14 years) dose is half.

Side effects include, abdominal pain, fever, dry mouth, insomnia, arthralgia, paresthesias, nightmares.

UNIT

4

Radiology

X-ray Chest (Normal and Abnormal)

NORMAL X-RAY CHEST

A chest X-ray is the common noninvasive investigation that helps not only in the diagnosis of respiratory disease but also in cardiovascular disease too, hence, should be performed routinely in these disorders.

An anteroposterior (AP view) X-ray chest is normally taken in emergency conditions mostly at the bed side; while the other view is posteroanterior (PA view) which is common in use in routine cases. These views in fact reflect the direction of the rays from the source to the plate. In PA view, the beam of rays falls from behind the patient and the heart size appears more or less normal; while in AP view the beam of rays falls from the front and the heart shadow appears as apparently enlarged.

The X-ray chest is read with respect to the following points:

1. View

Whether it is PA view or AP view.

2. Centralization or Centering

Look at the clavicles, if they are at the same level, then X-ray is centralized; and if not then it is poorly centralized.

3. Penetration/Exposure

If the bony cage, ribs and vertebral bodies are just visible through the cardiac shadow, then penetration is good. If they are too clearly visible, then it is over-penetrated and if not visible, then it is under penetrated (under exposed). In over-penetrated X-rays you are likely to miss low density lesions.

4. Sex

If breast shadows are visible, then X-ray belongs to the female patient.

5. Position of Diaphragm

The right dome of diaphragm is slightly higher than left due to presence of liver on the right. Both the costophrenic and cardiophrenic angles are clear.

6. Position of the Trachea

This is seen as a dark column representing the air within the trachea. Note whether trachea is central or displaced. This is seen in reference to central bony vertebral column behind it. The trachea may be deviated to the same side or opposite side in a number of conditions (Read the deviation of trachea in clinical methods).

7. Bony Cage

Note the central vertebral column and the horizontal ribs. Decide whether chest is symmetrical or any scoliosis present. Examine whether the ribs are unduly crowded (collapse or fibrosis) or widely separated (pleural effusion, pneumothorax) on one side than the other. Look for any cervical rib, bony erosion of the ribs.

8. Degree of Inspiration

To judge the degree of inspiration, count the number of ribs above the diaphragm. The anterior end of the 6th rib should be above the diaphragm as should be the posterior end of 10th rib. If more ribs are visible then the lung is hyperinflated. If fewer ribs are visible, then patient has not held the breath during full inspiration. It is important to note this because poor inspiration will make the heart size to look larger and cause the trachea to appear deviated to right.

9. Cardiac Shadow

It occupies the central part of the chest. Its right and left borders are defined:
  i. The right border is smooth, formed from above downwards by the superior vena cava, right atrium and inferior vena cava.
 ii. The left border is formed from above downwards by aortic knuckle, pulmonary conus (artery), left atrial appendage, and left ventricle.
iii. The cardiothoracic ratio is <50 per cent, i.e. the heart shadow is less than half of the maximum transthoracic diameter. If the cardiac shadow occupies >50 percent of the transthoracic diameter, then heart is said to be enlarged.

ABNORMALITIES ON CHEST X-RAY (PA AND AP VIEWS)

Abnormalities of the Cardiac Shadow

Causes of Prominent Aortic Knuckle

- Aortitis
- Aortic aneurysm
- Atherosclerosis of the aorta
- Post-stenotic dilatation.

Pulmonary Conus is Prominent in:

- Idiopathic dilatation of pulmonary artery
- Post-stenotic dilatation
- Pulmonary hypertension

The pulmonary artery shadow: It is absent in pulmonary valvular stenosis, pulmonary artery atresia, Fallot's tetralogy

Left atrial enlargement: It produces double atrial shadow and prominence of shadow of left atrial appendage and straightening of the left border. It is seen in mitralized heart. The right atrial enlargement produces straightening of the right border of the heart with double atrial shadow.

Ventricular enlargement: It produces enlargement of cardiac shadow in different directions. The right ventricular enlargement produces enlargement of cardiac shadow outwards; while left ventricular enlargement causes the heart shadow to enlarge down and out giving an appearance of *boot-shaped heart.*

The Lung Fields

For radiological purposes, the lung fields are divided into three zones. The **upper zone** extends from the apex to a transverse line drawn through the lower borders of the anterior ends of the 2nd costal cartilages. The **mid-zone** extends from this line to another line drawn through the lower borders of the 4th costal cartilage. The **lower zone** extends from this second line to the bases of the lungs or to the dome of diaphragm. Each zone is examined on both sides and compared with each other for any abnormal finding.

Chest X-ray (Lateral View)

This view is most useful in localising the lung lesion because interlobar fissures are clearly seen in this view. It should be examined in a systematic manner, i.e.

- Bony cage
- Position of trachea
- The diaphragm (as the level of the domes of diaphragm differs on the two sides, a double shadow may be seen).
- The lung fields. The lung fields are obscured by two relatively opaque shadows one above and behind due to shoulder joint and second below and in front due to the heart.

The abnormality on lateral view is detected by distortion of interlobar fissures which are seen as lines. The shrinkage of a lobe from collapse or fibrosis distorts these fissures/lines.

The Hilum

Look at the hilum. The left hilum is higher than the right though the difference is usually <2.5 cm. Compare the shape and density of the hila. They are concave in shape and look similar to each other.

CHEST X-RAY IN PULMONARY DISORDERS

Certain patterns encountered on chest X-ray in pulmonary diseases are;

Infiltrate

It is an abnormal shadow in the lung which does not have any pattern—a vague term (Fig. 4.1). If these infiltrates involve the alveoli such as in pneumonia and lymphoma, a homogeneous dense opacity is produced. When this opacity is confined to a lobe, it is called *lobar consolidation* and this is seen in bacterial pneumonia (Figs 4.2 and 4.3). An air bronchogram is also seen. Multiple such opacities when present in the lung constitute bronchopneumonia. The alveolar exudates may coalese to produce nodular opacities (Fig. 4.4) or large fluffy cottonwool like shadows (Fig. 4.5).

Fig. 4.1: Apical tuberculosis. There is infiltration in right upper zone without cavitation

Fig. 4.2: Consolidation right middle lobe
(chest X-ray PA view)

Fig. 4.3: Bilateral consolidation of lower lobes

Alveolar infiltrates are patchy, homogeneous and have an air bronchogram. They may be lobar or segmental

Contrary to this, interstitial infiltrates occur when there is involvement of interstitium as in viral pneumonias, interstitial pneumonitis and occupational disorders. The radiological patterns that arise from these infiltrates reflect as micronodular, reticular, reticulonodular and multiple linear shadows. On occasion both alveolar and interstitial infiltrates get superimposed on each other such as occur in pulmonary edema.

THE WHITENESS (OPACIFICATION) OF THE LUNGS

Acute Pulmonary Edema

In pulmonary edema, there is leakage of fluid from the pulmonary venous circulation into the alveoli and the lung interstitium producing haziness of the lungs from the center toward the periphery on both the sides. Acute pulmonary edema may be cardiogenic (heart size is enlarged due to left heart failure) or noncardiogenic (ARDS- type I respiratory failure) in which there is opacification of peripheral fields of the lung with normal cardiac size.

Radiological Findings

Radiological findings in the cardiogenic pulmonary edema (Fig. 4.6) are:

1. *Haziness of the lung.* Severe pulmonary edema due to LVF gives confluent alveolar shadowing (haziness) which spreads from the hilum towards periphery giving a *"bat's wing appearance"*. In ARDS, the haziness is more peripheral than central.

Fig. 4.4: Bilateral pulmonary tuberculosis. Note the bilateral infiltrates producing nodular opacities

Fig. 4.5: Bilateral fungal infection. Note the fluffy cotton-wool shadows

Fig. 4.6: Cardiogenic pulmonary edema. Chest X-ray (PA view) shows bilateral haze extending from the center to the periphery. There is enlargement of heart shadow

Bedside Medicine

2. *Upper lobe veins prominent.* In PA view in erect position, normal blood flow is greater in the lower lobes than the upper due to gravity, hence lower blood vessels are more prominent. In heart failure (pulmonary edema), the upper lobe veins are dilated due to diversion of blood flow – the first sign of the heart failure.
3. *Size of the heart.* Heart size is enlarged.
4. *Kerley's B lines.* These are caused by edema of the interlobular septa. They are horizontal, nonbranching white lines best seen at the periphery of the lungs just above the costophrenic angle.
5. Pleural effusion or hydrothorax. A small pleural effusion obliterating the costophrenic angle is common.

Differential Diagnosis of Pulmonary Edema (Bilateral Haze in the Lungs)

Two common causes of pulmonary edema (*cardiogenic* vs *noncardiogenic*) are compared in the Table 4.1.

Table 4.1: Radiological comparison of cardiogenic vs noncardiogenic pulmonary edema

Features	Cardiogenic edema (Fig. 4.6)	Noncardiogenic edema (Fig. 4.7)
Distribution of haze	Bilateral haze is more central than peripheral	Bilateral haze is more peripheral than central
Heart size	Enlarged	Normal
Upper lobe veins	Dilated and enlarged	Normal
Kerley B lines	Far more common	Less common
Pleural effusion	Common	Less common

Fig. 4.7: Noncardiogenic pulmonary oedema. Note the peripheral haze and normal cardiac shadow

Causes of ARDS (Noncardiogenic Pulmonary Edema)

ARDS is caused by any acute insult to either the alveolar or endothelial cells that result in loss of integrity of the junctions between these cells allowing fluid to leak into the alveoli. Causes include:
- Aspiration or inhalation of toxic gases
- Pneumonia
- Sepsis
- Drowning
- Hypersensitivity reaction
- Lung trauma
- Radiation
- Fat embolism (crush injury)
- Drug abuse
- Transfusion reaction

Pulmonary Embolism

It produces a wedge-shaped or triangular opacity situated in one of the periphery in a patient suffering from deep vein thrombosis (Fig. 4.8). The dome of the diaphragm may be raised on that side. It may lead to a small pleural effusion. There may be collapse or linear atelectasis. Pulmonary embolus can also lead to black area of underperfused lung which is difficult to detect on plain X-ray. CT scan and MRI are diagnostic. The enlargement of heart and prominent pulmonary conus suggests acute cor pulmonale.

Homogeneous Opacity Involving One Hemithorax

The causes are:
- Pleural effusion
- Consolidation

Fig. 4.8: Pulmonary embolism. There is an peripheral opacity (arrow) in the right lung. The pulmonary conus is prominent and heart shadow is not enlarged, probably due to emphysema

- Atelectasis
- Pulmonary agenesis
- Pneumonectomy.

Ipsilateral shift of the trachea and mediastinum, narrowing of the intercostal spaces, elevation of dome of diaphragm and compensatory emphysema of the uninvolved side indicate *atelectasis*, or collapse, fibrosis *pneumonectomy* and *pulmonary agenesis.* The collapse and fibrosis of the lung have been dealt separately.

The contralateral shift of the trachea and mediastinum, the homogeneous opacification in the peripheral lung field with concave border towards the lung, widening of the intercostal spaces, obliteration of costophrenic angle and nonvisibility of the dome of diaphragm on the involved side indicate pleural effusion (Figs 4.9A and B).

In mild pleural effusion, there may be just obliteration of costophrenic angle (Fig. 4.10); while a localised effusion produces a homogeneous opacification similar to a tumor with no shift of trachea or mediastinum (Fig. 4.11).

In massive consolidation, a rim of normal lung tissue at costophrenic angle may be seen. There may be no shift of trachea or mediastinum. No compensatory emphysema is seen.

A Lobar Homogeneous Opacity

A homogeneous opacity look like an area of white lung. If there is a patch of opacity, it could be due to collapse, pleural effusion or consolidation. If the opacity is uniform with a well demarcated border, then it is either a lobar collapse or pleural effusion which can be differentiated by shift of the trachea and mediastinum with crowding of the ribs and elevated dome of the diaphragm on the side involved in case of collapse but reverse will happen in pleural effusion (shift of trachea and mediastinum to opposite side, widening of the intercostal spaces and flattening of the dome of diaphragm). If the shadow is not uniform and the border is not well defined then it could be either consolidation or fibrosis. In fibrosis, the signs are similar to collapse of the lung. In consolidation (Fig. 4.12), note the followings:

- Presence of air-bronchogram within opacity (arrow) confirms the diagnosis of consolidation. In consolidation, the air spaces are filled with fluid or exudate making them appear as white whereas airways within opacity retain air, making them appear black. The areas of blackness within white background suggest air-bronchogram.
- The shadowing in consolidation gets denser as one moves down the lung because fluid sinks and makes the lower border denser and well defined.

Figs 4.9A and B: A. Homogeneous opacity of one hemithorax. Chest X-ray PA view showing pleural effusion, B. Bilateral pleural effusion. There is bilateral opacification of thorax besides the heart. There is no deviation of trachea or mediastinum

Coin-shaped Shadow

The term *coin lesion* is used to describe an area of whiteness situated within a lung field (Fig. 4.13). It needs not be strictly circular. The causes of single coin lesion are:

- Benign tumor, e.g. hematoma
- Malignant tumor, e.g. bronchial carcinoma, solitary secondary
- Infection, e.g. consolidation, abscess, tuberculosis (tuberculoma)
- Hydatid cyst
- Pulmonary infarction
- Rheumatoid nodule.

Fig. 4.10: Minimal pleural effusion. There is just obliteration of costophrenic angle (↑)

Fig. 4.11: Loculated pleural effusion. There is lobulated homogeneous opacity with no shift of trachea or mediastinum

Differentiating Features

- A speckled irregular or lobulated edge of the lesion suggests malignancy
- Calcification within the lesion indicates tuberculosis or infection
- More than one coin-shaped lesions suggest metastatic disease
- Air bronchogram suggests consolidation rather than a tumor
- Surrounding the lesion, the area of consolidation or collapse may indicate a tumor
- Malignant tumors are associated with mediastinal lymphadenopathy, rib erosion and pleural effusion.

Cavitatory Lung Lesion

A cavity is a walled off area of the lung which is darker in the center than the periphery (Fig. 4.14). Some coin-shaped lesions may cavitate. The causes of cavitating lung lesions are:
- Lung abscess (e.g. tubercular, pyogenic, malignant)
- Neoplasm with secondary degeneration and cavitation
- Cavitation around a pneumonia
- An infarct (rare)
- Rheumatoid nodule (rare)

Differential Features

- The cavity may contain a horizontal fluid level—a line within lesion. There will be whiteness (fluid) below the line with an area of blackness (air) above. This is common in pyogenic infection, i.e. lung abscess (Fig. 4.15A).

Fig. 4.12: Chest X-ray (PA view) showing consolidation of the right upper and middle lobe

Fig. 4.13: Chest X-ray (PA view) showing a coin-shaped lesion (arrow). The lesion is single and larger than a coin

437

Fig. 4.14: An apical tubercular cavity

Figs 4.15A and B: Chest X-ray PA view: A. A lung abscess in left lung (arrow); B. A cavity with fungal ball in left upper zone (←)

Fig. 4.16: Chest X-ray (PA view) showing multiple ring shadows suggesting bronchiectasis (←) of right lower lobe. In addition, there is superadded infection due to aspiration pneumonia

- If the walls of the cavity are thick (>5 mm) and irregular, infiltrating into the surrounding lung, then it is a neoplasm as opposed to an abscess. Staphylococcal abscess especially is a thin- walled called *pneumatocele*. This rule does not always hold true.
- A white ball within a cavity is characteristic of an aspergilloma which can be seen floating in the cavity (Fig. 4.15B).

Ring Shadows (e.g. Bronchiectasis)

Multiple ring shadows of any size upto 1 cm in diameter occurring in groups giving a honey-comb or "bunches of grapes" appearance on chest X-ray may suggest bronchiectasis (Fig. 4.16). Other lesions described in bronchiectasis are:

- *Tubular shadows.* These are thick white shadows upto 8 mm wide, represent bronchi filled with secretions (end-on bronchus).
- *Glove finger shadows.* These represent a group of tubular shadows seen head on and look like the finger of a glove.

The presence of any of these features suggests bronchiectasis but a normal chest X-ray does not however exclude the diagnosis. The CT scan is most sensitive diagnostic test available for bronchiectasis.

Causes of Bronchiectasis

1. *Structural* e.g. Kartagener's syndrome, obstruction (foreign body, a growth)
2. *Infection*, e.g. childhood pertussis or measles, tuberculosis, pneumonia
3. *Immune*, e.g. hypogammaglobulinemia, allergic bronchopulmonary aspergillosis
4. *Metabolic*, e.g. cystic fibrosis
5. *Idiopathic*, e.g. secondary to stasis.

Reticulonodular Shadows
(Fibrosis or Edema of the Lungs)

The reticulonodular shadowing which simply means a meshwork of lines that combines to form nodules and ring shadows of <5 mm in diameter. Sometime this meshwork is very fine giving a ground glass appearance, said to look like a thin veil over the lung. Later, it gives a more coarse appearance and is said to look like a honey-comb. Honey-combing is a feature of interstitial lung disease/pulmonary fibrosis. The causes of reticulonodular opacities are:

• Pulmonary edema
• Bronchopneumonia
• Lymphangitis carcinomatosis (Fig. 4.17).

Differentiating Features

• Bilateral basal reticulonodular shadowing could be either due to edema or fibrosis. Shadowing that is confined to midzone or apical region is more likely to be fibrosis
• The presence of small lungs indicates fibrosis rather than pulmonary/interstitial edema
• Shifting of the mediastinum to the side of shadowing is due to fibrosis rather than edema
• In fibrosis, heart border and diaphragm on the side involved appear blurred
• Vascular marking is less distinct in area of fibrosis.

Causes of Fibrosis

• Cryptogenic
• Occupational lung disease, e.g. extrinsic allergic alveolitis, asbestosis
• Infection, e.g. tuberculosis, psittacosis, aspiration pneumonia
• Collagen vascular disorders, e.g. rheumatoid arthritis, SLE
• Sarcoidosis
• Iatrogenic, e.g. amiodarone, busulphan, radiotherapy.

Miliary Shadowing

Miliary shadowing refers to small miliary opacities having similar density and size distributed in the lung(s) giving a spotted or mottled appearance. They sometimes can be confused with a ground glass appearance or normal vascular markings of the lung. To differentiate between them, move close to the X-ray and examine the shadowing carefully.

In miliary mottling, the opacities are discrete, small and have similar size and density, are mainly distributed in the peripheral lung fields (Fig. 4.18). The main causes of miliary mottling are;

Fig. 4.17: X-ray chest showing lymphangitis carcinomatosis

Fig. 4.18: Chest X-ray (PA view) showing miliary mottling appearance due to miliary tuberculosis

• Tuberculosis
• Sarcoidosis
• Disseminated metastases in the lungs
• Interstitial lung diseases.

Differentiating Features

- *Distribution of opacities:* In miliary tuberculosis, the opacities are most marked in the upper zone, in sarcoidosis, these are most marked in perihilar region and mid-zones; while in miliary metastases these are limited to lower zones.
- *Density:* Highly dense white opacities are likely to be due to dust related industrial/occupational disorders or calcified tuberculosis. Less dense changes could either be multiple secondaries or sarcoidosis or any other cause of miliary mottling.
- *Other associated signs:* Unilateral hilar enlargement suggests tuberculosis while bilateral hilar enlargement (lymphadenopathy) indicates sarcoidosis. Presence of subtle cavitating lesions suggest tuberculosis.

Collapse of the Lung

Collapse of the lung means an area of the lung devoid of air, hence, is detected as a white area within lung fields.

Radiological Features (Fig. 4.19)

1. *Lung fields:* Look at the lung fields. The right lung normally is larger than the left – if it is not, then suspect an area of right lung collapse.
2. *Position of diaphragm:* Normally, left dome should be lower than the right, if it is not (e.g. left dome elevated) then left lung collapse may be suspected.
3. *Position of the horizontal fissure:* Note the position of the horizontal fissure in the right lung. The horizontal fissure normally on the right should run from the centre of the hilum to the level of the 6th rib in the axillary line. If this is pulled up, it suggests right upper lobe collapse and if pulled down then right lower lobe collapse should be suspected.
4. *Position of the heart:* The heart shadow lies in the midline with one – third to the right and two – thirds to the left. The heart shadow gets deviated to the side of collapse.
5. *Heart borders:* Define the heart borders. Normally the borders are distinct. If the adjacent lung is collapsed, then the heart border will appear blurred. For example, if right heart border is blurred this indicates right middle lobe collapse; and if left is indistinct or blurred, then suspect lingular collapse.
6. *Position of trachea:* Normally trachea is central; it gets deviated if there is pathology in the upper lobes. Collapse of right or left upper lobe will pull the trachea towards the area of collapse (Figs 4.19A to D).

   Note. To determine the collapse of the lung both PA view and lateral chest X-rays must be taken and examined

Figs 4.19A and B: Collapse of right upper lobe: A. A chest X-ray (PA view) shows an area of opacification in the upper zone (1) of right lung. The horizontal fissure (2) is pulled upwards. There appears to be a large right upper hilar mass. The trachea (3) is shifted to right, i.e. same side of the mass. The ribs over the area of opacification are crowded with narrowing of intercostal spaces, B. Chest X-ray (lateral view) shows the area of opacification localised to upper most portion of the lung

Fig. 4.19C: Collapse of right middle lobe. It is difficult to spot. The right diaphragm may be raised (1), and horizontal fissure may be lower than usual. The lower zone of right lung shows a haze (3) with indistinct heart border. It is easier to detect on lateral film (not projected) where a triangular opacity with its apex towards hilum and its base running between sternum and diaphragm will be seen similar to collapse of left lower lobe (lingular collapse) in Figure 4.19D

Fig. 4.20: Pneumonectomy. Chest X-ray (PA view) shows that left hemithorax is white. The mediastinum lies in the left hemithorax and some of the right hypertrophied lung has herniated to the left side giving a slightly darker left apex (arrow) compared to base. This picture can be confused with collapse of left lung (whole)

7. *Lateral films:* Check the position of oblique and horizontal fissures. The horizontal fissure appears as faint white line which should pass horizontally from the hilum to the anterior chest wall. If this line is not horizontal, the fissure is displaced. The oblique fissure should pass obliquely downwards from the T4/T5 vertebrae, through the hilum, ending at the anterior third of the diaphragm.

Collapse of any of the lobes of the lungs gives a distinct appearance on X-ray (Figs 4.20 and 4.21).

Collapse of Whole Left Lung vs Pneumonectomy (Fig. 4.20)

The distinct features are:

1. In pneumonectomy, the left hemithorax is homogeneously opaque with no lung markings while in collapse, lung marking are visible.
2. In pneumonectomy, the whole mediastinum and even a portion of right lung lies in left hemithorax while in collapse only mediastinum is shifted.

Calcification in the Lung Fields

Causes

Parenchymal calcification

A. Diffuse

    i. Infection, e.g. tuberculosis, abscess, histoplasmosis, pneumonia

    ii. Tumors, e.g. hematomas, metastases

    iii. Unknown e.g. alveolar microliths, broncholitis

    iv. Silicosis

    v. Hemosiderosis (following hemoptysis in mitral stenosis)

Fig. 4.19D: Left lower lobe (lingular) collapse. Chest X-ray lateral view shows a triangular opacity with apex towards hilum and base between sternum and diaphragm

Figs 4.19A to D: Collapse of different lobes of the lungs on chest X-rays (PA and lateral views)

Figs 4.21A and B: Bronchogenic carcinoma.
Chest X-ray (PA) view shows;

A. Collapse of right upper lobe. Note the area of whiteness in upper zone of right lung. The horizontal fissure is elevated (1); there is shift of mediastinum to right side (2). The trachea is deviated to the right (3). The ribs over the area of whiteness are crowded. On lateral film, the increased whiteness in the uppermost part of the chest will be seen (not depicted).

B. Left upper lobe collapse. When it collapses, it causes haze to appear over the whole of the lung as it occupies major portion of the lung field on PA view. On the lateral film, an area of whiteness will be seen on the top of left lung (not shown). There is deviation of trachea and heart shadow towards the collapsed lung. The ribs spaces are narrowed on left side

B. Solitary
- Tuberculosis
- Histoplasmosis
- Hamartomas (pop-corn calcification)

Pleural calcification
Diffuse
- Tuberculosis (Fig. 4.22), empyema
- Asbestosis

Focal
- Asbestosis (Fig. 4.23)
- Talcosis

Fig. 4.22: Pleural calcification (diffuse) in tuberculosis on the left side of the lung (←)

Fig. 4.23: Asbestosis. Chest X-ray PA view shows bilateral opacities in the lower zones with pleural plaques of calcification

Egg-shell calcification (Fig. 4.24)
- Silicosis (most common)
- Coal-miner's pneumoconiosis
- Sarcoidosis

Mediastinal calcification
- Lymphadenopathy, e.g. sarcoidosis, tuberculosis, pneumoconiosis
- Tumors, e.g. teratoma, dermoid, thyroid adenoma.

Cardiac calcification
- Aortic arch (ring shaped or annular calcification in atherosclerosis)
- Pericardial calcification (adhesive or constrictive pericarditis)
- Calcification of mitral and aortic valves
- Thrombi and left atrial myxoma
- Calcification of coronary arteries

Chest wall calcification
- Soft tissue, e.g. cysticercosis, Guinea-worm
- Ribs (costal cartilage)
- Phleboliths

THE BLACK (HYPERTRANSLUCENT) LUNG FIELDS

Hypertranslucency

It refers to increased blackness of the lung fields due to trapping of air either in the pleural space or in the lungs. It may be unilateral or bilateral.

Caution

Before commenting on hypertranslucency, check the penetration of X-ray. If the vertebral bodies are just hardly visible behind the heart, it is a good quality X-ray while if they are clearly visible, then film is overpenetrated and makes the lungs appear black (hypertranslucent).

Causes of Hypertranslucency

Unilteral
- Pneumothorax
- Unilateral obstruction
- Bullae
- Eventration of the diaphragm

Bilateral
- Pneumothorax
- Bullous emphysema
- COPD
- Bronchial asthma
- Primary pulmonary hypertension (if vascular shadows disappear, the lung is replaced by air)
- Ebstein's anomaly
- Fallot's tetralogy

Chronic Obstructive Pulmonary Disease (COPD)

The radiological findings (Fig. 4.25) are due to hyperinflation of the lungs with constriction of the cardiac shadow.
- The lungs are large and voluminous due to hyperinflation which can be checked by counting the ribs anteriorly. If you can count more than 7 ribs above the diaphragm, then lungs are hyperinflated. This can be a normal finding in some individuals also.
- The domes of the diaphragm are low and flat instead of being convex due to hyperexpansion of the lungs.

Fig. 4.24: Egg cell calcification. Chest X-ray (PA view) shows an egg cell calcification in hilar lymph nodes in silicosis

Fig. 4.25: Chest X-ray showing COPD. Note all the characteristics described in the text

- The heart is tubular (elongated and narrow) due to overexpansion of both lungs. The heart, instead of sitting on the diaphragm often appears to "swing in the wind"
- Hypertranslucency of both the lungs is characteristic. Bullae (densely black areas of lung, usually round, surrounded by hairline shadows) may be seen which may compress the normal lung and distort the surrounding vasculature. Thus, to find out the bullae, look out for areas of decreased vascular markings.
- The lung vascular markings are reduced bilaterally (oligemic lungs) and fan out as straight lines from the hilum but stop two-thirds of the way out, i.e. peripheral pruning (peripheral fields appear without vascular markings).
- The ribs are more horizontal and the intercostal spaces appear widened.

Pneumothorax (Unilateral Black Lung)

Before commenting on unilateral blackness, check the technical quality of film. A rotated film (one clavicle is nearer the midline than the other) may make one side less dense than the other.

Radiological Features of Pneumothorax

- There is hypertranslucency of the lung in the periphery without vascular markings. This is due to air trapped in pleural space.
- There is sharply defined edge of the deflated lung, seen as a vertical line when X-ray is turned on its side which is convex towards periphery. In a large pneumothorax, deflated lung appears small towards the centre with convex borders (Fig. 4.26).
- The mediastinum is shifted away from the black lung indicating tension pneumothorax (Fig. 4.26) which returns to normal after removal of air an expansion of lung (Fig. 4.27).
- Differentiation between a bullae and pneumothorax is sometimes difficult and often impossible. However, if lung markings are seen either crossing the area of blackness or are limited to the periphery of the blackness, then it is a bullae rather than pneumothorax. Bullae are usually multiple if bullous disease is suspected.

Causes of Pneumothorax

- Spontaneous
- Iatrogenic/trauma, e.g. subpleural bleb rupture, transbronchial biopsy, central venous line insertion, ventilator-induced.
- Obstructive lung disease, e.g. asthma, COPD
- Infections, e.g. pneumonia, tuberculosis

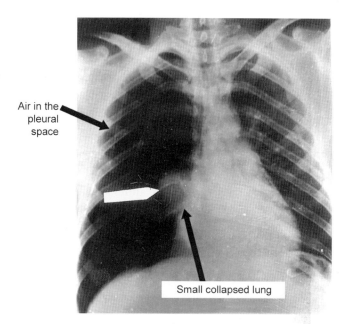

Fig. 4.26: Pneumothorax. Right sided tension pneumothorax. Chest X-ray (PA view) before compression shows;
- Right lung is blacker than left
- The lung is collapsed towards the hilum and its outline is demarcated by a thin pencil line indicated by a white arrow
- Mediastinum is shifted to left
- The black area of pneumothorax (→) is devoid of vascular marking

Fig. 4.27: After decompression by intercostal tube, the lung has expanded

- Cystic fibrosis
- Connective tissue diseases, e.g. Marfan's syndrome, Ehlers-Danlos syndrome.

Hydropneumothorax is the term that denotes a fluid level (a horizontal line) above which lies blackness of the lung without lung marking (pneumothorax) and below (Fig. 4.28) there is opacification due to fluid.

Bedside Medicine

444

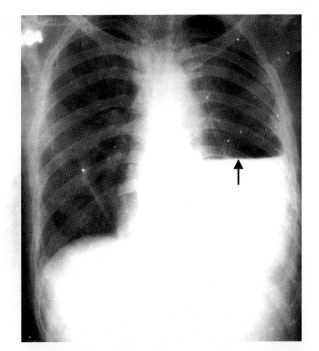

Fig. 4.28: Hydropneumothorax. Note the horizontal straight line (↑) between hypertranslucent area above and an opaque are below

Fig. 4.29: Chest X-ray (PA view) showing air under right dome of diaphragm (indicated by an arrow). The X-ray was taken from a patient with enteric perforation. There is a large air bubble below the left dome

THE ABNORMALITIES OF SUBDIAPHRAGMATIC REGION AND THE DIAPHRAGM

Finish your examination of chest X-ray by looking at the area under the diaphragm and the domes of diaphragm. The abnormalities in this area are:

1. Air under diaphragm
2. Elevation of diaphragm

Air under Diaphragm

The area immediately under the diaphragm will usually be white due to presence of solid structures (liver and spleen) except a darker round area under left diaphragm due to presence of air bubble in the stomach.

Air under the diaphragm is an important sign, since it indicates an intra-abdominal perforation (e.g. intestine, stomach, colon, etc.). The air leaks from the intestines or stomach and collects under the diaphragm when X-ray is taken in standing position. The air under the right dome of diaphragm can easily be recognised as a rim of blackness (Fig. 4.29) immediately under the diaphragm (╺). However, it is difficult to differentiate air under left dome from the normal stomach bubble as both produce blackness under diaphragm. The differences between the two are:

1. *Thickness of diaphragm:* The diaphragm appears as a thin white line between the white area below and the black lungs above. In the presence of air under left dome, this line becomes very thin (<5 mm) as it consists of diaphragm only. Normally due to the presence of air bubble in the stomach, this line is thicker (>5 mm) as it consists of diaphragm and the walls of the stomach.
2. *Length of air bubble:* Measure the length of air bubble. If it is longer than the half of the length of diaphragm, it is likely to be free air than stomach air bubble.
3. *Look at the other dome,* i.e. right hemidiaphragm: If there is air bubble below the right and left hemidiaphragm (Fig. 4.29), it is likely to be free air in the abdomen.

Elevation of Hemidiaphragm

The mid-point of right hemidiaphragm should be between the 5th and 7th ribs anteriorly; while the left dome is lower than right by about 3 cm. The diaphragm placed above the 5th rib is said to be elevated which may be unilateral or bilateral.

Causes

Unilateral elevation
- Subpulmonic pleural effusion (Fig. 4.30)
- Amebic liver abscess
- Subdiaphragmatic abscess or a tumor
- Basal pulmonary infarction
- Basal pulmonary atelectasis/collapse
- Eventration of the diaphragm (Fig. 4.31)
- Phrenic nerve palsy
- Gas in the colon or fundus of the stomach

Bilateral elevation
- Increased intra-abdominal pressure
- Pregnancy
- Obesity

Figs 4.30A and B: Subpulmonic pleural effusion: Chest X-ray (A) shows an abnormally elevated right dome of diaphragm with flattening (↑), gave a suspicion of diaphragmatic palsy or subpulmonic effusion, which revealed clearly a subpulmonic effusion (splash of fluid producing peripheral convex opacity with concavity toward lung) when chest X-ray (B) was taken in decubitus position

- Ascites
- Large abdominal masses
- Abdominal distension
- Infants
- Bilateral phrenic nerve palsy.

Clinically there is synchronous movements of the two hemidiaphragm. The paralysis of phrenic nerve is tested by sniff test, i.e. while sniffing, the paralysed diaphragm under fluoroscopy will move paradoxically upward due to negative intrathoracic pressure.

HILAR ENLARGEMENT (WIDENING OF HILUM)

Both the hila are similar in size and concave in shape. They have more or less same density. Abnormal hilum means either one hilum is bigger than the other or denser than the other. When hilum enlarges, its concave shape is lost – a first sign of hilar enlargement.

Causes of Hilar Enlargement

Unilateral (Fig. 4.32)

Due to Lymph Node Enlargement

- Infective, e.g. tuberculosis, histoplasmosis
- Sarcoidosis
- Neoplasm, e.g. lymphoma, metastasis from bronchial carcinoma

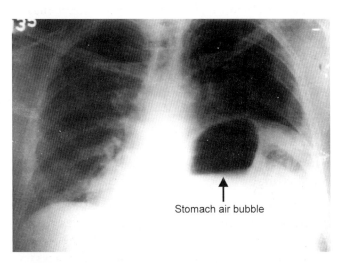

Stomach air bubble

Fig. 4.31: Chest X-ray (PA) view shows an elevated left hemidiaphragm due to eventration. Note the stomach air bubble in left hemithorax (↑), pushing the heart shadow to the right

Fig. 4.32: Chest X-ray (PA view) showing unilateral hilar enlargement due to lymphadenopathy (an arrow)

Due to Vascular Enlargement

• Pulmonary artery aneurysm
• Poststenotic dilatation of pulmonary artery

Bilateral

A. Bilateral lymph nodes enlargement (Fig. 4.33).
  • Infections, e.g. tuberculosis, histoplasmosis, AIDS, recurrent chest infections
  • Neoplasms, e.g. lymphoma, metastases
  • Occupational lung diseases, e.g. silicosis, berrylliosis
  • Sarcoidosis (a common cause)

Differential Features of Hilar Enlargement

1. Smooth enlargement of hilum is due to vascular lesion while lobulated appearance indicates lymphadenopathy and spiculated irregular or indistinct margins suggest malignancy.
2. Presence of calcification within the mass indicates lymph node enlargement usually tuberculosis. Egg-shaped calcification indicates lymphadenopathy due to silicosis.
3. Hilar enlargement due to malignant lung lesion is also associated with superior mediastinal lymphadenopathy
4. Look at the lung fields (for presence of tumor or tubercular infiltration) and bone/ribs for metastasis.

Mediastinal Shadow/Enlargement

The mediastinum comprises the central area between the two lungs and their pleural coverings. Laterally on either side, it is bounded by mediastinal pleura. It extends from the thoracic inlet (above) to the diaphragm (below) and from the sternum (front) to the spine (back). The structures present in the mediastinum include, lymph nodes, heart and great vessels (aorta and its branches), superior vena cava, thymus, oesophagus and fatty areolar tissue.

N.B. On PA view, measure the width of mediastinum (white area) at its maximum convexity and compare it to the width of the chest at that point; if it is >30 percent of the width of the chest, then mediastinum is said to be enlarged widened.

Causes of Mediastinal Widening (Enlargement)

1. *Lymphadenopathy*
  • Tuberculosis, sarcoidosis, lymphomas, leukemias, metastasis
2. *Aortic enlargement*
  • Aneurysm (Fig. 4.34)
  • Unfolding of aorta
3. *Thymus*
  • Thymoma
  • Thymic hyperplasia

Fig. 4.33: Hilar enlargement. Chest X-ray (PA view) shows widening of the mediastinum due to bilateral hilar enlargement

Fig. 4.34: Chest X-ray (PA view) showing widening of the mediastinum due to aortic arch aneurysm

4. *Cysts*
  • Dermoid; teratoma
  • Bronchogenic cyst
  • Pleuropericardial cyst
  • Meningocele
5. *Esophagus*
  • Cardia achalasia
  • Hiatus hernia
  • Enterogenous cyst

6. *Miscellaneous*
   - Lipoma
   - Mediastinal abscess
   - Ventricular aneurysm or cardiac tumor

Differentiating Radiological Features

1. *Site of enlargement/widening:* Look at the X-ray and note whether widening is at the top, in the middle or lower part of mediastinum.
   - Widening at the top could either be due to thyroid, thymus or innominate artery.
   - Widening of the middle or bottom of the mediastinum could be due to lymphadenopathy, aortic aneurysm, dilatation of esophagus (cardia achalasia) or a hiatal hernia.
   - If widening is at the top, then look at the position of the trachea.
   An enlarged thyroid will displace or narrow the trachea while tortuous innominate artery or thymus do not.
2. If you suspect an enlarged thyroid then look at the outline of the shadow.
   - A thyroid has a well defined shadow that tends to become less clear as one moves up to the neck.
3. Look at the right side of trachea. A white edge of trachea is 2-3 mm wide, its further widening suggest either enlarged superior vena cava or a paratracheal mass.
4. If you suspect widening of the aorta, follow the outer edge of the aorta downward, you may be able to detect a continuous edge which widens to form the edge of enlarged mediastinum. This would suggest that the widening is due to dilatation of the aorta.
5. Look at the calcification in the wall of aorta. If you detect a line of calcification then follow it. If it leads into an area of aortic knuckle, then this strongly suggests aortic aneurysm or atherosclerosis of aorta. If the line of calcification is separated from the edge of aortic shadow this strongly suggests aortic dissection.
6. To differentiate aortic aneurysm from unfolding of the aorta, follow both the edges of aorta and note for any widening which will suggest the aneurysm. Obtain a lateral film. If the edges of the aorta are parallel then you are probably dealing with unfolding of the aorta on the PA view of X-ray chest.

Surgical Emphysema (Fig. 4.35)

Collection of air in the soft tissue structure is called *surgical emphysema* because mostly it is due to either a complication of surgery or chest tube drainage.

Radiological Characteristics

- Look at the soft tissue shadow around the chest X-ray. Lozenge shaped areas of blackness which represent

Fig. 4.35: Chest X-ray (PA view) shows surgical emphysema. There is pocket of air outside the chest cage in the soft tissue indicated by an arrow (→) on left side

pockets of air in the soft tissue indicate surgical emphysema (Fig. 4.35). These areas lie in the same plane as the soft tissue structures. In severe cases, orientation of the planes is lost and dark and white lines are produced which cross a part or whole of the film.

Causes of Surgical Emphysema

- Trauma
- Iatrogenic, e.g. surgery, chest tube drainage
- COPD, asthma
- Oesophageal rupture
- Gas gangrene

ABNORMAL HEART SHADOW

The major part of the heart shadow may lie on the right side than left, indicates either shift of the mediastinum to the right or mesocardium (heart lies in the center) or dextrocardia (heart lies on the right-side instead of left).

Differential Radiological Features

1. First of all, always look for the radiographer marking, e.g. left or right at the top of X-ray. Incorrect marking can produce iatrogenic dextrocardia. If there is doubt, repeat the film.
2. Look for the trachea. Shift of the mediastinum indicates shift of the heart due to collapse, fibrosis, pneumonectomy.
3. If marking is correct, and trachea is central, look at the apex of the heart, if it lies on the right, then it is dextrocardia (Fig. 4.36). Dextrocardia will be further

Fig. 4.36: Dextrocardia. Note the followings
(i) Apex of heart lies on the right side
(ii) Aortic knuckle is absent on the left is present on the right side
(iii) Left dome of the diaphragm is elevated due to presence of liver on left. There is absence of stomach air bubble below left dome

confirmed by absence of aortic knuckle on the left side. It will be present on the right side.

4. Now look at the domes of diaphragm, higher left dome than right with air bubble below it confirms situs inversus.

The heart shadow is said to be enlarged if it occupies more than half of the transthoracic diameter.

Causes of Enlargement of Heart Shadow

1. Left to right shunt, e.g. ASD, VSD, PDA. This is associated with increased pulmonary plethora.
2. Ventricular enlargement. The shape of heart in ventricular enlargement has already been discussed.
3. Ventricular aneurysm.
4. Pericardial effusion.

Left to Right Shunt

Radiological Features (Fig. 4.37)

• Look at the X-ray for cardiomegaly. Confirm cardiomegaly by measurement described above.
• Look at the pulmonary conus, if full and convex, indicates pulmonary hypertension.
• Now look at the shape of the heart. See the apex of the heart which is rounded due to enlargement of right ventricle and is being lifted up clear off the diaphragm. As right atrium also enlarges in left to right shunt, the right border looks also rounded and fuller than normal.
• Determine the position of the heart with reference to position of the vertebrae. In left to right shunt (e.g.

ASD, VSD) the heart is sometimes shifted transversely to the left and so the right edge of the vertebral column is revealed.

• Pulmonary plethora. In left to right shunt, there is increased blood flow through pulmonary vessels leading to their dilatation called—*pulmonary plethora*. On X-ray, the vessels especially the pulmonary artery and lung vasculature are prominent (i.e. bronchovascular markings are visible up to the periphery) and increased pulsations of these vessels may be seen on fluoroscopy.
• Look at the aortic knuckle and arch of aorta. It is often smaller due to shunting of blood from left side to right side rather than passing through aorta.

Mitral Valve Disease

Mitral stenosis produces a combination of left atrial and right ventricular enlargement; while mitral regurgitation produces left atrial and left ventricular enlargement; other radiological signs are common to both. The heart in mitral valve disease is called *mitralized heart.*

Radiological Features (Fig. 4.38)

• Look at the cardiac shadow which is enlarged in mitral valve disease.
• Look at the left border. Straightening of the left border is due to left atrial enlargement. Sometimes the left atrium enlargement is so great (giant left atrium in mitral regurgitation) that this part of the heart bulges outward *(third mogul sign)*.
• Now look at the right border of heart. Look carefully for a double atrial shadow which is best seen in well penetrated film and is due to left atrial enlargement *(mitralized heart)*. The left atrium also causes the right

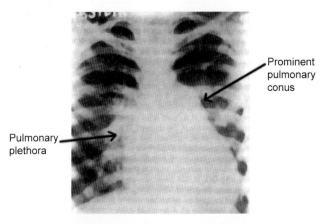

Prominent pulmonary conus

Pulmonary plethora

Fig. 4.37: Chest X-ray (PA view) shows features of left to right shunt. The X-ray was taken from a patient with ASD (atrial septal defect). There is mild cardiomegaly with large pulmonary artery and enlarged arteries in the hila with plethora in the lung fields. Aortic knuckle is small. The radiological appearance is suggestive of left to right shunt (ASD)

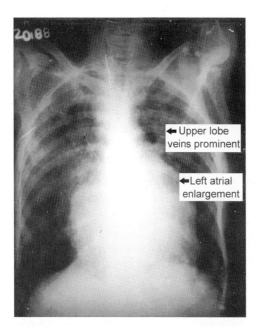

Fig. 4.38: Chest X-ray (PA) showing characteristic radiological features of mitral stenosis (mitralised heart). Heart size enlarged with prominent upper lobes veins, left atrial enlargement, double atrial shadow on the right side near the heart border, the apex is dipping into the diaphragm indicate mitralized heart

heart border to shift further over to the right than usual. For left atrial shadow, hold the X-ray in right hand in horizontal or oblique position infront of you in bright light, the double shadow, i.e. double right border will be visible as peripheral less opaque and inner dense opaque area.

- Look at the carina by following the tracheal shadow to its bifurcation into right and left bronchi. The angle between the two bronchi is <90°. Widening of this angle suggest left atrial enlargement.
- Look at the apex. If it is lifted up clear off the diaphragm, the heart enlargement is right ventricular type. If the heart lies on diaphragm (boot-shaped), then it is left ventricular enlargement.
- Look at the pulmonary area. Prominent pulmonary conus indicates pulmonary hypertension.
- Look at the lung fields and pulmonary vasculature. Prominent upper lobe veins *(inverted moustache sign)*, haziness of lung field from hilum towards periphery and the transverse Kerley's B line indicating interstitial edema indicate pulmonary venous hypertension and acute pulmonary edema or congestive heart failure.
- Look at the mitral valvular orifice area for flecks of calcification.

Left Ventricular Aneurysm

A left ventricular aneurysm is a cause of heart enlargement on chest X-ray. It can often cause generalised enlargement of left ventricle and be indistinguishable from left ventricular dilatation.

Radiological Features (Fig. 4.39)

- Heart shadow is enlarged
- Look at the left border of heart for a bulge. If a bulge is noticed, follow it to determine whether it imperceptibly merges with the heart border, if yes, then it is suggestive of ventricular aneurysm.
- Now look for calcification in this area. In long-standing aneurysm, a rim of calcification along the heart border may be seen.

Figs 4.39A and B: Chest X-ray (PA view) shows: A. Left ventricular aneurysm. There is enlarged cardiac shadow with a bulge on the lower left border of the heart B. Left ventricular enlargement. The heart is boot-shaped with prominent pulmonary conus (X-ray set for comparison). There is increased bronchovascular marking

Table 4.2: Causes of pericardial effusion

1. **Transudative**
   - Congestive cardiac failure
2. **Exudative**
   - Infection e.g. viral, bacterial (tuberculosis, pyogenic), amoebic (rupture of amoebic liver abscess into pericardium), fungal (actinomycosis, histoplasmosis)
   - Postmyocardial infarction
   - Neoplastic infiltration
   - Collagen vascular disorders e.g. rheumatoid arthritis, SLE
   - Trauma, postradiation
   - Iatrogenic, e.g. postcardiac surgery
   - Metabolic, e.g. uremia
   - Endocrine, e.g. myxedema
3. **Hemopericardium (blood in pericardial cavity)**
   - Trauma
   - Neoplastic infiltration
   - Aortic dissection
   - Bleeding diasthesis e.g. leukemia, anticoagulation

Pericardial Effusion

Pericardial effusion means collection of fluid in the pericardial sac leading to enlargement of cardiac shadow on chest X-ray.

Causes

They are given in the Table 4.2.

Radiological Features (Figs 4.40 and 4.41)

- *Cardiac shadow is enlarged:* Look at the X-ray and confirm the enlargement of cardiac shadow by measurements.
- *Money-bag appearance:* In contrast to chamber enlargement, the heart shadow is globular in shape with straightening of both the borders of the heart. Both the hila are covered by the heart shadow.
- *Lung fields:* In contrast to ventricular enlargement where lung fields are congested and vascular markings prominent near the hilum, the lung vasculature is normal or oligaemic in pericardial effusion.

Abdominal X-ray (Normal and Abnormal)

ABDOMINAL X-RAYS

How to Read an Abdominal X-ray?

Inspection of X-ray Film

Points to be noted are:
- **Technical assessment:** Assessment of date, name, date of birth, age and sex of the patient is essential. Further

Fig. 4.40: Chest X-ray (PA view) showing pericardial effusion. Note the money-bag appearance of the heart with oligemic lungs

Fig. 4.41: Pleuropericardial effusion. Note the pericardial effusion (heart shadow enlarged with oligemic lungs). In addition, there is peripheral convex opacity rising from the right costophrenic angle, merging with cardiac shadow and emerging above it as convex opacity with concavity towards lung indicating right pleural effusion

information gathered is ward No., name of the hospital which gives an idea about the problem of the patient being referred, i.e. gastrointestinal or genitourinary problem.

- **Projection of the film:** Every abdominal X-ray is an AP film because beam passed from the front to the back with the film behind the patient who is lying down with X-ray machine overhead. On demand, you can have an erect film or even decubitus views. Usually the radiographer will mark the film with a badge or write on it by hand "supine" or "erect" to guide you. Otherwise also, you can guess how a given film was taken from the relative positions of organs, fluid and gas, etc.

- **Penetration:** Under-penetration (film is less dark) is not a problem because if you can see the bones in the spine, the most of everything else you need to see will probably be visible as well. However, in any over-exposed film (excessively dark) areas on an X-ray must be inspected with a bright light behind them (there is provision in certain view boxes to see such area(s) or a separate device may be available). However in case of doubt, a good film after full preparation of the patient may be got done again because certain important information such as air under diaphragm which indicates an potential fatal condition is likely to be missed.

- **Shadows on the X-ray:** It is worth knowing that only five basic densities are visible such as;
    - i. Gas—Black
    - ii. Fat—Dark gray
    - iii. Soft tissue/fluid—Light grey
    - iv. Bone/calcification—White
    - v. Metal—Intense white

- **Visible structures on plain abdominal film**
  On X-rays, the abdominal structures outlined are:
    - i. Solid organs, e.g. liver, spleen, kidneys
    - ii. Hollow organs, e.g. gastrointestinal tract
    - iii. Bones

  These structure can be classified as:
    - Visible or not visible and therefore whether present or potentially absent
    - Too large or too small
    - Distorted or displaced
    - Abnormally calcified
    - Containing abnormal gas, fluid or discrete calculi.

Indications of Plain X-ray Abdomen

1. For stone and calcification in the genitourinary area, pancreas, solid organ, hematomas, abnormal mass (lymph nodes), vascular structures, etc.
2. Perforation of hollow organ, e.g. stomach, colon, appendix, etc. Erect film will show air under diaphragm.
3. Duodenal or paralytic ileus/or gallstone ileus. Dilated intestinal loops are seen.
4. Subdiaphragmatic pathology. An amebic liver abscess may push right dome of the diaphragm and a big spleen will push left dome. In ascites, both domes are raised on supine X-rays.

5. Eventration of diaphragm: The gastric contents are seen in thoracic cavity in eventration of left dome.
6. Certain soft tissue masses, e.g. psoas abscess, paravertebral abscess.

Importance of X-ray Abdomen

Look upon X-ray as an extension of physical examination and regard the radiological signs as equivalent to physical signs in clinical medicine.

Remember that the X-ray is only a snaps shot of the patient and that serious disease may still be present despite a normal initial X-ray. Follow up films are thus necessary to come at a correct diagnosis as the radiological signs evolve.

Never forget to get the X-ray reported by a radiologist because he/she is trained to see and extract the maximum amount of useful information from every film that can frequently help to optimize the care of your patient.

Always provide the radiologist with clear, full, legible and accurate clinical information. This will enhance the diagnostic value of the films you have requested and, thus, helps improve the quality of care of your patients.

Never try to subject the pregnant female to X-ray examination. If in doubt, either delay the investigation or use ultrasound to investigate the problem.

Normal Adult Supine AP X-ray Abdomen

This is the film frequently taken as it shows most of the structures to the best advantage. An X-ray should always be inspected on a view box as irregular illumination and reflection will prevent 10-20 percent of the useful information on it being visualized.

Look at the film (Fig. 4.42) for:
- Bones, e.g. spine, pelvis, lower ribs and the sacroiliac joints.
- The dark margins outlining the liver, spleen, kidneys, bladder and psoas muscles—this line is of an intra-abdominal fat.
- Gas in the body of the stomach and descending colon.
- The wide pelvis indicating the X-ray belong to a female.
- Pelvic phleboliths—a common normal finding.
- Joint spaces of the hip—look for any narrowing or any other abnormality.
- Always look for 'R' mark written anywhere on the film, usually low down on the right side. All references to right or left refers to patient's right and left.
- Lastly check that 'R' marker is compatible with visible anatomy, e.g.
    - Liver on the right
    - Left kidney higher than right
    - Stomach bubble on the left

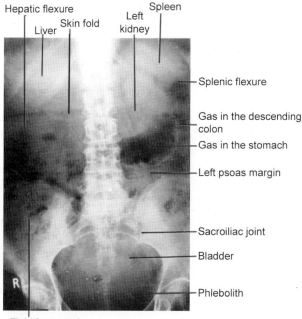

Fig. 4.42A: Plain X-ray abdomen of a normal adult (AP supine film) female

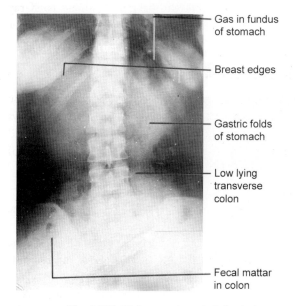

Fig. 4.42B: Plain normal erect abdominal X-ray in an adult female

Figs 4.42 A and B: Adult supine AP radiograph of a middle aged patient

- Spleen on the left
- Heart on the left if visible
- Dark skin fold going across the upper abdomen is normal.

Vertebral Column and Pevis

Look at the Bones and Sacroiliac Joint (Fig. 4.43)

Look at the X-ray (Fig. 4.44)

The bones (vertebral and pelvic bones) shows multiple dense foci. These are typical osteosclerotic secondaries (metastases) from carcinoma of prostate. The causes of increase bone density are given in Table 4.3.

Fig. 4.43: Osteomalacia. The X-ray pelvis taken from a patient of chronic renal failure. There is a decrease in bone density and thinning of the cortices. The pseudofractures or looser's zones (radiolucent bands) are indicated by arrows which are perpendicular to the bone

Fig. 4.44: Osteosclerotic secondaries from carcinoma prostate. The patient had IVP for hypercalcemia for renal stones, was found to have multiple dense foci in the pelvis and vertebrae, i.e. secondaries

Radiology

Table 4.3: Differential diagnosis of increased density of the bones

- Fluorosis—(Fig. 4.47)
- Chronic renal failure
- Paget's disease of the bone
- Osteosclerotic secondaries from prostate (Fig. 4.44)
- Milk-alkali syndrome

Look at the Spine (Figs 4.45 and 4.46)

Figure 4.45 shows biconcave vertebrae (cod-fish deformity). Figure 4.46 shows vertebral column looking like a bamboo-spine due to calcification of interspinal ligaments.

Kidneys

These are usually seen as bean-shaped objects of soft tissue density high in the abdomen. These are smooth in outline extending from the upper border of T_{12} on the left side to the lower border of L_3 on the right side, with the left kidney lying slightly higher than the right by about 1.5 cm. Both kidneys are inclined medially. Normally, they move down with inspiration and dropping several centimeters in the erect position. Usually, however, only parts of their outlines are visible and you have to make or deduce its outlines.

Preparation

For X-ray of urogenital system, the patient is put on low residue diet for 2-3 days. On the night previous to X-ray patient is given a purgative and a deflatulent, e.g. methyl polysiloxane or activated charcoal. Patients is kept on overnight fasting.

ABNORMALITIES OF KIDNEYS

A. Big Kidneys (Fig. 4.48)

- The kidney outlines are enlarged smoothly. The left kidney is slightly larger than the right, although duplex kidney (i.e. one with a double drainage system) may look bigger but histologically it is normal.
- The kidney may be enlarged on one side or on both side (read the causes in Table 4.4).
- The importance of detecting large kidneys is that they may be potential for recovery when this finding is associated with renal failure. Biopsy is required for confirmation of the diagnosis. Ultrasound is done to exclude renal obstruction and to assess renal parenchyma before biopsy.
- On the other hand, small kidneys (Table 4.5) represent to end-stage renal disease (e.g. irreversible state) making biopsy potentially hazardous, hence, small kidneys constitute contraindication for biopsy.

Fig. 4.45: Osteoporosis. There is cod-fish vertebral bodies (e.g. biconcave because of weakening of subchondral plates and expansion of intervertebral discs)

Fig. 4.46: Ankylosing spondylitis. Note the calcification of interspinous ligaments producing "Bamboo-spine"

Fig. 4.47: Skeletal fluorosis. A. X-ray spine shows increased bone density with calcification of interspinous ligaments. B. X-ray forearm shows calcification of interosseous membrane (→)

Table 4.4: Causes of enlarged kidneys

Bilateral	Unilateral
• Acute glomerulonephritis	• Acute obstruction
• Diabetic glomerulosclerosis	• Renal vein thrombosis
• Adult polycystic disease	• Acute pyelonephritis
• ATN	• Radiation nephritis
• Acute cortical necrosis	• Duplex system
• Bilateral acute pyelonephritis	• Compensatory hyper-
• Leukemic infiltration	trophy from contralateral
• Lymphomatous infiltration	nephrectomy or
• Amyloid kidneys	dysfunction
• Secondary renal disease	• Renal mass
• Excessive beer drinking	

Table 4.5: Causes of small kidneys

- Chronic glomerulonephritis
- Chronic renal ischemia (renal artery atherosclerosis)
- Chronic pyelonephritis
- Reflux nephropathy
- Infarctions of kidneys
- Senile atrophy
- Bilateral congenital hypoplasia

ABNORMALLY PLACED KIDNEY (FIG. 4.49)

Horse-shoe kidney tends to lie lower than the normal. The pathognomonic radiological sign is to see the renal cortices of the lower kidneys on plain X-ray crossing the margins of the psoas muscles medially to connect with the other side

Fig. 4.48: Plain X-ray abdomen showing large kidneys

- Look at the edges of the kidneys whether smooth or lobulated. Irregular kidney outlines indicates scarring of kidneys due to pyelonephritis or glomerulonephritis.

Fig. 4.49: IVP showing horse-shoe kidney (Lt)

with isthmus. The drainage system is malrotated forwards, best seen on the intravenous pyelography (Fig. 4.49).

The Hollow Organs

1. *Stomach* (X-ray to be taken in erect position-AP erect)

In the supine position, the gas in the stomach will rise anteriorly and the fluid in the stomach will pool posteriorly creating a circular outline which can be confused with gastric pseudotumor. This mass can be made to disappear by taking X-ray in upright or erect position. In the erect film, the gas bubble will be seen with a fluid level beneath the left dome of diaphragm.

Abnormalities

A Gastric Outlet Obstruction

Look at the X-ray and note:
- Abnormal large size of the gastric outline
- Excessive quantities of semidigested food in the stomach
- Small quantity of gas in the small bowel
- Two fluid levels, one on the left under the left dome of diaphragm and other on the right in the right hypochondriac region representing the duodenum. This double-bubble sign indicates high gut obstruction probably in the duodenum.

NB: This sign may also be seen in neonates with duodenal atresia.

The semidigested food residue and a fluid confirms obstruction.

NB: A bezoar (Fig. 4.50) looks like semidigested food, e.g. phytobezoar means retained vegetable matter and trichobezoar means hair ball in the stomach.

Q. What are causes of gastric outlet obstruction?
Ans. • Healed peptic ulcer
- Antral gastric carcinoma
- Lymphoma
- Gastritis
- Tuberculosis (lymph nodes producing obstruction from outside)
- Impacted foreign body
- Bezoar (hair ball, vegetable matter)
- Metastases producing compression from outside

Q. What are the clinical signs of pyloric obstruction?
Ans. The signs are:
- Increased peristalysis from left to right
- Abdominal distension
- Vomiting
- Succussion splash

Fig. 4.50: Trichobezoar. There is a mass of hair mixed with food particles retained in the stomach which is dilated due to outflow obstruction (double bubble sign indicates high gut obstruction)

Small Intestinal Obstruction/Paralytic Ileus

Small bowel pathology usually manifests itself on plain X-ray by abnormal accumulation of gas and fluid due to either functional (i.e. adynamic ileus) or truely mechanical (dynamic) obstruction. The differentiation between small bowel from large bowel obstruction is difficult on plain X-ray but following points help:

1. The large bowel obstruction is peripheral and contains faeces and gas; while small bowel obstruction is central and contains fluid and gas.
2. The more distal the obstruction (large bowel obstruction), the more distented loops will be seen.

Note:
i. Small fluid levels can be seen normally. Large fluid levels >3 indicate gut obstruction
ii. The longer the duration of the obstruction, the bigger the fluid levels.
iii. It is not necessary for obstruction to have fluid levels.

Caution: For fluid levels, always take either an erect or decubitus film